Male Sexual Dysfunction

Male Sexual Dysfunction

A Clinical Guide

EDITED BY

Suks Minhas MD, FRCS(Urol)

Consultant Urologist
University College Hospital
London, UK

John Mulhall MD, MSc, FECSM, FACS

Memorial Sloan-Kettering Cancer Center
New York, USA

WILEY Blackwell

This edition first published 2017 © 2017 by John Wiley & Sons Ltd

Registered Office
John Wiley & Sons Ltd, The Atrium, Southern Gate, Chichester, West Sussex, PO19 8SQ, UK

Editorial Offices
9600 Garsington Road, Oxford, OX4 2DQ, UK
1606 Golden Aspen Drive, Suites 103 and 104, Ames, Iowa 50010, USA

For details of our global editorial offices, for customer services and for information about how to apply for permission to reuse the copyright material in this book please see our website at www.wiley.com/wiley-blackwell.

Library of Congress Cataloging-in-Publication Data

Names: Minhas, Suks, 1966– editor. | Mulhall, John, editor.
Title: Male sexual dysfunction : a clinical guide / edited by Suks Minhas, John Mulhall.
Other titles: Male sexual dysfunction (Minhas)
Description: Oxford ; Ames, Iowa : John Wiley & Sons, Inc., 2017. | Includes bibliographical references and index.
Identifiers: LCCN 2016022487 (print) | LCCN 2016022873 (ebook) | ISBN 9781118746554 (cloth) | ISBN 9781118746448 (pdf) | ISBN 9781118746547 (epub)
Subjects: | MESH: Erectile Dysfunction | Penile Diseases | Sexual Dysfunction, Physiological–diagnosis | Sexual Dysfunction, Physiological–therapy
Classification: LCC RC889 (print) | LCC RC889 (ebook) | NLM WJ 709 | DDC 616.6/921–dc23
LC record available at https://lccn.loc.gov/2016022487

A catalogue record for this book is available from the British Library.

Wiley also publishes its books in a variety of electronic formats. Some content that appears in print may not be available in electronic books.

Cover image: © Don Farrall/Gettyimages

Set in 8.5/12pt Meridien by SPi Global, Pondicherry, India
Printed and bound in Singapore by Markono Print Media Pte Ltd

1 2017

Contents

List of contributors

James Bellringer
Parkside Hospital
London, UK

Catherine Benedict
Memorial Sloan Kettering Cancer Center
New York, USA

Pierre-Marc G. Bouloux
The Royal Free Hospital
London, UK

Gerald Brock
St Joseph's Health Sciences Centre; and Lawson Health Research Institute
London, ON, Canada

Culley Carson
University of North Carolina
Chapel Hill, NC, USA

Lizzie Chandra
St James Hospital, Leeds Teaching Hospitals NHS Trust
Leeds, UK

Kelly A. Chiles
George Washington University
Washington, DC, USA

Eric Chung
Princess Alexandra Hospital
Brisbane, Queensland, Australia

Giovanni Corona
Maggiore-Bellaria Hospital
Bologna, Italy

Victoria Dawson
University Hospital Southampton
Southampton, UK

Ian Eardley
Leeds Teaching Hospital Trust
Leeds, UK

Mark Emberton
University College Hospital
London, UK

Francisco J. Garcia
University of Western Ontario;
St Joseph's Health Sciences Centre;
Lawson Health Research Institute
London, ON, Canada

Angela Gregory
Nottingham University Hospital
Nottingham, UK

Geoffrey Hackett
University of Bedfordshire, Luton, UK
Good Hope Hospital,
Sutton Coldfield, UK

Paul K. Hegarty
Mater Private Hospital
Mahon, Cork, Ireland

Wayne J.G. Hellstrom
Tulane University
New Orleans, LA, USA

Graham Jackson
Guy's and St Thomas' Hospitals NHS Trust
London, UK

Salim Janmohamed
University College London
London, UK

Ates Kadioglu
Istanbul Faculty of Medicine, Istanbul University
Istanbul, Turkey

Jas Kalsi
Frimley Health NHS Foundation Trust and Imperial College Healthcare, London, UK

Oliver Kayes
St James Hospital, Leeds Teaching Hospitals NHS Trust
Leeds, UK

Mohit Khera
Baylor College of Medicine
Houston, TX, USA

Michael Kirby
The Prostate Centre
London, UK

Alex Kirkham
University College Hospital London
London, UK

Stephen Larsen
University College Hospital London
London, UK

Chi-Ying Li
University College Hospital London
London, UK

Marc Lucky
Aintree University Hospital
Liverpool, UK

Tom F. Lue
University of California
San Francisco, CA, USA

Mario Maggi
University of Florence
Florence, Italy

Martin Miner
Brown University
Providence, RI, USA

Suks Minhas
University College Hospital
London, UK

Caroline Moore
University College Hospital
London, UK

John Mulhall
Memorial Sloan Kettering Cancer Center
New York, NY, USA

Asif Muneer
University College Hospital London
London, UK

Christian J. Nelson
Memorial Sloan Kettering Cancer Center
New York, USA

Jalesh N. Panicker
The National Hospital for Neurology and Neurosurgery and
UCL Institute of Neurology
London, UK

Alexander W. Pastuszak
Baylor College of Medicine
Houston, TX, USA

Mark Paulos
Brown University
Providence, RI, USA

David Ralph
University College Hospital London
London, UK

Tina G. Rashid
Charing Cross Hospital
London, UK

Rowland Rees
University Hospital Southampton
Southampton, UK

Ashley Ridout
University College Hospital
London, UK

Emre Salabas
Istanbul Faculty of Medicine, Istanbul University
Istanbul, Turkey

Varun Sahdev
University College Hospital London
London, UK

Patrick Selph
University of Alabama at Birmingham
Birmingham, AL, USA

Majid Shabbir
Guy's Hospital
London, UK

Alan Shindel
UC Davis
Sacramento, CA, USA

C.J. Shukla
Western General Hospital, NHS Lothian
Edinburgh, UK

Vikram Soni
Baylor College of Medicine
Houston, TX, USA

Conrad von Stempel
University College Hospital
London, UK

Raanan Tal
Rambam Healthcare Campus
Haifa, Israel

Ronny B.W. Tan
Tan Tock Seng Hospital, Singapore

Phillip Thomas
Brighton and Sussex University Hospitals NHS Trust, Brighton, UK
Parkside Hospital, London, UK

Katarina Ivana Tudor
Department of Neurology, University Hospital Center Zagreb
Zagreb, Croatia

Linda Vignozzi
University of Florence, Florence, Italy

Marcel D. Waldinger
Drexel University College of Medicine
Philadelphia, PA, USA

Miles Walkden
University College Hospital
London, UK

Dan Wood
University College Hospital
London, UK

Michael Grant Wyllie
Global Pharma Consulting
Banbury, UK

Tet Yap
St George's Hospital
London, UK

Andrew Yates
Leeds & York Partnership NHS Foundation Trust
Leeds General Infirmary
Leeds, UK

Lindsay Yuh
UC Davis
Sacramento, CA, USA

Uwais B. Zaid
University of California
San Francisco, USA

Xiaoyu Zhang
University of California
San Francisco, USA

Foreword

This is a very important book. Its importance lies in the fact that male sexual health is these days central to very many men's quality-of-life. Male sexual dysfunction, resulting from aging or some disease process, such as diabetes, can therefore have serious, and often underestimated, repercussions. Men, particularly as they age, are extremely dependent on a lasting relationship with their partner for their well-being. In general, single or divorced men have a lower quality-of-life and higher risk of mortality than those who sustain their relationships in the longer term. Marital breakdown, which may be the consequence of male sexual dysfunction, can also have an impact on the next generation. The financial and emotional strains resulting from a fractured relationship may take a significant toll on the children, as well as on the two conflicted adults themselves.

As populations around the world age and increase, the incidence of male sexual dysfunction is set to rise and rise. Fortunately, as so well described in this book, its management has been transformed over the last 20 years by the advent of safe and effective pharmacotherapy, and, in selected cases, specialized andrological surgery. Viagra is still the world's most instantly recognizable pharmaceutical brand, and is now much more affordable in its generic form: sildenafil. However, counterfeit products, often containing hazardous ingredients, are unfortunately increasingly available, often over the internet, and have recently been associated with several deaths in the Far East. Intracavernosal injection therapy, pioneered originally by the impressive Professor Giles Brindley, has an increasingly important role to play in the more difficult-to-treat men, who are usually either post-pelvic surgery or longstanding diabetics. The third-line treatment for refractory cases of erectile dysfunction by implantation of inflatable or semi-rigid penile implants, which, provided that it is skillfully performed, can yield excellent results, is also well described in this excellent volume, along with other specialized surgical procedures for Peyronie's disease and other andrological conditions that can impact negatively on sexual function.

After many years in the wilderness "men's health" is at last beginning to take center stage. Sexual health is central to a man's self-esteem and well-being. I have high hopes that this book, edited by two of the world's leading experts in the specialty, which I whole-heartedly commend to you, will be widely read, not only by those with a special interest in male sexual health, but also by generalists and family practitioners, as well as nurse specialists. Only by improving the lamentably deficient knowledge about the safe and effective treatment options now available for the very many men who are affected by male sexual dysfunction, will their lives be improved and their relationships preserved. This is undoubtedly a most laudable ambition.

Roger Kirby
The Prostate Centre
London
W1G8GT

CHAPTER 1

Epidemiology of male sexual dysfunction

Raanan Tal

Rambam Healthcare Campus, Haifa, Israel

The broad term of sexual dysfunction includes erectile dysfunction, ejaculatory dysfunction, hypogonadism and low sexual desire, Peyronie's disease and other penile morphological alterations, and urinary incontinence associated with sexual function. Knowledge of the epidemiology of various sexual dysfunctions is important in designing sexual health programs and allocation of budget and healthcare resources, in patients' and partners' education, and in clinical assessment of individual subjects. There are numerous epidemiologic studies in the contemporary medical literature, comprehensively detailing the prevalence of sexual dysfunctions; however, reported epidemiologic data vary greatly. Several factors account for these inconsistent data. The main one is probably the definition used to define a particular sexual dysfunction. For example, in selected high-quality studies reporting on erectile function outcome in the post radical prostatectomy male population, more than 20 different definitions of favorable erectile function were used. Hence, the reported incidence of adequate erectile function varies, ranging from 25 to 78%.[1] Since the definition of sexual dysfunction is not unified, it is not unreasonable to expect variation in sexual dysfunction epidemiologic data: the higher the threshold for normal sexual function, the greater is the incidence of sexual dysfunction. Moreover, sexual dysfunction is commonly assessed using questionnaires. More objective modalities, such as hemodynamic assessment of the penis by Doppler ultrasound of the erect penis to establish a diagnosis of vasculogenic erectile dysfunction, or stopwatch-measured intravaginal ejaculatory latency time for establishing a diagnosis of premature ejaculation, are not commonly employed to define a sexual dysfunction. Not surprisingly, the type of questionnaire used in a certain study may also have an impact on epidemiologic findings.[2] Another issue in sexual function epidemiologic research is the study population, as the prevalence of sexual dysfunction varies greatly according to age, risk factors, demographic population characteristics, and other population-related factors.[3–8] An important consideration in the epidemiology of sexual dysfunction is the existence of specific risk factors in specific populations. There are many well-studied risk factors for sexual dysfunction.[9] Common risk factors include cardiovascular diseases, obesity, hypertension, hyperlipidemia, smoking, lower urinary tract symptoms, radical pelvic surgery and, of course, diabetes.[10–12] Radical pelvic surgery has a multifaceted impact on sexual function. For example, radical prostatectomy affects erectile function mainly by disruption of neural pathways, causing un-ejaculation resulting from removal of anatomic structures – the prostate and seminal vesicles – and increasing the risk of urinary incontinence during sexual activity owing to urinary sphincter weakness and even increasing the risk of penile morphologic changes, penile length loss, and Peyronie's disease.[13,14] There are also other, less commonly discussed but nonetheless important, factors that may be associated with the epidemiology of sexual dysfunction. It has been suggested that the prevalence of sexual dysfunction may be related to the availability of therapies and interventions for sexual dysfunction.[4] New therapies may increase patients' and partners' awareness and hence increase reporting of sexual dysfunction. In the light of these difficulties in measuring and reporting sexual dysfunction, epidemiologic data should be interpreted cautiously.

Male Sexual Dysfunction: A Clinical Guide, First Edition. Edited by Suks Minhas and John Mulhall.

Erectile dysfunction

Erectile dysfunction is the most commonly researched and discussed sexual dysfunction, and the most prevalent sexual dysfunction in older men. The first landmark study that looked at the epidemiology of erectile dysfunction was the Massachusetts Male Aging Study, by Feldman et al. and published in 1994.[15] This was a community-based observational study, and looked at a random sample of non-institutionalized men aged 40–70 years in the Boston area. Erectile function was assessed by a self-administered questionnaire, and the study's main findings were that the combined prevalence of minimal, moderate, and complete impotence was as high as 52%; subject age was the variable most strongly associated with impotence; and the prevalence of complete impotence tripled from 5 to 15% between subject ages 40 and 70 years.[15] Another pivotal erectile dysfunction epidemiologic study was the Cologne Male Survey by Braun et al., published in 2000.[10] This study looked at a European population, not a random sample but a representative sample of 8000 men, using a validated questionnaire. Results of this study were based on approximately 4500 evaluable questionnaires yielding a response rate of 56%. The prevalence of erectile dysfunction in this study was 19.2%, with a steep age-related increase (2.3 to 53.4%) and a high rate of conditions comorbid with erectile dysfunction – hypertension, diabetes, pelvic surgery, and lower urinary tract symptoms – corroborating findings of earlier studies of different populations. The most extensively studied risk factors for erectile dysfunction are cardiovascular risk factors, primarily diabetes, and other risk factors, including the metabolic syndrome and its components (abdominal obesity, dyslipidemia, hypertension, and impaired fasting glucose), smoking, ischemic heart disease, and peripheral vascular disease and other cardiovascular risk factors.[7,16,17] Recognition of these important risk factors, especially modifiable cardiovascular risk factors, may improve patient knowledge and awareness, and provide a window for cardiovascular disease diagnosis and early intervention in men with newly diagnosed erectile dysfunction, leading to not only better sexual health but also better overall health.[18–20] The main pathophysiologic link between erectile dysfunction and cardiovascular morbidity is probably endothelial dysfunction.[21] However, there are risk factors other than cardiovascular ones, both organic and psychological, that are associated with increased risk of erectile dysfunction. Among the significant organic non-vascular risk factors, is Peyronie's disease, an underdiagnosed condition in men presenting with newly diagnosed erectile dysfunction.[22] Peyronie's disease may contribute to the development of erectile dysfunction probably by altering the elastic properties of the penile tunica albuginea.[23] Another not uncommon risk factor for erectile dysfunction is testosterone deficiency (hypogonadism). It is well established that adequate testosterone levels are required not only for the penile vascular response during erection, but also to preserve penile structural integrity.[24,25] Erectile dysfunction is more prevalent in men with certain non-organic risk factors, such as emotional, couple related, and socioeconomic factors, creating a complex picture when the epidemiology of erectile dysfunction is discussed in certain specific populations.[8,26] A good example of an emotional risk factor for erectile dysfunction is depression. In a study by Shiri et al. the incidence of erectile dysfunction was 59/1000 person-years in men with depressive mood and 37/1000 person-years in those without depression.[27] Theses authors also found that the association of depression and erectile dysfunction is bidirectional: not only were men with depression at increased risk for erectile dysfunction, but also men with erectile dysfunction were at increased risk for depression.

In summary, the prevalence of erectile dysfunction is high and age-dependent, with more than half of men at age of 50 years or older being affected. There are many risk factors for erectile dysfunction, hence epidemiologic data in specific populations should be viewed with careful consideration of the specific characteristics of the population reviewed.

Premature ejaculation

Premature ejaculation is likely the most common sexual dysfunction in men across all age groups and populations, with a worldwide prevalence of approximately 30%.[28,29] For clinical research purposes the accepted definition of premature ejaculation is an intravaginal ejaculatory latency time (IELT) of 1–2 minutes; a prospectively stopwatch-measured IELT is preferred over self- or partner-reported IELT upon recall. While there is a definition of premature ejaculation for research purposes, in clinical practice there is no agreed definition. Waldinger et al. surveyed a population of 500 couples who were recruited from five countries, aged 18 years or older, had a stable heterosexual relationship for at least 6 months, with regular sexual intercourse. In their study, the median IELT was 5.4 minutes and the range was 0.55 to 41 minutes.[30] In their study, the median IELT decreased significantly with age, from 6.5 minutes in the 18–30 years group, to 4.3 minutes in the group older than 51 years, while other studies did not show this age-related increase in prevalence of premature ejaculation.[31,32] Regardless of whether the prevalence of premature ejaculation is clearly age-related or not, it is obvious that in younger men who are less likely to have other sexual dysfunctions such as organic erectile dysfunction, premature ejaculation is the most prevalent sexual dysfunction. In the real-world clinical setting, the use of stopwatch IELT to define premature ejaculation is definitely not a practical approach. Other ways to categorize men as having premature ejaculation are based on men self-reporting low or absent control over ejaculation irrespective of the duration of the ejaculation time, on the resulted distress for them or their sexual partner or both, or on patients' report that they "climax too soon." Indeed, in a Canadian web-based study of more than 3800 men, the prevalence of premature ejaculation (PE) ranged from 16% to 24% depending on the definition of PE utilized.[31] The etiology underpinning this high prevalence remains to be clarified, but current evidence reflects a shift from psychogenic theories to more neurobiological bases. While elucidation of the etiology of premature ejaculation is undoubtedly important for development of more effective therapies, it is clear that, whatever the cause of the condition, it is associated with a significant burden on psychological and overall health.[29] Generally, men with premature ejaculation are more likely to self-report other sexual dysfunctions (e.g., anorgasmia, low libido, erectile dysfunction) and psychological disturbances (e.g., depression, anxiety, excessive stress) than men without PE.[33] Similarly, as for other sexual dysfunctions, the epidemiology of PE may vary in special groups. Tang and Khoo showed that PE prevalence varied according to ethnicity.[32] It is worth mentioning that in their study, which included men in a primary care setting not a general population sample, the prevalence of PE was about 40%, significantly higher than in the general population. Shindel et al. looked at the prevalence of PE in another population of great interest, infertile couples, and found that about 50% of men reported that they ejaculated more rapidly than they wished. When men reported PE, their partners agreed with the diagnosis in 47% of cases. Female partners of men who did not report PE, reported PE in 11% of cases. Partner frustration related to PE was reported by 30% of men. Partners agreed that they were frustrated in 43% of these cases. Among the 70% of men who did not report partner frustration from PE, 93% of the partners agreed that they were not frustrated.

In summary, PE is hard to define exactly, yet it is the most prevalent sexual dysfunction and the most significant sexual dysfunction in young men.

Peyronie's disease

Peyronie's disease is commonly undiagnosed.[34] The main clinical symptom is penile curvature; however, men may have significant Peyronie's disease, manifested by penile plaques, erectile dysfunction, penile pain, and penile shortening, even without a curvature. Not uncommonly, the underlying cause of erectile dysfunction in poor responders to phosphodiesterase 5 inhibitors is Peyronie's disease. The diagnosis of Peyronie's disease in these men is established by physical examination and penile Doppler ultrasound in certain cases.[35] Moreover, in men who are not sexually active or in men who are sexually active without achieving erection and performing penetration, the penile curvature may not be seen and Peyronie's disease may exist but remain undiagnosed. Therefore, the reported prevalence of Peyronie's disease depends on the manifestations of this condition, on a high index of suspicion, and on patients, partners, and sexual health care providers' awareness. Epidemiological data on Peyronie's disease are limited. Prevalence rates of 0.4–9% have been published, but the majority of the medical literature supports a prevalence rate of 3–8% or 5–8%.[36,37] In the past, Peyronie's disease was considered a condition that is limited to older men. However, newer data show that Peyronie's disease does occur also in younger men and even in teenagers, but the prevalence in these very young men remains unknown.[38] Men younger than 40 years are more likely to present at an earlier stage of Peyronie's disease, to have diabetes, and to have more than one plaque at the time of presentation.[39] In certain populations at risk, the prevalence of Peyronie's disease is far greater. Diabetes, genetic predisposition, trauma of the penis, systemic vascular diseases, smoking, and alcohol consumption are all mentioned in the medical literature as risk factors for Peyronie's disease.[40,41] In diabetic men, not only is Peyronie's disease more prevalent, but also it tends to manifest in older age, and present with longer duration and greater severity: There is greater penile curvature and more pronounced penile deformity, and a greater prevalence of coexisting erectile dysfunction, probably resulting both from penile structural alterations due to Peyronie's disease itself and from diabetic vascular disease.[42] Tal et al. looked at the incidence of Peyronie's disease in a very distinct population consisting of men who had had radical prostatectomy as a monotherapy for prostate cancer, and calculated the 3-year post-prostatectomy incidence to be 16% and a mean time to presentation of 14 months after surgery.[14] Rhoden et al. conducted a case-control study to shed more light on Peyronie's disease risk factors, and found that race is a strong risk factor for Peyronie's disease, with an odds ratio of 8.5.[43] Interestingly, in this study, higher low-density lipoprotein (LDL)-cholesterol level (>130 mg/dL) and increased waist circumference (>102 cm) actually had a protective effect in Peyronie's disease, with an odds ratio of 0.5 for both. Moreno and Morgentaler investigated the association of testosterone deficiency and Peyronie's disease. Their study is of special significance since testosterone is a principal anabolic hormone in men and definitely has a major role in maintaining the health of penile tissues. In their pilot study, the severity of penile curvature correlated significantly with free testosterone level but not with total testosterone level, and a possible important association between testosterone deficiency and Peyronie's disease was suggested.[44] Besides the epidemiology of Peyronie's disease itself, sexual healthcare professionals should be aware of the epidemiology of emotional conditions in Peyronie's disease, which are under-represented in the medical literature and often under-diagnosed and treated in daily clinical practice. Consistent data from two leading sexual medicine centers in the United States show that the psychological burden in men with Peyronie's disease is great, possibly greater than in men with other sexual dysfunctions.[45,46] Overall very high rates of emotional burden and relationship problems attributable to Peyronie's disease were found: 81% and 54%, respectively, predictors of which were penile length-loss and inability to have intercourse. Using validated instruments, it was demonstrated that 48% of men with Peyronie's disease had clinically meaningful depression that would warrant medical evaluation. This high level of depression stayed consistent across time since diagnosis, suggesting that most men do not psychologically adjust to their diagnosis of Peyronie's disease; all men with Peyronie's disease should be considered for appropriate mental health screening. This high prevalence of psychological morbidity may be attributable to the fact that there is no fully effective treatment for Peyronie's disease, and men with symptomatic Peyronie's disease will never regain their pre-morbid penile function, appearance, and length.

In summary, the epidemiology of Peyronie's disease is intriguing: Its prevalence is higher and its age distribution is broader than previously thought; there are numerous suggested risk factors and a very high risk of associated psychological morbidity, inherent to changes in penile appearance and function, that should not be overlooked.

Hypogonadism

Hypogonadism (low testosterone) is under-diagnosed and under-treated. The significance of hypogonadism diagnosis and treatment cannot be over-emphasized, as androgen receptors and testosterone activity exist in most body tissues, organs, and systems. Testosterone deficiency effects are not limited to sexual function: besides desire and erection, it may also affect bone health, muscle mass, hematopoiesis, cognitive function, spermatogenesis and seminal fluid production, vascular and cardiac performance, lipid and glucose metabolism, and many other metabolic, primarily anabolic, processes. The key to diagnosis is awareness of the high prevalence of testosterone deficiency, identification of populations at risk, and early symptoms and laboratory evaluation. Worth mentioning is that symptoms of hypogonadism are not specific and can be attributed to other medical conditions, such as hypothyroidism or depression. Therefore, questionnaires are neither sensitive nor specific for hypogonadism screening or diagnosis, and must be combined with measured plasma testosterone levels.[47,48] Clinically, it was suggested that the findings that are best correlated with late onset hypogonadism are sexual symptoms (poor morning erection, low sexual desire, erectile dysfunction) and total testosterone level of less than 11 nmol/L (<320 ng/dL).[49] Epidemiologic questionnaire-based studies without testosterone measurement failed to correctly define the true prevalence of hypogonadism, yielding an overestimated prevalence of up to 80%.[50] Combining hypogonadism symptoms and plasma testosterone levels, Araujo et al. found that the overall prevalence of symptomatic testosterone deficiency in a random sample of men from the Boston Area Community Health Survey was 5.6%. In this study, symptomatic testosterone deficiency prevalence increased with age, yielding a prevalence of 18.4% in men over 70 years old.[51] Age-related increased prevalence of hypogonadism was also demonstrated in the Baltimore Longitudinal Study of Aging: the prevalence of hypogonadal testosterone levels was about 20% in men over 60 years old, 30% in men over 70 years old, and 50% in those over 80 years of age, using total testosterone criteria; the prevalence was even greater when free testosterone criteria were employed.[52] The prevalence of testosterone deficiency is increased in men with certain risk factors such as diabetes, cancer, lung disease, other systemic diseases, obesity, the metabolic syndrome, and erectile dysfunction, and in men with reduced mass and function of testicular tissue, for example, infertile men, men having varicocele, and men after unilateral orchiectomy.[53–55] Diabetes is a well-studied risk factor for testosterone deficiency: in a study by Corona et al. the prevalence of hypogonadism was 24.5% in diabetic men versus 12.6% in non-diabetic subjects, which was statistically significant after adjustment for age and body mass index (BMI).[56] Similar results were recently published by Al Hayek et al.: the prevalence of hypogonadism was 24.3% in diabetic and 8.3% in non-diabetic patients.[57] Hypogonadism also is common in men with erectile dysfunction, with a reported prevalence of approximately 30–40%.[58,59] Not uncommonly, erectile dysfunction is the presenting symptom. This population of men presenting with erectile dysfunction deserves special attention: it is a unique opportunity to impact men's health. Correct evaluation and management of testosterone deficiency and other cardiovascular risk factors may actually reduce future cardiovascular morbidity and mortality. Therefore, symptomatic treatment of erectile dysfunction in these men without in-depth risk factor identification should be discouraged.

Less discussed risk factors for hypogonadism include poorly functioning testicular tissue and/or reduced testicular mass. Hypogonadism is more common among infertile men, with an estimated prevalence of 20–30%.[60] Men with non-obstructive azoospermia, especially in Klinefelter's syndrome, are at even greater risk. Surgical sperm retrieval procedures may cause further testicular tissue insult and reduce Leydig cell mass and testosterone production. While azoospermia is uncommon in men (0.5–2%), varicocele is fairly common, with an incidence of 15% in the general male population and up to 40% in infertile men. Recent studies have shown that men with varicocele are at increased risk for low testosterone levels; furthermore, varicocele repair may increase testosterone levels and may be considered as a definitive treatment for hypogonadism.[61–63]

In summary, hypogonadism is a treatable cause of sexual dysfunction. While sexual dysfunction may be the presenting symptom, the benefits of testosterone level normalization are much broader. Awareness of the epidemiology of testosterone deficiency, especially in high-risk populations, is the key to diagnosis and treatment.

References

1 Tal R, et al. Erectile function recovery rate after radical prostatectomy: a meta-analysis. *J Sex Med* 2009;6(9):2538–46.

2 de Boer BJ, et al. Impact of various questionnaires on the prevalence of erectile dysfunction. The ENIGMA study. *Int J Impot Res* 2004;16(3):214–9.

3 Yang G, Pan C, Lu J. Prevalence of erectile dysfunction among Chinese men with type 2 diabetes mellitus. *Int J Impot Res* 2010;22(5):310–7.

4 Schouten BW, et al. Erectile dysfunction in the community: trends over time in incidence, prevalence, GP consultation and medication use – the Krimpen study: trends in ED. *J Sex Med* 2010;7(7):2547–53.

5 Paranhos M, et al. The prevalence of erectile dysfunction among Brazilian men screened for prostate cancer. *BJU Int* 2009;104(8):1130–3.

6 Bianco FJ Jr, et al. Prevalence of erectile dysfunction in men screened for prostate cancer. *Urology* 2009;74(1):89–93.

7 Teles AG, et al. Prevalence, severity, and risk factors for erectile dysfunction in a representative sample of 3,548 Portuguese men aged 40 to 69 years attending primary healthcare centers: results of the Portuguese erectile dysfunction study. *J Sex Med* 2008;5(6):1317–24.

8 Kupelian V, et al. Socioeconomic status, not race/ethnicity, contributes to variation in the prevalence of erectile dysfunction: results from the Boston Area Community Health (BACH) Survey. *J Sex Med* 2008;5(6):1325–33.
9 Lewis RW, et al. Epidemiology/risk factors of sexual dysfunction. *J Sex Med* 2004;1(1):35–9.
10 Braun M, et al. Epidemiology of erectile dysfunction: results of the 'Cologne Male Survey'. *Int J Impot Res* 2000;12(6):305–11.
11 Tan HM, et al. Prevalence and correlates of erectile dysfunction (ED) and treatment seeking for ED in Asian men: the Asian Men's Attitudes to Life Events and Sexuality (MALES) study. *J Sex Med* 2007;4(6):1582–92.
12 Guay AT. Sexual dysfunction in the diabetic patient. *Int J Impot Res* 2001;13 Suppl 5:S47–50.
13 Berookhim BM, et al. Prospective analysis of penile length changes after radical prostatectomy. *BJU Int* 2014;113(5b):E131–6.
14 Tal R, et al. Peyronie's disease following radical prostatectomy: incidence and predictors. *J Sex Med* 2010;7(3): 1254–61.
15 Feldman HA, et al. Impotence and its medical and psychosocial correlates: results of the Massachusetts Male Aging Study. *J Urol* 1994;151(1):54–61.
16 Heidler S, et al. Is the metabolic syndrome an independent risk factor for erectile dysfunction? *J Urol* 2007;177(2):651–4.
17 Selvin E, Burnett AL, Platz EA. Prevalence and risk factors for erectile dysfunction in the US. *Am J Med* 2007;120(2):151–7.
18 Glina S, Sharlip ID, Hellstrom WJ. Modifying risk factors to prevent and treat erectile dysfunction. *J Sex Med* 2013;10(1):115–9.
19 Kupelian V, et al. Relative contributions of modifiable risk factors to erectile dysfunction: results from the Boston Area Community Health (BACH) Survey. *Prev Med* 2010;50(1–2):19–25.
20 Baumgartner MK, et al. Patients' knowledge about risk factors for erectile dysfunction is poor. *J Sex Med* 2008;5(10): 2399–404.
21 Muller A, Mulhall JP. Cardiovascular disease, metabolic syndrome and erectile dysfunction. *Curr Opin Urol* 2006;16(6):435–43.
22 El-Sakka AI. Prevalence of Peyronie's disease among patients with erectile dysfunction. *Eur Urol* 2006; 49(3):564–9.
23 Raviv G, et al. Biochemical alterations of the tunica albuginea in impotence. *J Urol* 1997;158(5):1778–82.
24 Isidori AM, et al. A critical analysis of the role of testosterone in erectile function: from pathophysiology to treatment – a systematic review. *Eur Urol* 2014;65(1): 99–112.
25 Mirone V, et al. Androgens and morphologic remodeling at penile and cardiovascular levels: a common piece in complicated puzzles? *Eur Urol* 2009;56(2):309–16.
26 Laumann EO, et al. Prevalence and correlates of erectile dysfunction by race and ethnicity among men aged 40 or older in the United States: from the male attitudes regarding sexual health survey. *J Sex Med* 2007;4(1):57–65.
27 Shiri R, et al. Bidirectional relationship between depression and erectile dysfunction. *J Urol* 2007;177(2):669–73.
28 Carson C, Gunn K. Premature ejaculation: definition and prevalence. *Int J Impot Res* 2006;18 Suppl 1:S5–13.
29 Montorsi F. Prevalence of premature ejaculation: a global and regional perspective. *J Sex Med* 2005;2 Suppl 2:96–102.
30 Waldinger MD, et al. A multinational population survey of intravaginal ejaculation latency time. *J Sex Med* 2005;2(4):492–7.
31 Brock GB, et al. Canadian male sexual health council survey to assess prevalence and treatment of premature ejaculation in Canada. *J Sex Med* 2009;6(8):2115–23.
32 Tang WS, Khoo EM. Prevalence and correlates of premature ejaculation in a primary care setting: a preliminary cross-sectional study. *J Sex Med* 2011;8(7):2071–8.
33 Porst H, et al. The Premature Ejaculation Prevalence and Attitudes (PEPA) survey: prevalence, comorbidities, and professional help-seeking. *Eur Urol* 2007;51(3):816–23; discussion 824.
34 Miner MM, Seftel AD. Peyronie's disease: epidemiology, diagnosis, and management. *Curr Med Res Opin* 2014;30(1): 113–20.
35 Smith JF, et al. Penile sonographic and clinical characteristics in men with Peyronie's disease. *J Sex Med* 2009;6(10): 2858–67.
36 Hatzimouratidis K, et al. EAU guidelines on penile curvature. *Eur Urol* 2012;62(3):543–52.
37 Serefoglu EC, Hellstrom WJ. Treatment of Peyronie's disease: 2012 update. *Curr Urol Rep* 2011;12(6):444–52.
38 Tal R, et al. Peyronie's disease in teenagers. *J Sex Med* 2012;9(1):302–8.
39 Deveci S, et al. Defining the clinical characteristics of Peyronie's disease in young men. *J Sex Med* 2007;4(2): 485–90.
40 Arafa M, et al. The prevalence of Peyronie's disease in diabetic patients with erectile dysfunction. *Int J Impot Res* 2007;19(2):213–7.
41 Bjekic MD, et al. Risk factors for Peyronie's disease: a case-control study. *BJU Int* 2006;97(3):570–4.
42 Kendirci M, et al. Diabetes mellitus is associated with severe Peyronie's disease. *BJU Int* 2007;99(2):383–6.
43 Rhoden EL, et al. A cross-sectional study for the analysis of clinical, sexual and laboratory conditions associated to Peyronie's disease. *J Sex Med* 2010;7(4 Pt 1):1529–37.
44 Moreno SA, Morgentaler A. Testosterone deficiency and Peyronie's disease: pilot data suggesting a significant relationship. *J Sex Med* 2009;6(6):1729–35.
45 Smith JF, et al. Risk factors for emotional and relationship problems in Peyronie's disease. *J Sex Med* 2008;5(9): 2179–84.

46 Nelson CJ, et al. The chronology of depression and distress in men with Peyronie's disease. *J Sex Med* 2008;5(8):1985–90.

47 Chen W, et al. Are the Aging Male's Symptoms (AMS) scale and the Androgen Deficiency in the Aging Male (ADAM) questionnaire suitable for the screening of late-onset hypogonadism in aging Chinese men? *Aging Male* 2013;16(3):92–6.

48 Lackner JE, et al. Are there symptom-specific testosterone thresholds in aging men? *BJU Int* 2011;108(8):1310–5.

49 Wu FC, et al. Identification of late-onset hypogonadism in middle-aged and elderly men. *N Engl J Med* 2010;363(2): 123–35.

50 Trinick TR, et al. International web survey shows high prevalence of symptomatic testosterone deficiency in men. *Aging Male* 2011;14(1):10–5.

51 Araujo AB, et al. Prevalence of symptomatic androgen deficiency in men. *J Clin Endocrinol Metab* 2007;92(11): 4241–7.

52 Harman SM, et al. Longitudinal effects of aging on serum total and free testosterone levels in healthy men. Baltimore Longitudinal Study of Aging. *J Clin Endocrinol Metab* 2001;86(2):724–31.

53 Traish AM, et al. Testosterone deficiency. *Am J Med* 2011;124(7):578–87.

54 Dev R, et al. Association between hypogonadism, symptom burden, and survival in male patients with advanced cancer. *Cancer* 2014;120(10):1586–93.

55 Nord C, et al. Gonadal hormones in long-term survivors 10 years after treatment for unilateral testicular cancer. *Eur Urol* 2003;44(3):322–8.

56 Corona G, et al. Association of hypogonadism and type II diabetes in men attending an outpatient erectile dysfunction clinic. *Int J Impot Res* 2006;18(2):190–7.

57 Al Hayek AA, et al. The prevalence of hypogonadism among diabetic and non-diabetic men in Jordan. *J Diabetes Complications* 2014;28(2):135–40.

58 Martinez-Jabaloyas JM, DE-SDT Study Group. Testosterone deficiency in patients with erectile dysfunction: when should a higher cardiovascular risk be considered? *J Sex Med* 2014;11(8):2083–91.

59 Rabijewski M, et al. The high prevalence of testosterone deficiency in a population of Polish men over 65 years with erectile dysfunctions. *Aging Male* 2012;15(4):258–62.

60 Kim ED, et al. The treatment of hypogonadism in men of reproductive age. *Fertil Steril* 2013;99(3):718–24.

61 Hsiao W, et al. Varicocelectomy is associated with increases in serum testosterone independent of clinical grade. *Urology* 2013;81(6):1213–7.

62 Fisch H, Hyun G. Varicocele repair for low testosterone. *Curr Opin Urol* 2012;22(6):495–8.

63 Tanrikut C, et al. Varicocele as a risk factor for androgen deficiency and effect of repair. *BJU Int* 2011;108(9): 1480–4.

CHAPTER 2

Physiology of ejaculation

Marcel D. Waldinger
Drexel University College of Medicine, Philadelphia, PA, USA

Introduction

From the moment a man gets sexually aroused until he ejaculates there is a remarkable and very intriguing closely synchronized cooperation between his brain, his spinal cord, and his genital system. When a man starts to make love with his partner, his brain has to decipher the affective and erotic load of tactile impulses that come from the skin of various parts of his body, including the skin of his genitals. Indeed, in such circumstances the brain has to decipher the information that comes along with the notion of being touched by another person. The nervous system contains special nerve fibers that convey "affective" information when being touched and run from the skin to the central nervous system. This has only recently been discovered. These nerve fibers are called low threshold mechanoreceptive C tactile (CT) afferents.[1] They enable the brain to perceive with which "feelings" another person is touching the skin. However, research of these fibers in relation to erotic touch or sexuality is still in its infancy. These fibers are important not only for human beings but also for animals. By the activation of these affective peripheral nerve fibers an animal perceives the affective state of the other animal that is touching his or her hairy skin.

This chapter will describe the function of the anatomical structures that are required for ejaculation. Physiology is the term to denote this function.

The spinal cord and the brain of male rats

Ejaculation, that is, the rhythmic forceful expulsion of semen, results from a closely synchronized cooperation between different peripheral nerves, the spinal cord, and the brain. There are two successive phases during this synchronized coordination, emission and expulsion. The first phase starts in the spinal cord once the brain is informed that sexual activity is at hand.

Research in male rats has provided us with fundamental knowledge of what is actually happening during ejaculation at a physiological level. The synchronized coordination is mediated by a group of spinothalamic neurons in the lumbar part of the spinal cord. These neurons have been called the spinal generator of ejaculation (SGE).[2,3] They run from the spinal cord ("spino") to the thalamus ("thalamic") in the brain.

The spinal cord and the SGE

The SGE has been investigated in male rats since the 1980s.[2–4] In rodents it has been found that the SGE is located in lamina X and the medial part of lamina VII around the central canal, at the third and fourth lumbar (L3-L4) spinal segments. Afferent fibers in neurons from the genitals, conveying sensory information, terminate in the SGE. In the SGE these neurons contact interneurons that convey information to various other

Male Sexual Dysfunction: A Clinical Guide, First Edition. Edited by Suks Minhas and John Mulhall.

neurons. These interneurons contain the neuropeptides galanin, cholecystokinin, enkephalin, and gastrin-releasing peptide, and express neurokinin-1 (NK1), NMDA, and androgen receptors. A number of neurons of the SGE run to a very specialized area in the thalamus in the brain, the so-called parvocellular part of the subparafascicular nucleus of the thalamus. Therefore these neurons in the SGE are called lumbar spinothalamic (LSt) cells. Other neurons of the SGE make contact with spinal nuclei of the autonomic nervous system and somatic neurons.

The brain and the SGE

The SGE not only receives information from peripheral neurons and conveys their information to other neurons, but also its activity is mediated by the brain. The male rat brain contains a specific network for ejaculation (for review see Refs 5,6). As the localization of these specific neurons is bound to very tiny specific places in the brain, the names of their localization have become rather long and difficult to pronounce. They are located in the medial amygdala (posterodorsal part), the thalamus (parvicellular subparafascicular nucleus), the stria terminalis (posteromedial bed nucleus), the hypothalamus (posterodorsal and medial preoptic nuclei, paraventricular nucleus, and lateral hypothalamus), and the pons (raphe and gigantocellular nuclei). Neurons in these areas project to the medial preoptic area (MPOA), a key center in the control of ejaculation. The MPOA in turn contacts the caudal raphe and gigantocellular nuclei either directly or after relaying in periaqueductal gray[7] and the paraventricular nucleus of the hypothalamus (PVN).[8]

Peripheral nerves and ejaculation

In order to get an ejaculation integration of three sorts of nerve fibers has to be established: sympathetic neurons, parasympathetic neurons, and somatic nerves. These neurons originate in different areas of the spinal cord. Notably, when nerves convey information from the periphery (e.g., from the skin) to the central nervous system the nerve is called an afferent neuron. In contrast, when a nerve runs from the central nervous system to the periphery it is called an efferent neuron. In the case of ejaculation, both afferent and efferent neurons play a role in its neurophysiology.

Afferent neurons

The SGE receives information from the genitals through two afferent nerve pathways: the dorsal nerve of the penis and sympathetic neurons. These sensory afferent neurons terminate in the medial dorsal horn and the dorsal gray column of the spinal cord.[2,9]

The dorsal nerve of the penis

The dorsal nerve of the penis is the end branch of the pudendal nerve. It is a sensory nerve, which means that it only conveys sensory information from the penis to the spinal cord and the brain. It receives sensory information from sensory receptors in the penile skin, prepuce, and glans.[10,11] These sensory receptors are free nerve endings[12] and also encapsulated receptors (so-called Krause-Finger corpuscles) in the glans penis.[12] Stimulation of these Krause-Finger corpuscles facilitates the ejaculatory reflex.

Sympathetic nerves of the genitals

Sympathetic neurons from the genitals accompany the hypogastric nerve and, after passing through the paravertebral lumbosacral sympathetic chain, enter the spinal cord via thoracolumbar dorsal roots.[13]

Efferent neurons

From the SGE three sorts of neurons are sent to the genitals: sympathetic neurons, parasympathetic neurons, and somatic neurons.

Sympathetic neurons

The cell bodies of the sympathetic neurons are located in the thoracolumbar part of the spinal cord. The sympathetic neurons leave the spinal cord through the ventral roots. They first run to the paravertebral sympathetic chain. From this relay station they run directly via the splanchnic nerves to the intermesenteric ganglia (IMG), but may also reach the intermesenteric ganglia indirectly by first relaying in the celiac superior mesenteric ganglia (CSMG) to reach the IMG via intermesenteric nerves (IMN).[14]

Emanating from the IMG (which is called the superior hypogastric plexus in humans) are the hypogastric nerves. These sympathetic nerves join the parasympathetic nerves in the pelvic nerve and together they form the pelvic plexus.[14]

From the pelvic plexus both sympathetic and parasympathetic nerves innervate the anatomical structures that are involved in ejaculation.

Parasympathetic neurons

The cell bodies of the parasympathetic neurons are located in the sacral parasympathetic nucleus (SPN),[15] in the sacral spinal cord of a human. The parasympathetic neuron fibers travel in the pelvic nerve and are later joined by the sympathetic neuron fibers from the hypogastric nerves. Both the parasympathetic and sympathetic nerve fibers run to the pelvic plexus, which is called the inferior hypogastric plexus in humans. From this plexus the parasympathetic neuron fibers reach the pelvic anatomical structures that are involved in ejaculation.

Somatic neurons

In humans the cell bodies of somatic neurons are located in the sacral spinal cord (Onuf's nucleus). These somatic neurons proceed via the motor branch of the pudendal nerve to the pelvic floor striated muscles, including the bulbospongiosus and ischiocavernosus muscles.[16]

Emission and the autonomic nervous system

The emission phase

During the emission phase of ejaculation, the following genital anatomical structures play a major role: testis, epididymis, ductus deferens, vesica seminalis, prostate, bladder neck, and prostatic part of urethra. In addition, during emission, the functionality of particularly the autonomic (e.g., sympathetic and parasympathetic) centers in the thoraco-lumbar-spinal cord are essential.

Testis and epididymis

Spermatozoa are produced in the seminiferous tubules of the testes and translocated into the head of the epididymis. The epididymis, consisting of epithelial cells, connective tissue, and smooth muscle cells, consists of three parts: the head (caput), the body (corpus), and the tail (cauda). The spermatozoa in the seminiferous tubules and early epididymis are non-motile but become motile after maturation (18–24 hours) along the epididymis.[14] Mature spermatozoa are stored in the tail of the epididymis. During sexual arousal they are released in the ductus (or vas) deferens. The volume of spermatozoa is only less than 0.1 % of the total volume of the ejaculate.

Ductus deferens

The ductus deferens passes through the inguinal canal to enter the pelvic cavity. There it joins the excretory duct of the seminal vesicle forming the ejaculatory duct. The ejaculatory duct traverses the prostate and opens into the prostatic portion of the urethra via the verumontanum (a 2–3 mm high intraluminal urethral crest in humans). The last part of the ductus deferens is enlarged to form the ampulla.[14]

During the emission phase of ejaculation, strong peristaltic contractions of the ductus deferens bring spermatozoa into the ejaculatory duct and then into the urethra, where they are mixed with seminal fluids, excreted by the prostate and vesica seminalis.

Seminal vesicles

The seminal vesicles are two tubular glands lying between the posterior wall of the bladder base and the rectum. Each vesicle joins with the ductus deferens as it enters the prostate to form the ejaculatory duct. Epithelial cells of the inner layer of the seminal vesicles secrete 50–80% of the entire ejaculatory volume.[14]

The seminal vesicle secretions are thick, alkaline, and contain substances providing the spermatozoa with a protective and nutritive environment.[14]

During the emission phase of ejaculation, seminal vesicle fluid is expelled into the prostatic urethra via the excretory duct following contractions of smooth muscle cells of the gland.

Prostate

The prostate produces 15–30% of the total volume of sperm. Prostatic secretions are milky, slightly alkaline, and enhance spermatozoan survival. During the emission phase of ejaculation, muscular elements of the gland contract and eject the secretions into the prostatic urethra via the prostatic ducts and the utricle opening into the verumontanum.

Cowper's glands

The bulbourethral, or Cowper's glands are located posterolaterally to the membranous portion of the urethra at the level of the urogenital diaphragm. Bulbourethral gland excretory ducts extend forward through the urogenital diaphragm and open into the cavernous urethra. Bulbourethral clear thick secretions are poured into the urethra as sexual arousal increases. Their role is dual: neutralizing urine acidic residues and lubricating the urethra before sperm passes through.[14]

The seminal fluid with spermatozoa (semen) is poured into the posterior urethra via phasic contractions of the glands and their ducti while the bladder neck is firmly closed to prevent backflow into the bladder.

Expulsion and the somatic nervous system

During the expulsion phase of ejaculation, the following genital anatomical structures play a major role: urethra, pelvic floor striated muscles, bulbospongiosus muscle, and ischiocavernosus muscle. In addition, during expulsion, the functionality of particularly somatic spinal centers and nerves is important.

Somatic centers innervate the pelvic floor striated muscles, particularly the bulbospongiosus and ischiocavernosus muscles. The contractions of both muscles enable the expulsion of semen from the urethra. The bulbospongiosus muscle encompasses the median part of the penile root (bulb). The ischiocavernosus muscles surround the lateral roots of the penis (cura).

While the external urethral sphincter relaxes, intense rhythmic contractions of both muscles compress the urethra and corpus cavernosum. These contractions lead to the characteristic forceful pulsatile expulsion of sperm. Their intense contractions also contribute to further rigidity of the penis and probably also to the orgasmic feeling.

The central nervous system and ejaculation

In the SGE peripheral information from the genitals is integrated with information from the brain. his information can be summarized as either excitatory or inhibitory information affecting a spinal ejaculatory reflex. Actually, the extent of central serotonin (5-hydroxytryptamine, or 5-HT) neurotransmission and activity of certain 5-HT receptors determine whether the spinal ejaculatory reflex is inhibited or facilitated. This mechanism of action of serotonin is actually the mechanism by which selective serotonin reuptake inhibitors (SSRIs) modulate the duration of the intravaginal ejaculation latency time (IELT) in men and the ejaculatory latency (EL) in rodents.

However, it is in the brain that information from all the senses (visual, auditory, olfactory, gustatory, tactile) together with feelings, emotions, perceptions, and eroticism are integrated in cerebral (somato)sensory areas and also become integrated with motor centers that in turn provide descending information to the SGE.

Most detailed information of the brain areas involved in ejaculation is derived from studies of male rats. These animal studies were performed long before clinicians started to become interested in the neurobiology of ejaculatory disorders, for example, premature ejaculation. Particularly, studies using Fos protein expression as a marker for neuronal activity have contributed to our current knowledge on which brain areas are involved in ejaculation.[17]

The brain structures that play a specific role in ejaculation are medial amygdala (posterodorsal part) (MeApd), the thalamus (parvicellular subparafascicular nucleus) (SPFp), the stria terminalis (posteromedial bed nucleus) (BNSTpm), the hypothalamus (posterodorsal preoptic nucleus (PNpd), paraventricular nucleus, and lateral hypothalamus), and the pons (raphe and gigantocellular nuclei).[14]

Connections between these substructures and the medial preoptic area (MPOA) of the hypothalamus have been found to be essential for ejaculation.[17,18] Experiments have shown that emission and expulsion disappear after lesioning the MPOA,[19] or can be elicited by chemical[20,21] or electrical[22,23] stimulation. The MPOA has no direct connection with the SGE in the spinal cord. However, the MPOA affects the two ejaculatory phases by interconnecting with other areas in the brain that are involved in ejaculation: the paraventricular nucleus of the hypothalamus (PVN),[24] the periaqueductal gray (PAG),[25] and the paragigantocellular nucleus (nPGi) of the medulla oblongata.[26]

The parvocellular neurons of the PVN directly innervate autonomic neurons in the lumbosacral spinal cord[27,28] and the pudendal motoneurons located in the L5-L6 spinal segments in rats.[28] The PVN also has direct neuronal connections with the nPGi in the brainstem.[29]

Orgasm

In normal circumstances an ejaculation is accompanied by an orgasmic sensation. Orgasm is a complex neurophysiological process that consists of an intense cerebral discharge but also whole-body physiological changes.[14] The exact area in the brain where the orgasmic sensations are produced is not yet identified. However, in recent years brain imaging studies have provided new data about the areas that are activated and/or inhibited during orgasm. For example, in a positron emission tomography (PET) study in healthy male volunteers it was found that at the time of ejaculation, the strongest activation was found in the mesodiencephalic transition zone including the ventral tegmental area (VTA), SPFp, and medial and ventral thalamus. These thalamic areas are known to be associated with rewarding processes, visceral sensory responses, and control of pelvic floor motoneurons and sympathetic preganglionic neurons throughout the spinal cord.[14] This study and various other brain imaging studies have provided indications that the VTA is a key area of the neuronal substrate of orgasm.

References

1 Liljencrantz J, Olausson H. Tactile C fibers and their contributions to pleasant sensations and to tactile allodynia. *Front Behav Neurosci* 2014;8:37.

2 Truitt WA, Coolen LM. Identification of a potential ejaculation generator in the spinal cord. *Science* 2002;297:1566–9.

3 Borgdorff AJ, Bernabe J, Denys P, Alexandre L, Giuliano F. Ejaculation elicited by micro stimulation of lumbar spinothalamic neurons. *Eur Urol* 2008;54:449–56.

4 McKenna KE, Nadelhaft I. The organization of the pudendal nerve in the male and female rat. *J Comp Neurol* 1986;248:532–49.

5 Coolen LM. Neural control of ejaculation. *J Comp Neurol* 2005;493:39–45 [review].

6 Giuliano F, Clement P. Neuroanatomy and physiology of ejaculation. *Annu Rev Sex Res* 2005;16:190 216 [review].

7 Marson L. Lesions of the periaqueductal gray block the medial preoptic area-induced activation of the urethrogenital reflex in male rats. *Neuroscience Lett* 2004;367:278–82.

8 Simerly RB, Swanson LW. Projections of the medial preoptic nucleus: A *Phaseolus vulgaris* leucoagglutinin anterograde tract-tracing study in the rat. *J Comp Neurol* 1988;270: 209–42.

9 May AG, DeWeese JA, Rob CG. Changes in sexual function following operation on the abdominal aorta. *Surgery* 1969;65:41–7.

10 Johnson RD, Hubscher CH. Brainstem microstimulation differentially inhibits pudendal motoneuron reflex inputs. *NeuroReport* 1998;312:299–310.

11 Nordling J, Andersen JT, Walter S, Meyhoff HH, Hald T, Gammelgaard PA. Evoked response of the bulbocavernosus reflex. *Eur Urol* 1979;5:36–8.

12 Grundemar L, Hakanson R. Effects fo various neuropeptide Y/peptide YY fragments on electrically-evoked contractions of the rat vas deferens. *Br J Pharmacol* 1990;100:190–2.

13 Baron R, Janig W. Afferent and sympathetic neurons projecting into lumbar visceral nerves of the male rat. *J Comp Neurol* 1991;314:429–36.

14 Giuliano F, Clement P. Anatomy and physiology of ejaculation. In: Jannini EA, McMahon CG, Waldinger MD (eds), *Premature Ejaculation: From Etiology to Diagnosis and Treatment.* Milan: Springer, 2013; pp. 25–44.

15 Murphy AZ, Rizvi TA, Ennis M, Shipley MT. The organization of preoptic-medullary circuits in the male rat: evidence for interconnectivity of neural structures involved in reproductive behavior, antinociception and cardiovascular regulation. *Neuroscience* 1999;91:1103–16.

16 Saper CB, Loewy AD, Swanson LW, Cowan WM. Direct hypothalamo-autonomic connections. *Brain Res* 1976; 117:305–12.

17 Heeb MM, Yahr P. Anatomical and functional connections among cell groups in the gerbil brain that are activated with ejaculation. *J Comp Neurol* 2001;439:248–58.

18 Coolen LM, Peters HJ, Veening JG. Anatomical interrelationships of the medial preoptic area and other brain regions activated following male sexual behavior: a combined fos and tract-tracing study. *J Comp Neurol* 1998;397:421–35.

19 Arendash GW, Gorski RA. Effects of discrete lesions of the sexually dimorphic nucleus of the preoptic area or other medical preoptic regions on the sexual behavior of male rats. *Brain Res Bull* 1995;10:147–54.

20 Hoyle CHV. Transmission: purines. In: Burnstock G, Hoyle CHV (eds), *Autonomic Neuro Effector Mechanisms.* Harwood Academic, 1992; pp. 367–408.

21 Owman C, Stjernquist M. The peripheral nervous system. In: Bjorklund A, Hokfelt T, Owman C (eds), *Handbook of Chemical Neuroanatomy*. Amsterdam: Elsevier Science, 1988; pp. 445–544.

22 Kurokawa M, Tsunoo A. Parasympathetic depression of vas deferens contraction in the guinea-pig involves adenosine receptors. *J Physiol* 1998;407:135–53.

23 Marson L, McKenna KE. CNS cell groups involved in the control of the ischiocavernosus and bulbospongiosus muscles: a transneuronal tracing study using pseudorabies virus. *J Comp Neurol* 1996;374:161–79.

24 Shafik A, El Sibai O. Mechanism of ejection during ejaculation: identification of a urethrocavernosus reflex. *Arch Androl* 2000;44:77–83.

25 Redoute J, Stoleru S, Gregoire MC, et al. Brain processing of visual sexual stimuli in human males. *Hum Brain Mapp* 2000;11:162–77.

26 Murphy AZ, Hoffman GE. Distribution of gonadal steroid receptor-containing neurons in the preoptic-periaqueductal gray-brainstem pathway: a potential circuit for the initiation of male sexual behavior. *J Comp Neurol* 2001; 438:191–212.
27 Levin RJ. The mechanisms of human ejaculation – a critical analysis. *Sex Relationship Ther* 2005;31:123–31.
28 Rizvi TA, Ennis M, Shipley MT. Reciprocal connections between the medial preoptic area and the midbrain periaqueductal gray in rat: A WGA-HRP and PHA-L study. *J Comp Neurol* 1992;315:1–15.
29 Bancila M, Verge D, Rampin O, et al. 5-Hydroxytryptamine 2C receptors on spinal neurons controlling penile erection in the rat. *Neuroscience* 1999;92:1523–37.

CHAPTER 3

Physiology of penile erection

Uwais B. Zaid, Xiaoyu Zhang, and Tom F. Lue
University of California, San Francisco, USA

A better understanding of smooth muscle physiology, the nitric oxide pathway, neurophysiology, and functional penile anatomy has been instrumental in gaining a deeper understanding of erectile physiology. Knowledge of normal physiology aids in understanding the pathophysiology and developing potential therapeutics for erectile dysfunction.

Functional anatomy

Penile erectile tissues, vascular and cavernosal smooth muscle, and support structures are essential to tumescence. The human penis is composed of three cylindrical structures bound together by the tunica albuginea, ligaments, and muscles. There are the paired corpora cavernosa and a single corpus spongiosum, which houses the urethra. The complex yet tightly regulated interplay between these erectile tissues, vessels, and nerves is essential to penile erection and detumescence.

Tunica albuginea

The tunica albuginea (TA) is a bilayered structure composed of an inner circular layer and outer longitudinal layer. Additionally, it has multiple sublayers that surround and support the cavernosal tissues. Although its collagen fibers provide rigidity to support high pressures during erection, it is also flexible due to its elastin content. The inner layer is oriented in a circular fashion. From this layer, intracavernous pillars emanate and provide strength to the erectile tissues in addition to supporting the septum. The outer layer of the bilayered TA is oriented longitudinally and extends the length of the penis from the glans to the crura. These fibers are absent between the 5.00 and 7:00 positions, which is an area of relative weakness. Contrary to the corpora cavernosa, the corpus spongiosum lacks an outer longitudinal layer and intracorporeal supports, which leads to lower pressures during erection.

In addition to providing support for erectile tissues, the TA plays an essential role in tumescence by obstructing venous outflow. Emissary veins course between the inner and outer layers of the TA. With increasing intracorporeal pressures from arterial inflow, these veins are compressed between these layers, which diminishes venous outflow leading to higher pressure engorgement, the so-called veno-occlusive mechanism.

Erectile tissues

The paired corpora cavernosa are spongy cylinders containing erectile tissues encircled by the tough yet flexible TA and also surrounded by the ischiocavernosus muscle. Contraction of these muscles at the crus during erection further blocks venous outflow, leading to increased rigidity and further increases intracavernous pressures. Although the corpora cavernosa are separated by a septum, it is incomplete, and there is common flow distally. Within the corpora cavernosa there is a fibrous support skeleton composed of pillars from the TA and the incomplete septum. Furthermore, there are a series of interconnected sinusoids, which accommodate blood during erections. These are supported by elastic fibers and collagen and separated by smooth muscle trabeculae. Relaxation of these smooth muscles allows increased cavernosal engorgement.

In the flaccid state, blood slowly diffuses from central to peripheral sinusoids. Given this slow flow, blood gas levels are venous throughout the sinusoids.

Male Sexual Dysfunction: A Clinical Guide, First Edition. Edited by Suks Minhas and John Mulhall.

However, during erection, with rapid entry of arterial blood, central and peripheral sinusoidal blood gas levels approach that of arterial blood. Additionally, there are many endothelial-derived factors in the sinusoid and cavernosal smooth muscle cells that regulate vasoconstriction and dilation. These are discussed below.

The corpus spongiosum has larger sinusoids than the corpora cavernosa and is a lower pressure system given the lack of an outer longitudinal layer. This is completely absent in the glans penis as well. Additionally, the corpus spongiosum is surrounded by the bulbospongiosus muscle. During micturition, contraction helps to empty the urethra. During erections, contraction compresses the erectile tissue and deep dorsal vein leading to increased pressure and rigidity. Additionally, its rhythmic contraction assists with ejaculation.

Penile vasculature

Arterial supply

The internal pudendal artery, which is the terminal branch of the anterior trunk of the internal iliac artery, is usually the main source of blood to the penis. There is, however, significant variability in penile blood flow with accessory branches from the external iliac, obturator, vesical, and femoral arteries, which may often be the dominant source of blood. The internal pudendal artery terminates as the common penile artery, which branches into the dorsal, bulbourethral, and cavernous arteries. Distally these rejoin at the glans penis. The dorsal artery supplies blood to the glans, skin and subcutaneous tissue of penis. The bulbourethral artery supplies the corpus spongiosum and urethra. The cavernous artery gives off straight and helicine branches, which open directly into the sinusoids without intervening capillaries. During erection, when smooth muscle is relaxed, these are straight and dilated allowing arterial inflow; however, they become contracted and tortuous in the flaccid state, when smooth muscle is contracted, which decreases inflow.

Venous drainage

Penile venous drainage originates from tiny venules in the peripheral sinusoidal tissues, which travel in the trabeculae between the TA and peripheral sinusoids and form the subtunical venous plexus. These give rise to the emissary veins, which travel between the layers of the TA. During erection, compression of these by the TA limits venous outflow, which contributes to penile engorgement.

Neuroanatomy

Peripheral innervation

The penis is supplied by autonomic and somatic nerve fibers. Autonomic innervation to the corpora cavernosa and spongiosum is in the form of sympathetic and parasympathetic fibers via the cavernous nerves. Somatic fibers are both sensory and motor, allowing for cutaneous sensation and contraction of the bulbospongiosus and ischiocavernosus muscles.

Somatic innervation

Somatosensory innervation originates distally in sensory receptors of the skin, glans, and urethra. Additionally, sensory receptors are present in the corpora cavernosa. The glans is very highly innervated with thin myelinated A_d and unmyelinated C fibers. These sensory fibers form the dorsal nerve of the penis, which will coalesce with other fibers to become the pudendal nerve. The pudendal nerve enters the spinal cord at the S2-S4 levels. These fibers convey sensory information via the spinothalamic and spinoreticular tracts to the central nervous system. In addition to somatic functions, the dorsal nerve has autonomic functions, as evidenced by the presence of nerve bundles containing nitric oxide synthase (NOS). Onuf's nucleus, located in the S2-S4 segments, provides motor neurons that supply the pudendal nerve. These innervate the bulbospongiosus and ischiocavernosus muscles.

Autonomic innervation

Autonomic innervation is responsible for tumescence and detumescence. Specifically, sympathetic stimulation leads to detumescence whereas parasympathetic activation leads to erection. Thus, sacral parasympathetic fibers are responsible for tumescence and sympathetic thoracolumbar fibers are responsible for detumescence.

Sympathetic pathways

Penile sympathetic innervation to the pelvic plexus originates from T11 to L2 spinal segments. The presynaptic sympathetic cell bodies supplying these fibers are located in the lateral column between T10-T12 and L1-L2. These travel to the pelvic plexus via the hypogastric nerve. This forms the superior hypogastric plexus, which is formed from sympathetic fibers from the celiac plexus and lumbar splanchnic nerves, and the inferior mesenteric plexus.

Parasympathetic pathways

Parasympathetic fibers arise from presynaptic neuronal cells in the intermediolateral cell columns located between the S2 and S4 sacral spinal cord segments as pelvic splanchnic nerves and join the hypogastric nerves. These will join sympathetic fibers from the superior and inferior hypogastric plexuses and join the pelvic plexus. Recent studies demonstrate that many of these plexuses are a mix of sympathetic and parasympathetic nerves. From the pelvic plexus, autonomic nerve fibers that supply the penis form the cavernous nerves.

Central pathways

Spinal pathways

In the spinal cord, thoracolumbar sympathetic, sacral parasympathetic, and sacral pudendal motoneurons are involved with erections. The thoracolumbar center is generally inhibitory to erections whereas parts of the sacral and pudendal promote erections.

Supraspinal pathways

Centers in the brain play an essential role in initiation, inhibition, and maintenance of erections by integrating and processing multiple sensory inputs. Although multiple areas are involved in sexual function, including many areas of the forebrain, hypothalamus, brainstem, and midbrain, animal studies have demonstrated that penile sensory information is specifically relayed to the pons, brainstem, hypothalamic medial preoptic area (MPOA), paraventricular nucleus (PVN), thalamus, and cortex. MPOA stimulation causes erections via increased parasympathetic outflow. Additionally, the PVN also is pro-erectile when stimulated with apomorphine via dopaminergic receptors. However, in addition to these centers, there are many other areas in the brain responsible for regulation of erectile function.

These central structures are responsible for psychogenic, reflexogenic, and nocturnal erections. Psychogenic erections are penile erections from audiovisual stimulation. Central impulses activate the spinal centers to cause an erection. Reflexogenic erections are induced by genital stimulation. Sensory fibers will relay this information via ascending fibers to the brain, which processes this and activates autonomic centers to produce an erection. Nocturnal erections occur during rapid eye movement sleep. Functional studies show increased activity in the pontine area, amygdalae, and anterior cingulate gyrus. There is decreased activity in the prefrontal and parietal cortex.

Hemodynamics of penile erection and detumescence

Corpora cavernosa

Penile tumescence is ultimately controlled by vascular and corporeal smooth muscle regulation of blood flow. Erections result from relaxation of cavernosal and vascular smooth muscles, which leads to sinusoidal relaxation, arterial dilation, and venous compression. This leads to increased arterial inflow, decreased venous outflow, and ultimately penile engorgement. When the penis is flaccid, vascular and cavernosal smooth muscles are in a tonically contracted state. This limits the amount of arterial blood flow so that the partial pressure of oxygen (pO_2) approaches that of venous blood (35 mmHg). As a result of sexual stimulation, neurotransmitters are released from the cavernous nerve endings, leading to a cascade of events resulting in penile erection. The following events occur:

1. Smooth muscles in the arteriolar and arterial walls relax, leading to vascular dilation and increased blood flow to the penis.
2. With the influx of arterial blood and relaxation of smooth muscles, the cavernosal sinusoids expand and become engorged with trapped blood.
3. Sinusoidal expansion leads to mechanical compression of the subtunical venous plexus between the engorged sinusoids and tough TA. This leads to decreased venous outflow and increases sinusoidal blood trapping and engorgement.
4. As a result of this trapped blood, the TA stretches, leading to occlusion of the emissary veins between the layers of the TA, which further decreases venous outflow.
5. Consequently, penile blood pO_2 increases to 90 mmHg (closer to arterial oxygen levels) and the intracavernous pressure increases to 100 mmHg
6. The amalgamation of these events leads to penile erection, with the penis going from a flaccid state to the full erection phase.
7. Contraction of the ischiocavernosus muscle during erection further increases pressure during the rigid erection phase.

Detumescence occurs when arterial inflow decreases due to smooth muscle contraction. It has been described in three phases in the animal model:

1. Initially, a transient increase in intracorporeal pressure is noted due to smooth muscle contraction against a closed venous system during erection.

2 This leads to a slow decrease in corporeal pressure as venous channels reopen due to decreased mechanical compression.
3 Lastly, there is a rapid fall in pressure as venous outflow is completely restored.

Corpus spongiosum and glans penis

Although there is increased blood flow to the glans penis and corpus spongiosum during erection, due to the lack of a longitudinal TA layer and thinner TA, the pressure is one-third to one-half that in the corpora cavernosa. Engorgement of the glans during the full erection phase is due to partial compression of the deep dorsal and circumflex veins between Buck's fascia and the corpora cavernosa. Additionally, contraction of the ischiocavernosus and bulbospongiosus muscles promotes engorgement and increases pressure in the glans and spongiosum by compression of the spongiosum and penile veins during the rigid erection phase.

Neurophysiology of erections

Smooth muscle contraction and detumescence

Sympathetic activity is conveyed by α-adrenergic receptors. These are found throughout the cavernosal tissues and vasculature. Specifically, postsynaptic α1a and α1d receptors and presynaptic α2 receptors convey sympathetic stimulation to induce contraction of smooth muscles. Furthermore, norepinephrine seems to be the preferred neurotransmitter. The sympathetic nerves induce detumescence and maintain penile flaccidity by increasing sarcoplasmic free calcium (Ca^{2+}) levels, which promotes smooth muscle contraction. Presynaptic α2-adrenergic receptors increase extracellular calcium entry via membrane ion channels, and α1 receptors release sequestered intracellular calcium in addition to promoting entry of extracellular calcium. This leads to muscle contraction and maintenance of contractile tone, as discussed below.

Additionally, endothelin-1, which is synthesized and present in sinusoidal endothelial tissues, acts as a vasoconstrictor. It also potentiates the constrictor response to catecholamines on the sinusoidal endothelial tissue. These direct and indirect mechanisms suggest endothelin-1 is involved in detumescence. These effects are mediated by the ET-A and ET-B endothelin receptors; the former mediates contraction, whereas ET-B mediates relaxation.

Furthermore, constrictor prostanoids including prostaglandin I_2 (PGI_2), $PGF_{2\alpha}$, and thromboxane A_2 are produced by the cavernous tissues and may play a role in smooth muscle contraction, detumescence, and vasoconstriction. These also attenuate the dilatory effects of nitric oxide when released simultaneously, thus rendering it less effective. Additionally, angiotensin II, which is part of the renin-angiotensin system, is present in cavernosal endothelial and smooth muscle cells and mediates contraction via AT-I receptors. Thus, in the flaccid state, corporeal tissues are in a semicontracted state, which is attained through a combination of intrinsic muscle activity, adrenergic neurotransmission, and endothelium-derived factors.

Smooth muscle relaxation and tumescence

Parasympathetic nerve fibers release acetylcholine (ACh), vasoactive intestinal peptide (VIP), and nitric oxide (NO). The predominant neurotransmitter responsible for erections is NO, by causing smooth muscle relaxation. NO is released from non-adrenergic/non-cholinergic fibers within the erectile tissues. It is a gaseous molecule produced in nerve endings and endothelial tissues. NO is synthesized in nitrergic fibers and endothelial cells by nitric oxide synthase (NOS) via the conversion of L-arginine and oxygen to L-citrulline and NO. This reaction requires a pO_2 greater than 55 mmHg. NOS is present in endothelial cells (eNOS), neuronal cells (nNOS), and as an inducible form (iNOS). Although all three types are present in the corpora, eNOS and nNOS are primarily responsible for erections. NO catalyzes the conversion of guanosine-5′-triphosphate (GTP) to cyclic guanosine monophosphate (cGMP) via soluble guanylyl cyclase. cGMP leads to smooth muscle relaxation, as discussed below.

Additionally, cavernous tissue is rich in muscarinic receptors, which respond to ACh. Although this is not the primary neurotransmitter involved in tumescence, it may indirectly contribute to muscle relaxation by stimulating NO release and presynaptic inhibition of norepinephrine release from adrenergic neurons. Furthermore, although endothelium releases factors that promote vasoconstriction, it may also produce vasorelaxation via endothelium-derived hyperpolarization factor, PGI_2, and endothelin-1 via ET-B receptor activation.

Other neurotransmitters

Multiple other neurotransmitters may play a role in erectile function. Specifically, serotonergic receptors may inhibit sexual function, sexual drive, and erections, whereas dopaminergic input, via D1, D2, and D4 receptors, and adrenergic receptors promotes sexual function. For instance, apomorphine, which has D1 and D2 receptor activity, induces erection-absent sexual stimulation. Gamma-aminobutyric acid (GABA), cannabinoids, prolactin, and opioids may have an inhibitory role on sexual function and erectile function. Oxytocin, NO, and melanocortins promote erectile function.

Given the complexity of erectile function and regulation, there is significant cross-reactivity between tumescence and detumescence systems. For instance, noradrenergic receptors are modulated by nitrergic fibers and, conversely, adrenergic fibers regulate NO release via α2 presynaptic action. Additionally, there is communication at the level of the vascular smooth muscle as well.

Smooth muscle physiology

Smooth muscle contraction: penile flaccidity (Figure 3.1)

In the flaccid state, cavernous smooth muscle remains tonically contracted, which is termed the latch state. This allows maintenance of a basal tone with minimal energy expenditure. Studies have demonstrated spontaneous contractile activity in smooth muscle, which may also be activity induced. Smooth muscle contraction is regulated by sarcoplasmic Ca^{2+} levels. Ca^{2+} binds to calmodulin, a calcium-binding messenger protein, which triggers a cascade of events allowing myosin to crosslink to actin and contract the muscle.

Once Ca^{2+} binds to calmodulin, the affinity of the Ca^{2+}-calmodulin complex for myosin light chain kinase (MLCK), a serine/threonine-specific protein kinase, increases. MLCK is activated once bound by the Ca^{2+}-calmodulin complex. This leads to phosphorylation of

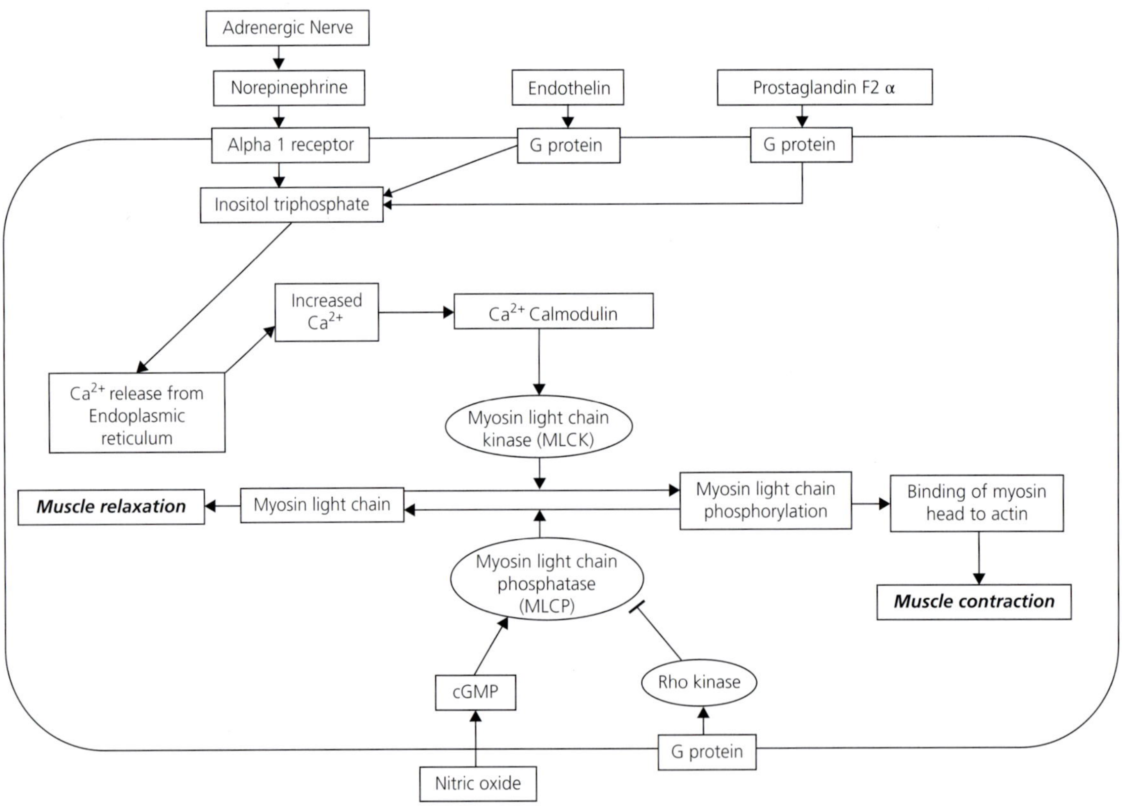

Figure 3.1 Pathways regulating smooth muscle contraction, which leads to detumescence.

myosin light chain (MLC) heads at the position 19 serine (Ser19), which activates the heads allowing crosslink formation with actin. Additionally, myosin-actin crosslinking activates ATPase activity of the myosin head region, which provides energy for subsequent cross-bridge cycles. The overall outcome of this process is muscle contraction. Adenosine triphosphate (ATP) provides the energy for this process.

Thus, for smooth muscle to contract, cytosolic Ca^{2+} needs to increase. During contraction, levels increase from 120–270 nM to 500–700 nM. This is accomplished via the action of different vasoconstrictor agents on their specific receptors, which activates a G-protein-coupled receptor (Gq). Activation of this leads to a downstream cascade that increases intracellular cytosolic calcium. Gq activates phospholipase C beta (PLC-β), a membrane-bound enzyme that hydrolyzes phosphatidylinositol 4,5-bisphosphate (PIP_2) to form inositol 1,4,5-trisphosphate (IP_3) and 1,2-diacylglycerol (DAG). IP_3 binds to the cellular smooth endoplasmic reticulum, leading to release of calcium to the cytoplasm. In addition to causing a release of calcium from the endoplasmic reticulum, IP_3 increases the ability of calcium to trigger the release of intracellular Ca^{2+} stores, leading to calcium-induced calcium release (CICR). To further increase intracellular calcium, constricting agents also open calcium-permeable non-selective channels, allowing entry of extracellular Ca^{2+} as well. All of these processes increase sarcoplasmic Ca^{2+} allowing it to interact with calmodulin and trigger smooth muscle contraction necessary to maintain flaccidity and cause detumescence.

There is some evidence that phasic contraction of penile smooth muscle results from increases in cytosolic Ca^{2+} and tonic contraction is from CICR pathways.

Smooth muscle relaxation: penile erection (Figure 3.2)

Smooth muscle relaxation is essential for erection. For smooth muscle to relax, MLC is dephosphorylated by myosin light chain phosphatase (MLCP). This dephosphorylation changes the conformation of the myosin head so it no longer crosslinks with actin. MLCP activity is regulated by the RhoA/Rho-kinase pathway. Rho-kinase, a serine/threonine kinase, and RhoA, a small GTPase protein, are expressed in penile smooth muscle cells, with concentrations significantly higher in cavernous smooth muscle than in vascular smooth muscle. Activated Rho-kinase inhibits the action of MLCP and promotes smooth muscle contraction.

Relaxation is also triggered by a decrease in sarcoplasmic Ca^{2+}, which leads to dissociation of the Ca^{2+}-calmodulin complex from MLCK. Additionally, Ser19 of myosin is dephosphorylated by MLCP, which leads to dissociation of the myosin-actin crosslink.

Smooth muscle relaxation results from several secondary messengers including cyclic adenosine monophosphate (cAMP) and cyclic guanylate monophosphate (cGMP). These activate specific protein kinases that phosphorylate downstream ion channels and proteins. This leads to cell hyperpolarization by opening membrane potassium channels, sequestration of calcium to the endoplasmic reticulum, and inhibition of membrane calcium channels. These events lead to decreased intracellular calcium, smooth muscle relaxation, and ultimately tumescence.

Cyclic adenosine monophosphate (cAMP)

cAMP is regulated by multiple molecules such as prostaglandins, adenosine, calcitonin gene-related peptides, and VIP. Its formation is catalyzed by the regulatory enzyme adenylyl cyclase (AC), which converts ATP to cAMP. The main receptor for cAMP is protein kinase A (PKA), also called cAMP-dependent kinase. Activation of PKA leads to phosphorylation of multiple downstream targets, with over 100 having been identified. PKA is composed of two regulatory and two catalytic subunits (R_2C_2). With cAMP binding, the regulatory subunits dissociate to $R_2(cAMP)_4$ with free catalytic subunits. This active enzyme then phosphorylates its downstream targets.

Cyclic guanylate monophosphate (cGMP)

cGMP is regulated by multiple molecules such as NO, carbon monoxide (CO), and natriuretic peptides. NO, a small gaseous molecule, is able to easily diffuse into cells where it interacts with soluble guanylyl cyclase (sGC). sGC catalyzes the conversion of GTP to cGMP. Guanylyl cyclase (GC) exists both in membrane-bound and soluble forms. It is, however, the soluble form (sGC), that is particularly involved in erectile function. sGC is composed of alpha and beta subunits. sGC links NO from NANC endings to cGMP. Protein kinase G (PKG), also known as cGMP-dependent kinase, is a serine/threonine-specific protein kinase that is activated by cGMP.

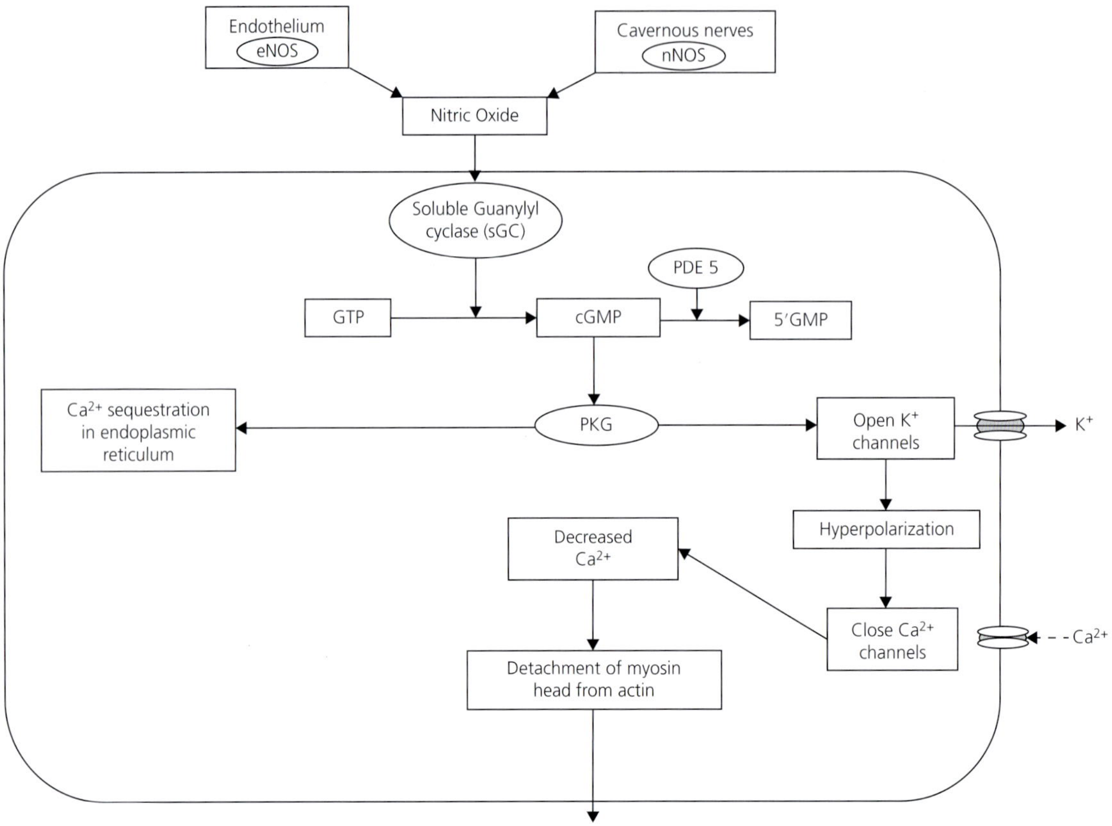

Figure 3.2 Cellular pathways regulating smooth muscle relaxation necessary for tumescence.

It leads to smooth muscle relaxation and erection by phosphorylating downstream targets.

Phosphodiesterase (PDE)

During signaling processes for erections, cGMP and cAMP levels rise two- to three-fold from baseline. To reverse the effects of these messengers, phosphodiesterases hydrolyze cAMP to adenosine monophosphate (AMP), and cGMP to guanylyl monophosphate (GMP). There are 11 families of PDE (PDE1-PDE11). All PDEs are found in the corporeal tissues except for PDE6, which is specific to the eye. However, PDE5 is the primary PDE that hydrolyzes cGMP and terminates its effect. It is the inhibition of this enzyme that has been used as a therapeutic for erectile dysfunction.

Summary

Thus, the complex interplay between the central and peripheral nervous systems, penile anatomy, and neurotransmitters tightly regulates tumescence and detumescence. Erections depend on the relaxation of cavernous and vascular smooth muscles from their tonically contracted state. This is mediated by many factors, particularly NO, which stimulates cGMP production, which in turn activates PKG leading to opening of potassium channels, which hyperpolarizes cells and closes calcium channels. This decrease in cytosolic calcium leads to smooth muscle relaxation. When cGMP is degraded by PDE, intracellular calcium increases and muscles contract.

Further reading

Andersson KE. Mechanisms of penile erection and basis for pharmacological treatment of erectile dysfunction. *Pharmacol Rev* 2011;63(4):811–59.

Andersson KE, Wagner G. Physiology of penile erection. *Physiol Rev* 1995;75(1):191–236.

Awad A, Alsaid B, Bessede T, Droupy S, Benoit G. Evolution in the concept of erection anatomy. *Surg Radiol Anat* 2011;33(4): 301–12.

Bosch RJ, Benard F, Aboseif SR, Stief CG, Lue TF, Tanagho EA. Penile detumescence: characterization of three phases. *J Urol* 1991;146(3):867–71.

Dean RC, Lue TF. Physiology of penile erection and pathophysiology of erectile dysfunction. *Urol Clin North Am* 2005;32(4):379–95, v.

Giuliano F. Neurophysiology of erection and ejaculation. *J Sex Med* 2011;8 (Suppl. 4):310–315.

Hong F, Haldeman BD, Jackson D, Carter M, Baker JE, Cremo CR. Biochemistry of smooth muscle myosin light chain kinase. *Arch Biochem Biophys* 2011;510(2):135–46.

Hsieh CH, Liu SP, Hsu GL, et al. Advances in understanding of mammalian penile evolution, human penile anatomy and human erection physiology: clinical implications for physicians and surgeons. *Med Sci Monit* 2012;18(7):RA118–25.

Janssen E. Sexual arousal in men: a review and conceptual analysis. *Horm Behav* 2011;59(5):708–16.

Lin CS, Xin ZC, Lin G, Lue TF. Phosphodiesterases as therapeutic targets. *Urology* 2003;61(4):685–91.

Lue TF. Erectile dysfunction. *N Engl J Med* 2000;342:1802–13.

Lue TF. Physiology of penile erection and pathophysiology of erectile dysfunction. In: Wein AJ (ed.), *Campbell-Walsh Urology*, 10th edn. Philadelphia, PA: Elsevier Saunders, 2012; pp. 688–707.

Mouras H, Stoleru S, Bittoun J, et al. Brain processing of visual sexual stimuli in healthy men: a functional magnetic resonance imaging study. *Neuroimage* 2003;20(2):855–69.

Pfitzer G. Invited review: regulation of myosin phosphorylation in smooth muscle. *J Appl Physiol (1985)* 2001;91(1): 497–503.

Qiu X, Villalta J, Lin G, Lue TF. Role of hydrogen sulfide in the physiology of penile erection. *J Androl* 2012;33(4):529–35.

CHAPTER 4

Anatomy of penile erection

Lindsay Yuh and Alan Shindel
UC Davis, Sacramento, CA, USA

Introduction

Penile erection is based on a complex interplay between physiologic, neurologic, endocrine, and vascular factors. Disruption of any of these components may lead to erectile dysfunction. Erectile dysfunction (ED) is defined as consistent or recurrent inability to achieve and maintain an erection sufficient for satisfactory sexual intercourse.[1–3] It has been estimated to affect 30 million men in the USA; up to 52% of men aged 40–70 have mild to complete ED.[4] The worldwide prevalence of ED is projected to increase to 322 million men by the year 2025.[5]

ED is associated with age and numerous medical illnesses. Recent advancements in our understanding of penile physiology and pathophysiology have revolutionized the approach to the man with ED. A thorough understanding of the normal mechanisms that mediate penile erection enables the provider to counsel and treat male patients with sexual concerns.

Penile anatomy

The penis is composed of three erectile bodies: two *corpora cavernosa* and one *corpus spongiosum*. The corpora cavernosa are located dorsally on the penis. They are attached via an incomplete midline septum composed of multiple strands of connective tissue; the septum becomes more complete towards the distal aspect of the penis.[6–8]

Each corpus cavernosum contains vascular sinuses (also known as lacunae) lined by endothelial cells. These lacunae engorge with blood during penile erection. A sheath of connective tissue called the *tunica albuginea* surrounds the lacunae. The tunica albuginea consists of multiple layers of collagen and elastic fibers, oriented in an inner circular and an outer longitudinal layer. This framework permits rigidity and axial strength during penile erection, and compliance and flexibility when the penis is flaccid.[9]

The corpus spongiosum contains the urethra and lies ventrally within the groove between two corpora cavernosa. Distally, the corpus spongiosum forms a broad cap of erectile tissue called the *glans penis,* which covers the tips of corpora cavernosa. The tunica albuginea surrounding the erectile tissue of the corpus spongiosum is much thinner than tunica albuginea of the corpora cavernosa and there is less erectile tissue present (Figure 4.1).[9–11]

The three erectile bodies and the tunica albuginea are surrounded (from deep to superficial) by penile fascia, Buck's fascia, superficial penile fascia (dartos fascia), and skin. The deep dorsal vein of the penis, dorsal arteries, and dorsal nerves are located on the superior aspect of the corpora cavernosa in Buck's fascia (Figure 4.2).

Vascular anatomy

The blood supply to the penis originates from the paired *penile arteries,* which are derived from the *internal pudendal arteries* and *internal iliac arteries.* The penile *arteries* travel along the medial border of the pubic rami and then continue along the urethra bulb. The *bulbourethral artery* is the first branch of the penile artery; the *dorsal artery of the penis* is the continuation of the common penile artery. The dorsal artery courses deep to dorsal penile vein and lateral to the cavernous nerves. The dorsal artery gives off circumflex branches around the lateral surface of the Corporal bodies.

Male Sexual Dysfunction: A Clinical Guide, First Edition. Edited by Suks Minhas and John Mulhall.

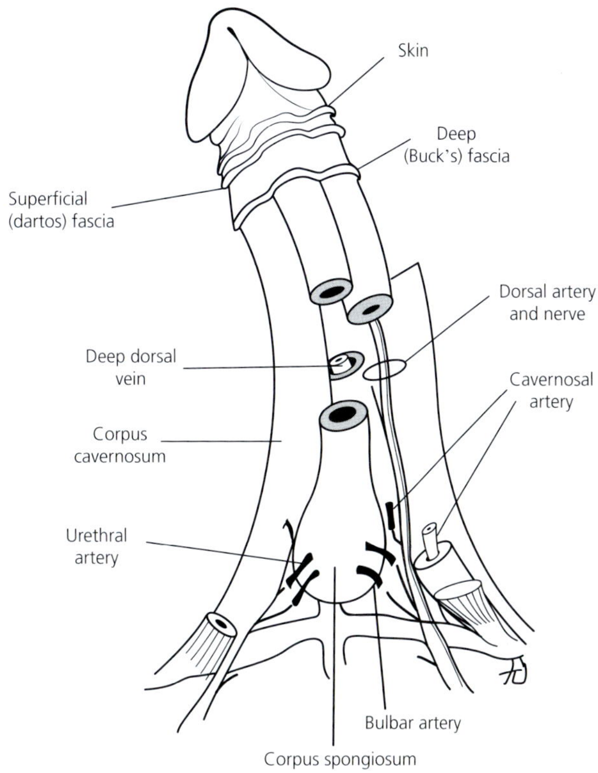

Figure 4.1 Ventral view of penile anatomy. The corpus spongiosum contains the urethra and lies within the groove between the two corpora cavernosa. The bulbar and urethral arteries are the first branches of the penile artery. The dorsal artery and nerve course lateral to the dorsal vein of the penis. Modified from Angermeier, KW. Surgical anatomy of the penis. In: *Operative Urology at the Cleveland Clinic*. Springer, 2006; pp. 377–83.

The terminal branch of the common penile artery is the *cavernosal artery*, which enters the corpus cavernosum at the hilum and runs the length of the penile shaft, giving off many helicine arteries inside the erectile tissue of the penis (Figure 4.1).

In some men, the cavernosal artery may arise from the pudendal artery; an accessory cavernosal artery from the pudendal artery is also present in some men. This is a normal anatomical variant and should be considered during pelvic surgery. The bulbourethral artery supplies the urethra and corpus spongiosum. The corpus spongiosum may also be supplied distally by collateral flow from distal branches of the dorsal artery of the penis.[8,12]

Neuroanatomy of penile erection

Autonomic nervous system regulation of erection

The penis is innervated by both autonomic (sympathetic and parasympathetic) and somatic (sensory and motor) nerves. The neurons in the spinal cord and peripheral ganglia merge via sympathetic and parasympathetic pathways to form the *cavernous nerves*. These autonomic fibers enter the corpora cavernosa and corpus spongiosum to control neurovascular events during erection and detumescence.[11]

The nerves involved in the sympathetic regulation of the penis emerge from the T11-L2 spinal levels. These nerve fibers exit the spine via sympathetic ganglia, through lumbar splanchnic nerves to the inferior mesenteric and superior hypogastric plexuses. These plexuses sit close to the aorta and are at risk for injury during retroperitoneal lymph node dissections; this may lead to retrograde ejaculation or anejaculation. The baseline sympathetic tone to the penis is mediated by adrenergic fibers that release norepinephrine. Sympathetic tone maintains the penis in the flaccid state and also triggers detumescence with resolution of sexual arousal.

The parasympathetic innervation to the penis arises from S2-S4 spinal segments, which join to form the inferior hypogastric plexus via the pelvic splanchnic nerves. The hypogastric plexus is approximately 4–5 cm

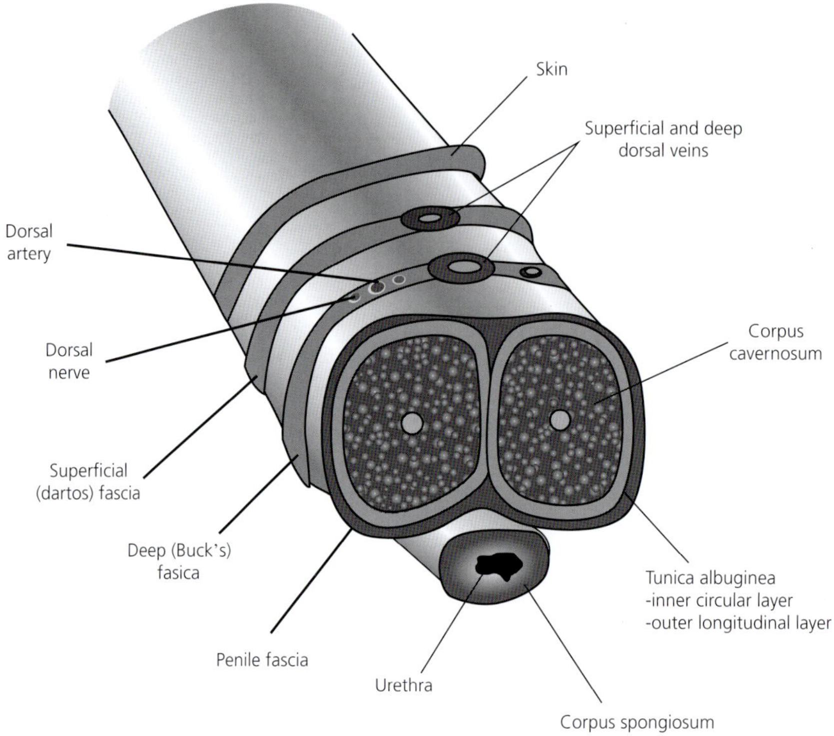

Figure 4.2 Cross-sectional view of penile anatomy. The three erectile bodies (two corpora cavernosa and midline corpus spongiosum) are surrounded by the tunica albuginea, which is composed of an inner circular layer and an outer longitudinal layer. The subsequent layers of the penis from deep to superficial are penile fascia, deep (Buck's) fascia, superficial (dartos fascia), and skin. The superficial dorsal vein courses through dartos fascia, and the deep dorsal vein runs through Buck's fascia. Modified from Angermeier, KW. Surgical anatomy of the penis. In: *Operative Urology at the Cleveland Clinic*. Springer, 2006; pp. 377–83.

long, located on both sides of the rectum. The midpoint of the hypogastric plexus lies at the level of the seminal vesicles, with a network of neurovascular structures coursing through it.[13,14] The most caudal portion of the pelvic plexus leads to the cavernous nerves that innervate the penis. Division of these vessels during operative dissection risks injury to the pelvic plexus and leads to postoperative erectile dysfunction.[13,15] The *cavernosal nerves* leave the endopelvic fascia, run along the posterior-lateral boarder of prostate, and branch medially and laterally before reaching the membranous urethra. Superficial branches travel on the lateral surface of urethral sphincter at 3 and 9 o'clock positions. As the cavernous nerves reach the hilum of the penis they join to form one of three discrete bundles at 1, 11, and 6 o'clock positions, superficial to the cavernous veins.[8] The cavernosal nerves pierce the corpora cavernosa and along with cavernosal arteries supply the erectile tissue. Small fibers also join the dorsal nerves of the penis as they course distally.

Stimulation of the pelvic plexus and cavernosal nerves induces erection, whereas stimulation of the hypogastric nerve or sympathetic trunk causes detumescence. This illustrates that sacral parasympathetic input is responsible for erections, and the thoracolumbar sympathetic pathway for detumescence.

Modulation of either the sympathetic or parasympathetic systems may contribute to penile erection. The specific contributions are apparent in spinal cord injured animals and humans. Suppression of sympathetic tone to the penis is thought to be the mechanism for mentally/psychologically provoked erections. In animal experiments where the spinal cord was removed below L4 or L5, exposure to a female in heat or stimulation of the medial preoptic area produced marked erections suggesting supraspinal mediation of tumescence. In this same sacral parasympathetic spinal cord injured model, erections were also elicited by stimulating the thoracolumbar sympathetic pathways. Human males who have suffered sacral spinal cord injury may retain psychogenic erections (i.e., penile erection in response to partner initiation, audiovisual stimulation, and/or fantasy) even through reflexogenic erections (penile erection in response to penile stimulation) may not be possible. Psychogenic erections in these patients may involve swelling and lengthening of the penis with variable degrees of rigidity.[9,16,17]

Psychogenic erections do not generally occur in patients with lesions above T10 level; this is consistent with knowledge that the sympathetic innervations of the penis are derived from the L2 spinal roots. In men with spinal cord injury above T10, impulses can still travel to the spinal cord by somatic and parasympathetic pathways; this contributes to reflexogenic erections in response to penile stimulation or contact.[9,18]

Although partial preservation of erection occurs in men with spinal lesions at various levels, maximal erection requires inhibition of the sympathetic tone of the penis and excitation of parasympathetic fibers.

Somatic nervous system regulation of erection

The somatosensory pathway originates from the sensory receptors in the penile skin, urethra, glans, and within the corpus cavernosum. These sensory fibers converge to form the dorsal nerve of the penis and then coalesce with the *pudendal nerve*. The pudendal nerve enters the spinal cord through S2-S4 nerve roots. Sensory information is transmitted to the spinal cord and from there to the brain for sensory processing. *Onuf's nucleus* is located in the sacral spinal segments and is the center for somatomotor penile signaling. Efferent nerves from this location will innervate the ischiocavernosus and bulbocavernosus muscles. Contraction of the ischiocavernosus muscle produces the rigid-erection state. Contraction of the bulbocavernosus muscle is necessary for ejaculation.[11]

Supraspinal regulation of erection

In animal models, the *medial preoptic area* and the *paraventricular nucleus of the hypothalamus* and hippocampus have been identified as important centers for sexual function and penile erections. Electrostimulation of these areas induced erections, and lesions at these sites limit copulatory behavior in male animals.[19]

With the advent of modern imaging techniques has come greater understanding of human brain activity during sexual arousal. Specific brain centers have been studied using positron emission tomography (PET) and magnetic resonance imaging (MRI) in men exposed to erotic stimuli (typically audiovisual sexual stimulation). Brain areas of note are the bilateral inferior temporal cortex (visual association area), right insula (somatosensory processing with motivational states), right inferior frontal cortex (sensory processing), left anterior cingulated cortex (autonomic and neuroendocrine function), right occipital gyrus (visual processing), right hypothalamus (male copulatory behavior), and left caudate (attention processing with responsiveness to new environmental stimuli).[20,21]

Hemodynamics and physiology of male erection

In a flaccid state, the arterial flow to the penis is minimal. The cavernosal smooth muscle as well as smooth muscle of the arterial wall are tonically contracted and the partial pressure of oxygen is about 35 mmHg.[9] The penile vasculature can contract even further as evidenced by shrinkage in cold weather and after phenylephrine injections. The contraction of penile smooth muscle appears to be mediated by actions of α-adrenergic agonists and endothelin-1 via ET-A endothelin receptors.[22–25]

Penile erection results from sexual stimulation (exposure to erotic material, penile contact, etc.), which triggers release of neurotransmitters that relax smooth muscle. The most important neurotransmitter in penile erection is nitric oxide (NO), which will be discussed later in this chapter.

Initial penile tumescence occurs by engorgement of the corpora cavernosa. The dilatation of arteries and arterioles supplying the corpora cavernosa causes up to a seven-fold increase in blood flow. The relaxation of sinusoidal smooth muscle within the corpora facilitates rapid filling and expansion of the sinusoidal system. The venous plexus located between sinusoids and the tunica albuginea is compressed, resulting in reduction of venous outflow. Further stretching of the tunica albuginea to capacity occludes veins between the inner circular and outer longitudinal layers, which further limits venous outflow. Blood is effectively trapped within the sinuses of the corpora cavernosa, increasing intracavernous pressure to around

100 mmHg and raising the penis from flaccid to the erect state (full erection phase).[26]

Arterial flow increases in the corpus spongiosum and glans penis in a similar manner; however, the pressure is only one-half to one-third the pressure in corpora cavernosa due to minimal occlusion from the thin tunica of the corpus spongiosum and glans penis. The glans penis and spongiosum may be just partially rigid during full erection; this structure may act as a large arteriovenous shunt. Increasing sexual arousal during sexual intercourse and/or masturbation triggers forceful contraction of ischiocavernosus muscles. With contraction of these muscles blood is forced into the corpus spongiosum and glans penis, causing maximal tumescence and potentially suprasystolic intrapenile pressures as high as several hundred mmHg. This is the rigid erection phase that typically occurs at high levels of arousal immediately before orgasm/ejaculation.[9–12,27–30]

After orgasm or resolution of sexual arousal, detumescence occurs. Detumescence is mediated by cessation of NO production, breakdown of molecular mediators of vasodilation, and sympathetic discharge during ejaculation.[31]

Molecular mechanisms of penile erection

Smooth muscle activity and calcium metabolism

The erectile tissue of the corpus cavernosum is composed of sinusoidal spaces interconnected and separated by smooth muscle surrounded by elastic fibers, collagen, and areolar tissue. Terminal nerves and arterioles are intimately connected through a smooth muscle network. Relaxation of sinusoids allows blood to fill the cavity; hence, penile erection is dependent on the compliance and relaxation of the smooth muscle. Nerves, neurotransmitters, and endothelium-derived substances control the relaxation of the penile smooth muscle.

The penis is kept in the flaccid state through tonic activity of adrenergic nerves causing smooth muscle contraction. Norepinephrine binds to smooth muscle receptors and this starts a signaling pathway (G-protein-coupled inositol trisphosphate) to release calcium from intracellular stores and to open calcium channels leading to influx of calcium from the extracellular space. This influx causes free cytosolic calcium to rise from resting levels. Ca^{2+} ions bind to calmodulin, and this calcium-calmodulin complex binds to myosin light chain kinase (MLCK) resulting in its activation. When active, MLCK phosphorylates myosin light chains, providing energy for actin cross-bridging and cycling of myosin attachments to actin. Cycling of the actin-myosin complex drives muscle contraction and vasoconstriction.[30]

Relaxation of smooth muscle and initiation of penile erection follows sequestration of free calcium into the sarcoplasmic reticulum. The dissociation of calmodulin from MLCK inactivates it, and myosin detaches from actin filaments. Intracellular second messengers mediating smooth muscle relaxation are cyclic adenosine monophosphate (cAMP) and cyclic guanosine monophosphate (cGMP). Contraction and relaxation of smooth muscle depends on intracellular levels of calcium. The regulation of calcium levels involves several mechanisms, which are discussed below.[32–34]

Nitric oxide/cyclic GMP

Nitric oxide (NO) is produced from oxygen and L-arginine under control of nitric oxide synthase (NOS) and serves many biological functions. Psychogenic and reflexive stimuli activate the parasympathetic neurons that initiate calcium entry into the cells and activation of neuronal NOS (nNOS), leading to a short-lived burst of NO.[35] NO diffuses into the cytoplasm of nearby smooth muscle cells to activate soluble guanylyl cyclase, which serves as its physiologic receptor. This binding causes a conformational change of guanylyl cyclase, activating the enzyme to catalyze the conversion of guanosine triphosphate (GTP) to cyclic guanosine monophosphate (cGMP). cGMP operates through cGMP-dependent protein kinase to regulate the contractile state of corporal smooth muscle. The downstream activities of cGMP include directing phosphorylation of proteins and ion channels (leading to opening potassium channels and membrane hyperpolarization) and sequestration of intracellular calcium. The net effect of these molecular events is a drop in cytosolic Ca^{2+} and relaxation of cavernosal smooth muscle (Figure 4.3).[32,34,36–38]

The vasorelaxant effects of NO cause increased blood flow and expansion of penile vasculature and sinusoidal spaces. Relaxation and shear stress through the vasculature endothelium activate phosphatidyl-inositol 2-kinase, which triggers a serine/threonine protein

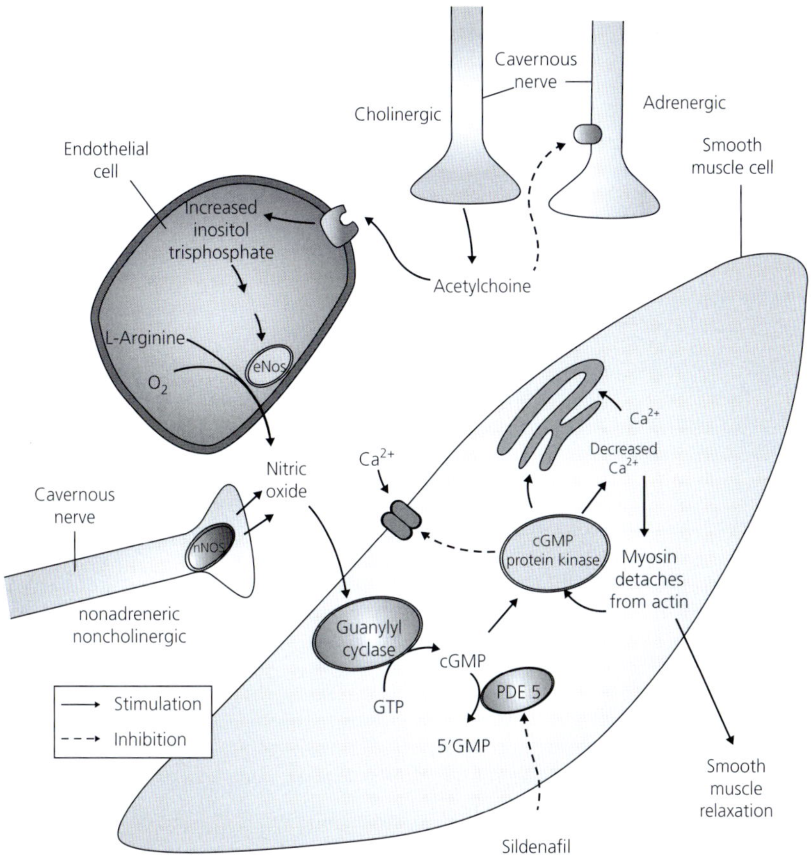

Figure 4.3 Molecular mechanisms of penile smooth muscle relaxation. Nitric oxide is released from endothelial cells (eNOS) and neurons (nNOS). NO diffuses to the cytoplasm of smooth muscle cells leading to activation of its intracellular receptor, guanylyl cyclase. This binding activates guanylyl cyclase leading to the conversion of guanosine triphosphate (GTP) to cyclic guanosine monophosphate (cGMP). Through cGMP-specific protein kinases cytosolic calcium levels decrease, leading to cavernosal smooth muscle relaxation. PDE5, phosphodiesterase type 5. Modified from Dean RC, Lue TF. Physiology of penile erection and pathophysiology of erectile dysfunction. *Urol Clin N Am* 2005;32:379–95.

kinase (AKT) to phosphorylate and activate endothelial NOS (eNOS) in endothelial cells.[32,39,40] This sustained increase in NO leads to maximal relaxation that does not require continuous neuronal depolarization and reduces calcium requirement for the maintenance of erection.

Gap junction channels interconnect the corpus cavernosum smooth muscle cells and allow them to function as a syncytium. Second messengers such as calcium ions and inositol trisphosphate are transported between corporal smooth muscle cells through these junctions allowing for synchronous myogenic activity. Cell-to-cell communication facilitates synchronization and integration of smooth muscle activity.[28,33]

Phosphodiesterase type 5

The phosphodiesterases (PDE) are a class of enzymes that degrade cyclic nucleotides such as cGMP and cAMP. There are over 50 isoenzymes identified to date, and PDE isoenzymes types 2, 3, 4, and 5 have been specifically located in the human corpora cavernosa. PDE type 5 (PDE5) is preferentially expressed in the corpus cavernosum and is selective for cGMP in the presence of bound zinc. PDE5 converts cGMP into inactive 5′-GMP; PDE5-mediated decrease in cellular cGMP opposes penile erection by potentiating vasoconstriction.[9,11,36,41,42]

PDE5 inhibitors (PDE5Is) are a class of drugs that competitively inhibit PDE5 and lead to elevated levels of cytosolic cGMP. The net result of increased cGMP is decreased intracellular calcium, smooth muscle relaxation, vasodilation, and penile erection. PDE5I (e.g., sildenafil, vardenafil, tadalafil, udenafil, avanafil, mirodenafil, and lodenafil) are the first-line agents of choice in the management of ED in the modern era.[25,43]

Rho/Rho-kinase pathway

Myosin light chain phosphatase (MLCP) dephosphorylates myosin and inactivates the actin-myosin cross-bridge movement. Normally, the contractile response is tightly associated with intracellular concentration of free Ca^{2+}; however, MLCP allows for increased force at low intracellular Ca^{2+} levels, or Ca^{2+} sensitization. The activity of MLCP is modulated by the RhoA/Rho-kinase pathway. RhoA is a small guanosine triphosphate (GTP)-binding protein involved in several cellular processes, with a 17-fold greater expression in cavernosal smooth muscle than in vascular smooth muscle. It is activated by G-protein and is regulated by GDP dissociation inhibitor (GDI), guanine nucleotide exchange factor (GEF), and GTPase. Activated RhoA has a variety of targets, including penile smooth muscle Rho-kinase. Rho-kinase inhibits MLCP, which inhibits the activity of the enzyme. When MLCP activity is low, MLC remains phosphorylated and smooth muscle contraction is maintained.[44,45]

Disruption of the RhoA-mediated activation of Rho-kinase promotes smooth muscle relaxation.[22,37,46–50] NO/cGMP-mediated vasodilation is also due in part to inhibition of the RhoA/Rho-kinase pathway. The pathway is upregulated in rat models with bilateral cavernous nerve injury, consistent with the ED phenotype common after pelvic surgery; this suggests a role for targeted therapy after radical prostatectomy.[22,45,48,51] This regulatory pathway is under investigation as a possible pharmacological target for management of ED.[49]

Other mediators

Other non-cholinergic parasympathetic neurotransmitters are capable of promoting smooth muscle relaxation and an erectile response, including calmodulin, vasoactive intestinal polypeptide (VIP), bradykinin, peptide histidine methionine, pituitary adenylate cyclase-activating polypeptide, helospectin, galanin, calcitonin gene-related peptide (CGRP), and prostaglandin E_1.[33,52] Prostaglandin E_1 by intracavernous injection is an approved therapy for ED. The relative importance of these other neuropeptides in the regulation of physiological erection remains fertile ground for further research.

Conclusions

Penile erection is the best understood aspect of the male sexual response. Our understanding of penile erection enables the contemporary provider to offer sound advice and treatment for men who have problems of penile erection. Familiarity with the mechanisms of penile erection is hence essential for healthcare providers who care for male patients.

References

1 National Institutes of Health. Impotence. *NIH Consens Statement Online* 1992 Dec 7–9; 10(4):1–33.
2 Montague DK, Jarow JP, Broderick GA, et al. Chapter 1: The management of erectile dysfunction: an AUA update. *J Urol* 2005;174(1):230–9.
3 Montorsi F, Adaikan G, Becher E, et al. Summary of the recommendations on sexual dysfunctions in men. *J Sex Med* 2010;7(11):3572–88.
4 Feldman HA, Goldstein I, Hatzichristou DG, Krane RJ, McKinlay JB. Impotence and its medical and psychosocial correlates: results of the Massachusetts Male Aging Study. *J Urol* 1994;151(1):54–61.
5 Ayta IA, McKinlay JB, Krane RJ. The likely worldwide increase in erectile dysfunction between 1995 and 2025 and some possible policy consequences. *BJU Int* 1999;84(1):50–6.
6 Hsieh CH, Liu SP, Hsu GL, et al. Advances in understanding of mammalian penile evolution, human penile anatomy and human erection physiology: clinical implications for physicians and surgeons. *Med Sci Monit* 2012;18(7): RA118–25.
7 Hsu GL, Hsieh CH, Wen HS, et al. Anatomy of the human penis: the relationship of the architecture between skeletal and smooth muscles. *J Androl* 2004;25(3):426–31.
8 Yiee JH, Baskin LS. Penile embryology and anatomy. *TheScientificWorldJOURNAL* 2010;10:1174–9.
9 Dean RC, Lue TF. Physiology of penile erection and pathophysiology of erectile dysfunction. *Urol Clin N Am* 2005; 32(4):379–95, v.
10 Hsu GL. Hypothesis of human penile anatomy, erection hemodynamics and their clinical applications. *Asian J Androl* 2006;8(2):225–34.
11 El-Sakka AI, Lue TF. Physiology of penile erection. *TheScientificWorldJOURNAL* 2004;4 Suppl 1:128–34.
12 Simonsen U, Garcia-Sacristan A, Prieto D. Penile arteries and erection. *J Vasc Res* 2002;39(4):283–303.
13 Walsh PC, Schlegel PN. Radical pelvic surgery with preservation of sexual function. *Ann Surg* 1988;208(4):391–400.
14 Walsh PC. Preservation of sexual function in the surgical treatment of prostatic cancer—an anatomic surgical approach. *Important Adv Oncol* 1988:161–170.

15 Walsh PC, Brendler CB, Chang T, et al. Preservation of sexual function in men during radical pelvic surgery. *Md Med J* 1990;39(4):389–93.

16 Courtois FJ, Macdougall JC, Sachs BD. Erectile mechanism in paraplegia. *Physiol Behav Apr* 1993;53(4):721–6.

17 Giuliano F, Rampin O. Neural control of erection. *Physiol Behav* 2004;83(2):189–201.

18 Allard J, Edmunds NJ. Reflex penile erection in anesthetized mice: an exploratory study. *Neuroscience* 2008;155(1):283–90.

19 Temel Y, van Lankveld JJ, Boon P, Spincemaille GH, van der Linden C, Visser-Vandewalle V. Deep brain stimulation of the thalamus can influence penile erection. *Int J Impot Res* 2004;16(1):91–4.

20 Arnow BA, Desmond JE, Banner LL, et al. Brain activation and sexual arousal in healthy, heterosexual males. *Brain* 2002;125(Pt 5):1014–23.

21 Mouras H, Stoleru S, Bittoun J, et al. Brain processing of visual sexual stimuli in healthy men: a functional magnetic resonance imaging study. *Neuroimage* 2003;20(2):855–69.

22 Mills TM, Lewis RW, Wingard CJ, Linder AE, Jin L, Webb RC. Vasoconstriction, RhoA/Rho-kinase and the erectile response. *Int J Impot Res* 2003;15 (Suppl 5):S20–4.

23 Andersson KE. Pharmacology of penile erection. *Pharmacol Rev* 2001;53(3):417–50.

24 Andersson KE. Neurophysiology/pharmacology of erection. *Int J Impot Res* 2001;13 (Suppl 3):S8–S17.

25 Andersson KE. Mechanisms of penile erection and basis for pharmacological treatment of erectile dysfunction. *Pharmacol Rev* 2011;63(4):811–59.

26 Lue TF. Neurogenic erectile dysfunction. *Clin Auton Res* 2001;11(5):285–94.

27 Carrier S, Brock G, Kour NW, Lue TF. Pathophysiology of erectile dysfunction. *Urology* 1993;42(4):468–81.

28 Christ GJ. The penis as a vascular organ. The importance of corporal smooth muscle tone in the control of erection. *Urol Clin North Am* 1995;22(4):727–45.

29 Miyata Y. Penile erection occurs when penile vascular resistance is decreased and corporal smooth muscle is relaxed. *Eur Urol* 2007;52(1):259.

30 Saenz de Tejada I, Angulo J, Cellek S, et al. Physiology of erectile function. *J Sex Med* 2004;1(3):254–65.

31 Bosch RJ, Benard F, Aboseif SR, Stief CG, Lue TF, Tanagho EA. Penile detumescence: characterization of three phases. *J Urol* 1991;146(3):867–71.

32 Burnett AL. Nitric oxide regulation of penile erection: biology and therapeutic implications. *J Androl* 2002;23(5):S20–6.

33 Kandeel FR, Koussa VK, Swerdloff RS. Male sexual function and its disorders: physiology, pathophysiology, clinical investigation, and treatment. *Endocr Rev* 2001;22(3):342–88.

34 Rajfer J, Aronson WJ, Bush PA, Dorey FJ, Ignarro LJ. Nitric oxide as a mediator of relaxation of the corpus cavernosum in response to nonadrenergic, noncholinergic neurotransmission. *N Engl J Med* 1992;326(2):90–4.

35 Bredt DS, Hwang PM, Snyder SH. Localization of nitric oxide synthase indicating a neural role for nitric oxide. *Nature* 1990;347(6295):768–70.

36 Corbin JD. Mechanisms of action of PDE5 inhibition in erectile dysfunction. *Int J Impot Res* 2004;16 (Suppl 1):S4–7.

37 Mills TM, Lewis RW, Wingard CJ, Chitaley K, Webb RC. Inhibition of tonic contraction – a novel way to approach erectile dysfunction. *J Androl* 2002;23(5):S5–9.

38 Lue TF. Erectile dysfunction. *N Engl J Med* 2000;342(24): 1802–13.

39 Cartledge J, Minhas S, Eardley I. The role of nitric oxide in penile erection. *Expert Opin Pharmacother* 2001;2(1): 95–107.

40 Priviero FB, Leite R, Webb RC, Teixeira CE. Neurophysiological basis of penile erection. *Acta Pharmacol Sin* 2007;28(6):751–5.

41 Kuthe A, Magert H, Uckert S, Forssmann WG, Stief CG, Jonas U. Gene expression of the phosphodiesterases 3A and 5A in human corpus cavernosum penis. *Eur Urol* 2000;38(1):108–14.

42 Lue TF, Lee KL. Pharmacotherapy for erectile dysfunction. *Chin Med J (Engl)* 2000;113(4):291–8.

43 Burnett AL. Phosphodiesterase 5 mechanisms and therapeutic applications. *Am J Cardiol* 2005;96(12B):29M–31M.

44 Jin L, Burnett AL. RhoA/Rho-kinase in erectile tissue: mechanisms of disease and therapeutic insights. *Clin Sci (Lond)* 2006;110(2):153–65.

45 Gratzke C, Strong TD, Gebska MA, et al. Activated RhoA/Rho kinase impairs erectile function after cavernous nerve injury in rats. *J Urol* 2010;184(5):2197–204.

46 Mills TM, Chitaley K, Lewis RW, Webb RC. Nitric oxide inhibits RhoA/Rho-kinase signaling to cause penile erection. *Eur J Pharmacol* 2002;439(1–3):173–4.

47 Wang H, Eto M, Steers WD, Somlyo AP, Somlyo AV. RhoA-mediated Ca2+ sensitization in erectile function. *J Biol Chem* 2002;277(34):30614–21.

48 Sauzeau V, Le Jeune H, Cario-Toumaniantz C, et al. Cyclic GMP-dependent protein kinase signaling pathway inhibits RhoA-induced Ca2+ sensitization of contraction in vascular smooth muscle. *J Biol Chem* 2000;275(28):21722–9.

49 Dai Y, Chitaley K, Webb RC, Lewis RW, Mills TM. Topical application of a Rho-kinase inhibitor in rats causes penile erection. *Int J Impot Res* 2004;16(3):294–8.

50 Chitaley K, Webb RC, Mills TM. RhoA/Rho-kinase: a novel player in the regulation of penile erection. *Int J Impot Res* 2001;13(2):67–72.

51 Hannan JL, Albersen M, Kutlu O, et al. Inhibition of Rho-kinase improves erectile function, increases nitric oxide signaling and decreases penile apoptosis in a rat model of cavernous nerve injury. *J Urol* 2013;189(3):1155–61.

52 Saenz de Tejada I. Molecular mechanisms for the regulation of penile smooth muscle contractility. *Int J Impot Res* 2002;14 (Suppl 1):S6–10.

CHAPTER 5

Endocrinology of male sexual dysfunction

Salim Janmohamed[1] and Pierre-Marc G. Bouloux[2]

[1] *University College London, London, UK*

[2] *The Royal Free Hospital, London, UK*

Introduction

Male sexual dysfunction (MSD) encompasses disturbances of libido, erectile function, ejaculation, orgasm, and detumescence, and affects up to 10% of middle-aged or older men.[1] MSD may be an initial manifestation of important underlying systemic disorders that can affect and, indeed, dominate wider well-being and clinical management.

Endocrine disorders should be considered in this context, although non-endocrine factors, particularly psychosexual ones, may be more important. Endocrinopathies can be associated with a range of other non-specific, non-sexual symptoms, such as fatigue and weight disturbance. Of all hormonal disorders, diabetes mellitus (DM) is, worldwide, the most common and important cause of organic erectile dysfunction (ED), increasing the risk three-fold compared to men without a history of DM.[2] By comparison,,male hypogonadism, a clinical syndrome resulting from subphysiological testosterone levels due to a perturbation of the hypothalamo-pituitary-testicular (HPT) axis at one or more levels, is a far less common cause of sexual dysfunction. Decreased production of spermatozoa by the testicular germinal epithelium can represent an additional component of hypogonadism but may not be clinically relevant in many men. Other endocrine disturbances, including pituitary, thyroid, and adrenal dysfunction and calcium disorders may give rise to, *inter alia*, psychosexual and erectile dysfunction.

In this chapter, we consider the central organization of sexual function, the regulation of the hypothalamo-pituitary-testicular axis, the role of androgens in sexual function, and finally the different pathologies of the endocrine system that impact on male sexual function.

Central organization of sexual function

Hypothalamic and limbic areas are of fundamental importance with regard to sexual desire, motivation, and arousal, particularly outputs from the medial preoptic area to the ventral tegmentum, and efferent dopaminergic projections to limbic, prefrontal, and anterior cingulate cortical areas, the nucleus accumbens, and amygdala. Androgen effects on sexual function may in part result from enhancement of reward-seeking circuit activity and be mediated by the effects of testosterone on dopaminergic receptors in the medial preoptic area, both directly and after aromatization to estradiol.[3] The highest density of androgen receptor expression is found in hypothalamic nuclei known to participate in sexual and reproductive behavior, as well as other brain regions with important hypothalamic afferents. The anterior pituitary contains receptors for all sex steroid hormones.

In addition to androgens and other sex steroids, a range of peptides and neurotransmitters, often with important inter-dependent effects on synthesis, release,

Male Sexual Dysfunction: A Clinical Guide, First Edition. Edited by Suks Minhas and John Mulhall.

and signaling, are involved in sexual function. Gonadotropin-releasing hormone (GnRH) is the key regulator of luteinizing hormone (LH) and follicle-stimulating hormone (FSH) secretion. Neurotransmitter inputs to GnRH neurons include dopamine, serotonin, neuropeptide Y, and the predominantly excitatory effects of norepinephrine and glutamate and dominant inhibitory drive of GABA and endogenous opioid peptides.

Opioid, serotonergic, and endocannabinoid systems exert inhibitory effects on excitatory systems. Opioids (e.g., β-endorphin) and analogs can directly inhibit release of hypothalamic GnRH, and thereby LH and testosterone release, and also mediate and modulate sex steroid feedback on GnRH neurons (Figure 5.1). Melanocortin signaling via MCR4 receptors can increase sexual desire and, in healthy men, erectile activity, effects first described with the agent bremelanotide. This signaling pathway has previously been described in small mammals.[4] Gonadal steroids and inhibin B are responsible for negative feedback inhibition of gonadotropin secretion.

The kisspeptin-GPR54-neurokinin B pathway and regulation of GnRH release

Kisspeptin, a hypothalamic peptide encoded by *KISS1*, is an important neuromodulator that acts on GPR54 receptors to regulate GnRH release.[5] Kisspeptin axons form dense pericapillary plexuses in the human infundibular stalk, the site of neurosecretion of GnRH. Kisspeptin expression is regulated by testosterone and estradiol.[6] Sensitivity to sex steroid feedback, which may also underlie the switch from negative to positive feedback of estrogen in females, and metabolic cues,

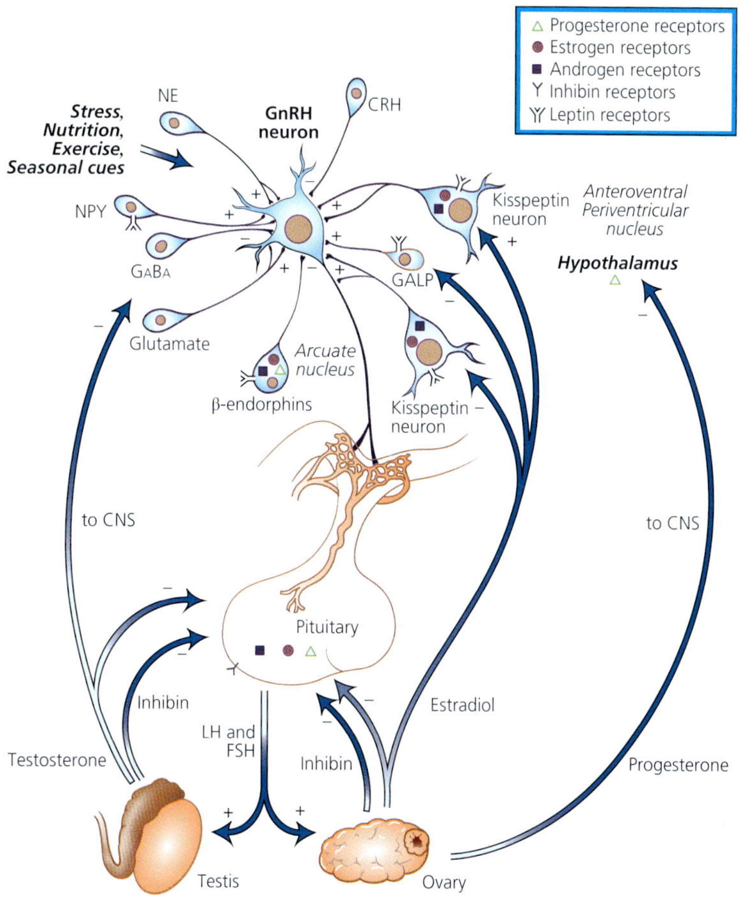

Figure 5.1 Schematic diagram of the hypothalamic-pituitary-gonadal axis showing neural systems that regulate gonadotropin-releasing hormone (GnRH) secretion and feedback of gonadal steroid hormones at the level of the hypothalamus and pituitary. CNS, central nervous system; CRH, corticotropin-releasing hormone; FSH, follicle-stimulating hormone; GABA, gamma-aminobutyric acid; GALP, galanin-like peptide; LH, luteinizing hormone; NE, norepinephrine; NPY, neuropeptide Y. Source: Low M. Chapter 7, Neuroendocrinology. In: Melmed S, Polonsky KS, Larsen PR, Kronenberg HM (eds), *Williams Textbook of Endocrinology*, 13th edn. Elsevier 2016. Reproduced with permission of Elsevier.

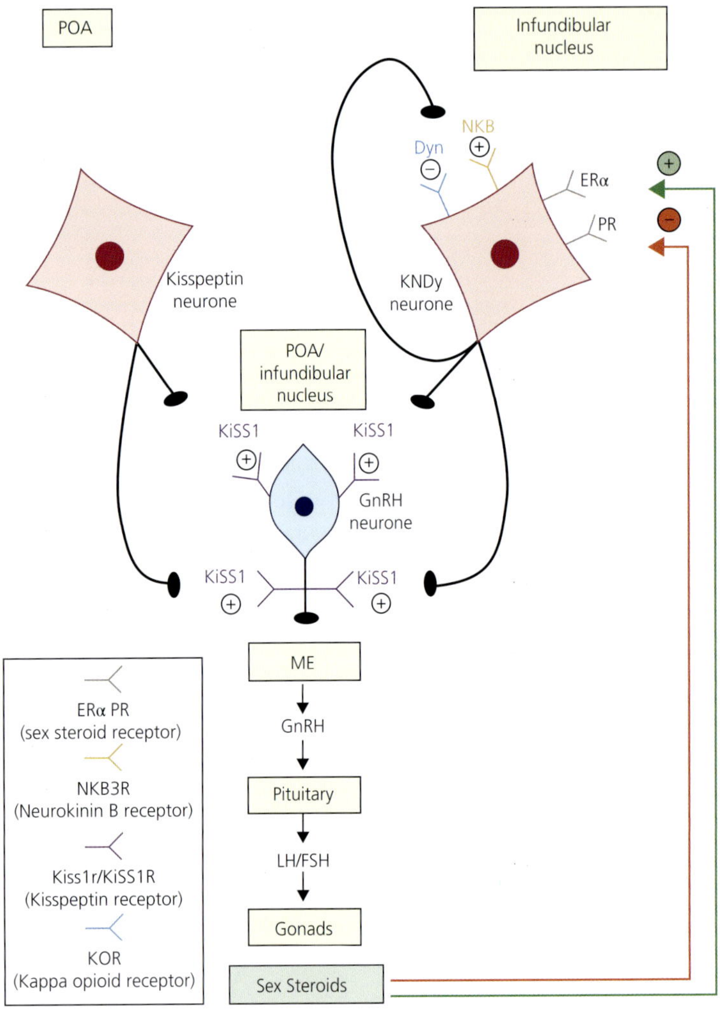

Figure 5.2 Schematic diagram showing the neuroanatomy of the kisspeptin-GnRH pathway and the relationship between KNDy neurons and GnRH neurons in humans. Kisspeptin signals directly to the gonadotropin-releasing hormone (GnRH) neurons, which express kisspeptin receptor. The location of kisspeptin neuron populations within the hypothalamus is species specific, residing within the preoptic area (POA) and the infundibular nucleus in humans. Kisspeptin neurons in the infundibular nucleus co-express neurokinin B and dynorphin (KNDy neurons), which via neurokinin B receptor and kappa opioid peptide receptor autosynaptically regulate pulsatile kisspeptin secretion, with neurokinin B being stimulatory and dynorphin inhibitory. In humans, KNDy neurons in the infundibular nucleus relay both negative (red) and positive (green) sex steroid feedback. The role of the POA kisspeptin population in mediating sex steroid feedback in humans is incompletely explored. ME, median eminence; –, stimulatory; 2, inhibitory; ERα, estrogen receptor alpha; PR, progesterone receptor; Kiss1/KiSS1, kisspeptin; NKB, neurokinin B; Dyn, dynorphin. LH, luteinizing hormone; FSH, follicle-stimulating hormone. Adapted and reproduced with permission from Skorupskaite et al. (2014).[6]

enable regulation of sex-hormone-mediated secretion of gonadotropins, and control of puberty and fertility (Figure 5.2). The primacy of this pathway in modulating GnRH release is evidenced by the hypogonadotropic hypogonadism that ensues with loss-of-function mutations in kisspeptin, its receptor GPR54, and neurokinin B and its receptor in humans.

Effect of gonadotropins at testicular level

Testosterone, produced directly by the testes, or following conversion from androstenedione (largely of adrenal and testicular origin) and dehydroepiandrosterone (DHEA, and DHEA sulfate, adrenal origin), is biologically the most important androgen. Luteinizing hormone is the key regulator of Leydig cell function, and the principal hormone stimulating Leydig cell steroidogenesis (intramitochondrial conversion of cholesterol into pregnenolone) and, thereby, testosterone synthesis in adult males. A variety of local (paracrine) testicular regulators appear to modulate secretion of testosterone from Leydig cells. These include activin, inhibin, insulin-like growth factor 1 (IGF1), transforming growth factor α (TGFα), and TGFβ, and epidermal growth factor (EGF). Testosterone production totals between 5 and 7 mg in the adult male. In per day, testosterone acts as a prohormone and is converted into its 5-alpha reduced metabolite dihydrotestosterone, which has 10 times the potency of testosterone at the androgen receptor. Loss-of-function mutations in the enzyme that mediates the conversion of testosterone (T) to dihydrotestosterone (DHT) in the developing phallus, scrotum, and prostate – 5-alpha reductase isoform 2 – leads to a disorder of male sexual development with microphallus and unfused scrotal folds.

Testosterone exerts its action on the androgen receptor, either directly or, as discussed above, after local tissue conversion by 5-alpha reductase to DHT. Other physiological effects of testosterone are mediated by the estrogen receptor, following aromatization to estradiol, and by more rapid, non-genomic mechanisms (Figure 5.3). It is now recognized that the androgen receptor is polymorphic with respect to the number of polyglutamic acid $(CAG)_n$ and polyglycine $(GGN)_n$ repeats expressed at the N-terminus of the protein. Long GAG repeats decrease the sensitivity of androgen action and *vice versa*.

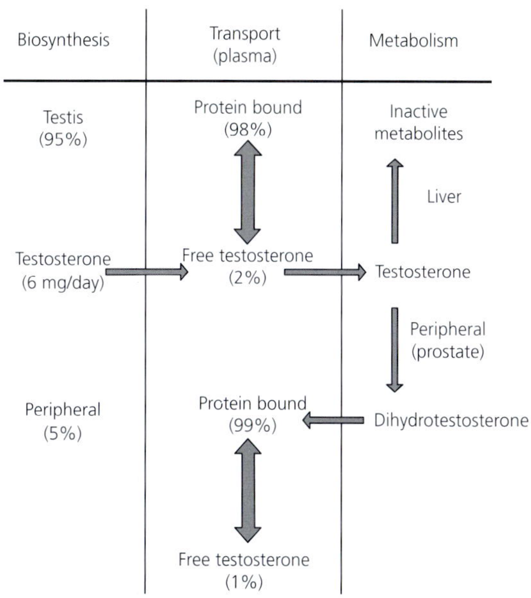

Figure 5.3 Production, transport, and metabolism of biologically active androgens. Testosterone is predominantly derived from the testis and is mainly bound to transport proteins in the circulation. In peripheral tissues it is metabolized or converted to other active steroids such as dihydrotestosterone or estradiol. Reproduced and adapted with permission from Nieschlag E, Behre HM. *Testosterone: Action, Deficiency, Substitution*, 4th edn. Cambridge University Press, 2012; Chapter 2.

Testosterone action in male sexual function

Testosterone has multiple central and peripheral effects related to sexual function. These include promotion of (spontaneous) sexual thoughts, desire, erections, and regulation of ejaculate volume, but it is not a key determinant of orgasms per se. The broader role of testosterone metabolites such as estradiol and DHT is unclear; previous studies had suggested that estradiol production through aromatization was an important prerequisite for normal sexual function in males,[3] but a recent study has challenged this view by showing that percutaneous DHT administration at a dose that suppressed gonadotropin, testosterone, and estradiol production, did not have an adverse effect on sexual function.[3,7]

Testosterone has trophic and regulatory effects on penile (cavernous smooth muscle) nitric oxide synthase (NOS) generation, effects mediated by conversion to DHT. Nitric oxide generation is essential for the vasorelaxation that leads to erection (Figure 5.4). Importantly, testosterone is essential for non-stimulus-related tumescence, notably REM-sleep-related or nocturnal penile tumescence, positively affecting the frequency, duration, and magnitude of erections.

Erections in response to erotic stimuli can occur without testosterone; however, testosterone is necessary for maximal tumescence and maintenance of arousal and full erection following withdrawal of any sexual stimulus.[8] Sexual interest declines with experimental induction of androgen deficiency using GnRH antagonists or prolonged use of GnRH agonists. Treatment of men with androgen deficiency results in corresponding improvements in sexual symptoms, with restoration of sexual interest being apparent within 1–2 weeks.

Endocrine disorders

A wide range of endocrine disorders, either in isolation or in conjunction with other conditions, can give rise to sexual/erectile dysfunction (Table 5.1). Endocrinological assessment is required when endocrine disorder is suspected based on history, physical findings, or test results.

If hypogonadism is identified, it is helpful to differentiate whether it is primary (testicular or hypergonadotrophic) or secondary (central or hypogonadotrophic) in nature as this will directly guide elucidation of

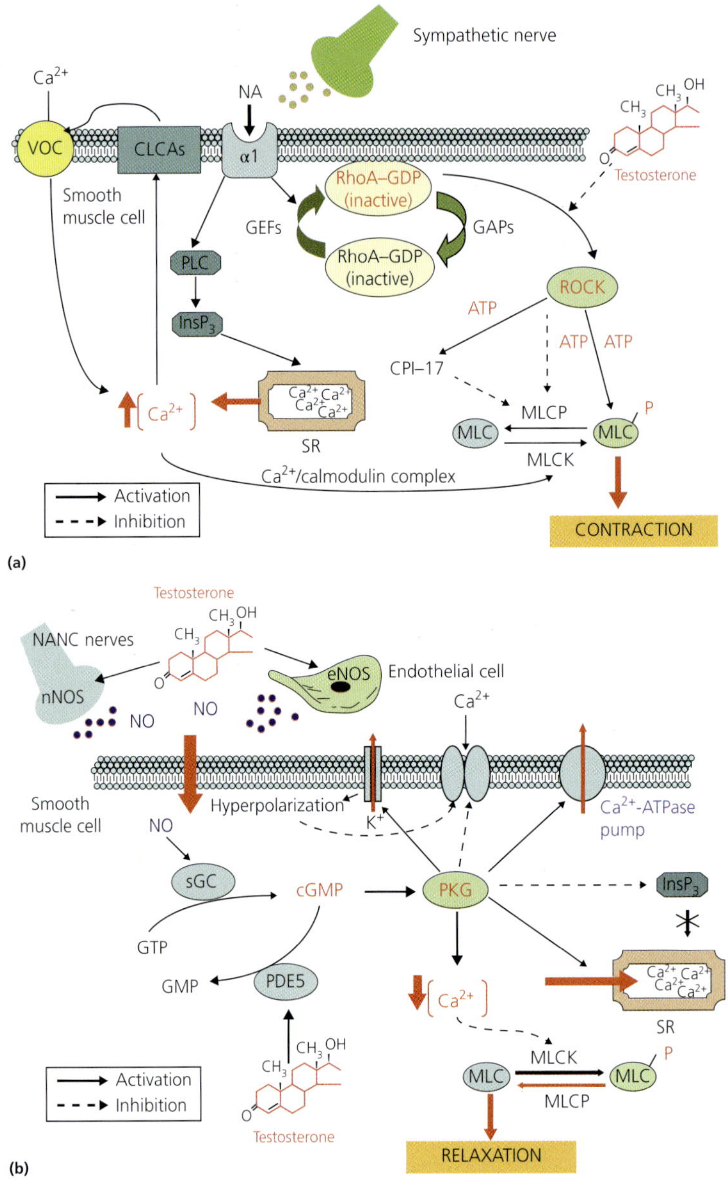

Figure 5.4 Schematic representation of the biochemical events leading to **a)** penile flaccidity or **b)** erection. **a)** Penile flaccidity: Noradrenaline (NA) binding generates inositol 1,4,5-trisphosphate ($InsP_3$), which, by increasing intracellular calcium (Ca^{2+}) levels, activates Ca^{2+}-sensitive chloride channels (CLCAs), resulting in membrane depolarization with the diffusion of the stimulus to the neighboring cells and the opening of voltage-operated channels (VOC). The increased Ca^{2+} flow promotes, through calmodulin, activation of myosin light chain (MLC) kinase (MLCK) and cell contraction. Cell contraction is also obtained by altering the Ca^{2+} sensitivity through a NA-induced activation of a second pathway, RhoA/ROCK, which increases, through a series of kinase activations, the sensitivity of MLC to Ca^{2+}. Testosterone is considered to negatively regulate the latter event. **b)** Penile erection: Nitric oxide (NO) diffuses into smooth muscle cells (SMC) and activates a soluble guanylate cyclase (sGC), which in turn transforms guanosine triphosphate (GTP) into cyclic guanosine monophosphate (cGMP). Cyclic GMP activates protein kinase G (PKG), which through the indicated pathways, finally decreases intracellular Ca^{2}+ levels, leading to relaxation. Phosphodiesterase type 5 (PDE5) metabolizes cGMP into GMP, thereby limiting its effects. Testosterone enhances PDE5 activity. Other abbreviations: CPI-17, protein phosphatase 1 regulatory, subunit 14A; eNOS, endothelial nitric oxide synthase; GAP, GTPase activating protein; GEF, guanine nucleotide exchange factor; MLCP, myosin light chain phosphatase; nNOS, neuronal nitric oxide synthase; PLC, phospholipase C; RhoA, Ras homolog gene family member A; ROCK, Rho-associated coiled-coil containing protein kinase; SR, sarcoplasmic reticulum.

Table 5.1 Classification of disorders that may be associated with endocrine and sexual dysfunction.

Hypogonadism

Primary* (hypergonadotrophic) – reduced serum testosterone and elevated gonadotrophins & testicular pathology
- Trauma, torsion, cryptorchidism
- Orchitis, HIV
- Klinefelter's syndrome (karyotype 47XXY), XYY syndrome, gonadal dysgenesis
- Chemotherapy

Secondary* (hypogonadotrophic hypogonadism, or HH) *with or without hyperprolactinemia* – inappropriately normal or low gonadotrophins
- Hypothalamo-pituitary disease or damage:
  - Tumor (e.g., pituitary adenoma, craniopharyngioma), developmental cysts, hypophysitis
  - Genetic, syndromic: often isolated HH, e.g., Kallmann's syndrome, Prader–Willi, Laurence–Moon–Biedl
  - Infiltration, e.g., sarcoid, hemochromatosis (iron overload)
  - Infection, e.g., histiocytosis, TB
  - Head injury, irradiation (inc. cancer therapy in childhood), vascular injury
- Obesity(usually when severe)
- Type 2 diabetes (T2DM): multiple factors including low SHBG/serum testosterone
- Other acute and chronic systemic disorders: organ failure (liver, kidney, lung, heart), rheumatoid arthritis, starvation/malnutrition, acute and critical illness
- Endurance exercise
- Pharmacotherapy:
  - Drugs elevating serum prolactin (e.g. anti-psychotics, and other agents with dopamine antagonist effects)
  - Androgenic anabolic steroids (AAS) and other recreational drugs
  - GnRH agonist or antagonist (androgen deprivation therapy)
  - Glucocorticoid excess
  - HIV therapy (reduced bioavailable serum testosterone)
  - Chronic opioid analogue therapy
  - Immune checkpoint inhibitors (hypophysitis)

Some conditions may cause combined primary and secondary hypogonadism, e.g., hemochromatosis, thalassemia, old age

Phenotypic heterogeneity with potential for spontaneous improvement in some variants

Other endocrine causes
- Thyroid dysfunction
- Hypercalcemia
- Cushing's syndrome
- Rare disorders: e.g., aromatase deficiency, androgen insensitivity; other genetic disorders, e.g., DAX1 mutation, androgen resistance

underlying pathology and further management (Figure 5.5). For example, suspected hypogonadotrophic hypogonadism may warrant pituitary imaging and testing of other aspects of pituitary function, as well as influence the approach to replacement therapy when fertility is required.[9]

Central hypogonadism is uncommon, both in absolute terms and in comparison to primary testicular dysfunction, but the likelihood may be greater in subjects with marked hypotestosteronemia (<4.5 nmol/L).[10] In general, gonadotroph function is affected early in the course of pituitary failure relative to other pituitary end-organ axes. Central hypogonadism should be considered in individuals who have undergone cranial irradiation for non-pituitary tumors as it is more prevalent than suspected.[11] Some conditions may result in a mixture of both types of hypogonadism (e.g., hemochromatosis, hemoglobinopathy, *DAX-1* mutations, aging, childhood cancer treatment with chemotherapy and/or irradiation).[12,13]

Clinical evaluation

The clinical history should ideally include an interview with the sexual partner, with a focus on the nature of sexual difficulty, psychological factors (stress, depression, quality of relationship with sexual partner), risk factors for ED (e.g., type 2 diabetes mellitus (T2DM), cardiovascular, neurological, drug therapy) and factors that might have a bearing on subsequent management (e.g., drug-drug interactions, coagulopathy). Full penile

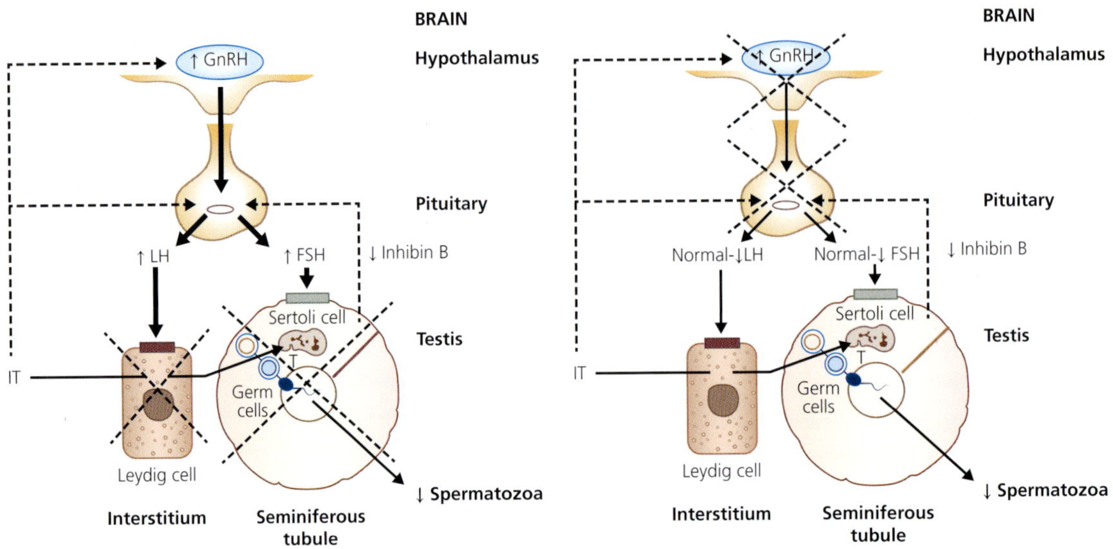

Figure 5.5 Hypogonadism due to alterations in the hypothalamic-pituitary-testicular axis. **a)** Primary hypogonadism due to testicular disease. Classically, this results in both androgen deficiency and impairment of sperm production and elevated luteinizing hormone (LH) and follicle-stimulating hormone (FSH) levels (hypergonadotrophic hypogonadism) due to loss of negative feedback regulation of gonadotropins. GnRH, gonadotropin-releasing hormone; T, testosterone. **b)** Secondary hypogonadism due to hypothalamic and/or pituitary disease. This manifests as both androgen deficiency and impairment of sperm production and inappropriately normal or low LH and FSH levels (hypogonadotrophic hypogonadism). Source: Matsumoto A, Bremner W. Testicular disorders. In: Melmed S, Polonsky KS, Larsen PR, Kronenberg HM (eds), *Williams Textbook of Endocrinology*, 13th edn. Elsevier, 2016; Chapter 19. Reproduced with permission of Elsevier.

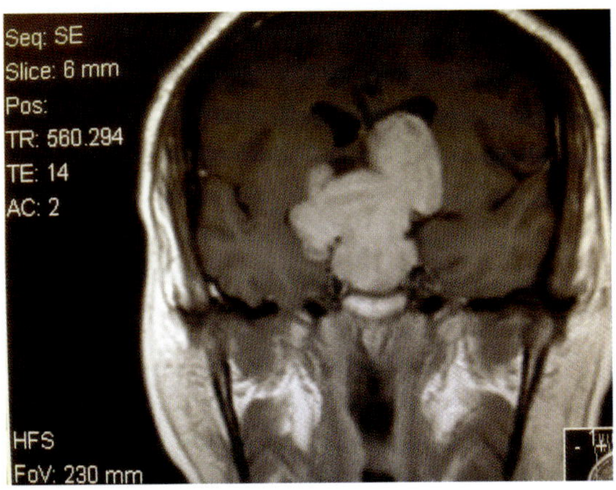

Figure 5.6 Macroadenoma of the pituitary, with large suprasellar extension, causing secondary hypogonadism, and other features of hypopituitarism.

tumescence under any circumstances (e.g., masturbation) suggests intact endocrine, neurological, and vascular function, implying that a complaint of erectile dysfunction is more likely to be psychogenic. By contrast, reduced spontaneous (i.e., unrelated to coitus) erectile activity is suggestive of organic disease, although this may be a feature of longstanding psychogenic dysfunction.

Suspected hypogonadism warrants enquiry about family history, sexual development, changes in secondary sexual characteristics, pointers to testicular pathology, symptoms of a pituitary mass and dysfunction, and history of infertility. The possibility of adrenal, thyroid, and other endocrine disease should also be considered (Figure 5.6).

In addition to reduced sexual function, including spontaneous erections and fertility, androgen deficiency may be clinically suspected on the basis of the following features: a history of hot flushes; osteoporosis; disordered sexual development (delay, eunuchoidism, small penile size); hypogonadal (youthful) facies (i.e., pale skin with decreased wrinkling and sebum production); reduced androgen-dependent body hair (axillary, pubic, facial); reduction in shaving frequency; gynecomastia; reduced testicular volume and consistency; and low-volume ejaculate (Figure 5.7). Other features, for example, reduced physical performance, alterations in

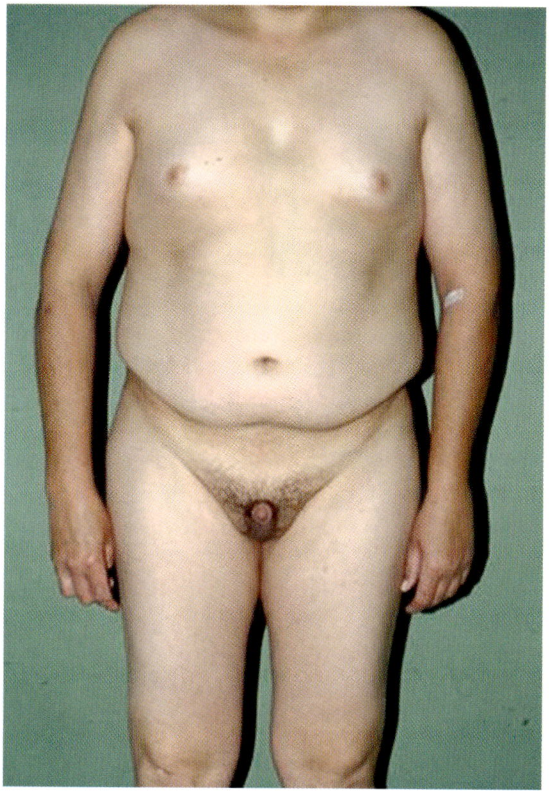

Figure 5.7 Clinical features of hypogonadism. A 32-year-old man with severe androgen deficiency caused by Kallmann's syndrome (hypogonadotrophic hypogonadism and anosmia) who presented with poor sexual function, sparsity of body hair, and poorly developed secondary sexual characteristics and 3 cc testes. Luteinizing hormone <1.0; follicle-stimulating hormone 0.4; testosterone level 1.2 U/L.

body composition (reduced muscle bulk, increased fat),[14] and effects on mood and psychological and general well-being are less specific and, from a diagnostic perspective, should be weighted accordingly.

Physical examination

Physical examination is directed to evaluating the differential diagnosis based on the history and ascertaining the presence of systemic disease, and pointers to vasculogenic, neurological, and endocrinological disorder. In particular, examination of secondary sexual characteristics, testicular volumes and consistency, visual fields, examination of breast tissue for gynecomastia and galactorrhea, should be undertaken. Examination of height and span may give valuable insights into the likely time of origin of the hypogonadism. Eunuchoid segments (span>height by 3 cm) is characteristically seen with a pubertal origin of hypogonadism.

Investigations

Careful investigation is aimed at confirming the etiology of sexual dysfunction suspected from clinical assessment. Endocrine investigations for possible hypogonadism should initially comprise early morning serum testosterone (replicate values, preferably not during acute illness) in view of diurnal variation resulting in an early morning peak and potential underestimation of serum testosterone later in the day,[15] LH and FSH (gonadotropins), and serum prolactin as a minimum. The circadian rhythmicity in testosterone is generally lost after the age of 60. The prevalence of repeatedly low serum testosterone and/or hyperprolactinemia in 1022 unselected men with ED was found to be 4% and 9%, respectively below and above the age of 50 years.[16] Similarly, a low overall prevalence of significant structural hypothalamo-pituitary lesions (6.9%, 95% confidence interval 2.9–10.5%) has been found in men with erectile failure and secondary hypogonadism, albeit from a time in which both CT (limited sensitivity) and MRI were used; pituitary macroadenomas and hypothalamic lesions were observed solely in men with extremely low (≤3.5 nmol/L) total serum testosterone values.[10]

Total, bioavailable, and free testosterone

Reference ranges for serum testosterone are generally uncorrected for age, resulting in a substantial number of older men with testosterone levels falling below the lower limit. Circulating testosterone is predominantly (45–50%) bound to sex hormone-binding globulin (SHBG) and considered unavailable for uptake by tissues. A substantial fraction (35–40%) is also bound to serum albumin but may be bioavailable. A much smaller fraction (~2%) circulates as free testosterone. In routine clinical practice, unless otherwise specified, all these fractions are assayed and reported as total serum testosterone. If there is doubt about the reliability of total serum testosterone in reflecting the clinical situation, for example due to possible effects on circulating SHBG (Table 5.2), bioavailable or free plasma testosterone may be of greater diagnostic value; these can be measured or calculated, the latter requiring total testosterone, SHBG, and albumin concentrations[17] (http://www.issam.ch/freetesto.htm). Assay of free testosterone by commercial methods involving radioimmunoassay is subject to poor

Table 5.2 Conditions associated with alterations in sex hormone-binding globulin (SHBG) concentrations.

Reduced SHBG levels	Increased SHBG levels
Obesity (moderate or severe)	Aging
Type 2 diabetes mellitus	Liver disease – cirrhosis, hepatitis
Nephrotic syndrome	HIV disease
Glucocorticoids, progestogens	Estrogens
Hypothyroidism	Thyrotoxicosis
Acromegaly	Anticonvulsants
Familial SHBG deficiency	

accuracy, sensitivity, and inter-laboratory comparability versus the gold standard method, equilibrium dialysis; however, the latter technique is not generally available outside the research setting.[18]

Androgen deficiency

Hypogonadism is an important and treatable cause of sexual dysfunction, yet it is a relatively uncommon underlying cause. Secondary disorders of sexual desire are most commonly associated with psychogenic factors (desire deficiency and performance anxiety) rather than androgen deficiency. A minimal level of serum testosterone appears necessary for sexual desire and non-erotic stimulus driven erections. However, the relationship is less clear in ostensibly healthy, aging men. Similarly, the commonest ejaculatory disorder, premature ejaculation, is not usually related to endocrine or other organic disease. Androgen deficiency is not known to cause isolated orgasmic dysfunction.

By contrast, androgen deficiency is a well-known potential cause of ED, particularly sleep-related (nocturnal) erections, which may be related to decreased descending noradrenergic tone and night-time peaks in serum testosterone.[19] However, the prevalence of hypotestosteronemia may be similar in men with and without ED.[20] Testosterone deficiency may also result in reduced ejaculate volume and other manifestations such as altered body composition, including reduced bone density (and increased fracture risk) and muscle mass.[21–23] There are conflicting reports concerning the effects of hypogonadism and testosterone replacement therapy on cardiovascular events and mortality in elderly men, with some studies suggesting that hypogonadism is associated with excess mortality,[24–28] and that testosterone replacement confers a beneficial effect, potentially via cardiovascular protection.[29–31] In contrast, other data suggest that exogenous testosterone has uncertain, neutral, or adverse effects on cardiovascular risk factors and health,[32–34] and may impair survival, as described further below.

Late-onset hypogonadism

Various age-related changes in well-being, including reduced virility, erectile dysfunction, and changes in body composition, have long been ascribed to declining testicular function. The prevalence of erectile dysfunction is well known to increase with age, affecting up to 50% of men by age 70 years.[2] Nocturnal penile tumescence has been quantified and appears to decline by 25% overall between adolescence and the eighth decade.[35] Serum total testosterone declines with age by approximately 0.124 nmol/L/year.[36] Similarly, between the ages of 40 and 70 years, free- and albumin-bound testosterone decrease annually by about 1.3% and 0.4% respectively.[37–39]

This modest decline in serum testosterone with age, by contrast with menopausal declines of serum estradiol in women, has been variably described as late-onset hypogonadism (LOH), andropause, and androgen deficiency of the aging male (ADAM). The basis for the observed age-related reduction in serum testosterone appears to be multifactorial. In part, this may be due to an increase in SHBG, resulting in lower serum free testosterone. In addition, there is also evidence of reduced Leydig cell numbers[40] and hypothalamic-pituitary function,[20] independent of but also possibly related to obesity, manifesting as a relatively blunted rise in serum gonadotropins with age, that is, progressive primary and secondary hypogonadism.

Whether the aforementioned clinical features of a transitional phase in aging human adult males and progressive hypotestosteronemia are causally related is controversial. The European Male Ageing Study of approximately 3000 community-dwelling men aged 40–79 years in eight European countries evaluated 32 possible symptoms of hypogonadism. Only nine symptoms were shown to be related to low total or free circulating testosterone. These comprised three sexual (decreased sexual interest and morning erections and erectile dysfunction), three physical (an inability to engage in vigorous activity, an inability to walk more than 1 km, and an inability to bend, kneel, or stoop), and three psychological symptoms (loss of energy, sadness, and fatigue).

Using a definition of late-onset hypogonadism based on the presence of three (sexual) symptoms considered relatively specific for androgen deficiency plus low serum testosterone (total serum testosterone < 11 nmol/L and free testosterone < 225 pmol/L), the study population prevalence of LOH was found to be 2.3%. Moderate and severe LOH, defined by the degree of hypotestosteronemia, was significantly associated with multiple end-organ deficits consistent with androgen action: lower hemoglobin, mid-upper arm circumference, bone mineral density (BMD), and physical function (measured by Short Form-36 questionnaire), slower gait speed, and poorer general health.[21]

It is unclear whether treatment of older men with modestly subnormal serum testosterone per se (e.g., 8–11 nmol/L, but dependent on normative range for assay) with androgen replacement carries a positive benefit-to-risk ratio in general; unequivocal efficacy has not been demonstrated, and there is concern about the potential to cause or exacerbate conditions that are more prevalent in older men, for example, benign prostatic hyperplasia[41] and lower urinary tract symptoms (LUTS) or coronary heart disease,[42] as described further below.

In summary, the relationship between age-related decline in serum testosterone and sexual dysfunction is not invariable, and there is no clear treatment-related sexual benefit, unless there is unequivocal clinical and biochemical (e.g., < 6 nmol/L, dependent on assay reference range) evidence of androgen deficiency.[43] Therefore, in men with ED, underlying androgen deficiency should only be definitively diagnosed in the presence of compatible clinical features and at least two clearly subnormal early morning serum testosterone values,[44] in order to minimize the risk of misdiagnosis, unduly raising treatment expectations, and inappropriate androgen therapy.

Hyperprolactinemia

Hyperprolactinemia is a relatively infrequent cause of erectile failure and reduced libido in men. However, these are the commonest manifestations of hyperprolactinemia, in contrast to galactorrhea, and generally respond well to normalization of serum prolactin.[45,46] A raised serum prolactin without clear cause, such as dopamine antagonist therapy, should prompt a screen for macroprolactin, a multimeric molecular variant that raises measured total prolactin but is biologically inactive (in contrast to monomeric prolactin), especially in the absence of clear-cut androgen deficiency. In this setting, true, monomeric hyperprolactinemia is generally associated with pituitary disease, either related to a prolactinoma or due to pituitary stalk disruption (disconnection) reducing tonic dopaminergic inhibition of lactotrophs (Figure 5.8). Very rarely, it occurs as a consequence of profound hypothyroidism, which itself can be associated with sexual dysfunction.

Hyperprolactinemia causes central hypogonadism by reducing hypothalamic GnRH secretion, as well as pituitary responsiveness to this peptide, thereby diminishing testicular production of testosterone. This is unlikely to be the sole mechanism in operation, since libido is rarely responsive to testosterone administration alone unless hyperprolactinemia has been corrected. Alternatively, it may occur in varying degrees on top of direct structural damage to pituitary gonadotrophs by the physical presence of underlying hypothalamo-pituitary disorder (e.g., a mass compressing the hypothalamo-pituitary structure).

Type 2 diabetes mellitus (T2DM)

Diabetes mellitus is the commonest endocrine disorder associated with sexual dysfunction, including ejaculatory dysfunction and ED in particular. In men with T2DM, serum total and free testosterone is more likely to be slightly lower than in men who are not diabetic. In respect of total serum testosterone, the relationship may be indirectly related via a lower SHBG associated with obesity. Gonadotrophins are not typically elevated, and this has been interpreted as reflecting hypogonadotrophic hypogonadism.[47] The increased adiposity in T2DM with greater aromatization of testosterone yielding higher estradiol levels with subsequent feedback inhibition of gonadotropins has been suggested as one mechanism of the hypogonadism.

Overall, ED may be twice as common in men with DM as those without. However, the rising incidence of T2DM, and of both conditions with age, may also mean that the coexistence of both conditions in any individual may not always be causally related. Nonetheless, the absence of clear alternative causes of ED, and the coexistence of micro- and macrovascular complications, particularly in the context of poor glycemic control and longer duration of diabetes,[48] is suggestive of a causative role for T2DM in any individual with such symptoms.

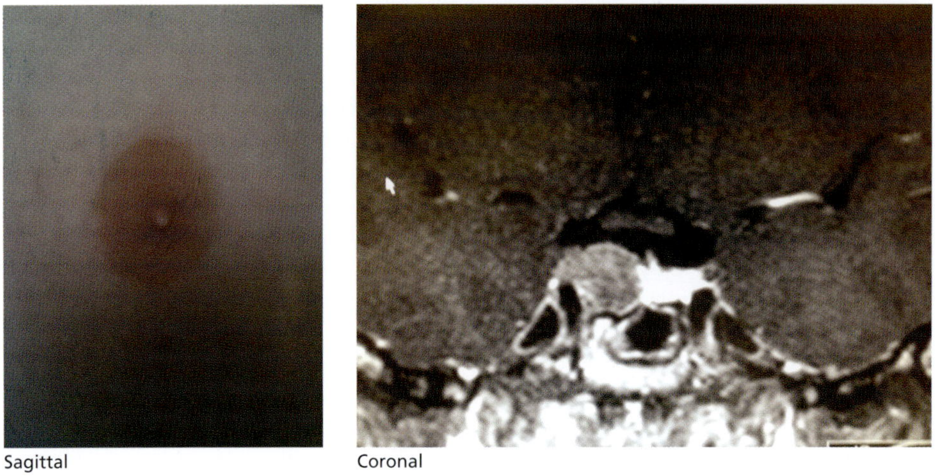

Figure 5.8 Right-sided macroprolactinoma with extension into the right cavernous sinus causing a right sixth nerve palsy, and galactorrhea. Prolactin 33,400 mU/L (nomolar range <360).

Sexual dysfunction, particularly ED, should routinely be enquired about during clinical assessment of subjects with DM.

Multiple factors associated with sexual dysfunction in DM include: psychosexual problems related to chronic disease; atherosclerotic peripheral vascular disease and treatment (e.g., betablockade); autonomic neuropathy (may be relevant to ejaculatory dysfunction also); endothelial (eNOS) and smooth muscle (RhoA/Rho-kinase abnormalities) dysfunction; and Peyronie's disease.[49]

Thyroid dysfunction

Male patients with thyroid disease do not commonly complain of symptoms of sexual dysfunction. This may be due to a failure to elicit such symptoms given the predominance of classical, systemic symptoms of thyroid dysfunction, possible attribution to neuropsychiatric disturbance, and sparsity of research data concerning males, consistent with the greater frequency of thyroid disease in women.

Thyrotoxicosis

Thyroid hormone excess is associated with increased SHBG and, therefore, elevated total (but with lower free) serum testosterone. In addition, total and free estradiol levels may be elevated,[50] and hyperestrogenism occasionally results in gynecomastia. The lower affinity of estradiol for SHBG may lead to a reduced free testosterone:estradiol ratio, which will accentuate the gynecomastia. Circulating gonadotropins, though generally normal, sometimes demonstrate an elevation of LH. Sexual dysfunction may manifest as reduced libido, potentially due to effects on mood and adrenergic and serotonergic transmission.[51] In one small observational study of Italian patients, premature ejaculation and ED were noted to affect 50% and ~15% of thyrotoxic subjects, respectively; symptoms of sexual dysfunction tended to be reversible upon attainment of euthyroidism.[52]

Hypothyroidism

Hyper- and hypogonadotrophic hypogonadism,[53] as well as normal serum gonadotropins, have been described in adult males with thyroid underactivity. In the aforementioned Italian study, improvement in reduced libido, delayed ejaculation, and ED, evident in 9 out of 14 men at baseline, was noted in a substantial proportion of individuals who achieved euthyroidism with thyroid hormone replacement. The pathophysiological basis for these sexual symptoms is uncertain, but may involve defects of mood and serotonergic transmission.

Pharmacotherapy

Drug-induced sexual dysfunction

This is under-recognised. In addition to better known examples, such as androgen deprivation therapy (Figure 5.9), drug-induced hyperprolactinemia and ED due to beta-blockers, the effects of emergent, illicit, and undeclared drugs, and less well appreciated impacts of established therapies should be entertained.

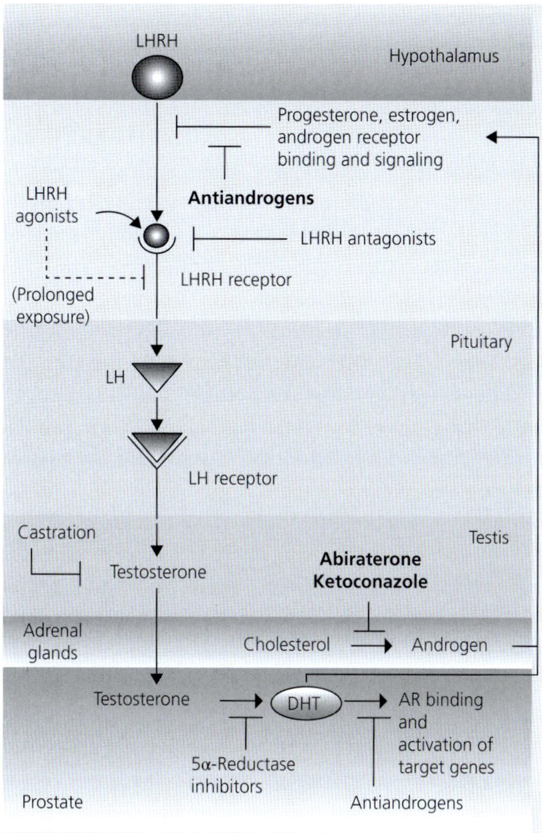

Figure 5.9 Hypothalamo-pituitary-testicular axis and potential sites of therapeutic disruption. AR, androgen receptor; DHT, dihydrotestosterone; LH, luteinizing hormone; LHRH, luteinizing hormone releasing hormone. Reproduced and adapted with permission from Nieschlag E, Behre HM. *Testosterone: Action, Deficiency, Substitution*, 4th edn. Cambridge University Press, 2012; Chapter 2.

HIV therapy

Over and above direct adverse effects of HIV on gonadal axis function,[54] treatment with a number of antiretroviral agents can be associated with a decline in bioavailable testosterone and sexual function in the face of a normal total serum testosterone, due to induction of SHBG production, as noted above. A 20% incidence of androgen deficiency has been noted in men with HIV receiving highly active antiretroviral therapy (HAART).[55] In the presence of possible symptoms of hypogonadism, a trial of testosterone therapy can be considered, although efficacy cannot be assumed.

Opioid analogs

Chronic use of opioid analogs is associated with hypogonadotrophic hypogonadism and is greatly underappreciated, particularly in the setting of the functional decline associated with sarcopenia. It is important to ascertain as it is potentially amenable to a therapeutic trial of androgen supplementation.[56]

Androgenic anabolic steroids (AAS)

The use of AAS in certain sports is widespread and should be considered in the context of certain occupations and hobbies.[57] AAS may be used unwittingly in "exercise supplements," intermittently, in supraphysiological doses (causing acne, gynecomastia, testicular atrophy, and infertility), and as part of a cocktail (stacking). In particular, use of pharmacological doses of testosterone may lead to grossly elevated levels of estradiol, occasionally with the appearance of gynecomastia ("bitch tits"). Use is often deliberately undeclared. AAS may not cross-react in assays for serum testosterone and, therefore, will not be detected unless sought using specialist testing such as urine mass spectrometry.

AAS-induced feedback inhibition of the HPT axis results in hypogonadotrophic hypogonadism and low serum testosterone; that is, the HPT axis is downregulated or switched off. Restoration and normalization of HPT activity, using one of the approaches noted below, may be slow and confounded by intermittent re-use of AAS, and some regimens incorporate anastrozole or tamoxifen to expedite recovery of the HPT axis.

Treatment of sexual dysfunction associated with endocrinopathy

General considerations

Since ED is often multifactorial, especially in older men, it is important to address all remediable factors, including relationship factors (psychosexual counselling), depression, drug effects, and cardiovascular risk factors, as well as specific management of endocrinopathy.

Erectile dysfunction unrelated or unamenable to androgen therapy can be managed with a trial of a selective oral phosphodiesterase type 5 (PDE5) inhibitor. If that is not feasible due to a contraindication, or inadequacy of response, for example in subjects with diabetes mellitus, alternatives such as local vasodilator therapy using an intra-urethral or intra-cavernosal method of delivery, typically of prostaglandin E1 (PGE_1), or vacuum therapy may be tried according to availability, preference, and medical considerations (e.g., desire for fertility). PDE5 therapy is efficacious in the treatment of men with T2DM but may be less so compared to use in psychogenic or vasculogenic ED. Efficacy may be improved when PDE5 therapy is used in combination with testosterone.[58,59] In men with DM, vascular dysfunction may necessitate use of higher doses (20–40 µg) of intra-cavernosal PGE_1.

In contrast to PDE5 inhibitors, there is a paucity of evidence supporting adequate efficacy and acceptable safety of certain centrally acting therapies (generally used "off-label") in the management of ED, notably trazodone (a selective serotonin reuptake inhibitor (SSRI) possessing antagonistic effects at $5\text{-}HT_{2c}$ and alpha 1 receptors of Adrenergic),[60] yohimbine (inhibitor of monoamine oxidases and alpha-2 adrenoceptor antagonist),[61] and apomorphine (dopamine agonist).[62] Agents with dopaminergic, and noradrenergic activity (including dopamine agonists, trazodone, bupropion, and venlafaxine) have been associated with adverse effects of increased sexual desire, and have been used (off-label) to induce improvements in libido. Ejaculatory dysfunction, which is not uncommon in men with T2DM, may respond to pharmacotherapeutic agents (used off-label), such as midodrine, ephedrine, and imipramine, although the evidence for efficacy is very limited.[63] Therapeutic approaches for ED in development include potassium channel modulators and gene and stem cell therapy.

Testosterone therapy

Men with unequivocal hypogonadism should be treated with androgen replacement (supplementation), generally indefinitely for most pathologies, unless fertility is also required in the setting of secondary gonadal failure. In this situation, testosterone therapy should be avoided as it results in inappropriately low intra-testicular testosterone concentrations, which impairs spermatogenesis; an approach relying on testicular stimulation of both testosterone production and spermatogenesis should be employed instead. Treatment options in this setting include oral clomifene citrate, parenteral human chorionic gonadotropin (hCG) with or without human menopausal gonadotropin (hMG), and pulsatile GnRH delivered subcutaneously by pump.

Testosterone therapy is contraindicated in men with breast or prostate cancer. Preceding specialist evaluation is indicated in the presence of suspected prostate cancer (e.g., uncharacterized prostatic abnormality such as nodule or elevated PSA), severe LUTS, erythrocytosis, untreated severe obstructive sleep apnea, or poorly controlled heart failure, due to the possibility of exacerbation by androgen treatment. In highly selected hypogonadal patients with a remote history (>1 year) of fully resected prostate cancer (prostate-specific antigen (PSA) < 0.1 ng/dL), testosterone replacement therapy has been cautiously administered with benefit and without evidence of PSA recurrence.[64]

Dosing with testosterone should be based on the degree of androgen deficiency, consideration of comorbidities, and clinical response, guided by biochemical monitoring. It should be initiated cautiously, especially in cases of severe and longstanding hypogonadism, to minimize the risk of adverse events (see below). A trial of testosterone therapy might be considered in men with putative LOH, targeting the lower end of the referent range (e.g., ≤ 14 nmol/L) and recognizing that there may be a limited response, if at all. An algorithm to guide investigation and management of suspected hypogonadism is depicted in Figure 5.10.

Evidence concerning the utility of androgen replacement therapy is largely drawn from studies of testosterone in hypogonadal men.[65] These have demonstrated improvements in overall sexual activity, including domains related to overall satisfaction, sexual desire and thoughts, frequency and magnitude of spontaneous (nocturnal) erections, erectile scores, and intercourse frequency. There is also some evidence of promotion of response to PDE5 inhibitors by androgen therapy, possibly by induction of penile NOS, in men who have failed to respond to sildenafil.[66] In one meta-analysis that included hypogonadal men, testosterone was significantly more likely than placebo to restore erectile function (575 vs 16.7%). Further, the response rate was notably higher in men with erectile dysfunction due to primary hypogonadism compared to those with secondary causes (64% vs 44%), and also in men treated by the transdermal route compared to intramuscular or oral administration (80.9%, 51.3%, and 53.2%, respectively).[67]

In addition to improvement in sexual function, there are other important benefits of androgen therapy.[44] These include improvement of vitality and well-being,

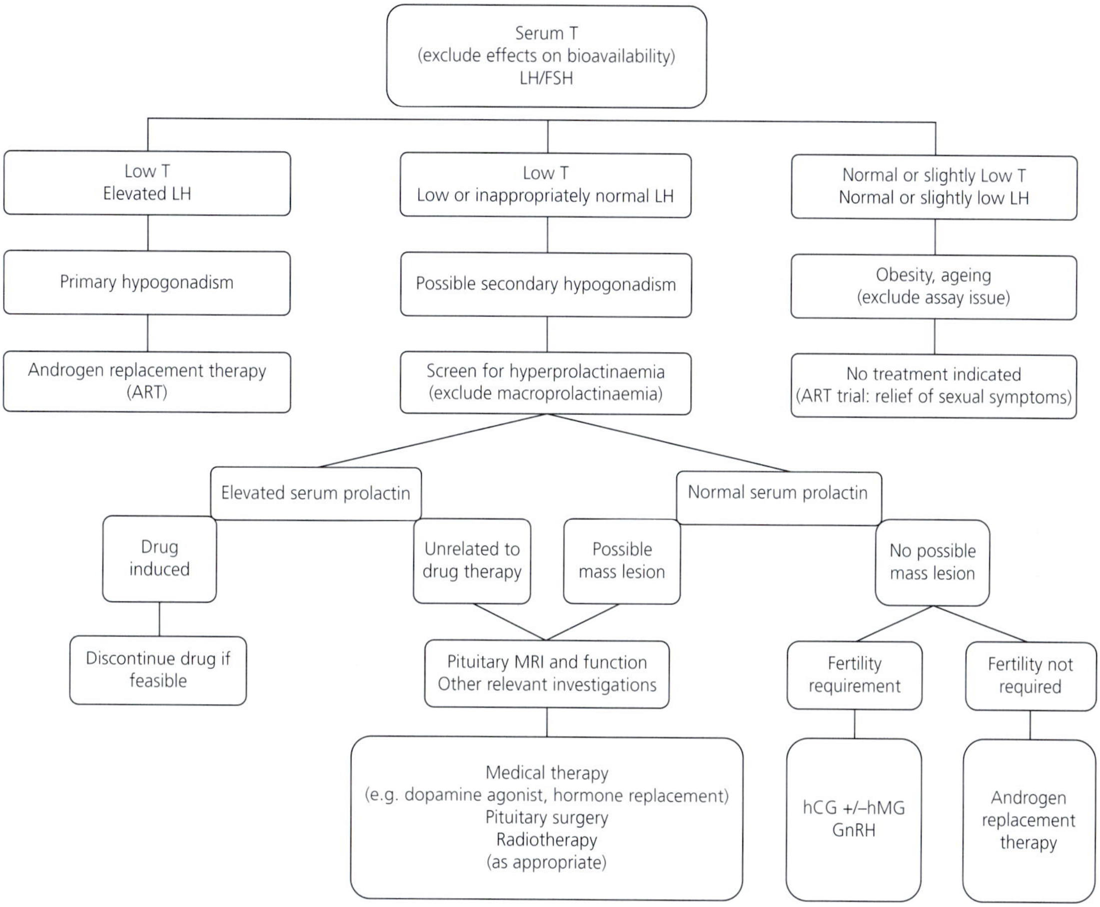

Figure 5.10 Investigation and management of suspected hypogonadism. FSH, follicle-stimulating hormone; GnRH, gonadotropin-releasing hormone; hCG, human chorionic gonadotropin; LH, luteinizing hormone; MRI, magnetic resonance imaging; T, testosterone.

and body hair, body composition and function (muscle mass and strength, fat-free mass, and bone mineral density).[68–74]

Choice of preparation

Various options for androgen replacement therapy exist, differing largely in their route of administration, formulation, and pharmacokinetics, giving rise to variable durations of effect, and differences in peak and trough (waning) effects, convenience, and cost.[75]

One of the earliest approaches, and one still commonly employed, entails intramuscular injections of testosterone esters every 1–3 weeks (e.g., cypionate, enanthate); convenience has been improved since the availability of a castor oil formulation of testosterone undecanoate that can be given every 2–3 months. Another potentially convenient method involves the use of testosterone pellets, implanted subcutaneously under local anesthesia. Clinical efficacy is maintained for 3–6 months, depending on dose (e.g., 400–1000 mg) and is not subject to the peak and trough effects apparent with intramuscular injections of standard formulations of testosterone esters.

Transdermal formulations of testosterone have become increasingly popular over the past few decades,[65] largely because of convenience. Whilst transdermal patches, which vary in required site of application (genital or non-genital skin), are ostensibly convenient, they are not always well tolerated because of local irritation and lack of reliable adhesion. Topical testosterone gels, which require daily self-application, and enable ready dose titration, are very widely used. Patients should be warned of potential risk of passive transfer, particularly to female intimates, and should take precautions to minimize this according to instructions in the package insert.

Daily, oral administration of testosterone undecanoate formulated in castor oil (and other excipients including medium-chain triglycerides) arguably offers the most convenient means of treating androgen deficiency. However, its use results in a non-physiologically high ratio of dihydrotestosterone to testosterone, and there may be significant inter- and intra-individual variation in absorption via lymphatics. For these reasons, use of this formulation is relatively limited in endocrine clinical practice. Buccal preparations of testosterone are also available.

Adverse effects

The nature of potential adverse events should clearly be discussed in advance of treatment. Risk minimization requires standardized, regular surveillance for changes in prostate health (evaluation of LUTS severity, PSA, digital rectal examination), hematocrit,[41,76] lipids (including reduced HDL, although improvements in total cholesterol are also reported),[77] and adverse effects on other aspects of well-being (e.g., behavior, tender gynecomastia due to aromatization to estrogen, acne, male pattern alopecia), and systemic comorbidities.[78]

A widely advocated surveillance schedule is 1, 3, 6, and 12 months after initiation of testosterone therapy and annually thereafter,[44] reflecting the time course of attainment of stable serum testosterone, and measures of efficacy and adverse events. A rise in serum PSA by 1 ng/dL or a PSA velocity of 0.4 ng/dL or more per year over at least 2 years warrants urological assessment. Erythrocytosis requires temporary cessation of testosterone therapy and investigation for other potential underlying causes. In the absence of any such cause, resumption of testosterone treatment at a lower dose may be considered. Recurrent polycythemia can sometimes be managed by concomitant periodic venesection.

Recently, a few observational studies in men have suggested that androgen supplementation may carry a heightened risk of major adverse cardiovascular events, particularly in older men or those with a history of heart disease,[79] supporting a qualitatively similar finding in an earlier trial of androgen therapy that was discontinued before completion.[80] Further substantial, high quality, prospective clinical trial data characterizing the cardiovascular safety profile of androgen therapy, including in older men with age-related decline in androgen levels, are required before conclusive evidence of a causal relationship can be assumed.[81] Until these become available, middle-aged and older men should be counseled about this issue.[42]

Other medical therapies

Hyperprolactinemia due to prolactinoma is generally highly susceptible to effective treatment with dopamine agonist therapy.[82,83] In selected hypogonadal patients, particularly those with central hypogonadism and/or infertility, specialist treatments other than testosterone may be required. Clomiphene citrate, an oral selective estrogen receptor modulator, may have limited therapeutic impact on erectile dysfunction in individuals with hypogonadotrophic hypogonadism.[84] Specialist supervision is required for therapy with human chorionic gonadotropin (hCG) (subcutaneous, once or twice weekly), and pulsatile GnRH. Selective androgen receptor modulators (SARMs), which may offer an improved benefit-risk profile in comparison to testosterone therapy, are still undergoing development.[85]

References

1 Laumann EO, Paik A, Rosen RC. Sexual dysfunction in the United States: prevalence and predictors. *JAMA* 1999;281(6):537–44.

2 Feldman HA, Goldstein I, Hatzichristou DG, Krane RJ, McKinlay JB. Impotence and its medical and psychosocial correlates: results of the Massachusetts Male Aging Study. *J Urol* 1994;151(1):54–61.

3 Carani C, Rochira V, Faustini-Fustini M, Balestrieri A, Granata AR. Role of oestrogen in male sexual behaviour: insights from the natural model of aromatase deficiency. *Clin Endocrinol (Oxf)* 1999;51(4):517–24.

4 Van der Ploeg LHT, Martin WJ, Howard AD, et al. A role for the melanocortin 4 receptor in sexual function. *PNAS* 2002;99(17):11381–6.

5 Seminara SB, Kaiser UB. New gatekeepers of reproduction: GPR54 and its cognate ligand, KiSS-1. *Endocrinology* 2005;146(4):1686–8.

6 Skorupskaite K, George JT, Anderson RA. The kisspeptin-GnRH pathway in human reproductive health and disease. *Hum Reprod Update* 2014;20(4):485–500.

7 Sartorius GA, Ly LP, Handelsman DJ. Male sexual function can be maintained without aromatization: randomized placebo-controlled trial of dihydrotestosterone (DHT) in healthy, older men for 24 months. *J Sex Med* 2014;11: 2562–70.

8 Carani C, Granata AR, Bancroft J, Marrama P. The effects of testosterone replacement on nocturnal penile tumescence and rigidity and erectile response to visual erotic stimuli in hypogonadal men. *Psychoneuroendocrinology* 1995;20(7): 743–53.

9 Coviello AD, Matsumoto AM, Bremner WJ, et al. Low-dose human chorionic gonadotropin maintains intratesticular testosterone in normal men with testosterone-induced gonadotropin suppression. *J Clin Endocrinol Metab* 2005;90(5): 2595–602.

10 Citron JT, Ettinger B, Rubinoff H, et al. Prevalence of hypothalamic-pituitary imaging abnormalities in impotent men with secondary hypogonadism. *J Urol* 1996;155(2):529–33.

11 Appelman-Dijkstra NM, Kokshoorn NE, Dekkers OM, et al. Pituitary dysfunction in adult patients after cranial radiotherapy: systematic review and meta-analysis. *J Clin Endocrinol Metab* 2011;96(8):2330–40.

12 Schmiegelow M, Lassen S, Poulsen HS, et al. Gonadal status in male survivors following childhood brain tumors. *J Clin Endocrinol Metab* 2001;86(6):2446–52.

13 McDermott JH, Walsh CH. Hypogonadism in hereditary hemochromatosis. *J Clin Endocrinol Metab* 2005;90(4):2451–5.

14 Finkelstein JS, Lee H, Burnett-Bowie SA, et al. Gonadal steroids and body composition, strength, and sexual function in men. *N Engl J Med* 2013;369(11):1011–22.

15 Brambilla DJ, Matsumoto AM, Araujo AB, McKinlay JB. The effect of diurnal variation on clinical measurement of serum testosterone and other sex hormone levels in men. *J Clin Endocrinol Metab* 2009;94(3):907–13.

16 Buvat J, Lemaire A. Endocrine screening in 1,022 men with erectile dysfunction: clinical significance and cost-effective strategy. *J Urol* 1997;158(5):1764–7.

17 Vermeulen A, Verdonck L, Kaufman JM. A critical evaluation of simple methods for the estimation of free testosterone in serum. *J Clin Endocrinol Metab* 1999;84(10):3666–72.

18 Rosner W, Auchus RJ, Azziz R, Sluss PM, Raff H. Utility, limitations, and pitfalls in measuring testosterone: an Endocrine Society position statement. *J Clin Endocrinol Metab* 2007;92(2):405–13.

19 Hirshkowitz M, Moore CA, O'Connor S, Bellamy M, Cunningham GR. Androgen and sleep-related erections. *J Psychosom Res* 1997;42(6):541–6.

20 Korenman SG, Morley JE, Mooradian AD, et al. Secondary hypogonadism in older men: its relation to impotence. *J Clin Endocrinol Metab* 1990;71(4):963–9.

21 Tajar A, Huhtaniemi IT, O'Neill TW, et al. Characteristics of androgen deficiency in late-onset hypogonadism: results from the European Male Aging Study (EMAS). *J Clin Endocrinol Metab* 2012;97(5):1508–16.

22 LeBlanc ES, Nielson CM, Marshall LM, et al. The effects of serum testosterone, estradiol, and sex hormone binding globulin levels on fracture risk in older men. *J Clin Endocrinol Metab* 2009;94(9):3337–46.

23 Vanderschueren D, Vandenput L, Boonen S, Lindberg MK, Bouillon R, Ohlsson C. Androgens and bone. *Endocrine Rev* 2004;25(3):389–425.

24 Shores MM, Matsumoto AM, Sloan KL, Kivlahan DR. Low serum testosterone and mortality in male veterans. *Arch Intern Med* 2006;166(15):1660–5.

25 Laughlin GA, Barrett-Connor E, Bergstrom J. Low serum testosterone and mortality in older men. *J Clin Endocrinol Metab* 2008;93(1):68–75.

26 Hyde Z, Norman PE, Flicker L, et al. Low free testosterone predicts mortality from cardiovascular disease but not other causes: the Health in Men Study. *J Clin Endocrinol Metab* 2012;97(1):179–89.

27 Khaw KT, Dowsett M, Folkerd E, et al. Endogenous testosterone and mortality due to all causes, cardiovascular disease, and cancer in men: European prospective investigation into cancer in Norfolk (EPIC-Norfolk) Prospective Population Study. *Circulation* 2007;116(23):2694–701.

28 Araujo AB, Dixon JM, Suarez EA, Murad MH, Guey LT, Wittert GA. Endogenous testosterone and mortality in men: a systematic review and meta-analysis. *J Clin Endocrinol Metab* 2011;96(10):3007–19.

29 Shores MM, Smith NL, Forsberg CW, Anawalt BD, Matsumoto AM. Testosterone treatment and mortality in men with low testosterone levels. *J Clin Endocrinol Metab* 2012;97(6):2050–8.

30 Muraleedharan V, Marsh H, Kapoor D, Channer KS, Jones TH. Testosterone deficiency is associated with increased risk of mortality and testosterone replacement improves survival in men with type 2 diabetes. *Eur J Endocrinol* 2013;169(6):725–33.

31 Oskui PM, French WJ, Herring MJ, Mayeda GS, Burstein S, Kloner RA. Testosterone and the cardiovascular system: a comprehensive review of the clinical literature. *J Am Heart Assoc* 2013;2(6):e000272.

32 Wu FCW, von Eckardstein A. Androgens and coronary artery disease. *Endocrine Rev* 2003;24(2):183–217.

33 Ruige JB, Ouwens DM, Kaufman JM. Beneficial and adverse effects of testosterone on the cardiovascular system in men. *J Clin Endocrinol Metab* 2013;98(11):4300–10.

34 Schooling CM. Testosterone and cardiovascular disease. *Curr Opin Endocrinol Diabetes Obes* 2014;21(3):202–8.

35 Kandeel FR, Koussa VKT, Swerdloff RS. Male sexual function and its disorders: physiology, pathophysiology, clinical investigation, and treatment. *Endocrine Rev* 2001;22(3):342–88.

36 Harman SM, Metter EJ, Tobin JD, Pearson J, Blackman MR. Longitudinal effects of aging on serum total and free testosterone levels in healthy men. Baltimore Longitudinal Study of Aging. *J Clin Endocrinol Metab* 2001;86(2):724–31.

37 Wu FC, Tajar A, Pye SR, et al. Hypothalamic-pituitary-testicular axis disruptions in older men are differentially linked to age and modifiable risk factors: the European Male Aging Study. *J Clin Endocrinol Metab* 2008;93(7):2737–45.

38 Orwoll E, Lambert LC, Marshall LM, et al. Testosterone and estradiol among older men. *J Clin Endocrinol Metab* 2006;91(4):1336–44.

39 Gray A, Feldman HA, McKinlay JB, Longcope C. Age, disease, and changing sex hormone levels in middle-aged men: results of the Massachusetts Male Aging Study. *J Clin Endocrinol Metab* 1991;73(5):1016–25.

40 Neaves WB, Johnson L, Porter JC, Parker CR Jr, Petty CS. Leydig cell numbers, daily sperm production, and serum gonadotropin levels in aging men. *J Clin Endocrinol Metab* 1984;59(4):756–63.

41 Marks LS, Mazer NA, Mostaghel E, et al. Effect of testosterone replacement therapy on prostate tissue in men with late-onset hypogonadism: a randomized controlled trial. *JAMA* 2006;296(19):2351–61.

42 The risk of cardiovascular events in men receiving testosterone therapy. An Endocrine Society Statement. Endocrine Society, February 7, 2014. Available at: https://www.endocrine.org/membership/email-newsletters/endocrine-insider/2014/february-20-2014/society-statement-risk-of-cardiovascular-events-in-men-receiving-testosterone-therapy-available

43 Kaufman JM, Vermeulen A. The decline of androgen levels in elderly men and its clinical and therapeutic implications. *Endocrine Rev* 2005;26(6):833–76.

44 Bhasin S, Cunningham GR, Hayes FJ, et al. Testosterone therapy in men with androgen deficiency syndromes: An Endocrine Society Clinical Practice Guideline. *J Clin Endocrinol Metab* 2010;95(6):2536–59.

45 De RM, Zarrilli S, Vitale G, et al. Six months of treatment with cabergoline restores sexual potency in hyperprolactinemic males: an open longitudinal study monitoring nocturnal penile tumescence. *J Clin Endocrinol Metab* 2004;89(2):621–5.

46 Colao A, Vitale G, Cappabianca P, et al. Outcome of cabergoline treatment in men with prolactinoma: effects of a 24-month treatment on prolactin levels, tumor mass, recovery of pituitary function, and semen analysis. *J Clin Endocrinol Metab* 2004;89(4):1704–11.

47 Dhindsa S, Prabhakar S, Sethi M, Bandyopadhyay A, Chaudhuri A, Dandona P. Frequent occurrence of hypogonadotropic hypogonadism in type 2 diabetes. *J Clin Endocrinol Metab* 2004;89(11):5462–8.

48 Fedele D, Coscelli C, Santeusanio F, et al. Erectile dysfunction in diabetic subjects in Italy. Gruppo Italiano Studio Deficit Erettile nei Diabetici. *Diabetes Care* 1998;21(11):1973–7.

49 El-Sakka AI, Tayeb KA. Peyronie's disease in diabetic patients being screened for erectile dysfunction. *J Urol* 2005;174(3):1026–30.

50 Krassas GE, Poppe K, Glinoer D. Thyroid function and human reproductive health. *Endocrine Rev* 2010;31(5):702–55.

51 Jannini EA, Ulisse S, D'Armiento M. Thyroid hormone and male gonadal function. *Endocrine Rev* 1995;16(4):443–59.

52 Carani C, Isidori AM, Granata A, et al. Multicenter study on the prevalence of sexual symptoms in male hypo- and hyperthyroid patients. *J Clin Endocrinol Metab* 2005;90(12):6472–9.

53 Donnelly P, White C. Testicular dysfunction in men with primary hypothyroidism; reversal of hypogonadotrophic hypogonadism with replacement thyroxine. *Clin Endocrinol (Oxf)* 2000;52(2):197–201.

54 Sellmeyer DE, Grunfeld C. Endocrine and metabolic disturbances in human immunodeficiency virus infection and the acquired immune deficiency syndrome. *Endocrine Rev* 1996;17(5):518–32.

55 Rietschel P, Corcoran C, Stanley T, Basgoz N, Klibanski A, Grinspoon S. Prevalence of hypogonadism among men with weight loss related to human immunodeficiency virus infection who were receiving highly active antiretroviral therapy. *Clin Infect Dis* 2000;31(5):1240–4.

56 Vuong C, Van Uum SHM, O'Dell LE, Lutfy K, Friedman TC. The effects of opioids and opioid analogs on animal and human endocrine systems. *Endocrine Rev* 2010;31(1):98–132.

57 Basaria S. Androgen abuse in athletes: detection and consequences. *J Clin Endocrinol Metab* 2010;95(4):1533–43.

58 Shabsigh R, Kaufman JM, Steidle C, Padma-Nathan H. Randomized study of testosterone gel as adjunctive therapy to sildenafil in hypogonadal men with erectile dysfunction who do not respond to sildenafil alone. *J Urol* 2004;172(2):658–63.

59 Greenstein A, Mabjeesh NJ, Sofer M, Kaver I, Matzkin H, Chen J. Does sildenafil combined with testosterone gel improve erectile dysfunction in hypogonadal men in whom testosterone supplement therapy alone failed? *J Urol* 2005;173(2):530–2.

60 Lance R, Albo M, Costabile RA, Steers WD. Oral trazodone as empirical therapy for erectile dysfunction: a retrospective review. *Urology* 1995;46(1):117–20.

61 Ernst E, Pittler MH. Yohimbine for erectile dysfunction: a systematic review and meta-analysis of randomized clinical trials. *J Urol* 1998;159(2):433–6.

62 Gontero P, D'Antonio R, Pretti G, et al. Clinical efficacy of apomorphine SL in erectile dysfunction of diabetic men. *Int J Impot Res* 2005;17(1):80–5.

63 Master VA, Turek PJ. Ejaculatory physiology and dysfunction. *Urol Clin North Am* 2001;28:363–75.

64 Agarwal PK, Oefelein MG. Testosterone replacement therapy after primary treatment for prostate cancer. *J Urol* 2005;173(2):533–6.

65 Snyder PJ, Peachey H, Berlin JA, et al. Effects of testosterone replacement in hypogonadal men. *J Clin Endocrinol Metab* 2000;85(8):2670–7.

66 Aversa A, Isidori AM, Spera G, Lenzi A, Fabbri A. Androgens improve cavernous vasodilation and response to sildenafil in patients with erectile dysfunction. *Clin Endocrinol (Oxf)* 2003;58(5):632–8.

67 Jain P, Rademaker AW, McVary KT. Testosterone supplementation for erectile dysfunction: results of a meta-analysis. *J Urol* 2000;164(2):371–5.

68 Bhasin S, Storer TW, Berman N, et al. Testosterone replacement increases fat-free mass and muscle size in hypogonadal men. *J Clin Endocrinol Metab* 1997; 82(2):407–13.

69 Behre HM, Kliesch S, Leifke E, Link TM, Nieschlag E. Long-term effect of testosterone therapy on bone mineral density in hypogonadal men. *J Clin Endocrinol Metab* 1997;82(8): 2386–90.

70 Schroeder ET, Zheng L, Ong MD, et al. Effects of androgen therapy on adipose tissue and metabolism in older men. *J Clin Endocrinol Metab* 2004;89(10):4863–72.

71 Page ST, Amory JK, Bowman FD, et al. Exogenous testosterone (T) alone or with finasteride increases physical performance, grip strength, and lean body mass in older men with low serum T. *J Clin Endocrinol Metab* 2005; 90(3):1502–10.

72 Katznelson L, Finkelstein JS, Schoenfeld DA, Rosenthal DI, Anderson EJ, Klibanski A. Increase in bone density and lean body mass during testosterone administration in men with acquired hypogonadism. *J Clin Endocrinol Metab* 1996; 81(12):4358–65.

73 Tracz MJ, Sideras K, Boloña ER, et al. Testosterone use in men and its effects on bone health. A systematic review and meta-analysis of randomized placebo-controlled trials. *J Clin Endocrinol Metab* 2006;91(6):2011–16.

74 Finkelstein JS, Klibanski A, Neer RM, et al. Increases in bone density during treatment of men with idiopathic hypogonadotropic hypogonadism. *J Clin Endocrinol Metab* 2012;69(4):776–83.

75 Bhasin S, Cunningham GR, Hayes FJ, et al. 2010 Testosterone therapy in men with androgen deficiency syndromes: An Endocrine Society clinical practice guideline. *J lin Endocrinol Metab* 2010;95(6):2536–59.

76 Calof OM, Singh AB, Lee ML, et al. Adverse events associated with testosterone replacement in middle-aged and older men: a meta-analysis of randomized, placebo-controlled trials. *J Gerontol A Biol Sci Med Sci* 2005;60(11):1451–7.

77 Malkin CJ, Pugh PJ, Jones RD, Kapoor D, Channer KS, Jones TH. The effect of testosterone replacement on endogenous inflammatory cytokines and lipid profiles in hypogonadal men. *J Clin Endocrinol Metab* 2004;89(7):3313–8.

78 Rhoden EL, Morgentaler A. Risks of testosterone-replacement therapy and recommendations for monitoring. *N Engl J Med* 2004;350(5):482–92.

79 Vigen R, O'Donnell CI, Baron AE, et al. Association of testosterone therapy with mortality, myocardial infarction, and stroke in men with low testosterone levels. *JAMA* 2013;310(17):1829–36.

80 Basaria S, Coviello AD, Travison TG, et al. Adverse events associated with testosterone administration. *N Engl J Med* 2010;363(2):109–22.

81 The Testosterone Trial in Older Men. ClinicalTrials.gov identifier: NCT00799617.

82 Gillam MP, Molitch ME, Lombardi G, Colao A. Advances in the treatment of prolactinomas. *Endocrine Rev* 2006;27(5): 485–534.

83 Melmed S, Casanueva FF, Hoffman AR, et al. Diagnosis and treatment of hyperprolactinemia: an Endocrine Society clinical practice guideline. *J Clin Endocrinol Metab* 2011;96(2):273–88.

84 Guay AT, Bansal S, Heatley GJ. Effect of raising endogenous testosterone levels in impotent men with secondary hypogonadism: double blind placebo-controlled trial with clomiphene citrate. *J Clin Endocrinol Metab* 1995; 80(12):3546–52.

85 Negro-Vilar A. Selective androgen receptor modulators (SARMs): A novel approach to androgen therapy for the new millennium. *J Clin Endocrinol Metab* 1999;84(10): 3459–62.

CHAPTER 6

Pharmacology of drugs used for the treatment of erectile dysfunction

Ian Eardley

Leeds Teaching Hospital Trust, Leeds, UK

Introduction

Drugs have been used increasingly for the treatment of men with erectile dysfunction (ED) since the 1980s. While oral agents such as yohimbine were used in those early days, their efficacy was relatively poor and the discovery in the mid-1980s that intracavernosal injection of vasoactive agents was both feasible and effective made that approach the most commonly used means of treating men with ED, until the late 1990s. In 1998, oral sildenafil was approved in the United States for the treatment of men with ED, and subsequently a number of similar compounds have been made available for clinical use. These compounds have proven to be effective and safe and remain the most widely used pharmacological agents for men with ED. However, a number of other oral and topical agents have subsequently been licencsed and used with varying degrees of success. This chapter will describe the clinical pharmacology of these drugs, with an emphasis upon those agents that are used in clinical practice today.

Oral agents

The launch of sildenafil in 1998 fundamentally changed the management of men with ED. Prior to that date, for most men, either intracavernosal or intraurethral administration had been required for drugs to be effective. Sildenafil was the first of a class of effective oral agents that became known as the PDE5 (phosphodiesterase type 5) inhibitors, although both prior to the launch of sildenafil and subsequently, other oral agents have been used in the treatment of men with ED with varying degrees of success. This section deals with the clinical pharmacology of the oral agents.

Phosphodiesterase type 5 (PDE5) inhibitors

The primary neurotransmitter that mediates penile erection in the human male is nitric oxide. It is released from parasympathetic nerve endings within the penis in response to a sexual stimulus, and is augmented by release of nitric oxide from the vascular endothelium of the corpus cavernosum. After penetrating the smooth muscle cells of the corpus cavernosum and the penile vasculature, nitric oxide stimulates the soluble enzyme guanylate cyclase to convert guanosine triphosphate (GTP) to cyclic guanosine monophosphate (cGMP), which is the active second messenger that stimulates smooth muscle relaxation. Downstream effects include activation of protein kinase G, alterations in the function of cellular ion channels, and reduction in the intracellular calcium with consequent smooth muscle relaxation, vasodilatation, and penile erection. The effects of cGMP are terminated in the penis by the enzyme phosphodiesterase type 5 (PDE5), which converts the cGMP into linear 5-GMP.[1,2] Inhibitors of PDE5 therefore, in the presence of a sexual stimulus, will maintain higher levels of intracavernosal smooth muscle cGMP, thereby potentiating the smooth muscle relaxation and as a consequence improving the erectile response. In the absence of a sexual stimulus, given that the level of nitric oxide is low, the PDE5 inhibitors will have no effect at all upon penile erection.

Male Sexual Dysfunction: A Clinical Guide, First Edition. Edited by Suks Minhas and John Mulhall.

Affinity and selectivity of the PDE5 inhibitors

PDE5 inhibitors are competitive inhibitors of the enzyme, and compete for the catalytic binding site on the enzyme where cGMP is usually bound. Several of the drugs have a structural similarity to cGMP but bind to this site with higher affinity than cGMP. This affinity is assessed pharmacologically by measurement of the IC_{50}, which is the dose of the drug that is required to produce 50% inhibition of the enzyme. Therefore, the lower the IC_{50}, the more potent the compound. As can be seen in Table 6.1, the IC_{50} of the commercially available PDE5 inhibitors are all in the nanomolar range. That they are not degraded by the enzyme itself may be significant, since those drugs that bind most tightly to the enzyme might have a prolonged effect because of this.[3]

Phosphodiesterase type 5 is only one of 11 types of phosphodiesterase that have differential activity for cGMP and for cAMP, differential tissue distribution (Table 6.2), and different physiological functions. PDE5 is found in high concentrations within the corpus cavernosum, but is also found in other tissues including vascular smooth muscle, smooth muscle of the upper gastrointestinal tract, and the nasopharyngeal mucosa. In addition to having a high affinity for PDE5, clinically useful inhibitors should also have a low affinity for the other PDEs, thereby avoiding unwanted pharmacological effects. The degree to which the clinically available compounds actually achieve this is summarized in Table 6.1.

Table 6.1 Affinity and selectivity of the phosphodiesterase type 5 (PDE5) inhibitors.

Inhibitor	IC_{50} for PDE5	PDE selectivity
Sildenafil[4,5]	3.7 nM	Low activity against PDE6 (16-fold difference)
Tadalafil[4,5]	1.8 nM	Low activity against PDE11 (25-fold difference)
Vardenafil[4,5]	0.91 nM	Low activity against PDE6 (21-fold difference)
Avanafil[5,6]	1 nM	Very low activity against PDE6 (121-fold difference)
Udenafil[7]	5.84 nM	Low activity against PDE3 (8.9-fold difference) Low activity against PDE6 (9.1-fold difference)
Mirodenafil[8]	0.33 nM	Low activity against PDE6
Lodenafil[9]	<10 nM	Low activity against PDE1 (IC_{50} = 31.6 nM) Low activity against PDE10 (IC_{50} = 36.2 nM)

IC_{50} = median inhibitory concentration.

Table 6.2 Tissue distribution of the phosphodiesterase enzymes.

PDEA1	Smooth muscle, heart, lung, brain, sperm
PDE1B	Neurons, lymphocytes, smooth muscle
PDE1C	Brain, proliferating human smooth muscle, spermatids, olfactory epithelium
PDE2A	Adrenal medulla, brain, heart, platelets, macrophages, endothelial cells
PDE3A	Heart, vascular smooth muscle, platelets, oocyte, kidney
PDE3B	Vascular smooth muscle, adipocytes, hepatocytes, kidney, β cells, developing sperm, T lymphocytes, macrophages
PDE4A	Widely expressed with mRNA found in many tissues especially olfactory system, immune cells, and testis
PDE4B	High levels of mRNA detected in a variety of tissues especially immune cells and brain
PDE4C	Lung, testis, and several cell lines mainly of neuronal origin
PDE4D	Widely distributed and found in a variety of tissues
PDE5A	Platelets, vascular smooth muscle, brain, lung, heart, kidney, skeletal muscle
DE6A/ PDE6B	Rod cells of the photoreceptor layer of retina; also found in pineal gland
PDE6C	Cone cells of the photoreceptor layer of retina; also found in pineal gland
PDE7A	Immune cells, heart, skeletal muscle, endothelial cells
PDE7B	Brain, heart, liver, skeletal muscle, pancreas, testis
PDE8A	Many tissues especially testis, spleen, small intestine, ovary, colon, and kidney
PDE8B	Brain and thyroid
PDE9A	Highest levels in kidney, brain, spleen, various gastrointestinal tissues, and prostate
PDE10A	Highest expression in brain, testis, heart, and thyroid
PDE11A	Skeletal muscle, prostate, testis, salivary gland, thyroid gland, liver

The clinically encountered side effects of the PDE5 inhibitors probably reflect inhibition of PDE5 in other tissues. The most prominent of these are headache, nasal congestion, indigestion, and slight lowering of blood pressure.[10,11] Cross-reactivity with PDE6, a feature of sildenafil and to a lesser degree of vardenafil, potentially causes visual side effects, since PDE6 is located in the retina. Indeed, visual side effects are an occasional dose-related consequence of treatment with sildenafil,[12] although there only seems to be a modest and reversible effect upon the electroretinogram associated with a bluish tinge to vision.[13] Tadalafil has minor activity against PDE11. While the physiological role of PDE11 is unknown it is found in skeletal muscle, prostate, heart, testis, and the anterior pituitary. It is not thought that the effect of tadalafil upon PDE11 has any significant functional consequence.

Pharmacokinetics of the PDE5 inhibitors

While all the commercially available PDE5 inhibitors have a high affinity for PDE5 and reasonably good selectivity for PDE5 over the other isoenzymes, there are differences in their kinetics that differentiate the compounds clinically. These characteristics are summarized in Table 6.3 and reflect the kinetics of the drugs when used in on demand.

The T_{max} to a large extent predicts the onset of clinical activity, with most of the drugs having data demonstrating efficacy in some patients within an hour.[11] Although there are differences between the T_{max} of the different compounds, the nature of the clinical trials means that it is impossible to say whether one of the drugs is "faster" than the others, however. On the other hand, the $T_{½}$ of two of the compounds, namely tadalafil and udenafil, is substantially longer than the other compounds and this predicts a longer duration of action.[10,11] It also allows these drugs to be used differently on a regular dosing basis. The kinetics of tadalafil, when used on a daily dosing basis, show that steady state is reached within around 5 days, with exposure being approximately 1.6-fold greater than after a single dose.[14]

Food will delay the absorption of all the PDE5 inhibitors, although the effect is less marked for tadalafil, in part because it is the slowest to be absorbed anyway.

The PDE5 inhibitors are metabolized in the liver, with inhibitors of the CYP3A4 enzyme system potentiating and prolonging the PDE5 inhibitory effect.

Drug interactions of the PDE5 inhibitors

Given the metabolism within the liver, this class of drugs typically interact with drugs that affect the CYP3A4 system. Drugs such as rifampicin, which induce CYP3A4, will decrease PDE5 inhibitor levels, while inhibitors of CYP3A4 such as erythromycin, ketoconazole, and protease inhibitors such as ritonavir, will increase the plasma levels of the PDE5 inhibitors.

The other major interactions of this class of compounds relate to action on the systemic vasculature. Organic nitrates interact significantly with all these drugs, and in severe cases can result in severe hypotension, which can be lethal if not recognized.[18,19] As such, concurrent use of PDE5 inhibitors with nitrates or nitric oxide donors is absolutely contraindicated. There are similar but less marked interactions with alpha-adrenoceptor blocking agents,[20] where again when taken concurrently there can be significant postural hypotension. However, if there is a 6-hour time delay between using the two medications this interaction is not seen, meaning

Table 6.3 Pharmacokinetics of the PDE5 inhibitors.

Inhibitor	C_{max} (ng/mL)[a]	T_{max} (h)	$T_{½}$ (h)	Bioavailability
Sildenafil[4]	450 (100 mg)	0.8	3–5	40%
Tadalafil[14]	378 (20 mg)	2	17.5	Not reported in humans
Vardenafil[4]	20.9 (20 mg)	0.7–0.9	4–5	14.5%
Avanafil[15]	Not reported	0.5–75	5	Not reported in humans
Udenafil[16]	416.2 (100 mg)	0.8–1.3	7.3–12.1	Not reported
Mirodenafil[17]	373.4 (100 mg)	1.26	1.96	Not reported
Lodenafil[9]	157 (160 mg)	1.2	2.4	Not identified

[a]Values in brackets denote the dose of the drug that was used in the study where the values of C_{max} were calculated.

that these two classes of drugs can be used together in clinical practice, providing that this precaution is taken.

Clinical effects of the PDE5 inhibitors

The PDE5 inhibitors are effective treatments for ED when used orally. Those that are clinically available have similar efficacy,[10,11] with around 70% from a broad population of men with ED having a good response to therapy. Some patients respond better than others; notably men who have developed ED following radical prostatectomy have a poor response rate because with the damage to the cavernosal nerves there is no neuronal release of nitric oxide, and without such release the PDE5 inhibitors will be ineffective. Similarly poor response rates are seen in diabetic men, where it is presumed that the severe endothelial dysfunction that underlies the pathophysiology of ED explains the poor response.[10,11] To date, there has been no evidence of tachyphylaxis with the PDE5 inhibitors.[10]

As outlined above, the chief side effects are headache, flushing, indigestion, and nasopharyngeal congestion.[10] These side effects are seen to some extent with all the PDE5 inhibitors and probably reflect inhibition of PDE5 in other parts of the body. With sildenafil there are occasional visual side effects, reflecting the interaction with PDE6. With tadalafil, muscular cramps or back pain are an occasional side effect. As discussed earlier, while it was hypothesized that this reflected inhibition of PDE11, there is no evidence for this and it may simply reflect the long duration of action of tadalafil. The side-effect profile of tadalafil when used on a daily dosing basis (at a dose of 5 mg daily) is not substantially different from the profile when used on demand, where the doses used are higher (10–20 mg).

Apomorphine

Apomorphine is a mixed D1/D2 receptor dopaminergic agonist that has a high affinity for D2-like receptors (D2, D3, and D4) that are thought to be important for the initiation of penile erection within the paraventricular nucleus.[21] In animal studies, apomorphine administration appears to activate oxytocinergic neurons that project from the hypothalamus to the spinal cord and which appear to stimulate penile erection.[22]

Ineffective when swallowed, apomorphine has been developed as a sublingual formulation for men with ED. When administered sublingually it results in detectable plasma concentrations within 10 min, with a T_{max} of around 0.74 hours and a $T_{½}$ of 2.7–4.2 hours. Although apomorphine is highly bound to plasma proteins, it is also highly lipid soluble and therefore able to cross the blood–brain barrier, such that brain concentrations are around six times higher than those seen in plasma. After metabolism, most apomorphine is excreted in the urine.[21] Although both 2 mg and 3 mg formulations have been licensed, the lower dose should be used in men with either renal or hepatic impairment. (Note: The availability of this drug is now variable in different countries. It was licensed in the UK, for instance, but is no longer available there.)

Efficacy was demonstrated at both the 2 mg and the 3 mg dosage for men with ED, with a side-effect profile that included nausea, headache, and dizziness.[10] A few patients developed syncope, although this was relatively rare. Although higher doses were used in the clinical trials the frequency of adverse events precluded licensing of those higher doses.[23] It was also recommended that caution be exercised when apomorphine was administered in combination with antihypertensive medication and with nitrates.[21] In a single trial comparing apomorphine with sildenafil in men with ED, the latter demonstrated considerably greater efficacy,[24] and the use of apomorphine has subsequently diminished considerably.

Other oral agents

Yohimbine is an alpha-2 adrenoceptor antagonist that has been used for many years for the treatment of ED. It was used prior to the advent of intracavernosal injection therapy, although it had relatively poor efficacy. Since the launch of the PDE5 inhibitors it has had only a very minor role in the therapeutic armamentarium. Quite how it works has remained somewhat elusive. Initially thought to act centrally as an alpha-2 adrenoceptor antagonist that "switched off" pathways that inhibit erections, there is increasing evidence that it may act peripherally to block vasoconstriction of the penile arteries.[11,25] Orally active, at doses of 5–15 mg, it has a T_{max} of just over 1 hour, with a $T_{½}$ that is only just longer.[26] The duration of activity is, however, somewhat longer at around 12 hours, reflecting the production of an active metabolite.[25,26] There is evidence of modest efficacy in men with ED,[27] but there is an extensive side-effect profile including symptoms of increased sympathetic activity (anxiety, nausea, restlessness, agitation, sleeplessness, tachycardia, palpitations, and diarrhea).[11]

An oral preparation of phentolamine underwent clinical trials in the late 1990s.[28] The pharmacology of phentolamine is discussed more fully below, but the oral formulation never reached clinical practice.

Intracavernosal agents

Intracavernosal application of drugs for the treatment of ED was first described in the early 1980s by Brindley[29] and Virag.[30] Their pioneering work led to widespread clinical use of a variety of intracavernosal agents for men with ED, all of which had a common mechanism of action, namely relaxation of the cavernosal smooth muscle. The drugs achieved this by a variety of pharmacological mechanisms, which are described in detail below. Cavernosal smooth muscle relaxation, usually allied with arterial vasodilatation, results in tumescence, and ultimately, when accompanied by closure of the veno-occlusive mechanism (see Chapter 3) in a rigid penile erection. The need to apply these drugs intracavernosally reflects their potential to cause systemic vasodilatation if administered intravenously. The most plausible explanation for the ability of a localized injection within the corpus cavernosum to produce generalized tumescence throughout the penis with subsequent erection involves the spread of electric current and ions between penile smooth muscle cells via gap junctions.[31] At the present time, the only drugs used in clinical practice (either alone or in combination) are prostaglandin E_1 (alprostadil), papaverine, phentolamine, and vasoactive intestinal polypeptide (VIP).

Alprostadil (prostaglandin E_1/PGE_1)

Alprostadil is a synthetic form of prostaglandin E_1, which itself is a naturally occurring prostaglandin found in particularly high concentration in semen. PGE_1 is licensed for intracavernosal, intraurethral, and topical use. It is a smooth muscle relaxant within the penis, with its effect being mediated via activation of specific receptors on the smooth muscle cell, which stimulate adenylate cyclase to produce increased levels of intracellular cyclic AMP (cAMP). Downstream effects are entirely analogous to those seen with increased levels of cGMP following PDE5 inhibition. Additional mechanisms may involve the inhibition of noradrenaline release from sympathetic nerve terminals and suppression of angiotensin II secretion from the corpus cavernosum.[25] The actual mechanism of breakdown of PGE_1 within the penis is poorly understood, although it is known to have a short duration of action and to be extensively metabolized.[32] Excretion is mainly in the urine. Following intracavernosal administration of doses of between 5 and 40 μg, an erectile response occurs within 10–15 minutes and persists typically for up to an hour. Response rates vary according to the population being treated, but generally 70–80% of men will achieve a good erectile response.[11] The major side effects are penile pain, which occurs in up to 50% of men, and prolonged erections, which are relatively uncommon.[10] Erections that last longer than 3–4 hours require specific treatment, since erections that last longer than this can result in permanent penile damage.

Papaverine

Papaverine is a non-specific phosphodiesterase inhibitor that was first used as a treatment for erectile dysfunction by Virag.[30] Pharmacologically it has been shown to relax both cavernosal smooth muscle and penile arteries.[25] Used at doses between 30 and 110 mg it is an effective treatment for men with ED, but its clinical use is limited by the relatively high rate of prolonged erection and penile fibrosis.[11] Although it was once used widely, it is not actually licensed for this indication.

Phentolamine

Phentolamine is a non-selective competitive antagonist of the alpha-adrenoceptors with similar affinity for the alpha-1 and alpha-2 receptors, although there are possible additional effects as a serotoninergic antagonist, as an activator of nitric oxide synthase, and as a mast cell activator.[25] As a single agent, when administered intracavernosally it has limited efficacy and is most commonly administered either in combination with papaverine or with VIP.

Vasoactive intestinal polypeptide (VIP)

VIP is a naturally occurring polypeptide that has been proposed as a putative neurotransmitter mediating penile erection. It is co-localized within penile nerves with acetylcholine and with nitric oxide.[33,34] Its actions, which include vasodilatation, are mediated via stimulation of membrane-bound adenylate cyclase with increased levels of intracellular cAMP. Following intracavernosal injection it has a short plasma half-life and on its own does not produce an erection.[35] Its main use has been in combination with phentolamine.[36]

Combination therapy

The combination of papaverine and phentolamine was the earliest combination treatment used for intracavernosal injection therapy. A typical combination used 1 mg phentolamine with 30 mg papaverine,[11] and indeed such a combination was marketed in some European countries. As a combination the potential advantages over single drug administration are increased (synergistic) efficacy and reduced side effects, although the potential for prolonged erections and penile fibrosis remains.[10]

More recently the combination of phentolamine and VIP has been extensively investigated as an intracavernosal therapy.[36,37] Again, the efficacy of the two agents combined appears to be significantly greater than for either of the two agents when used independently. The side-effect profile is relatively benign, although one notable difference from other intracavernosal formulations is the presence of systemic vasodilation and flushing, which reflects the effects of VIP within the general circulation. Although it has been licensed as a combination therapy for men with ED, it has not been extensively marketed.

Finally the other combination that has been widely used, particularly in North America, is so-called "trimix," which combines papaverine, phentolamine, and prostaglandin E_1.[11] Although there is little clinical trial evidence, the combination appears to have considerable efficacy, albeit with a relatively high rate of prolonged erection. The combination has never been licensed and local reconstitution within a hospital pharmacy is required. Although the proportions of the different drugs used vary, a typical combination is 40 µg of PGE_1, 1 mg of phentolamine, and 30 mg of papaverine.[11]

Other agents

Intraurethral therapy

Alprostadil has also been administered intraurethrally for men with ED, and for a time, just prior to the launch of sildenafil, this proved to be a widely used and reasonably effective therapy. The cellular mechanism of action of alprostadil is described above. When administered intraurethrally, the alprostadil is absorbed via the urethral mucosa into the corpus spongiosum, and then passes retrogradely via venous channels into the corpus cavernosum.[38] There is significant "spillage" into the systemic circulation such that much higher doses are required (between 125 and 1000 µg) for efficacy to be achieved and such that there is a low but definite incidence of flushing and systemic hypotension.[39] The clinical effect occurs within 5–10 min and the duration of effect is around 1 hour. Clinical trials have demonstrated modest efficacy,[32,39] but less so than intracavernosal injection therapy.[40] It is less convenient than oral therapy and its clinical usage is limited nowadays.[10,11]

Topical therapy

Alprostadil has also been formulated in a topical preparation that can be used for men with ED.[41,42] Recently marketed in North America and in Europe, the pharmacological mode of action has been described above. Absorption through the skin is improved by the skin permeation enhancer 2-dimethyl-amino-propionic acid dodecyl ester (DDAIP). Once absorbed through the skin, access to the corpus cavernosum is achieved by retrograde venous flow in a way analogous to the intraurethral preparation. Following application inside the distal urethra, T_{max} is achieved in 0.6–1 hour, with a $T_{½}$ of 3–5 hours. The clinical effect occurs within 5–30 min. Again, due to loss into the systemic circulation, large doses of 100–300 µg are required for clinical efficacy. Efficacy rates appear substantially lower than the PDE5 inhibitors.

Summary

A variety of drugs have been used for the treatment of ED, with a range of pharmacological actions. To date, drugs that work peripherally within the penis have been more successful than centrally acting agents, although they either have to be administered locally or there has to be some "special" mechanism to achieve tissue specificity. The way in which the PDE5 inhibitors achieve this is via the requirement for neuronal release of nitric oxide within the penis, which can only occur in the presence of a sexual stimulus. The efficacy and safety of the PDE5 inhibitors have made them the market leaders, and their role in the management of men with ED will be described in Chapter 19. Centrally acting drugs have to date been disappointing, with their side-effect profiles limiting the dose of the drug that can safely be used.

References

1 Corbin JD, Francis SH. Molecular biology and pharmacology of PDE5 inhibitor therapy for erectile dysfunction. *J Androl* 2003;24(6 Suppl.):S38–41.

2 Corbin JD, Francis SH. Pharmacology of phosphodiesterase-5 inhibitors. *Int J Clin Pract* 2002;56(6):453–9.

3 Francis SH, Morris GZ, Corbin JD. Molecular mechanisms that could contribute to prolonged effectiveness of PDE5 inhibitors to improve erectile function. *Int J Impot Res* 2008;20(4):333–42.

4 Francis SH, Corbin JD. Molecular mechanisms and pharmacokinetics of phosphodiesterase-5 antagonists. *Curr Urol Rep* 2003;4(6):457–65.

5 Kotera J, Mochida H, Inoue H, et al. Avanafil, a potent and highly selective phosphodiesterase-5 inhibitor for erectile dysfunction. *J Urol* 2012;188(2):668–74.

6 Wang R, Burnett AL, Heller WH, et al. Selectivity of avanafil, a PDE5 inhibitor for the treatment of erectile dysfunction: implications for clinical safety and improved tolerability. *J Sex Med* 2012;9(8):2122–9.

7 Doh H, Shin CY, Son M, et al. Mechanism of erectogenic effect of the selective phosphodiesterase type 5 inhibitor, DA-8159. *Arch Pharmacol Res* 2002;25(6):873–8.

8 Lee J, Yoo HH, Rhim KJ, Sohn DR, Kim DH. Metabolism and excretion of 5-ethyl-2-{5-[4-(2-hydroxyethyl)piperazine-1-sulfonyl]-2-propoxyphenyl}-7-propyl-3,5-dihydropyrrolo[3,2-d]-pyrimidin-4-one (SK3530) in rats. *Rapid Commun Mass Sp* 2007;21(7):1139–49.

9 Glina S, Fonseca GN, Bertero EB, et al. Efficacy and tolerability of lodenafil carbonate for oral therapy of erectile dysfunction: a phase III clinical trial. *J Sex Med* 2010;7(5): 1928–36.

10 Eardley I, Donatucci C, Corbin J, et al. Pharmacotherapy for erectile dysfunction. *J Sex Med* 2010;7(1 Pt 2):524–40.

11 Porst H, Burnett A, Brock G, et al. SOP conservative (medical and mechanical) treatment of erectile dysfunction. *J Sex Med* 2013;10(1):130–71.

12 Luu JK, Chappelow AV, McCulley TJ, Marmor MF. Acute effects of sildenafil on the electroretinogram and multifocal electroretinogram. *Am J Ophthalmol* 2001;132(3):388–94.

13 Jagle H, Jagle C, Serey L, et al. Visual short-term effects of Viagra: double-blind study in healthy young subjects. *Am J Ophthalmol* 2004;137(5):842–9.

14 Forgue ST, Patterson BE, Bedding AW, et al. Tadalafil pharmacokinetics in healthy subjects. *Brit J Clin Pharmacol* 2006;61(3):280–8.

15 Kyle JA, Brown DA, Hill JK. Avanafil for erectile dysfunction. *Ann Pharmacother* 2013;47(10):1312–20.

16 Kim BH, Lim HS, Chung JY, et al. Safety, tolerability and pharmacokinetics of udenafil, a novel PDE-5 inhibitor, in healthy young Korean subjects. *Brit J Clin Pharmacol* 2008;65(6):848–54.

17 Shin KH, Kim BH, Kim TE, et al. The effects of ketoconazole and rifampicin on the pharmacokinetics of mirodenafil in healthy Korean male volunteers: an open-label, one-sequence, three-period, three-treatment crossover study. *Clin Ther* 2009;31(12):3009–20.

18 Webb DJ, Freestone S, Allen MJ, Muirhead GJ. Sildenafil citrate and blood-pressure-lowering drugs: results of drug interaction studies with an organic nitrate and a calcium antagonist. *Am J Cardiol* 1999;83(5A):21C–8C.

19 Kloner RA, Hutter AM, Emmick JT, Mitchell MI, Denne J, Jackson G. Time course of the interaction between tadalafil and nitrates. *J Am Coll Cardiol* 2003;42(10):1855–60.

20 Kloner RA, Jackson G, Emmick JT, et al. Interaction between the phosphodiesterase 5 inhibitor, tadalafil and 2 alpha-blockers, doxazosin and tamsulosin in healthy normotensive men. *J Urol* 2004;172(5 Pt 1):1935–40.

21 Argiolas A, Hedlund H. The pharmacology and clinical pharmacokinetics of apomorphine SL. *BJU Int* 2001;88(Suppl 3):18–21.

22 Andersson KE. Pharmacology of penile erection. *Pharmacol Rev* 2001;53(3):417–50.

23 Dula E, Bukofzer S, Perdok R, George M, Apomorphine SLSG. Double-blind, crossover comparison of 3 mg apomorphine SL with placebo and with 4 mg apomorphine SL in male erectile dysfunction. *Eur Urol* 2001;39(5):558–3; discussion 64.

24 Eardley I, Wright P, MacDonagh R, Hole J, Edwards A. An open-label, randomized, flexible-dose, crossover study to assess the comparative efficacy and safety of sildenafil citrate and apomorphine hydrochloride in men with erectile dysfunction. *BJU Int* 2004;93(9):1271–5.

25 Andersson KE. Mechanisms of penile erection and basis for pharmacological treatment of erectile dysfunction. *Pharmacol Rev* 2011;63(4):811–59.

26 Le Corre P, Dollo G, Chevanne F, Le Verge R. Biopharmaceutics and metabolism of yohimbine in humans. *Eur J Pharm Sci* 1999;9(1):79–84.

27 Ernst E, Pittler MH. Yohimbine for erectile dysfunction: a systematic review and meta-analysis of randomized clinical trials. *J Urol* 1998;159(2):433–6.

28 Goldstein I. Oral phentolamine: an alpha-1, alpha-2 adrenergic antagonist for the treatment of erectile dysfunction. *Int J Impot Res* 2000;12(Suppl 1):S75–80.

29 Brindley GS. Cavernosal alpha-blockade: a new technique for investigating and treating erectile impotence. *Brit J Psychiat* 1983;143:332–7.

30 Virag R. Intracavernous injection of papaverine for erectile failure. *Lancet* 1982;2(8304):938.

31 Christ GJ. Gap junctions and ion channels: relevance to erectile dysfunction. *Int J Impot Res* 2000;12(Suppl 4):S15–25.

32 Hanchanale V, Eardley I. Alprostadil for the treatment of impotence. *Expert Opin Pharmacother* 2014;15(3):421–8.

33 Vanhatalo S, Parkkisenniemi U, Steinbusch HW, de Vente J, Klinge E. No colocalization of immunoreactivities for VIP and neuronal NOS, and a differential relation to cGMP-immunoreactivity in bovine penile smooth muscle. *J Chem Neuroanat* 2000;19(2):81–91.

34 Hedlund P, Ny L, Alm P, Andersson KE. Cholinergic nerves in human corpus cavernosum and spongiosum contain nitric oxide synthase and heme oxygenase. *J Urol* 2000;164(3 Pt 1):868–75.

35 Kiely EA, Bloom SR, Williams G. Penile response to intracavernosal vasoactive intestinal polypeptide alone and in combination with other vasoactive agents. *Brit J Urol* 1989;64(2):191–4.

36 Sandhu D, Curless E, Dean J, et al. A double blind, placebo controlled study of intracavernosal vasoactive intestinal polypeptide and phenotolamine mesylate in a novel auto-injector for the treatment of non-psychogenic erectile dysfunction. *Int J Impot Res* 1999;11(2):91–7.

37 Dinsmore WW, Gingell C, Hackett G, et al. Treating men with predominantly nonpsychogenic erectile dysfunction with intracavernosal vasoactive intestinal polypeptide and phentolamine mesylate in a novel auto-injector system: a multicentre double-blind placebo-controlled study. *BJU Int* 1999;83(3):274–9.

38 Bschleipfer T, Cimniak HU, Beckert R, Hauck EW, Weidner W, Sparwasser C. Possible hemodynamic pathways of intraurethral prostaglandin-E1 (MUSE). *Int J Impot Res* 2004;16(4):365–8.

39 Padma-Nathan H, Hellstrom WJ, Kaiser FE, et al. Treatment of men with erectile dysfunction with transurethral alprostadil. Medicated Urethral System for Erection (MUSE) Study Group. *N Engl J Med* 1997;336(1):1–7.

40 Shabsigh R, Padma-Nathan H, Gittleman M, McMurray J, Kaufman J, Goldstein I. Intracavernous alprostadil alfadex is more efficacious, better tolerated, and preferred over intraurethral alprostadil plus optional actis: a comparative, randomized, crossover, multicenter study. *Urology* 2000;55(1):109–13.

41 Steidle C, Padma-Nathan H, Salem S, et al. Topical alprostadil cream for the treatment of erectile dysfunction: a combined analysis of the phase II program. *Urology* 2002;60(6):1077–82.

42 Rooney M, Pfister W, Mahoney M, Nelson M, Yeager J, Steidle C. Long-term, multicenter study of the safety and efficacy of topical alprostadil cream in male patients with erectile dysfunction. *J Sex Med* 2009;6(2):520–34.

CHAPTER 7

Pharmacology of drugs used in premature ejaculation

Michael Grant Wylie
Global Pharma Consulting, Banbury, UK

In several urological disorders, particularly the lower urinary tract symptoms (LUTS) associated with both overactive bladder (OAB) and benign prostatic hyperplasia (BPH), the textbooks would have us believe that the pharmacology and/or pathophysiology underlying clinical benefit is well understood. This is particularly true of the dogma relating the utility of sildenafil in erectile dysfunction (ED) to an exclusive action in the periphery on one isoenzyme of phosphodiesterase. The actuality may be completely different, with contributions from other isoenzymes not only at peripheral autonomic neuroeffector junctions but also within the central nervous system (CNS) potentially making contributions. Our understanding of the pharmacology of drugs used in the treatment of premature ejaculation is even poorer due to a combination of factors:

1. Evidence-based support for the clinical utility of most drugs is somewhat limited compared to that available for other urological and sexual health disorders/dysfunctions.
2. The polypharmacology of "effective" agents.
3. The lack of proven animal models of both the ejaculatory reflex and the pathophysiology of premature ejaculation.

However, the most obvious starting point is an examination of the three major classes of agents that have achieved some degree of approved or "off-label" utility: neurotransmitter uptake inhibitors; locally acting agents; and centrally active agents (e.g., opioids, as exemplified by tramadol, and oxytocin antagonists).

"Selective" neurotransmitter reuptake inhibitors

Like many drug discovery programs the impetus arose form chance clinical observation where one man's side effect is another man's benefit; that is, the well-documented side effect of certain antidepressants is delay of ejaculation. In terms of exploitation of this side effect, there is a plethora of published data from carefully controlled clinical trials (see, e.g., Ref. 1) and the resultant meta-analyses showing that there is some degree of clinical benefit in the long-term use of reuptake inhibitors, particularly those that inhibit the serotonin reuptake system. From double-blind, placebo-controlled studies there is little doubt that some degree of clinical benefit can be achieved in the absence of obtrusive side effects. This includes the demonstration of significant changes in objective endpoints, particularly intravaginal ejaculatory latency (IELT), and patient-reported outcomes (PROs), such as the index of premature ejaculation (IPE) and premature ejaculation profile (PEP). Over the last decade, driven perhaps by commercial considerations rather than serious scientists, it has become the dogma that selectivity for this monoamine over the catecholamines (dopamine and norepinephrine) is particularly advantageous. Hence a certain cachet is attached to any drug labeled as a selective serotonin reuptake inhibitor (SSRI). Unfortunately some of the more clinically effective reuptake inhibitors, such as clomipramine, are not particularly selective for the

Male Sexual Dysfunction: A Clinical Guide, First Edition. Edited by Suks Minhas and John Mulhall.

serotonin reuptake system, and truly selective agents have not made it into clinical evaluation. Clinical validation would be dependent on evaluation of much more selective agents, for example, panuramine.[2] However, it remains that drugs that inhibit serotonin reuptake are effective, so one can assume that this neurotransmitter is involved in the modulation of the ejaculatory reflex and contributes to some degree to the clinical profile of drugs such as dapoxetine[3] (Figure 7.1).

However, given the medical need and size of the commercial opportunity it is somewhat surprising that a second generation dapoxetine has not been developed. In an attempt to define the pharmacology of PE it is important to understand the history of dapoxetine. In the late 70s dapoxetine failed in Lilly's hands as an antidepressant at least in part due to poor pharmacokinetics (short half-life not achieving steady state), an attribute that was subsequently claimed to make it near ideal for PE – a half-life of 3–4 h was considered optimal for "on demand" use. However, as discussed in detail elsewhere,[4] there is a paradox. In essence all selective reuptake inhibitors (SRIs) appear to take several weeks of continuous steady-state dosing to become fully effective. In other words the benefit in PE mirrors the time to onset of their clinical antidepressant action and is actually dependent on an adaptive post-junctional change involving not only 5-HT receptors but other receptor types. The requirement for induction of such changes is the achievement and maintenance over several weeks of steady-state plasma concentrations of the drug. A drug with a short half-life like dapoxetine could only steady state if taken five or six times a day. Thus, assuming dapoxetine is actually consistently effective on the first dose this would indicate that there was another component to its action; if it merely represents an acute inhibition of serotonin reuptake other SSRIs would also be expected to be effective on the first dose. Perhaps not surprisingly, faced with the relative lack of understanding of the precise mechanism of action of dapoxetine, the pharmaceutical industry has shown little ability or desire to improve on its clinical profile.

What would normally happen within industry at this point is that programs would be mounted to improve on the clinical profile particularly directed toward

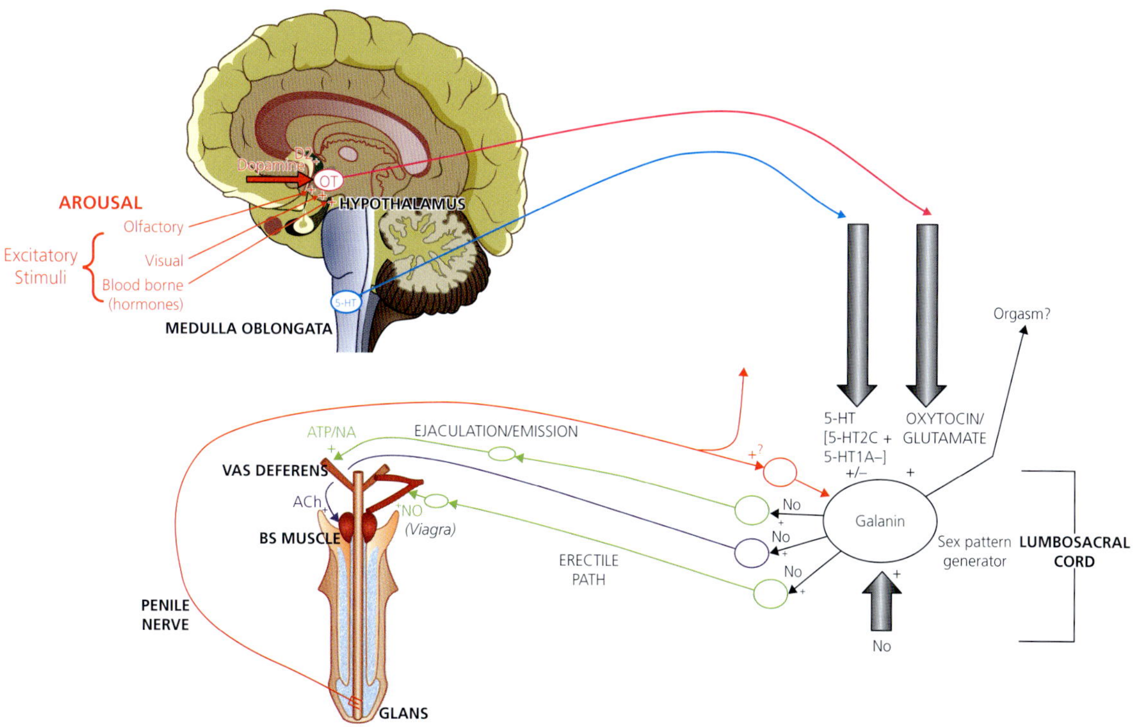

Figure 7.1 The neurophysiology of ejaculation in the human male. ACh, acetylcholine; Bulbospongiosus muscle; D2, dopamine D2 receptors; 5-HT, 5-hydroxytryptamine (serotonin) receptors; NA; NO, nitric oxide; OT, oxytocin receptors.

increasing the benefit:risk ratio. Indeed, much more selective agents have been synthesized and have entered late-stage clinical development. Returning, however, to dapoxetine. At least in the eyes of the Food and Drug Administration (FDA), the regulatory body in the United States, there were concerns about the relatively narrow therapeutic window and in particular the long-term CNS manifestations. There was deemed to be a potential risk, given the relatively young age group, of suicidal ideation.

The key question in terms of improving on the clinical profile of dapoxetine lies in understanding the precise mechanism of action of the drug. Although much elegant research has been conducted by inter alia Marcel Waldinger[5] and François Guiliano[6] leading to hypotheses round the importance of various changes in pre- and post-junctional 5-HT effects, the conclusions are constrained by the lack of a definitive animal model. Animal models can only be validated by correlation between data from that particular model with a well-defined clinical profile. This must include relative rank order of potency in both human and animal and evaluation of drugs with high pharmacological selectivity or preferably site specificity. This has not been the case, and the relationship between autonomic and central dysfunction in the rat and ejaculatory (and indeed erectile) function/dysfunction is at best equivocal. This does not imply that Waldinger's conclusions, largely based on molecular biology and phenotypic and genotypic analysis, are incorrect only that they can only be proved with the advancement of selective pharmacological agonists and antagonists into humans for full clinical profiling. Unless gene therapy becomes acceptable in non-life-threatening conditions, the molecular biologist will never be able to prove unequivocally a link between a receptor or enzyme and a disease process. Correlation of clinical phenomenon and molecular mechanism is best achieved by using drugs of known pharmacology. The development and subsequent evaluation of subtype selective (A, B, and D) alpha-1-adrenoceptor antagonists in BPH would represent the classical pharmaceutical industry approach. Intriguingly this actually demonstrated that most of our original hypothesis that the alpha-blocker class acts to alter perurethral tone was invalid and the action was more likely to be a vascular one on attenuation of bladder ischemia.[7] Likewise, the development of selective drugs for muscarinic receptor subtypes has also increased our understanding of the pathophysiology of OAB; ironically, however, it is difficult to conclude that there has been much of an improvement in clinical performance beyond that achieved with the original subtype non-selective drug, oxybutynin. It is particularly difficult to unravel the pharmacology of a clinical action when the tools involved are relatively blunt instruments. Even the most neurotransmitter-selective SSRI will activate a variety of serotonin receptor types (subtypes). The primary action on the reuptake system is manifest by the altered synaptic 5-HT interacting with a multiplicity of serotonin receptors. The situation is further complicated by the knowledge that the initial elevation of synaptic 5-HT produced not only an acute change at the receptor level but also a secondary or adaptive change; at least in the case of the use of SSRIs in depression it is this adaptive change that is considered more relevant.[4] Although several agonists and antagonists with some degree of selectivity for subtypes have been synthesized, none has been evaluated in PE. As the development and clinical evaluation of these or even more selective 5-HT agonists/antagonists[8] is unlikely to happen in PE, all we can really conclude based on clinical evidence is that modulation of serotoninergic systems can influence ejaculatory latency and provide reasonably effective treatment of PE. We cannot conclude with any degree of certainty exactly where anatomically serotonin is important or which receptor type(s) are involved. Even more so than usual given the relative lack of agents that have entered clinical development, humans are the ultimate experimental animals and particularly complex ones at that. The situation is exacerbated by the poorly characterized polypharmacology of the serotonin reuptake inhibitors that have shown clinical benefit. Unfortunately there appears to be little incentive for the pharmaceutical industry to develop more selective SSRIs, and/or serotonin agonists or antagonists, for any clinical indication including PE.

Use of locally active agents

Prior and indeed subsequent to the approval of dapoxetine there was widespread use not only of the selective reuptake inhibitors described above but also of locally applied agents. These are often described as anesthetic gels or desensitizing agent, which can be both accurate and inaccurate descriptors. In terms of composition they do invariably contain local anesthetics and not surprisingly can produce localized penile anesthesia and/or desensitization. However, importantly, clinical benefit can be achieved in the absence of obtrusive desensitization.

The most widely used preparation is EMLA (eutectic mixture of local anesthetics). Although it is effective there are limitations insofar as it has to be applied for 30–40 min before use, a condom must be used to avoid transfer to the partner, and there is a high incidence of penile desensitization. To circumvent these deficits a novel drug combination, PSD502, was developed and has gained regulatory approval in the European Union (EU).

Prilocaine and lidocaine in base form were chosen as the local anesthetic agents for the PSD 502 formulation because, when mixed, they exhibit eutectic-like properties, which are required for the development of a metered dose spray formulation. In addition to these unique physico-chemical properties, they possess similar and desirable pharmacological properties.[9]

Pharmacologically, prilocaine and lidocaine have a rapid onset of action (5–10 min) and a moderate duration of action (30–60 min), which are not altered when the agents are combined. These features are considered to be optimal for the treatment of PE. Both drugs belong to the amide group of local anesthetics, which, unlike the ester group, are associated with a negligible risk of local hypersensitivity – an important factor in choosing drugs for repeated topical application. Both drugs have the same pK_a (7.7), meaning they have the same absorption characteristics, and they have similar potency (lidocaine is 1.27-fold more potent than prilocaine).

Prilocaine and lidocaine are normally crystalline at room temperature, with melting points of 37–38 °C and 68–69 °C, respectively. Combination of prilocaine with lidocaine results in a lowering of the melting point of the mixture in comparison to the melting points of the individual components. Development of EMLA cream has relied on the eutectic properties of combining prilocaine and lidocaine. It is the exploitation of this eutectic property that has enabled the:

1 development of the formulation of PSD502, which is chemically stable for long periods of time;
2 production at larger scale of PSD502;
3 utility of PSD502 to be formulated as an aerosol treatment.

Rationale for use of base forms of prilocaine and lidocaine

Various formulations and combinations of prilocaine and lidocaine are used as anesthetic therapies but most, if not all, use the ionized, lipid-insoluble HCl salt form. The salt forms are readily soluble in aqueous solution and so are suitable for preparation of injectable systemic preparations; but as they are not lipid soluble they do not readily penetrate epithelial surfaces and are not suitable for topical delivery. In contrast, as base forms are not ionised, they are absorbed and as a result, in the optimal state to provide clinical benefit to PE patients.

Two large-scale phase III clinical trials have been completed on PSD502, with over 26,000 exposures.[10,11] They showed highly significant changes in IELT and all domains of the PROs used for both patients and their partners. There was no evidence of tachyphylaxis (pharmacological tolerance) and indeed benefit increased with time, presumably as the relationship improved. It has been hypothesized that in these situations the drug may not be required on every occasion. There was only minimal evidence of partner transfer and/or penile desensitization. This led to approval by EMA in November 2013.

The clinical data would tend to support the proposition that benefit in PE can be achieved with locally acting agents without producing obtrusive penile desensitization. One possible explanation for the overall clinical profile is that PE patients may be experiencing penile hypersensitivity.[12] PSD502 is acting to normalize the sensitivity. An analogy is that antihypertensive drugs can reduce high blood pressure to normalize but do not consistently produce hypotension. The formulation and actuation pattern of PSD502 was developed specifically to optimize clinical performance. Other products lack either the rigorous clinical supportive data or are actually marketed as "desensitizing agents."

The advantage of the PSD502-based approach is that there is no assumption about the etiology of PE. In clinical trials almost 90% of patients respond, with approximately 50% entering the normal range of IELT after p.r.n. use over 9 months. This high responder rate is likely to be a consequence of an action on a pathway that is fundamentally involved in ejaculatory control, that is, within the afferent-efferent reflex arc.

Although comparator trials have not been conducted, the equivalent data on dapoxetine show a much lower responder rate (defined as the number of patients achieving an increase in IELT of at least 1 minute); this would indicate that although serotonin plays a role, it may well be only in a subset of patients.

In terms of an understanding of the pharmacology of PE, PSD502 provides only limited insight. The product, like all local anesthetics, is acting on sodium channels, presumably altering a local afferent-efferent reflex initiated at the level of the glans penis. Target organ selectivity has been achieved not by pharmacological manipulation but by pharmacokinetic means. There is no evidence at the molecular level that there is a specific Na channel that could give improved clinical benefit beyond that achieved with PSD502. On that basis it would be difficult to develop Structure activity relationship (SAR) leading to clinical improvement with respect to either efficacy or the benefit-risk profile. The advantage of this type of approach is that there is no real assumption of the etiology and as such a fairly wide spectrum of PE patients may receive benefit. One could speculate that approaches based on pharmacologically selective agents, although potentially effective, could have their benefit restricted to patient subsets.

Other potential "broad spectrum" approaches

There is some clinical evidence that tramadol can delay ejaculation.[13] It is likely that a large component of this is due to its action on opioid receptors, but little is known about the selectivity for individual opioid receptor subtypes. Equally the drug's site of action is unknown as drugs of this (opioid) class can have central, spinal, and peripheral actions. It is, however, well documented that at almost every synapse studied opioids inhibit neurotransmitter release; the issues are what synapse, which opioid receptor subtype, and what neurotransmitter is relevant to the observed clinical profile. Potentially if some of these could be unraveled this could represent a fertile starting point for de novo development of drugs for PE. The SAR round opioid receptor types, being developed as novel analgesics and drugs for irritable bowel syndrome (IBS), OAB, and neuroprotection, is well characterized and several prototypes have already been used in humans.[14] However, a major issue will be the regulatory authority's reaction to chronic administration of an opioid for the treatment of PE.

Overall, therefore, most of the drugs that are used, either with regulatory approval or "off label," have achieved clinical utility based on clinical observation rather than rational drug design based on detailed knowledge of their pharmacology and development of an appropriate structure activity relationship (SAR). There is no evidence that the pharmaceutical industry is interested in basic R&D in PE, and this is likely to remain the case until a regulatory route map for approval in the United States becomes apparent. The FDA requires clinical trial data to be accrued using a validated PRO. The agency definition of validated is unrelated to the degree of "validation" acceptable for publishing, even in the best peer group-reviewed journals.

Coming next?

The finding that oxytocin has been implicated in the control of male sexual behavior and ejaculation (see Figure 7.1) has led to the evaluation of selective oxytocin antagonists in non-clinical animal models and clinical trials. The original studies in rats led the authors to conclude: "Targeting OT receptors with a highly selective approach seems a promising approach to treatment of premature ejaculation."[15] This conclusion was based on subtle changes in a variety of physiological endpoints in the rat, considered to be surrogate predictors of clinical response. Unfortunately, in a "gold standard" double-blind controlled study there was no evidence for the same OT antagonist, epelsiban, producing any change in IELT or in any of the endpoints of either of the PROs used in the study.[16] The dissociation between clinical and non-clinical findings must raise issues about the relevance of animal models of premature ejaculation, or at least the interpretation of data generated thereby.

Summary

In summary, although many neurotransmitters have been implicated in the control of ejaculation and in the pathophysiology of PE (Figure 7.1) it is not possible to unambiguously define precisely the process requiring modulation. It is likely that as the defect is multifactorial a polypharmacological approach may be required. That said, patient subsets may be responsive to specific pharmacological approaches, as exemplified by SRIs or oxytocin. The alternative is to manage the symptoms rather than attach too much importance to understanding the science, as with, for example, PSD502. Effective symptomatic improvement is achievable but we cannot expect a "cure."

References

1 McMahon CG, Althof SE, Kaufman JM, et al. Efficacy and safety of dapoxetine for the treatment of premature ejaculation: integrated analysis of results from five phase 3 trials. *J Sex Med* 2011;8:524–39.

2 Blurton PA, Broadhurst AM, Cross JA, et al. Panuramine, a selective inhibitor of uptake of 5-hydroxytryptamine in the rat. *Neuropharmacology* 1984;23:1049–52.

3 Andersson K-E, Mullhall JP, Wyllie MG. Pharmacokinetic and pharmacodynamic features of dapoxetine, a novel drug for on-demand treatment of premature ejaculation. *BJU Int* 2006;97:311–15.

4 Wyllie MG. The dapoxetine paradox. *BJU Int* 2010;105: 1041–2.

5 Janssen PK, Schaik RV, Olivier B, et al. The 5-HT2c receptor gene Cys23Ser polymorphism influences the intravaginal ejaculation latency time in Dutch Caucasians with lifelong premature ejaculation. *Asian J Androl* 2014;16:607–14.

6 Facchinetti P, Giuliano F, Laurin M, et al. Direct brain projections onto the spinal generator of ejaculation in the rat. *Neuroscience* 2014;272:207–16.

7 Pingeraa GM, Mitterberger M, Pallwein L, et al. Alpha-blockers improve chronic ischaemia of lower urinary tract in patients with lower urinary tract symptoms. *BJU Int* 2008;101:319–24.

8 Fletcher A, Cliffe IA, Dourish CT. Silent 5-HT1A receptor antagonists: utility as research tools and therapeutic agents. *Trends Pharmacol Sci* 1993;14:441–8.

9 Henry R, Morales A, Wyllie, MG. TEMPE: topical eutectic-like mixture for premature ejaculation. *Expert Opin Drug Deliv* 2008;5:251–61.

10 Dinsmore WW, Wyllie MG. PSD502 improves ejaculatory latency, control and sexual satisfaction when applied topically 5 min before intercourse in men with premature ejaculation: results of a phase III, multicenter, double-blind, placebo-controlled study. *BJU Int* 2009:103:940–9.

11 Carson C, Wyllie MG. Improved ejaculatory latency, control and sexual satisfaction when pSD502 is applied topically in men with premature ejaculation: results of a phase III double-blind, placebo-controlled study. *J Sex Med* 2010;7: 3179–89.

12 Wyllie MG, Hellstrom WTG. The link between penile hypersensitivity and premature ejaculation. *BJU Int* 2011;107: 452–7.

13 Salem EA, Wilson SK, Bissada NK. Tramadol HCl has promise in on-demand use to treat premature ejaculation. *J Sex Med* 2008:5:188–93.

14 Dietis N, Rowbotham DJ, Lambert DG. Opioid receptor subtypes: fact or fiction. *Br J Anaesth* 2011;107:8–18.

15 Clement P, Bernabe J, Compagnie S, et al. Inhibition of ejaculation by the non-peptide oxytocin receptor antagonist GSK 577296 a multi-level site of action. *Br J Pharmacol* 2013:169:1477–85.

16 Shinghai R, Barnes A, Mahar KM. Safety and efficacy of epelsiban in the treatment of men with premature ejaculation: a randomized, double-blind, placebo-controlled, fixed-dose study. *J Sex Med* 2013;10:2506–17.

CHAPTER 8

Cardiovascular risk and erectile dysfunction

Graham Jackson
Guy's and St Thomas' Hospitals NHS Trust, London, UK

Erectile dysfunction (ED) is common and increases with increasing age. It is defined as the recurrent or consistent inability to maintain or obtain a penile erection sufficient for satisfactory sexual intercourse. Occasional failures occur usually due to social circumstances, for example, too much alcohol. It is estimated that 20–40% of men aged 60–69 and 50–100% of men over 70 years of age suffer from ED.[1] However, it has become apparent that though ED is less frequent in men in their 40s and 50s it is a marker of significant increased risk.[2] In a study of 1400 men aged 40–75 years of age with no known coronary artery disease and followed up for 10 years, ED at baseline in the age group 40–49 years predicted a 50-fold increase in CAD events per 1000 patient years compared to men who at baseline had no ED (Table 8.1). The risk in the 50–59 age group was increased five times, and in the 60–69 age group two-fold, with no increased risk in those aged over 70.

The Second Princeton Consensus on Sexual Dysfunction and Cardiac Risk concluded that the recognition of ED as a warning sign for cardiovascular disease has led to the concept of a man with ED and no cardiac symptoms being considered a cardiac (or vascular) patient until proven otherwise.[3] The recognition that ED predicts both all-cause mortality and significant cardiovascular events reinforces this approach.[4]

Erectile dysfunction and cardiovascular disease: examining the link

Endothelial dysfunction represents a common denominator for both ED and vascular disease (ED = ED). In several studies Vlachopoulos and colleagues have shown that ED is associated with increased inflammatory and endothelial prothrombotic activation in men with and without coronary artery disease (CAD), with ED conferring an incremental unfavorable impact on the circulating levels of these markers when combined with CAD.[5–7] They believe that low-grade systemic inflammation could be an important element of the association between ED and CAD. In turn, they believe that measuring inflammatory activation may improve the diagnostic approach to patients with suspected ED, particularly with regard to establishing those at higher risk of CAD.

As we understand it, the endothelium is a major regulator for vascular homeostasis, producing several signaling molecules, most notably nitric oxide, which promotes vasodilation, inhibits platelet aggregation/adhesion, and exerts antifibrotic effects.[6] Endothelial dysfunction is characterized by an increased permeability to plasma constituents including low-density lipoproteins and impaired nitric oxide synthesis/degradation. Such events lead to vasoconstriction, platelet aggregation, and white blood cell adhesion. Consequently, endothelial dysfunction is considered to be an early marker of vascular disease, contributing to the development of atherosclerotic lesions and later clinical complications.[8]

Given that the endothelium is the same throughout the arterial tree, it follows that if there is a problem at one part of the circulation (ED) there could be a problem elsewhere, which need not be symptomatic (e.g., "silent" CAD or carotid disease). The artery size hypothesis seeks to explain the differing presentations of the

Male Sexual Dysfunction: A Clinical Guide, First Edition. Edited by Suks Minhas and John Mulhall.

Table 8.1 Erectile dysfunction (ED) predicts coronary events.[2] The younger the age group, the greater the cardiovascular risk from ED. In men in their 40s who have ED at baseline, cardiovascular risk over a 10-year follow-up is 50-fold greater than men who have normal erections.

Age group 1400 men with no known CAD: 10-year follow-up	ED at baseline CAD events per 1000 patient years with CI intervals	No baseline ED CAD events per 1000 patient years with CI intervals
40–49	48.52 (1.23–269.26)	0.94 (0.02–5.21)
50–59	27.15 (7.40–69.56)	5.09 (3.38–7.38)
60–69	23.97 (11.49–44.10)	10.72 (7.62–14.66)
70+	29.63 (19.37–43.75)	23.30 (17.18–30.89)

CAD, coronary artery disease; CI, confidence interval.

Table 8.2 Artery size and atherothrombosis. A significant restriction to flow in the penile arteries may be subclinical in larger vessels.

Artery	Diameter (mm)	Clinical event
Penile	1–2	ED
Coronary	3–4	Ischemic heart disease
Carotid	5–7	TIA/stroke
Femoral	6–8	Claudication

TIA, transient ischemic attack.

same pathology and why ED could be a marker for silent disease elsewhere.[9]

Artery size varies according to location within the vascular system (Table 8.2). For example, the lumen of the penile arteries is considerably smaller (1–2 mm) compared with that of the coronary (3–4 mm), carotid (5–6 mm), and femoral (6–8 mm) arteries. Because of their smaller size and greater surface area the same level of plaque burden and/or endothelial dysfunction has a greater effect on blood flow through the penile arteries than through the coronary, carotid, and femoral arteries. Therefore the clinical manifestations of penile endothelial dysfunction may become evident before the consequences of coronary or peripheral vascular disease. By the time the lumina of the larger arteries become significantly obstructed (>50%) the penile blood flow may have already decreased considerably, which explains why so many men with CAD have ED.

Thus on the basis of the artery size hypothesis a malfunction in the penile arteries causing ED may be a predictor of silent subclinical cardiovascular disease. In addition, because an acute coronary syndrome often arises as a result of the rupture of a subclinical plaque, the presence of ED may also be an early warning sign of an acute coronary event including mortality.[10]

In support of this concept a series of 300 patients with acute chest pain and angiographically proven CAD were evaluated with a semi-structured interview to assess their medical and sexual histories prior to presentation.[11] The prevalence of ED among these patients was 49% ($n = 147$). In these 147 men with both ED and CAD, ED was experienced before CAD symptoms in 99 patients (67%). The mean time interval between the occurrence of ED and the occurrence of CAD was 38.8 months (range 1–168 months). Interestingly, all men with ED and type 1 diabetes developed sexual dysfunction before the onset of CAD symptoms.

ED is more frequent in diabetic patients with silent CAD than in those without. In a study of men with type 2 diabetes ($n = 260$) the incidence of ED (IIEF questionnaire) was significantly higher in the population with asymptomatic CAD than in the population without CAD (33.8% vs 4.7%; $p < 0001$).[12] ED not only predicted CAD independently of other risk factors, but also was the strongest predictor of silent CAD in this study.

The large Prostate Cancer Prevention Trial provided the first evidence of a strong association between ED and the subsequent development of clinical cardiovascular events.[13] ED at entry or that developed during follow-up was found to predict significantly any cardiac event with a hazard ratio of 1.45 ($p < 0.001$; 95% confidence interval (CI): 1.25–1.69). The data also showed that the cardiovascular risk associated with incident ED (that is developed during follow-up) was at least as great as the risk associated with a family history of myocardial infarction, current smoking, or hypercholesterolemia.

Box 8.1 Case history.

A 59-year-old gentleman married with three children and two grandchildren presented with erectile dysfunction on a background of treated hypertension for the previous three years. He was completely asymptomatic for coronary artery disease, enjoying his golf, playing it regularly, and suffering no restrictive symptoms such as chest pain or breathlessness. He was on no cardioactive medication other than his hypertensive medication and his resting ECG was normal with a completely normal examination. He had a responsible position as a director of several companies. Given his important position, he attended a medical screening session routinely. He was not significantly overweight, and was a lifelong non-smoker; the only cardiovascular risk factor that he had was ED, and his cholesterol on simvastatin 10 mg daily was 2.5 mmol/L with the LDL 0.78. As part of his executive screen he had a treadmill exercise ECG which demonstrated a good ability at 12 minutes of exercise but there were some inferior ST changes, which were suspicious for ischemia. A coronary CT angiogram was therefore arranged, which was surprisingly abnormal. There was extensive confluent calcification with a score of 1505, and invasive angiography was advocated to clarify the diagnosis.

This revealed a 50% lesion in the left anterior descending coronary artery, and a lesion of approximately 95% stenosis in the right coronary artery (Figure 8.1). A coronary angioplasty and stent to the right coronary artery was successful (Figure 8.2).

At follow-up he has returned to a normal full and active life with blood pressure 133/60 mmHg, normal blood glucose, LDL cholesterol 0.78 mmol/L, and he remains completely symptom-free. He continues to use tadalafil to good effect for his erectile dysfunction.

Comment

This case exemplifies the difficulty of proceeding in the best interest of the patient. These patients do not figure in any of the comparative studies so there are no guidelines to the value of the intervention. However, we do know that erectile dysfunction predicts mortality (presumably due to acute plaque rupture) so currently it is reasonable to intervene to stabilize the plaque in the hope that mortality and acute cardiac events can be reduced.[14] The patient has this fully explained to them.

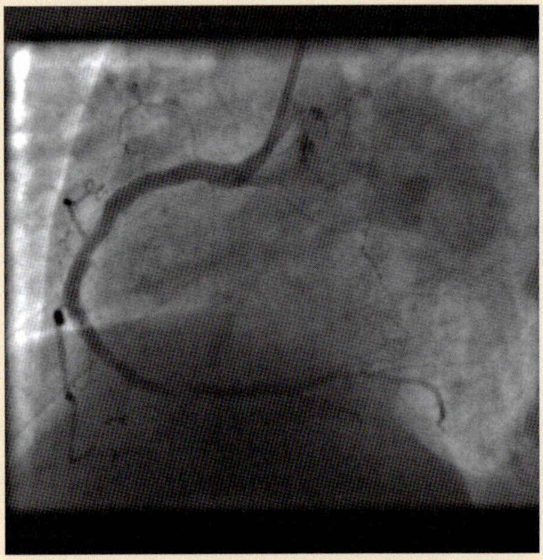

Figure 8.1 Angiogram identifies critical right coronary artery stenosis.

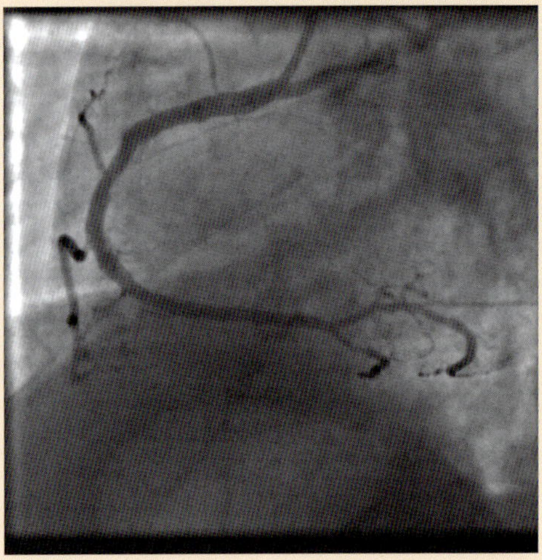

Figure 8.2 Successful stent insertion into right coronary artery as shown in Figure 8.1.

The temporal relationship

Several studies suggest that there is a strong temporal relationship between ED and CAD, with ED preceding a cardiovascular event by at least 2–5 years.[15] This temporal relationship was investigated in a questionnaire-based study that included 207 patients with CVD attending cardiovascular rehabilitation programs and 165 age-matched controls from general practice in the UK. Patients completed up to four questionnaires including the IIEF. Of the individuals with CVD, 56% were experiencing symptoms of ED at the time of the study and had done so for a mean of 5 ± 5.3 years. In contrast, 37% of individuals in the control group had ED symptoms for a mean of 6.6 ± 6.8 years. This interesting finding in the controls reflects the importance of asking about ED routinely.

In the AssoCiation Between eRectile dysfunction and coronary Artery disease (COBRA) trial, 93% of patients with a chronic coronary syndrome reported ED symptoms before the onset of angina pectoris, with a mean interval of 24 (range 12–36) months.[16] This finding further reinforces the concept of a lead time of at least 2–5 years between the development of ED and symptomatic CAD. The time intervals (range) for patients with one-, two-, and three-vessel disease were 12 (9.5–24), 24 (16.5–36), and 33 (21–47) months, respectively. There was a significant relationship between the length of time from ED to CAD onset and the number of vessels involved ($p=0.016$). Importantly, given that men with ED may be at cardiovascular risk, this long lead time provides an early opportunity for cardiovascular risk reduction.[17]

Prediction of CVD events and mortality

The correlation between ED and CVD was first discussed in 1999.[18] Subsequently the question of ED predicting silent obstructive coronary artery disease was the result of case presentations in 2001.[19] In this report patient 1 had developed ED 2 months before an acute anterior infarction; and patient 2, investigated largely due to his ED, angiographically had coronary artery disease documented. These findings were reinforced by a paper later that year concerning erectile dysfunction being a marker for cardiovascular disease.[20] It became apparent that erectile dysfunction offered us a window of opportunity for preventing vascular disease.[21]

Two recent meta-analyses have greatly helped our assessment of the link between ED and the prediction of CVD and mortality.[1,10] Prior to these analyses studies had evaluated the effect of age on the ED link to increased cardiovascular risk, identifying the importance of ED as an especially powerful predictor of CVD events in young and middle-aged men (ages 30–60 years) where CVD preventive resources should be maximized.

A study of 1400 men aged 40–75 years with no known CAD were prospectively followed for 10 years.[2] As can be seen from Table 8.1 men in their 40s with ED have a 50-fold increase in CAD events per 1000 patient years compared with men with normal erectile function, whereas there is a five-fold increase for men in their 50s (is there a more powerful risk factor?). In a retrospective study from Western Australia over 10–15 years, men in their 20s and 30s were more than seven times more likely to have a CVD event if they had ED,[22] and Riedner and colleagues found in a coronary angiographic study that CAD was 2.3 times higher in men under 60 years of age with ED.[23] In all three studies the ED/CAD link became less marked with age over 70 years.

Dong et al. performed a meta-analysis from 12 prospective studies involving 36,744 men.[24] In Table 8.3 the relative risks for men with ED are seen to be significantly increased for CVD, CAD, stroke, and all-cause mortality. Importantly, the ED risk was independent of conventional risk factors, and the mortality increase fits in with the rupture of a vulnerable plaque, as previously discussed.

Vlachopoulos and colleagues (Table 8.3) included 14 studies involving 92,757 men, with similar findings to the Dong meta-analysis.[10] However, of especial importance is that they found the relative risk to be higher in younger men and intermediate risk groups (5–20% 10-year conventional risk).

Both meta-analyses confirmed that the presence of ED increases the risk for future CVD events, myocardial infarction (MI), stroke, and all-cause mortality. ED should therefore be incorporated into routine clinical practice as a diagnosis needing treatment as well as a diagnosis that could trigger an aggressive CVD risk reduction strategy.[4]

In a review of the literature looking specifically at the association between ED and CAD the relationship

Table 8.3 Relative risk of increased events and mortality: erectile dysfunction (ED vs no ED).

	Meta-analysis 16 ($n=92{,}757$)	Meta-analysis 27 ($n=36{,}744$)
Pooled endpoints	1.44*	1.48*
Cardiovascular disease mortality	1.19	n/a
Myocardial infarction	1.62*	1.46*
Stroke	1.39*	1.35*
All-cause mortality	1.25*	1.19

*All significant except cardiovascular disease mortality.

of ED to systemic endothelial dysfunction is emphasized, but from a clinical standpoint though ED may precede CVD it can be used as an earlier marker to identify men at high risk of CVD events including mortality.[25] The review concludes that ED patients at high risk of cardiovascular disease should undergo a detailed cardiological assessment and receive intensive treatment of risk factors.

In addition, the Princeton III Consensus recommendations for the management of ED and cardiovascular disease have emphasized that, given the link between ED and CVD (which may be asymptomatic), patients could benefit from cardiovascular risk reduction.[26] Finally, Martin Miner and colleagues have concluded that all men with vasculogenic erectile dysfunction require a cardiovascular work-up.[27] The body of evidence, therefore, supports cardiovascular risk reduction and risk factor management in all men with vasculogenic ED.

In a prospective study I addressed the fundamental question in men with ED and no cardiac symptoms as to whether there is CVD, especially asymptomatic CAD, and how to detect it.[28] Exercise electrocardiography depends on identifying flow-limiting lesions of at least 50–70% stenosis, as does stress echocardiography or myocardial perfusion scanning. As most men with ED have subclinical cardiac disease it is not surprising that stress testing failed to identify their problem, with the potential for false reassurance. This is important given that ED predicts acute coronary syndromes and all-cause mortality, which in 50–60% of cases are not associated with any preceding cardiac symptoms. ED becomes the missing marker of increased risk especially in younger men at intermediate risk (5–20% 10-year risk) and is simple to enquire about.[29]

In this study outpatient multidetector computed tomography (MDCT) demonstrated asymptomatic CAD in 60 of 65 men, with non-calcified plaques in seven men. This fits with the pathophysiological concept of plaque rupture explaining the acute events and mortality, and establishes ED as a cardiovascular equivalent, with a man with ED and no cardiac symptoms being considered a CVD patient until proven otherwise.

Of concern is the failure of exercise electrocardiography in detecting the significantly severe cases that lead to stent insertion or coronary bypass surgery. It can be argued that in the absence of ischemic symptoms or inducible ischemia a conservative risk reduction approach was indicated. The problem is that these ED patients fall outside previously studied groups and action is taken based on the known event and mortality increase over time. A randomized trial of conservative versus anatomically appropriate interventional treatment with a baseline MDCT and exercise electrocardiograph is now clinically indicated, especially as this is an increasingly prevalent condition (see Box 8.1).

Depending on location not every man with ED will have access to MDCT. A reasonable approach is to use calcium screening (1–2 mSU X-rays compared with CXR 0.02) in those most at risk, especially men aged 30–60 years, but preferably MDCT (5–20 mSU) to detect soft and/or non-calcified plaque. Alternatively, a policy of aggressive risk reduction in all identified men with ED (ask routinely) and elective investigation when clinically appropriate could be pursued, but this demands detailed and regular follow-up. An ideal algorithm is provided in Figure 8.3.

Methods of evaluating the risk

The exercise electrocardiogram has been shown to be unsatisfactory in identifying silent coronary artery disease because the lesions are frequently less than 50% stenosis.[30] MDCT may be able to address this shortcoming and be used in patients with a normal exercise test to identify early subclinical plaque disease, which is vulnerable to rupture and may lead to increased mortality and increased cardiac events in asymptomatic men with ED.

The assessment of vascular risk in men with ED and the role of the cardiologist and general physician has recently been reviewed.[31] Again, the emphasis on the link is documented and the risks in the various age groups identified (Table 8.1). Furthermore, in my recent study looking at ED and asymptomatic CAD detected by computed tomography coronary angiography, the MDCT was substantially superior to exercise testing and reinforces the fact that subclinical disease may not present symptomatically or by exercise electrocardiography.

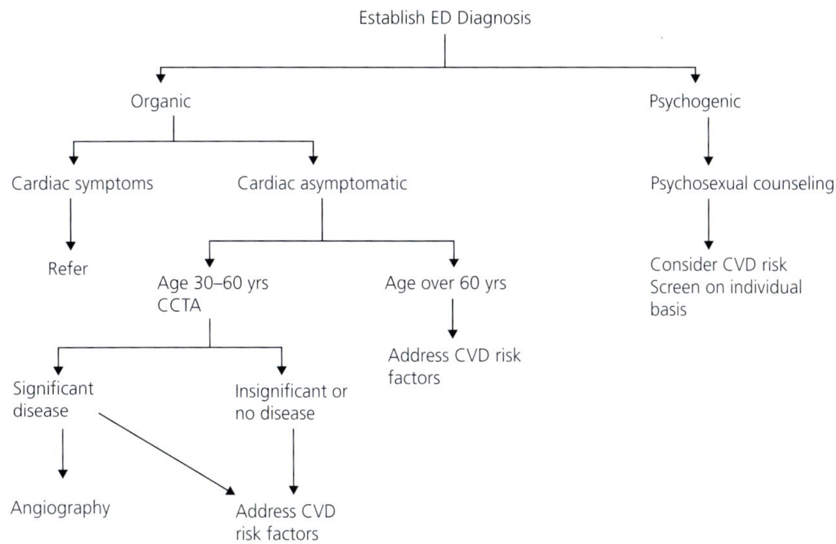

Figure 8.3 Algorithm for assessing cardiovascular disease (CVD) following a diagnosis of erectile dysfunction. Cardiac Computed Tomography Angiograph (CCTA).

Whilst it is certainly true that biomarkers have an important role to play, with the advent of MDCT, a relatively non-invasive outpatient approach to the anatomy of the coronary arteries, I believe the way forward is that all men with erectile dysfunction should undergo this outpatient procedure.

Conclusion

Erectile dysfunction should be considered a vascular disease until proven otherwise. Because data show that the occurrence of ED symptoms often precedes a cardiovascular event by 2–5 years, it provides a unique window of opportunity for risk mitigation. Thorough risk assessment of men presenting with ED and no cardiac symptoms is imperative. Traditional risk factors such as smoking, hypertension, and hypercholesterolemia should always be assessed. Furthermore, a question on ED should be included in all cardiovascular risk assessments and be incorporated into risk assessment guidelines. A cardiologist or other clinician with relevant expertise plays a particularly important role in evaluating the CVD risk in men with ED who may have subclinical CVD. Increased recognition of the potential for CVD in men with ED, followed by appropriate preventive action, can improve and may save lives.

A final thought...

However, these powerful theoretical and clinically relevant arguments and practical comments become irrelevant if we do not talk about sex.[32] The cardiologist's role and the general physician's role is to open up the discussion, proactively raising the question as part of a common sense approach to coronary artery disease and quality of life.

References

1 Johannes CB, Araujo AB, Feldman HA, Derby CA, Kleinman KP, McKinlay JB. Incidence of erectile dysfunction in men 40 to 69 years old: longitudinal results from the Massachusetts male aging study. *J Urol* 2000;163:460–3.
2 Inman BA, Sauver JL, Jacobson DJ, et al. A population-based, longitudinal study of erectile dysfunction and future coronary artery disease. *Mayo Clin Proc* 2009;84:108–13.
3 Jackson G, Rosen RC, Kloner RA, Kostis JB. The second Princeton consensus on sexual dysfunction and cardiac risk: new guidelines for sexual medicine. *J Sex Med* 2006;3:28–36; discussion 36.
4 Jackson G. Prediction of coronary artery disease by erectile function status: evidence based data. *Sex Med Rev* 2013;1:104–7.
5 Vlachopoulos C, Ioakeimidis N, Terentes-Printzios D, Stefanadis C. The triad: erectile dysfunction-endothelial dysfunction-cardiovascular disease. *Curr Pharm Des* 2008;14:3700–14.

6 Vlachopoulos C, Rokkas K, Ioakeimidis N, Stefanadis C. Inflammation, metabolic syndrome, erectile dysfunction, and coronary artery disease: common links. *Eur Urol* 2007;52:1590–600.
7 Vlachopoulos C, Aznaouridis K, Ioakeimidis N, et al. Unfavourable endothelial and inflammatory state in erectile dysfunction patients with or without coronary artery disease. *Eur Heart J* 2006;27:2640–8.
8 Solomon H, Man JW, Jackson G. Erectile dysfunction and the cardiovascular patient: endothelial dysfunction is the common denominator. *Heart* 2003;89:251–3.
9 Montorsi P, Montorsi F, Schulman CC. Is erectile dysfunction the "tip of the iceberg" of a systemic vascular disorder? *Eur Urol* 2003;44:352–4.
10 Vlachopoulos CV, Terentes-Printzios DG, Ioakeimidis NK, Aznaouridis KA, Stefanadis CI. Prediction of cardiovascular events and all-cause mortality with erectile dysfunction: a systematic review and meta-analysis of cohort studies. *Circ Cardiovasc Qual Outcomes* 2013;6:99–109.
11 Montorsi F, Briganti A, Salonia A, et al. Erectile dysfunction prevalence, time of onset and association with risk factors in 300 consecutive patients with acute chest pain and angiographically documented coronary artery disease. *Eur Urol* 2003;44:360–4; discussion 4–5.
12 Gazzaruso C, Solerte SB, Pujia A, et al. Erectile dysfunction as a predictor of cardiovascular events and death in diabetic patients with angiographically proven asymptomatic coronary artery disease: a potential protective role for statins and 5-phosphodiesterase inhibitors. *J Am Coll Cardiol* 2008;51:2040–4.
13 Thompson IM, Tangen CM, Goodman PJ, Probstfield JL, Moinpour CM, Coltman CA. Erectile dysfunction and subsequent cardiovascular disease. *JAMA* 2005;294: 2996–3002.
14 Jackson G. Erectile dysfunction increases cardiovascular risk: time to reduce it. *Trends in Urology and Men's Health* 2014;5:28–30.
15 Hodges LD, Kirby M, Solanki J, O'Donnell J, Brodie DA. The temporal relationship between erectile dysfunction and cardiovascular disease. *Int J Clin Pract* 2007;61: 2019–25.
16 Montorsi P, Ravagnani PM, Galli S, et al. Association between erectile dysfunction and coronary artery disease. Role of coronary clinical presentation and extent of coronary vessels involvement: the COBRA trial. *Eur Heart J* 2006;27:2632–9.
17 Jackson G. The importance of risk factor reduction in erectile dysfunction. *Curr Urol Rep* 2007;8:463–6.
18 Jackson G. Erectile dysfunction and cardiovascular disease. *Int J Clin Pract* 1999;53:363–8.
19 O'Kane PD, Jackson G. Erectile dysfunction: is there silent obstructive coronary artery disease? *Int J Clin Pract* 2001;55:219–20.
20 Kirby M, Jackson G, Betteridge J, Friedli K. Is erectile dysfunction a marker for cardiovascular disease? *Int J Clin Pract* 2001;55:614–8.
21 Jackson G. Erectile dysfunction: a window of opportunity for preventing vascular disease? *Int J Clin Pract* 2003; 57:747.
22 Chew KK, Finn J, Stuckey B, et al. Erectile dysfunction as a predictor for subsequent atherosclerotic cardiovascular events: findings from a linked-data study. *J Sex Med* 2010;7:192–202.
23 Riedner CE, Rhoden EL, Fuchs SC, et al. Erectile dysfunction and coronary artery disease: an association of higher risk in younger men. *J Sex Med* 2011;8:1445–53.
24 Dong JY, Zhang YH, Qin LQ. Erectile dysfunction and risk of cardiovascular disease: meta-analysis of prospective cohort studies. *J Am Coll Cardiol* 2011;58:1378–85.
25 Gandaglia G, Briganti A, Jackson G, et al. A systematic review of the association between erectile dysfunction and cardiovascular disease. *Eur Urol* 2014;65:968–78.
26 Nehra A, Jackson G, Miner M, et al. The Princeton III Consensus Recommendations for the Management of Erectile Dysfunction and Cardiovascular Disease. *Mayo Clin Proc* 2012;87:766–78.
27 Miner M, Nehra A, Jackson G, et al. All men with vasculogenic erectile dysfunction require a cardiovascular workup. *Am J Med* 2014;127:174–82.
28 Jackson G. Erectile dysfunction and asymptomatic coronary artery disease: frequently detected by computed tomography coronary angiography but not by exercise electrocardiography. *Int J Clin Pract* 2013;67:1159–62.
29 Miner M, Seftel AD, Nehra A, et al. Prognostic utility of erectile dysfunction for cardiovascular disease in younger men and those with diabetes. *Am Heart J* 2012;164:21–8.
30 Jackson G, Padley S. Erectile dysfunction and silent coronary artery disease: abnormal computed tomography coronary angiogram in the presence of normal exercise ECGs. *Int J Clin Pract* 2008;62:973–6.
31 Jackson G, Nehra A, Miner M, et al. The assessment of vascular risk in men with erectile dysfunction: the role of the cardiologist and general physician. *Int J Clin Pract* 2013;67:1163–72.
32 Jackson G. Let's talk about sex. *Clin Res Cardiol* 2013;102:327–8.

CHAPTER 9

The evaluation of the patient with erectile dysfunction

Geoffrey Hackett
University of Bedfordshire, Luton, UK; and Good Hope Hospital, Sutton Coldfield, UK

Introduction

Several studies have shown, that despite the advent of effective therapies, the average man suffers from erectile dysfunction (ED) for an average of 2 years before seeking help,[1] usually at the insistence of a partner. Most often we are attempting to save a second relationship, as ED has often caused the failure of the major relationship in that man's life. Few studies have fully evaluated the true social and economic impact of ED. The reasons for late presentation have been investigated,[2] and common problems are embarrassment, the feeling that it will "go away," and the failure to appreciate the association of ED with important medical conditions.

In recent years, the evaluation of patients has commenced in chronic disease assessments, particularly in diabetes, where the nurse is ideally placed to ask the question as part of a structured management protocol. In the UK there is current NICE (National Institute for Health and Care Excellence) guidance for primary care physicians to ask about ED and offer appropriate lifestyle advice.[3] The evaluation of the patient with ED should ideally commence before the patient would normally raise the issue.

Using the right language

A suggested comment to start the process is: "Many patients with your medical condition [e.g., diabetes, hypertension, etc.] have problems with erections. Could it be that you have difficulty?" Even if this results in initial denial, permission has been given, the first step of the PLISSET model, taught by psychosexual therapists.[1]

It is vitally important that we use the appropriate terms for individual patients. Patients often confuse the term "libido" with erection problems. It is important to talk about "loss of interest in sex" and "absence of sexual thoughts" and be aware that men might avoid sex because of fear of failure rather than suffering from a true lack of desire. We need to ask precisely what happens with each erection and whether it is loss of erection or early ejaculation, or indeed both, that terminates sexual activity. We need to ask questions such as "what would you like to achieve from your therapy?" and "what does your partner think of your problem?" It is a fault of many health commissioning systems that the man alone is referred as he is a "unit of health care," often attending without the partner. In many ways the primary care physician is ideally placed as usually he or she will be responsible for the care of the entire family.

We need to avoid terms such as "psychogenic" and "organic" as over 80% of men will have features of both.[1] Analogies can be helpful if they are relevant, and appropriate humor can aid communication in certain circumstances.

Sexual history

A detailed description of the problem, including the duration of symptoms and original precipitants, should be obtained.[1] Other factors that should be identified and recorded are:

- Original precipitating factor or factors (if identified).
- Predisposing factors (if identified).
- Maintaining factors (if identified).
- Any subsequent investigations.

Male Sexual Dysfunction: A Clinical Guide, First Edition. Edited by Suks Minhas and John Mulhall.

- Treatment interventions along with the response achieved.
- An expression of tumescence and rigidity with quality of morning awakening erections, and spontaneous, masturbatory, or partner-related activity erections.
- Sexual desire, ejaculatory and orgasmic dysfunction.
- Previous erectile capacity.
- Issues around any sexual aversion or sexual pain.
- Partner issues, e.g., physical illness or disability, menopause, or vaginal pain.

Concurrent medical, psychiatric, and surgical history should also be recorded, as should the current relationship status (single, married, in a long-term relationship, etc.) and a history of previous sexual partners and relationships. Issues of sexual orientation and gender identity should also be noted. Finally, the patient should be asked about alcohol, smoking, and illicit drug misuse.

The physical examination

All men with ED should have a full cardiovascular risk assessment, including BP and pulse, even if there seems to be an obvious cause.[1] A genital examination is recommended, and this is essential if there is a history of rapid onset of pain, deviation of the penis during tumescence, the symptoms of hypogonadism, or other urological symptoms (past or present). A digital rectal examination (DRE) of the prostate is not mandatory in ED but should be conducted in the presence of genitourinary or protracted secondary ejaculatory symptoms.[1] Blood pressure, heart rate, waist circumference, and weight should be measured.

Questionnaires

The use of validated questionnaires, particularly the International Index of Erectile Function (IIEF) or the validated shorter version of the Sexual Health Inventory for Men (SHIM), may be helpful to assess sexual function domains as well as the impact of treatments and interventions.[4] The Ageing Male Symptom (AMS) score is useful to detect the symptoms of possible hypogonadism,[5] and the Hospital Anxiety and Depression Scale (HADS) can detect underlying depression,[6] which is frequently underdiagnosed in men. The International Prostate Symptom Score (IPSS) can be helpful to detect associated lower urinary tract symptoms (LUTS)/benign prostatic hyperplasia (BPH),[7] which might be important in management. It can be very useful for the patient to complete these scores in the waiting room prior to consultation. These scores can help in the writing of a detailed report and assessing change on follow-up consultations but they are not a replacement for a thorough history and medical examination.

Current guidelines

Although 16 years after the first license of phosphodiesterase type 5 inhibitors (PDE5Is), there is still no NICE guidance on ED; current NICE guidance on type 2 diabetes and the 2013 Quality Outcome Framework (QOF) recommend that all men should be asked annually about ED, assessed, and offered oral treatment with the lowest acquisition cost.[3]

Since the initial publication of the British Society for Sexual Medicine (BSSM) guidelines in 2008 and the European Association of Urology (EAU) guidelines in 2007,[1] several reviews have been made in the light of recent research and expert opinion. These changes relate predominantly to the recognition of the important predictive value of ED for underling coronary heart disease (CHD) and the importance of diagnosing and treating associated hypogonadism.[8] Recent guidelines from cardiologists have focused on the importance of risk factor medication in the management of ED.[8]

The risk factors for ED (sedentary lifestyle, obesity, smoking, hypercholesterolemia and the metabolic syndrome, type 2 diabetes, and hypogonadism) are very similar to the risk factors for cardiovascular disease[1,8] that are regularly managed in primary care. A recent publication from the European Male Ageing Study (EMAS) suggested that the presence of ED and a morning total testosterone (TT) of less than 8 nmol/L increased cardiovascular and all-cause mortality five-fold.[9]

Several recent expert review papers have confirmed that ED is an important marker for cardiovascular risk and that the detection and modification of risk factors,[1] especially in younger men,[6] is at least as important as treating the underlying condition. The recent Princeton III guidelines[8] suggest that questioning about ED is an essential component of all male medical health assessments. These guidelines also clarify the assessment of fitness for sexual activity (Figure 9.1), which is important for all patients, not just those on oral therapy.

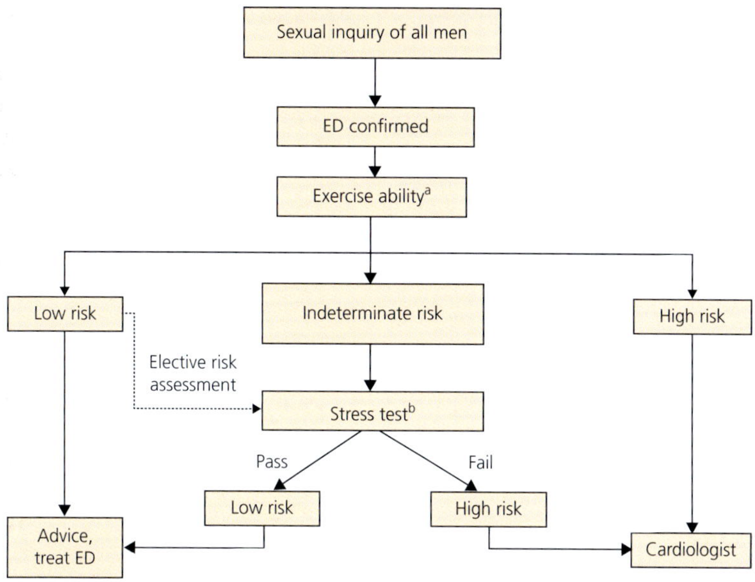

Figure 9.1 Management of erectile dysfunction (ED) in all men with ED, especially those with known cardiovascular disease. [a]Sexual activity is equivalent to walking 1 mile on the flat in 20 minutes or briskly climbing two flights of stairs in 10 seconds. [b]Sexual activity is equivalent to 4 minutes of the Bruce treadmill protocol.

Table 9.1 Relative risks for men with erectile dysfunction.

	Relative risk	95% Confidence interval	*p* Value
Overall	1.48	1.25–1.74	<0.001
Coronary heart disease	1.46	1.31–1.63	<0.001
Stroke	1.35	1.19–1.54	<0.001
All-cause mortality	1.19	1.05–1.34	0.005

In addition to the risk factors for ED, ED itself is a cardiovascular risk factor conferring a risk equivalent to a current moderate level of smoking. ED confers a 1.46 increased risk (Table 9.1) for cardiovascular disease,[3] especially in younger men under 40, where the magnitude of risk may be up to 50-fold.[10]

Laboratory investigations in the man presenting with ED: the key role of the GP

These should involve:[1]

1 Serum lipid profile as high total cholesterol and low HDL independently predict ED.
2 Fasting glucose and HbA1c or the International Federation of Clinical Chemistry (IFCC) protocol as the early accurate diagnosis of diabetes has important management and prescribing implications.
3 Morning (before 11 am) serum total testosterone (TT) and ideally sex hormone-binding globulin (SHBG) and calculated free testosterone (FT).

Current opinion is that men with a mean TT of less than 8 nmol/L on two occasions (or FT <180 pmol/L) and with bothersome symptoms, are candidates for testosterone replacement therapy (TRT), and that men with levels of 8–12 nmol/L (FT 180–225 pmol/L) should be considered, especially if they have not responded to oral therapy. At the time of the second blood test luteinizing hormone (LH) and prolactin (mandatory if TT <5.2 nmol/L) should be checked to distinguish between primary and secondary hypogonadism and to rule out the rare possibility of a pituitary adenoma.[11]

BSSM guidelines do not recommend routine prostate specific antigen (PSA) unless clinically indicated or if testosterone therapy is contemplated. Informed consent is required to ensure the patient understands the implications and possible follow-up of any abnormal result.

Specialist investigations

With the advent of oral therapy, specialist investigations are less often required, on the basis that the findings will not influence the management.[1] Under some medical systems, there may be an expectation that investigations will be conducted for "thoroughness." There is a small group of patients who insist that a cause for their ED is scientifically confirmed and physicians need to be aware of this (Table 9.2).

Nocturnal penile tumescence and rigidity (NPTR)

Nocturnal and early awakening erections are a normal physiological event in all men and are associated with the REM pattern of sleep. This test measures a natural event, free from the confines of needles and a radiology department, which may cause patient anxiety and a subsequent artificial result. The major use is in medico-legal cases to establish if a functional erection is possible. The disadvantage is that it often requires hospital admission.

Intracavernous injection (ICI) test

This outpatient test involves the injection of prostaglandin E_1 into the corpora cavernosa of the penis and to assess penile rigidity after 10 minutes. Its use as a diagnostic test for ED is limited as a positive result can be found in both normal patients and those with mild vascular disease. The main use of this test is in the assessment of penile deformities. Before the advent of oral therapy, the ICI was routinely conducted and caution was required with dose selection due to the risk of priapism. Nowadays the ICI is conducted only after failure of oral therapy, pre-selecting a group with likelihood of more severe vascular disease. In diabetic patients, where the pathology of the ED is multifactorial, ICI might help to differentiate between predominantly neurogenic and vascular disease, which can save many months of trying multiple medications. Another advantage of diagnostic ICI is that, in patients with a negative outlook, it can demonstrate that there is a therapy that has efficacy, promoting a positive outlook. Patients need to be warned of the possible risk of priapism with a plan for intervention if necessary but most clinics do not insist on formal written consent.

Colour duplex ultrasound (CDU) of penile arteries

This radiological investigation measures blood flow and gives an excellent assessment of the penile vasculature in response to an injection of a vasoactive agent.Major indications are penile plaques, fibrosis, deformity, or curvature where surgery might be complicated. Younger men with vascular trauma or severe ED where the etiology is unclear are candidates for CDU. There is usually little value in men over 55 because of the mixed pathology involved in the ED. Some patients insist on investigation to establish a firm diagnosis, and in some countries CDU is performed as part of a general workup of the man with ED, with little consideration as to how the findings might influence management. Intracavernosal injection is required with risk of prolonged erection if too high a dose is chosen (see above). Sometimes excessive anxiety can reduce

Table 9.2 Further investigations to evaluate the man with erectile dysfunction (ED).

Investigation	Rationale	Indication
Intracavernous injection test		Assessment of penile deformities
Color Doppler ultrasound	Assesses vascular integrity	Young patients being considered for surgical intervention
Phalloarteriography	To clarify vascular abnormality	Arterial abnormality found on Doppler ultrasound
Cavernosometry/cavernosography	Assesses venous occlusive mechanism	When primary venous leakage suspected in young man
Nocturnal penile tumescence	Assesses nocturnal erections when smooth muscle relaxed. Reduces false positive investigation rate	When other investigations inconclusive or prior to surgery

the response and compromise the validity of the test. Measurements are taken at the proximal third of the penile shaft at time 0, 2, 5, 10, 15, 20, and 25 minutes. A peak systolic velocity of over 35 cm/s is regarded as normal, and less than 25 cm/s suggests severe vascular disease. With increasing intracavernosal pressure, there should be diminishing flow in diastolic. This indicates an appropriate venous response. Assuming that adequate arterial flow is obtained then persistent significant end-diastolic flow is typical when there is venous leakage. Sustained end-diastolic flow (EDF) greater than 5–7 cm/s is regarded as evidence of venous incompetence.

Arteriography

These are highly specialized investigations that are only performed in specific circumstances. Arteriography should only be performed when an arterial lesion has been found on duplex Doppler evaluation. After catheterization of a femoral artery and intracavernosal injection, the internal iliac arteries and branches can be assessed. The major indication is younger men with lifelong ED where a possible arteriovenous (AV) malformation is detected on CDU. In some cases embolization may be possible under X-ray control. Recently, a few interventional cardiologists have reported cases with isolated vascular lesions that may be amenable to stenting and localized vascular procedures.

Dynamic infusion cavernosometry or cavernosography

Cavernosometry is an uncomfortable investigation occasionally used to diagnose primary venous pathology in young men suggested by prior CDU. The procedure involves the insertion of a large-gauge butterfly needle into the corpora followed by a vasoactive injection and subsequently contrast media. The site and size of venous abnormalities can be determined prior to planned venous surgery. Unfortunately the high recurrence rates associated with venous leak surgery means that this procedure is now used less frequently.

Radionuclide scanning

Various agents have been used in an attempt to obtain absolute flow rates but at considerable expense. Current opinion is that such scans add little to standard and less expensive procedures.

Neurophysiological testing

Occasionally patients vehemently complain of persistent numbness often in spite of adequate erection obtained with therapy. These patients need to be assessed for causes of a generalized neuropathy as well as focused pelvic assessment.

Penile abnormalities

Surgical problems that cause erectile dysfunction, for example, phimosis, tight frenulum, and penile curvatures, should be diagnosed clinically and are usually treated surgically. These patients should also have a full assessment as other risk factors need to be addressed to facilitate the resolution of ED.

Many of these men are diagnosed and treated by physicians who have limited background knowledge and clinical experience of ED. This can be a problem because the proper assessment of men presenting with ED can:[1]

- Uncover diabetes – as ED may be the first symptom in up to 20%.
- Detect dyslipidemia, which might not otherwise dictate treatment according to primary coronary prevention guidelines but may be the major reversible component in the patient's ED.
- Reveal the presence of hypogonadism, a reversible cause of ED, which can sometimes be managed without the need for specific ED therapy and which has other long-term health implications (Figure 9.2).
- Identify occult cardiac disease; ED in an otherwise asymptomatic man may be a marker for underlying coronary artery disease.
- Identify partner and relationship issues that may need to be addressed in addition to medical management.

Despite the likely presence of such underlying conditions, many men with ED may undergo little or no evaluation before treatment, particularly if they seek help from sources such as the internet.[12] Men do not readily visit their GP with medical problems, and a consultation for ED may represent a vital opportunity for health intervention. Currently GPs receive extra remuneration for female-related health issues; ED would be an ideal topic for enhanced payment.[11]

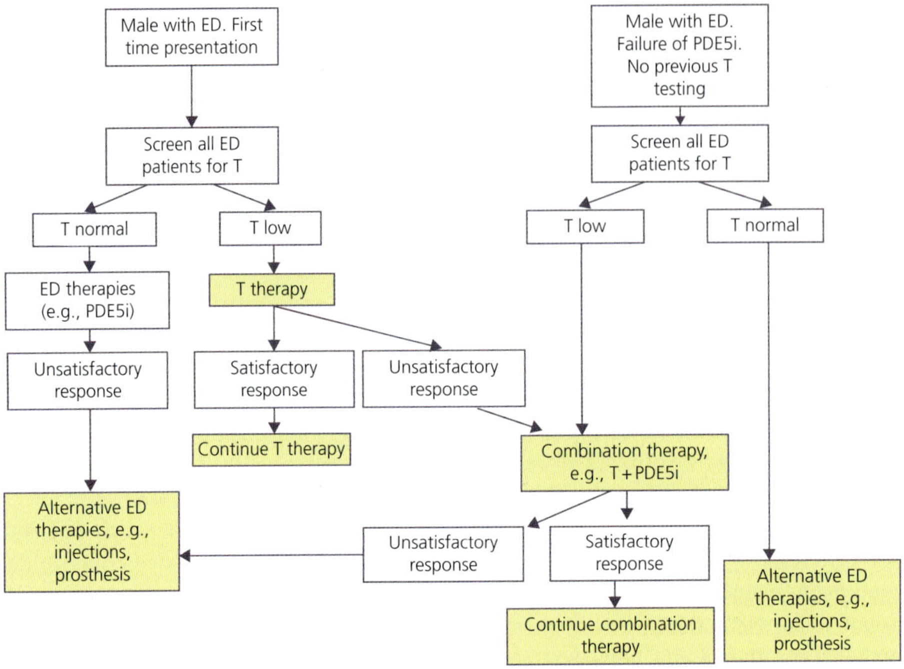

Figure 9.2 Algorithm for androgen therapy in a man presenting with erectile dysfunction (ED). PDE5I, phosphodiesterase type 5 inhibitor; T, testosterone.

Patient/partner education – consultation and referrals

The primary reason for referral to the clinician should be elicited. In particular, it is useful to know if the referral was initiated by the patient, the partner, both, or another healthcare professional. The motivating factors and expectations should be clarified as well as the intention, or otherwise, of the partner to accept any specific pharmacological, physical, or psychological therapies. An understanding by the patient and partner of basic anatomy and physiology and the purpose of blood and specialist investigations is helpful. An explanation of the principles of the treatment options is valuable. Provision of information, initially by a leaflet and followed up by some other source of information (such as videos or internet pages) is valuable reinforcement for patients.

Indications for secondary referral

Most patients do not need referral for further investigations[1] unless specifically indicated. However, some patients wish to know the etiology of their ED and should be investigated appropriately. Other indications for specialist investigations include:

- Young patients (under 40 years old) especially those who have always had difficulty in obtaining and/or sustaining an erection.
- Patients with a history of trauma, including possible cycling-related ED.
- Where an abnormality of the testes or penis is found on examination.
- Patients unresponsive to medical therapies that may desire surgical treatment for ED.

Specialist laboratory investigation is rarely required unless surgical intervention is contemplated.

Problems associated with prescribed drugs

Around 65% of men with hypertension will suffer from ED, and those on thiazide diuretics or beta-blockers are at increased risk.[1] ACE inhibitors (ACEIs) and calcium channel blockers are probably neutral but there is now considerable evidence that angiotensin receptor blockers (ARBs) can significantly improve erections.[1,13] Studies have shown positive effects with valsartan, losartan, and irbesartan, and there are no longer cost implications in prescribing ARBs in preference to ACEIs. If men are routinely asked about ED and problems are detected early, change to an ARB may resolve the issue. In cases with established atherosclerotic disease, switching therapy is unlikely to be beneficial.[1] Recent evidence suggests that statins,[14] when prescribed early improve erections, but in complex patients with established CHD, they may have adverse effects on erectile function, predominantly through effects on androgen levels.

Selective serotonin reuptake inhibitor (SSRI) antidepressants cause ED, and desire and ejaculatory disorders, and many prescriptions can be reduced or stopped if the ED is treated.[1] Patients often complain that their ED treatment might not be working when, in effect, the problem might be related to a recent SSRI prescription. Psychotropic medications may cause hyperprolactinemia and low testosterone with reduced response to ED therapies. It can sometimes be difficult to negotiate with colleagues in psychiatry, who often do not understand the impact of sexual dysfunction on the patient.

Recent publications have highlighted the high prevalence of ED (80%) in men taking long-term opiate-containing analgesics,[15] such as codeine and tramadol. Over 70% of men taking such analgesic drugs for over 3 months had TTs of less than 8 nmol/L.

Men on long-term anticonvulsant drugs have been shown to be at high risk of ED through drug interaction and lowered androgen levels.

Alpha-blockers, particularly tamsulosin, cause ejaculatory problems in over 30% of men on direct questioning, which can be extremely important in view of the strong association between LUTS/BPH and ED and the recent licensing of daily PDE5Is to treat LUTS.[16]

The role of lifestyle modification

Recent studies on men without severe cardiovascular risk factors[17] have shown modest three-point improvement of the EF domain of the IIEF after 2 years of intensive diet and exercise modification.[18] These findings suggested that lifestyle modification could play an important role in ED management, such that in the UK primary care physicians are required to show that smoking cessation, diet, and exercise advice has been issued to all men with ED and diabetes. Unfortunately no study has looked at the impact of lifestyle modification in ED associated with multiple, often combined risk factors. Physicians need to be aware that a three-point improvement over 2 years with intensive intervention might not be relevant to men with severe ED, especially as they are unlikely to be receiving the intensive support provided in studies.

Recent studies have also shown that weight loss can raise testosterone levels in hypogonadal men, leading many to recommend diet and exercise as the mainstay of management for the hypogonadal man.[19] The EMAS study evaluated 2395 (mean BMI 27.6) men over a mean of 4.4 years[20] and found that a 10% reduction in weight produced a 2.2 nmol/L increase in testosterone, with weight gain resulting in a corresponding decrease in TT. FT was only significantly reduced with 15% weight loss, and smoking cessation was associated with a slight fall in testosterone independent of weight change. The effect was less marked in men with diabetes, and in the entire cohort an equal number of men gained weight over the 4.4 years as achieved weight loss. The same group also reported that a TT of less than 8 nmol/L was associated with a five-fold increased hazard ratio and double the mortality risk compared with those with normal levels. If the patient experienced sexual symptoms – ED, loss of morning erection, lack of desire – the mortality risk was increased three-fold.[9] They concluded that "detection of low T in men presenting with sexual symptoms offered an opportunity to identify a small subgroup of men at particularly high risk of dying."

These studies raise the issue as to whether relying on lifestyle advice for the man with ED and low testosterone is ethical, based on the fact that diet might have previously failed despite the best efforts of skilled healthcare practitioners (HCPs), and improvements might take years, during which time he will be exposed to mortality risk and undertreated ED. The possible impact on his relationship of a 4-year treatment strategy needs to be considered, although some might prefer to address their problem predominantly with lifestyle change. Recent studies consistently show that TRT is associated with significantly greater weight reduction over 5 years, with corresponding metabolic benefits[21] and prompt improvement in sexual function.[22] Recent retrospective studies suggest a possible reduction in mortality with TRT,[23,24] although a recent publication showing similar findings came to a different conclusion, but was the subject of markedly flawed analysis.[25]

Current prescribing issues in ED

During the consultation, the physician will have assessed the needs and expectations of the patient and their partner, and treatment needs to be tailored to achieve this within the limitation of their means and the healthcare system. Lifestyle modification should have been addressed, along with optimal management of risk factors. Current guidelines list oral therapy, and possibly a vacuum device, as first-line therapy, with sexual counseling for couples with important psychological and relationship issues.[1]

There are currently three PDE5Is available, sildenafil, tadalafil, and vardenafil, with others to follow. Frequent exposure to the full dose of oral therapy on at least eight occasions is required, accompanied by direct stimulation.[1]

In June 2013 the patent on sildenafil expired and the cost has fallen to under £1 per tablet. On this basis, there is little justification for restricting the quantity of medication, especially on private prescription. Many patients previously obtaining medication from hospital on a "severe distress" basis should be re-evaluated because a private prescription may be a better financial option for the patient, especially when travel and parking costs are considered, plus the huge saving on unnecessary referrals.[26] This is also a "safer" practice in view of the potential for contraindicated medication being prescribed when medications are provided from different sources. The patent expiry of sildenafil is an excellent opportunity to defeat the internet counterfeiters and treat men with important cardiovascular risk factors in the appropriate primary care setting. The 1998 UK Department of Health (DoH) guidance on ED,[3,26] based on cost implications, has become outdated and potentially wasteful of secondary care resources. As a result, in 2014, the DoH allowed generic sildenafil and alprostadil to be prescribed for all men with ED, but the 1998 regulations will still apply to older drugs. The stated objectives behind these decisions were to allow more men to present to GPs and have appropriate risk factor management and reduce the number of men seeking potentially dangerous counterfeit medication from the internet.

Recently tadalafil 5 mg daily, having already proved a popular option to treat ED without the need for "on demand therapy," has been licensed to treat BPH/LUTS as a UK National Health Service (NHS) prescribed drug. Current theories suggest that LUTS are related to pelvic vascular disease, insulin resistance, and sympathetic overactivity rather than simply an issue of prostate size.[27] Alpha-blockers are known not to influence disease progression, and long-term studies of PDE5Is will be of interest.[27]

Data suggest that efficacy in LUS/BPH is similar to that of tamsulosin. As both ED and LUTS coexist in around 70% of cases,[27] it would be logical to use one drug to treat both conditions, especially as tamsulosin causes sexual adverse events in over 30%,[10] and product labeling still suggests "caution" in using the two drugs together.[27] If we consider a man with bothersome LUTS funding his own ED therapy, he might well appreciate a consultation facilitating a switch to daily therapy that might treat both problems. If the man has ED and a small prostate, and an alpha-blocker is ineffective, then the next action might be a transurethral resection of prostate (TURP), which would then qualify him for NHS ED therapy. Substitution or addition of tadalafil 5 mg daily might deal with both issues and avoid surgery. These issues raise ethical concerns as to whether our role as GPs is to advise what might be in the best interest of the patient or primarily consider the local prescribing issues.[26]

The role of testosterone replacement in ED

The BSSM[2] and Endocrine Society[11] guidelines recommend TT measurement in *all* men with ED and treatment of low testosterone (≤8 nmol/L) prior to a PDE5 inhibitor (Figure 9.2). Clearly if the patient also had established CVD risk factors then a PDE5I will also be required. Recent long-term studies have shown considerable sexual and metabolic benefits associated with TRT.[21] Many studies focus solely on erectile function, whereas sexual function (desire, ejaculation, orgasm, intercourse, and overall satisfaction) are significantly improved when hypogonadal men are treated with TRT.[22] Morning erections are highly androgen dependent, and many men value this as being as important as achieving a firm erection once a week for intercourse. If we do not ascertain what the patient is looking for, it is less likely that we will deliver the outcome they desire. If offered the choice, many men will opt for testosterone therapy as it is usually covered by a healthcare or reimbursement system, whereas PDE5Is are not.

TRT is usually considered to be lifelong[11] unless profound weight loss is achieved, as this may be associated with an elevation of natural testosterone levels. There are considerable funding and long-term monitoring issues associated with this approach and these need to be integrated into models of diabetes and cardiovascular care.

Conclusion

The BSSM-ED guidelines were reviewed in 2013 to include recent publications. It is firmly established that ED is an important marker for cardiovascular disease and should be included routinely in men's health assessment. The management of associated cardiovascular risk is at least as important as the management of the erection problem. The availability of low cost generic sildenafil should make treatment more readily available and affordable, enabling men with cardiovascular disease to be diagnosed and treated and avoid health risks associated with counterfeit internet medication.

References

1 Hackett G, Kell P, Ralph D. British Society for Sexual Medicine guidelines on the management of erectile dysfunction. *J Sex Med* 2008;5(8):1841–65.

2 Haro JM, Beardsworth A, Casariego J, et al. Treatment-seeking behavior of erectile dysfunction patients in Europe: Results of the Erectile Dysfunction Observational Study. *J Sex Med* 2006;3(3):530–40.

3 Home P, Mant J, Diaz J, Turner C, on behalf of the Guideline Development Group. Management of type 2 diabetes: summary of updated NICE guidance. *BMJ* 2008;336:1306–8

4 Rosen RC, Riley A, Wagner G, Osterloh IH, Kirkpatrick J, Mishra A. The International index of erectile function (IIEF): a multidimensional scale for assessment of erectile dysfunction. *Urology* 1997;49:822–30.

5 Heineman LA, Zimmermann T, Vermeulen A, Theil C. A new Aging Male Symptom rating scale (AMS). *Aging Male* 1999;2:105–14.

6 Zigmond AS, Snaith RP. The Hospital Anxiety and Depression Scale. *Acta Psychiatr Scand* 1983;67:361–70.

7 Bosch JL, Hop WC, Kirkels WJ, et al. The International Prostate Symptom Score in a community-based sample of men between 55 and 74 years of age: prevalence and correlation of symptoms with age, prostate volume, flow rate and residual urine volume. *Br J Urol* 1995;75(5):622–30.

8 Nehra A, Jackson G, Miner M, et al. The Princeton III Consensus Recommendations for the Management of Erectile Dysfunction and Cardiovascular Disease. *Mayo Clin Proc* 2012;87(8):766–78.

9 Pye SR, Huhtaniemi IT, Finn JD, et al. Late onset hypogonadism in elderly men. *J Clin Endocrin Metab* 2014;99:1357–66.

10 Inman BA, Sauver JL, Jacobson DJ. A population-based, longitudinal study of erectile dysfunction and future coronary artery disease. *Mayo Clin Proc* 2009;84(2):108–13.

11 Bhasin S, Cunningham GR, Hayes FJ. Testosterone therapy in men with androgen deficiency syndromes: an Endocrine Society clinical practice guideline. *J Clin Endocrinol Metab* 2010;95(6):2536–59.

12 Jackson G, Boon N, Eardley I, Dean J, Hackett G. Erectile dysfunction and coronary artery disease prediction: evidence-based guidance and consensus. *Int J Clin Pract* 2010;64(7):848–57.

13 Bohm M, Baumhakel M, Teo K, ONTARGET/TRANSCEND Erectile Dysfunction Substudy Investigators. Erectile dysfunction predicts cardiovascular events in high-risk patients receiving telmisartan, ramipril, or both: the ONgoing Telmisartan Alone and in combination with Ramipril Global Endpoint Trial/ Telmisartan Randomized AssessmeNt Study in ACE iNtolerant subjects with cardiovascular Disease (ONTARGET/ TRANSCEND) Trials. *Circulation* 2010;121(12):1439–46.

14 Gazzaruso C, Solerte SB, Pujia A. Erectile dysfunction as a predictor of cardiovascular events and death in diabetic patients with angiographically proven asymptomatic coronary artery disease: a potential protective role for statins and 5-phosphodiesterase inhibitors. *J Am Coll Cardiol* 2008;51(21):2040–4.

15 Rubinstein AL, Carpenter DM, Minkoff JR. Hypogonadism in men with chronic pain linked to the use of long-acting rather than short-acting opioids. *Clin J Pain* 2013;29:840–5.

16 Rosen RC, Wei JT, Althof SE, et al. Association of sexual dysfunction and lower urinary tract symptoms of BPH and BPH medical therapies: results from the BPH registry. *Urology* 2009;73:562-6.

17 Derby CA, Mohr BA, Goldstein I, Feldman HA, Johannes CB, McKinlay JB. Modifiable risk factors and erectile dysfunction: can lifestyle changes modify risk? *Urology* 2000;56:302–6.

18 Esposito K, Giugliano F, Di Palo C, et al. Effect of lifestyle changes on erectile dysfunction in obese men: a randomized controlled trial. *JAMA* 2004;291:2978–84.

19 Grossman M. Low testosterone in men with type 2 diabetes: significance and treatment. *J Clin Endocrinol Metab* 2011;96:2341–53.

20 Camacho EM, Huhtaniemi IT, O'Neill TW, et al. Age-associated changes in hypothalamic-pituitary-testicular function in middle-aged and older men are modified by weight and lifestyle factors: longitudinal results from the European Male Age in Study. *Eur J Endocrinol* 2013;168:445–55.

21 Traish AM, Haider A, Doros G, Saad F. Long-term testosterone therapy in hypogonadal men ameliorates elements of the metabolic syndrome: an observational, long-term registry study. *Int J Clin Pract* 2014;68:314–29.

22 Hackett G, Cole N, Bhartia M, et al. Testosterone replacement therapy improves metabolic parameters in hypogonadal men with type 2 diabetes but not in men with coexisting depression: The BLAST Study. *J Sex Med* 2014;11:840–56.
23 Shores MM, Smith NL, Forsberg CW, Anawalt BD, Matsumoto AM. Testosterone treatment and mortality in men with low testosterone levels. *J Clin Endocrinol Metab* 2012;97:2050–8.
24 Muraleedharan V, Marsh H, Kapoor D, Channer KS, Jones TH. Testosterone deficiency is associated with increased risk of mortality and testosterone replacement improves survival in men with type 2 diabetes. *Eur J Endocrinol* 2013; 169:725–33.
25 Vigen R, O'Donnell CI, Barón AE, et al. Association of testosterone therapy with mortality, myocardial infarction, and stroke in men with low testosterone levels. *JAMA* 2013; 310:1829–36.
26 Hackett GI. Schedule 11 – impact on treating erectile dysfunction. *Br J Diabetes Vasc Dis* 2002;2:315–18.
27 Uckert S, Oelke M. Phosphodiesterase (PDE) inhibitors in the treatment of lower urinary tract dysfunction. *Br J Clin Pharmacol* 2011;72(2):197–204.

CHAPTER 10

Endocrinological investigation of men with erectile dysfunction

Giovanni Corona[1], Linda Vignozzi[2], and Mario Maggi[2]
[1] *Maggiore-Bellaria Hospital, Bologna, Italy*
[2] *University of Florence, Florence, Italy*

Introduction

Sexual activity involves a complex array of behaviors, bringing together two separate partners, in the majority of cases of opposite genders, communicating their reciprocal sexual interest in reproduction or just in having fun. Hence, communication is the cornerstone of sexual activity. There are several languages used for sexual communication, but the most common is hormones, messages sent from dedicated glands into the bloodstream for recipient targets. Therefore, when sexual communication is problematic, such as in the case of erectile dysfunction (ED), understanding endocrine causes and consequences is mandatory. Hormone alterations can be involved in determining ED or can be the consequence of ED, often with a bidirectional interconnection.[1–4]

The prevalence of endocrine disorders in subjects consulting an outpatient clinic for ED is reported in Figure 10.1. The most common disorders are those affecting the ability of the testis to secrete the main male hormone, testosterone (T). Also metabolic disorders are often observed in men with ED and, in particular, obesity and type 2 diabetes mellitus (T2DM). Another endocrine disorder occurring less frequently, but with specific sexual correlates, is hyperprolactinemia. Thyroid disorders are not uncommon, but their specific contribution to ED is more questionable. All these conditions will be analyzed in the following sections. Note that more than 70% of the consulting individuals resulted were positive for at least one of the conditions depicted in Figure 10.1.

Hypogonadism

Male hypogonadism is defined as the failure of the testes to produce germ cells, sex steroids (T being the most abundant), or both. It may be the result of either an absent or inadequate secretion of hypothalamic gonadotropin-releasing hormone (GnRH) or of pituitary gonadotropin or, finally, of a testicular deficiency in sex steroid/sperm production.[1–5] The latter condition is termed primary hypogonadism (hypergonadotropic), while the former ones are known as secondary or central (hypogonadotropic) hypogonadism. All the forms of hypogonadism can be acquired or, less frequently, congenital. Among the latter, Klinefelter's syndrome (KS) is the most common form of primary hypogonadism, occurring in 1:500 individuals. Idiopathic hypogonadotropic hypogonadism (IHH) is the most commonly observed form of congenital secondary hypogonadism and is 100-fold less prevalent than KS. A hypogonadism-like syndrome can also result from reduced sensitivity, or insensitivity, to T or because of reduced bioavailability of T, due to an increase in its carrier protein, sex hormone-binding globulin (SHBG).

The aforementioned classification of hypogonadism (i.e., primary/secondary) does not take into consideration T deficiency-related symptoms. It is well known that both primary and secondary hypogonadism symptoms and signs are dictated more by the age of onset of the testicular failure than by the cause of this failure.[3,4] In fact, whereas early-onset hypogonadism is associated with severe symptoms and signs, the form with an adult

Male Sexual Dysfunction: A Clinical Guide, First Edition. Edited by Suks Minhas and John Mulhall.

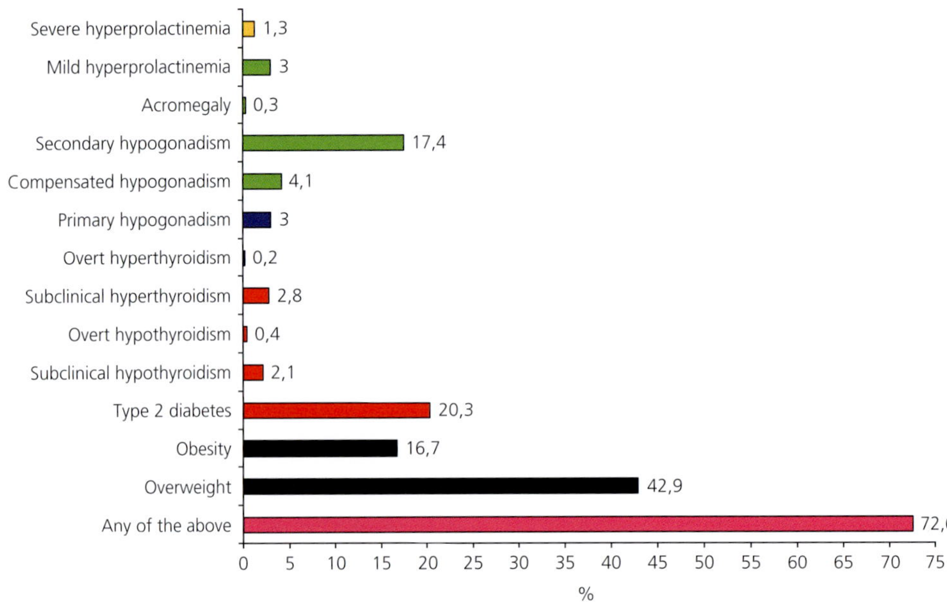

Figure 10.1 Prevalence of endocrinological problems as derived from a consecutive series of 4388 subjects seeking medical care for sexual dysfunction at our unit between 2000 and 2013. Hyperprolactinemia (circulating prolactin levels >420 mU/L or 20 ng/mL) was considered mild (prolactin levels 420–735 mU/L, or 20–35 ng/mL) or severe (prolactin levels >735 mU/L, or 35 ng/mL) as previously reported.[18,19] Gonadal status was identified according to the European Male Aging Study criteria: normal or eugonadal (testosterone ≥10.5 nmol/L and luteinizing hormone ≤9.4 U/L); secondary hypogonadism (testosterone <10.5 nmol/L and luteinizing hormone ≤9.4 U/L); primary hypogonadism (testosterone <10.5 nmol/L and luteinizing hormone >9.4 U/L); and compensated hypogonadism (testosterone ≥10.5 nmol/L and luteinizing hormone >9.4 U/L).[9] Subclinical hypo- and hyperthyroidism were defined when TSH values were outside the reference ranges (0.4–4.5 mU/L) with normal free thyroid hormones. Overt hypo- and hyperthyroidism were defined when both TSH and free thyroid hormone values were outside the reference ranges.

onset is less clinically apparent and is known as late-onset hypogonadism (LOH). Increased visceral adiposity and metabolic derangements, including T2DM and metabolic syndrome (MetS), are the most common morbidities associated with LOH.[6,7]

The prevalence of different forms of LOH in the general population has been analyzed in the European Male Aging Study (EMAS) – a survey of more than 3400 community-dwelling, middle-aged and older men.[8,9] Low T (<10.4 nmol/L) was detected in 13.8% of the cohort, with the secondary form of LOH (luteinizing hormone, LH ≤9.4 U/L) more prevalent (11.8%) than the primary one (2%), which is characterized by increased LH levels (LH >9.4 U/L). The same study reported that 9.5% of the European population could be classified as having compensated hypogonadism, that is, with T in the normal range (≥10.5 nmol/L), but with inappropriately high LH (>9.4 U/L).[9] The clinical significance of compensated hypogonadism is still a matter of debate.[9]

Considering that T production from the testis is progressively reduced by 0.4–2% per year from the third decade onward,[7] distinguishing pathological conditions underlying LOH from a physiological T decline is not easy In addition, recognizing hypogonadism in adult subjects complaining of, and consulting for, sexual dysfunctions is an increasingly difficult task, because sexual problems are, per se, the most common symptoms associated with the LOH condition. In fact, in the aforementioned European survey, it was established that hypoactive sexual desire, and loss of spontaneous and sex-related erections are the three correlates most closely associated, in a syndromic way, with a low T level[8] (see below). Other physical and psychological symptoms and signs often considered as being associated with LOH are reported in Table 10.1 (for review see Refs 1,2,10). In the EMAS study, three physical symptoms (inability to engage in vigorous activity, inability to walk for a long distance, and an inability to bend) and three psychological symptoms (loss of energy, sadness, and

Table 10.1 More and less specific clinical, biochemical, and instrumental parameters associated with hypogonadism.

	Sexual symptoms	Physical symptoms	Psychological symptoms	Clinical signs	Biochemical and/or instrumental signs
More specific	Reduced sexual desire (libido) Erectile dysfunction Decreased spontaneous erections	Decreased vigorous activity Difficulty walking >1 km Inability to bend	Sadness Loss of energy Fatigue	Increased body fat, body mass index Very small (especially <5 mL) or shrinking testes Decreased prostate size	Oligozoospermia/azoospermia Reduced prostate specific antigen (PSA) Osteoporosis
Less specific	Decreased frequency of intercourse Decreased autoeroticism Delayed ejaculation	Hot flushes, sweats Decreased energy, motivation, initiative, and self-confidence Reduced muscle bulk and strength Diminished physical or work performance	Poor concentration and memory Sleep disturbance, increased sleepiness	Loss of body (axillary and pubic) hair, reduced shaving Gynecomastia	Mild anemia (normochromic, normocytic, in the female range)

fatigue) were apparently associated with low T.[8] However, differences in T levels between symptomatic men and asymptomatic men were minimal, reflecting the weak overall association between physical and psychological symptoms and T levels in that cohort. Interestingly, in another EMAS study on compensated hypogonadism, in a confounder-adjusted model, only physical symptoms and not the sexual ones were associated with the condition.[9] It is important to note that only the syndromic association between sexual symptoms and low T were dose-dependent and confirmed in the EMAS validation set, in which the strengths of the association between symptoms and low T levels determined the minimum criteria necessary for identifying LOH. Hence, according to the EMAS study, only the simultaneous presence of three sexual symptoms combined with a total T level of less than 11 nmol/L and a free testosterone level of less than 220 pmol/L can be considered the minimum criteria for the diagnosis of LOH.[8] Similar thresholds were proposed by the International Society for Sexual Medicine, that is, total T below 12 nmol/L and free T below 225 pmol/L, if typical symptoms are present.[10] Therefore in a population of aged subjects seeking medical care for sexual dysfunction, a dedicated medical history, an accurate physical examination, and an appropriate biochemical evaluation are mandatory for identifying LOH subjects and for assessing the correct therapeutic intervention (see also Figure 10.2).

Medical history

To help clinicians in collecting the most relevant information for recognizing hypogonadism, several questionnaires have been developed (for review see Refs 1–5). All these instruments have demonstrated a good sensitivity in cross-sectional surveys; however, their relative specificity is rather low.[1,2,10] In addition, they are not specifically designed for subjects with sexual dysfunction. We previously developed and validated a brief (12 items) structured interview (ANDROTEST) specifically designed for the screening of hypogonadism in subjects with sexual dysfunctions.[4] The patient's answer is codified on a 0–3 Likert scale by the interviewer, who does not need any specific training. The final score can range from 1 to 32. A higher score identifies a higher prevalence of hypogonadism-related symptoms and signs. In the validation sample, we reported that an ANDROTEST score higher than 8 has an almost 70% sensitivity and specificity in detecting low total or free T.[4] The structured interview investigates sexual symptoms (ED, hypoactive sexual desire, and delayed ejaculation), as well as the presence of the most common hypogonadism-related comorbidities. More recently, we also reported that the combination of ANDROTEST with the detection of psychological symptoms as derived from the Middlesex Hospital Questionnaire, modified (MHQ) further improves its ability in detecting hypogonadism.[11]

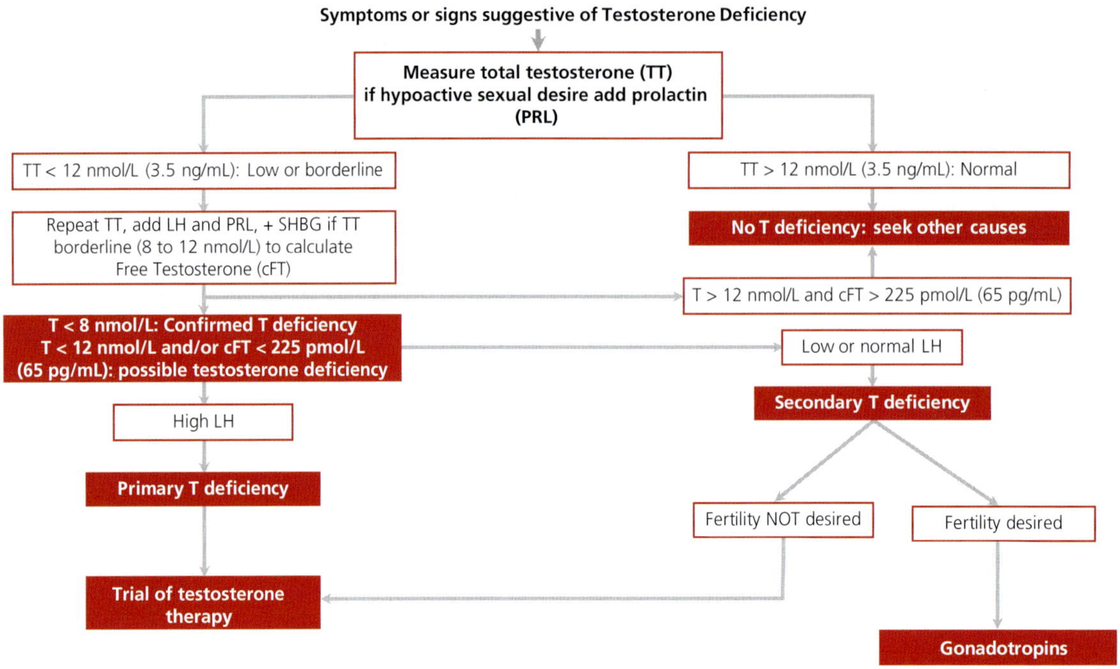

Figure 10.2 Algorithm for the diagnosis of testosterone deficiency. PRL, prolactin; cFT, calculated free testosterone; TT, total testosterone; LH, luteinizing hormone; SHBG, sex hormone-binding globulin.

Physical examination

Examining testis volume (TV) by using the Prader orchidometer is mandatory in every patient with sexual dysfunction. We found that higher TV is positively associated with T and gonadotropin levels but also with overweight/obesity, smoking, alcohol abuse, and hypertension, most probably because the latter conditions might affect testicular microcirculation and decrease the T secretory capacity of the testis; hence more LH is needed to compensate the reduced T secretion.[12] Gynecomastia is another sign frequently associated with hypogonadism.[13]

According to the Standard Operating Procedures in Sexual Medicine,[14] a correct physical examination should also include digito-rectal examination (DRE) of the prostate. This relatively easy medical procedure can exclude the presence of suspected peripheral prostatic nodules or glandular inflammation and provide useful information on the state of prostate growth. The presence of an enlarged prostate can be suggestive of benign prostatic enlargement (BPE). In addition, because the prostate represents one of the main targets of androgen action, a reduced prostate volume may be suggestive of hypogonadism.[15]

Biochemical evaluation

Approximately 2% of circulating T is free (or binding protein unbound), whereas the rest is either tightly bound to SHBG or loosely bound to albumin (bioavailable T). Circulating SHBG (and thereby total T) levels are decreased by androgens and glucocorticoids and increased by estrogens and thyroxine. Other determinants of circulating SHBG are upregulation by acute or chronic liver disease and androgen deficiency, and downregulation by obesity, insulin, and growth hormone (GH) deficiency. The majority of immunoassays (IAs) show good accuracy in the estimation of high (adult male) total T levels; however, they usually overestimate low T concentration, reducing the specificity and sensitivity for diagnosing hypogonadism. Recently, the EMAS group compared different measurement methods for T, namely, a common validated platform IA (Modular Analytics E170 electrochemiluminescence, Roche Diagnostics) and a gas chromatography mass spectrometry (GC-MS) method.[16] Although the two methods show an overall high correlation ($r=0.93$, $p<0.001$), the IA was less robust in the hypogonadal range (<11 nmol/L; $r=0.72$, $p<0.001$). Nonetheless, the conclusion was that validated IA platforms can be as good as GC-MS in the clinically important discrimination between eugonadal and hypogonadal men, especially when combined with the clinical signs of androgen deficiency.

Measurements of free T (FT) and non-SHBG-bound T are cumbersome and direct methods are unreliable. The gold standard for non-SHBG-bound T measurement is ammonium sulfate precipitation, and for FT the dialysis technique. However, these methods are non-automated, time-consuming, and require expensive techniques and, therefore, are not routinely used in most laboratories. A MS-based assessment of FT in ultrafiltrates was proposed as a candidate comparison method.[1,2,10] Since SHBG concentrations can be influenced by many factors, the calculation of free T with available web algorithms – including the Vermeulen (http://www.issam.ch/freetesto.htm) and Sodergard formulae – should be preferred in clinical practice, because they are readily available and have been validated by comparison with the equilibrium dialysis assay, at least for the Vermeulen formula. These algorithms assume that when the concentrations of total T, SHBG, and albumin, and the constants for the binding of T to SHBG and albumin are known, FT and bioavailable T can be calculated. However, values reported for albumin and SHBG binding constants are relatively variable (almost one log unit) and, in addition, calculated results rely on the robustness of the measurements of SHBG and total T. The free androgen index (FAI), which is obtained as the quotient 100T/SHBG, is a surrogate of the previous calculations and is simpler and more rapid. Because the relationship between SHBG and T is relatively linear in the lowest T range, but exponential for higher values and solved by a second-degree equation, this formula might be useful for females, but it is totally inapplicable in male individuals. A comparison of FAI and free T (determined by centrifugal ultrafiltration) yielded a correlation coefficient of 0.858 for 20 adult females but only 0.435 for 19 adult males.[1,2,10] Hence, we suggest systematically using calculated FT (cFT), by using the Vermeulen equation (http://www.issam.ch/freetesto.htm). Concerning the threshold for cFT, we suggest using 225 pmol/L, as indicated by several guidelines[1,2,10] and essentially validated in the EMAS study.[8]

We recently proposed that prostate specific antigen (PSA) could represent a marker of T bioactivity.[15,17] In those studies, the relationship between circulating T and PSA was better described by an exponential curve (power model) with a sharp rise in the hypogonadal range and a flat plateau in the eugonadal one, according to the previously formulated "saturation hypothesis" of the biological effect of T.[15,17,18] After adjusting for age, low PSA was associated with hypogonadism-related features (i.e., delayed puberty, lower testis volume, and gynecomastia) and associated conditions, such as MetS and cardiovascular diseases (CVD). Furthermore, low PSA was associated with impaired sex- and sleep-related erections and less frequent intercourse. Hence, low PSA could help in identifying a low T state. The best sensitivity and specificity for detecting TT of less than 8 nmol/L was at PSA less than 0.65 ng/mL (65.2% and 55.5%, respectively).[15]

Prolactin

In contrast to the well-known role of prolactin (PRL) in female reproduction (i.e., promoting breastfeeding), the physiological effect of PRL on male reproductive fitness is unknown, although several data have demonstrated a marked inhibitory effect of hyperprolactinemia on sexual desire,[19] most probably acting on hypothalamic GnRH (and therefore on T production) and/or dopamine production and turnover. Conversely, the effect of hyperprolactinemia on erectile function is more questionable (see below).

Prolactin modification and erectile function

Both hyperprolactinemia and, more recently, reduced prolactin (PRL) levels have been associated with the impairment of erectile function. The specific evidence will be analyzed in the following sections.

Hyperprolactinemia

In men seeking medical care for sexual dysfunction, the prevalence of mild hyperprolactinemia (MHPRL, defined as PRL >420 mU/L or >20 ng/mL) is quite variable, ranging from more than 13% to less than 2%.[19] In contrast, severe hyperprolactinemia (SHPRL, defined as PRL >735 mU/L or >35 ng/mL) is a relatively rare event (<1%).[19] We report here similar results in a large series (>4000) of subjects seeking medical care for sexual dysfunction (see Figure 10.1). Previous findings have shown that among patients with MHPRL, repeat blood sampling reveals normal PRL values in 50% of cases, most probably due to venepuncture stress.[20] In addition, SHPRL underlines an organic problem in the hypothalamic-pituitary region in two-thirds, and a drug-induced condition in almost one-third of cases.[20] In particular, drugs blocking dopaminergic (antipsychotic and antiemetic) or increasing serotoninergic (antidepressants) transmission represent the most common causes of iatrogenic hyperprolactinemia.[19,20]

It has been reported that a severely reduced libido is associated with a ten-fold greater chance of having SHPRL, while no association was observed with MHPRL.[20,21] Similar data were observed in a more recent study involving more than 3700 male patients with sexual dysfunction.[21] SHPRL impairs physiological pulsatile gonadotropin secretion leading to the development of secondary hypogonadism. The latter has been considered the most important pathogenic mechanism involved in the SHPRL-induced reduced libido.[19,20] However, it has been suggested that PRL also plays a direct role in the control of male sexual desire.[19,20] Accordingly, among hypogonadal subjects with hyperprolactinemia, prolactin-lowering drugs are able to restore both T levels and libido, while TRT is not as effective.[19,20]

The relationship between hyperprolactinemia and erectile function is under debate. Some authors have suggested a possible pathogenetic link between severe ED and SHPRL[22,23] (for review see Ref. 19). However, in our studies we were unable to confirm the latter association after adjustment for confounders including T levels.[20,21] Hence, it can be speculated that SHPRL-induced hypogonadism could explain, at least partially, the association between ED and SHPRL.[19]

Hypoprolactinemia

In apparent contrast with the aforementioned findings, we previously reported that in subjects with sexual dysfunction low PRL was associated with arteriogenic ED.[24] We more recently confirmed this observation in the general European population.[25] Some experimental studies indicated that acute, but not chronic, pharmacological elevation of brain PRL is associated with a facilitated, rather than an impaired, sexual behavior, including increased penile erection, mounting, and intromission activity.[26] Similar results have been reported in men.[27]

All these findings indicate that PRL might have a more positive, rather than negative, effect on initiating or maintaining sexual behavior. It is still unclear how PRL may facilitate male sexual behavior. Different mechanisms can be advocated to explain these associations. In fact low PRL in the peripheral circulation could mirror, within the hypothalamus, either increased dopaminergic or decreased serotonergic signaling. The latter, however, represents the most intriguing hypothesis.[19,24,25]

Determination of prolactin

Since hyperprolactinemia represents quite a rare condition in patients seeking medical care for sexual dysfunction, current guidelines do not recommend widespread evaluation of PRL levels in ED patients.[19] On the other hand, PRL should be measured in all subjects complaining of reduced sexual desire or in the presence of low T levels. Conversely, gynecomastia does not represent a pathognomonic sign of hyperprolactinemia, since patients with gynecomastia do not always have hyperprolactinemia.[19,28] Most probably, hyperprolactinemia acts through a suppression of the pituitary-testis axis, more than through a direct action on the breast tissue. When PRL levels are required, current blood must be sampled fasting and at rest to reduce the stress linked to venepuncture. In case of results exceeding 20 ng/mL (400 mU/L), the test should be repeated after discontinuation of any drug interfering with PRL secretion and, if possible, after insertion of a catheter.[19] This will eliminate almost 50% of MHPRLs found at first assay. If not already checked, serum T and thyroid-stimulating hormone (TSH; because TSH-releasing hormone is a PRL-stimulating factor) should be measured at the same time. In case of non-drug-induced SHPRL associated with normal T and TSH levels, screening for these biologically inactive variants of PRL with high molecular weight, which constitute "false hyperprolactinemia or macroprolactinemia," is recommended.[19,28] This may be done by means of PRL chromatography or, in a cheaper way, by precipitation with polyethylene glycol. Macroprolactinemia accounts for 10 to 22% of all causes of hyperprolactinemia, and is found in about 1% of the general population.[28] In case of SHPRL and reduced T levels, after excluding a drug-induced form, computed tomography (CT) scan, or better, a magnetic resonance image (MRI) of the hypothalamic-pituitary area should be performed, in order to exclude hypothalamic-pituitary tumors.[19,28]

Thyroid hormones

Hyperthyroidism is a quite common endocrine disease, with a prevalence of 0–2% in men and an incidence of 20/1,000,000/year in the general population and a male:female ratio of 1:5.[19] Hypothyroidism is one of the most common chronic endocrine disorders in the Western population, with annual incidence rates of 2 in 10,000 for males.[19] Subclinical disorders represent other common clinical conditions present in about 2–5% of the general population. They are characterized by normal thyroid hormones and elevated (5–10 mU/L: *subclinical hypothyroidism*) or suppressed (<0.2–0.1 mU/L: *subclinical hyperthyroidism*) TSH levels. Similar figures have been observed in subjects consulting for ED (see Figure 10.1).

While subclinical thyroid diseases are in the vast majority of cases totally asymptomatic, overt hypo- and hyperthyroidism are often clinically manifest. Hyperthyroid symptoms include palpitation, trembling, unexplained weight loss, sleep disturbances, diarrhea, and fatigue. These individuals may become irritable and easily upset. When hyperthyroidism is severe, patients can suffer shortness of breath, chest pain, and muscle weakness. Usually the symptoms of hyperthyroidism are so gradual in their onset that patients do not recognize the symptoms until they become more severe. This means the symptoms may continue for weeks or months before patients fully realize that they are sick. In older people, some or all of the typical symptoms of hyperthyroidism may be absent, and the patient may just lose weight or become depressed.

The signs and symptoms of hypothyroidism vary, depending on the severity of the hormone deficiency. But in general, problems tend to develop slowly, often over a number of years. Fatigue, increased sensitivity to cold, constipation, dry skin, and unexplained weight gain are frequently associated with milder problems at the beginning, while advanced hypothyroidism, known as myxedema, is rare, but when it occurs it can be life-threatening.

Thyroid hormones and erectile function

Although thyroid dysfunction is often highlighted as a common ED-associated condition, only a few evidence-based reports have investigated this aspect (for review see Ref. 19). We recently evaluated the relationship between thyroid hormone and erectile function in a large series ($n = 3203$) of subjects seeking medical care for sexual dysfunction at our unit and in subjects from the EMAS study.[29] We found that in both samples overt hyperthyroidism – but not hypothyroidism or subclinical conditions – was associated with an increased risk of severe ED.[29] However, although our study showed that ED was a symptom frequently observed in patients with overt hyperthyroidism (>60%), the latter was an infrequent (<1%) clinical condition in patients seeking medical care for ED[29] (see also Figure 10.1). Thyroid hormone receptors have been described in human corpora cavernosa.[30] Studies in animal models of hyperthyroidism indicate an impairment of nitric oxide-dependent relaxation of corpora cavernosa.[19] It is therefore possible that hyperthyroidism-associated ED could be due to a direct effect of thyroid hormones on their cognate receptors.[19] Accordingly, a small uncontrolled Italian study documented that the restoration of euthyroidism might improve ED.[31]

Determination of thyroid hormones

Since thyroid diseases are rarely detected in patients seeking medical care for sexual dysfunction, current guidelines do not recommend the evaluation of thyroid hormones in ED patients, unless specific symptoms or signs are observed or in the presence of ejaculatory problems.[19] Accordingly, associations between delayed ejaculation, premature ejaculation, and hypo- and hyperthyroidism, respectively, have been extensively documented[32,33] (for review see Ref. 19). In addition, hyperthyroidism is a well accepted cause of acquired premature ejaculation.[19] Screening for thyroid dysfunction can be performed using any of several serum thyroid function tests. However, the isolated determination of TSH is usually recommended, because it can detect abnormalities before other tests become abnormal. When used to confirm suspected disease in patients referred to a specialty endocrine clinic, the TSH test has a sensitivity above 98% and a specificity greater than 92% for clinical and functional diagnoses.[34] Free triiodothyronine (FT_3) and thyroxine (FT_4) should be checked only when TSH is outside the reference range.[34]

Other hormones

Adrenal hormones

Adrenal insufficiency is a rare clinical condition, due to hypothalamic-pituitary defects (secondary adrenal insufficiency) or to several conditions affecting primarily the adrenal gland (primary adrenal insufficiency). The latter, also called Addison's disease, affects 1–4 in every 100,000 people, in all age groups and both sexes.[19] The symptoms of adrenal insufficiency usually begin gradually and include worsening fatigue, muscle weakness, loss of appetite, and weight loss. Hyperpigmentation, or darkening of the skin, can occur in Addison's disease but not in secondary adrenal insufficiency. Because the symptoms progress slowly, they are often ignored until a stressful event like an illness or accident causes them to worsen.

Fatigue and muscle weakness also characterize the excess of adrenal cortisol production commonly known as Cushing's syndrome (CS). An estimated 10 to 15 of every million people are affected every year by CS, which is more prevalent in females, accounting for about 70% of all cases. Other symptoms of CS include weight gain, fatty tissue deposits (particularly in the face, known as moon face, and between the shoulders, known as buffalo hump), and skin changes, such as pink or purple stretch marks (striae) on the skin of the abdomen, thighs, breasts, and arms; thinning, fragile skin; and slow-healing cuts, insect bites, and infections.

The prevalence of sexual dysfunction in patients with secondary adrenal insufficiency is unknown. However, Granata et al., in a small uncontrolled study,[35] recently reported that subjects with a first diagnosis of primary autoimmune adrenal insufficiency are characterized by worse sexual function, and improved by cortisol and aldosterone supplementations. Adrenal insufficiency has been traditionally treated with glucocorticoids alone or with mineralocorticoids (for the primary condition), while treating the concurrent androgen deficiency with dehydroepiandrosterone (DHEA) has not yet attained standard of care, due to the presence of conflicting results.[19]

An age-dependent reduction of circulating DHEA sulfate has been reported. DHEA and its sulfate, DHEAS, have been implicated in a broad range of biological abnormalities including obesity, diabetes, osteoporosis, sexual dysfunction, cancer, and mental disorders.[19] However, the results of several small DHEA supplementation studies are rather inconclusive, if not negative.[19] We recently confirmed these data in a meta-analysis of the available placebo-controlled studies.[36]

In men, Cushing's syndrome has been frequently associated with decreased libido, decreased fertility, and ED.[19] However, it is not known yet whether ED is due to the excess of cortisol production or secondary to the related hypogonadism or a consequence of fat accumulation.[19]

Growth hormone

The most common disease of growth hormone (GH) excess is due to a GH-secreting pituitary adenoma, causing a syndrome known as acromegaly, a relatively rare condition, with an estimated prevalence of 20–60 cases per million.[19] Symptoms develop insidiously, taking years to decades to become apparent, with a mean duration of symptom onset to diagnosis of 12 years.[19] Although impotence and decreased libido are often reported as a symptom of acromegaly in textbooks,[19] it is still unclear if this is due to the excess of GH or to compression by the GH-producing tumor of neighboring gonadotropin-producing cells. In fact, secondary hypogonadism is a relatively common feature of acromegaly, due to an excess of PRL, to mixed hyperproduction of GH and PRL, or to compression of the pituitary stalk.[19]

Considering that, in the aging male, a progressive reduction of release of GH and of its downstream hormone, insulin growth factor I (IGF-I), has been described, the effect of GH, with and without T supplementation, has been tested, although in limited series and without any positive effects.[19]

In conclusion, due to limited evidence, the determination of adrenal hormones as well as GH or IGF-I, is not recommended in subjects with ED. The evaluation of these specific hormones should be requested only in the presence of specific symptoms and signs.

Obesity

Definition

Obesity is an excessive accumulation of body fat mass relative to lean body mass, usually due to an unbalanced diet and sedentary lifestyle.[37] The usual definition of obesity is based on body mass index (BMI), a simple index of weight-per-height (a person's weight in kilograms divided by the square of their height in meters) (http://www.who.int/topics/obesity/en/). According to BMI, obesity is categorized as follows:[37]

- grade 1: BMI 30 to <35;
- grade 2: BMI 35 to <40;
- grade 3: BMI ≥40.

Overweight and obesity is now considered to be a global epidemic, on the rise not only in Western societies, but also in developing countries. Obesity causes concern because it is a risk factor for developing CVD, cancer, and common chronic diseases, such as diabetes mellitus, hypertension, and dyslipidemia, all conditions that can lead to a reduced quality of life and premature death.[37] For obesity-associated morbidities it is now clear that the distribution of fat is another relevant factor, one that is not computed in BMI. In fact, BMI does not take into account the accumulation of visceral fat, which characterizes the most pathogenic form of obesity: abdominal or central obesity, which can be easily quantified by waist circumference (WC). The WC is easily measured with a flexible tape placed on a horizontal plane at the level of the iliac crest. The superiority of WC over BMI in the prediction of CVD and diabetes is remarkable, considering that measurement of WC has a lower reproducibility than that of BMI. BMI may overestimate the degree of obesity in individuals who are overweight but with expanded lean mass (e.g., professional athletes or body-builders); on the other hand, in subjects with reduced muscle mass (e.g., the elderly), excess body fat can occur within the normal BMI range; this is so-called "sarcopenic obesity," which is associated with a particularly relevant burden of obesity-related complications. Two action levels of WC were determined in Western countries to identify men whose health risks were increasing (action level 1: >94 cm), or high (action level 2: >102 cm).37 Action levels based on WC measurements were shown to be a valuable and simple method for alerting people with an increased risk of CVD, who might benefit from weight management.[37] People at action level 1 are 1.5–2-fold more likely to have one or more major CV risk factors; people with WC above action level 2 are 2.5–4.5-fold more likely to have one or more major CV risk factors.

In adult men, it is well known that T and SHBG decline as a function of obesity class.[7,37,38] The relationship between low T and fat accumulation is a bidirectional one, because it has been demonstrated that inducing hypogonadism is associated with an increase in (visceral) adiposity and that an increase in visceral adiposity is associated with low T, most probably because of a decreased GnRH neuron function.[7,39] However, the association between ED and increased WC is apparently independent from obesity-associated comorbidities and hypogonadism. In fact, in two distinct cohorts from Florence, Italy, reflecting a general and a symptomatic (ED) cohort, the association between ED and central obesity was confirmed even after adjusting for total T and known obesity-associated comorbidities, and was more dependent on organic than psychological and relational problems.[37] In line with these data, in a rabbit model of MetS-induced increased visceral adiposity, non-alcoholic steatohepatitis, and ED, we recently demonstrated that treatments aimed at reducing liver and circulating tumor necrosis factor α (TNFα) levels or neutralizing TNFα action significantly improve penile responsiveness to acetylcholine.[40] Hence, obesity-related factors other than T seem to play a direct role in the pathogenesis of ED. For all these reasons, BMI and, more importantly, waist line should be measured in all patients seeking medical care for ED.

Type 2 diabetes mellitus

Type 2 diabetes (T2DM) is a complex metabolic disorder characterized by hyperglycemia, relative deficiency of insulin secretion, and a reduced response of target tissues to insulin (insulin resistance), strictly associated with overweight and obesity. The dramatic worldwide increase in the prevalence of T2DM is posing a massive health problem in both developed and developing countries.[37] Sexual health is greatly impaired by DM.[37–41] It has been reported that ED occurs in at least 35–90% of men with DM, with the onset of ED occurring at an earlier age (10–15 years before) than in those without DM.[41] Common multifactorial complications such as peripheral neuropathy, atherosclerosis of large blood vessels, and endothelial dysfunction of arterioles are all involved in the pathogenesis of DM-associated ED. The possibility that hypogonadism might contribute to DM-related sexual dysfunction has also been envisaged.[37,41] A large body of evidence indicates that ED can be considered as a useful sign for the screening of silent myocardial ischemia in diabetic subjects.[42,43] In addition, it has also been emphasized that even prediabetic states, including impaired glucose tolerance (IGT) and impaired fasting glucose (IFG), are clinical conditions characterized by an increased prevalence of arteriogenic ED and ED-related hypogonadism. Hence, diagnosing such conditions could be of dramatic relevance for the correct management of ED.[44,45]

Laboratory criteria

According to the standard operating procedures of the International Society for Sexual Medicine,[14] and the European Association of Urology,[46] fasting plasma glucose (FPG) should be evaluated in all subjects complaining of ED.

Impaired glucose tolerance is defined as 2-h plasma glucose on oral glucose Tolerance test of between 7.8 and

11.0 mmol/L (140–199 mg/dL).[47] The IGT category was introduced in the late 1970s, whereas IFG, defined by fasting glucose concentrations of between 6.1 and 6.9 mmol/L (110–125 mg/dL), was proposed for the first time only in 1997 by the American Diabetes Association (ADA).[47] In 2003, the ADA recommended that this diagnostic threshold of FPG should be lowered to 5.6 mml/L (100 mg/dL).[47] This change was based on receiver operating characteristics (ROC) curve analysis in detecting DM over a period of 5 years from Pima Indian, Mauritius, San Antonio, and Hoorn Study data.[47] However, this decision has been questioned by several associations.[47] Finally it should be recognized that in the presence of IFG, OGTT is recommended to exclude undiagnosed DM.[47]

For decades, the diagnosis of diabetes has been based on glucose criteria, either the FPG or the 75-g OGTT. These include the FPG ≥126 mg/dL (7 mmol/L) or 2-h PG ≥200 mg/dL (11.1 mmol/L).[47] Recent data indicated that, assuming universal screening of the undiagnosed, the glycated hemoglobin (HbA1c) cut point of ≥6.5% identifies one-third fewer cases of undiagnosed diabetes than a FPG cut point of ≥126 mg/dL.[47] Additionally, patients with severe hyperglycemia, such as those who present with severe classic hyperglycemic symptoms or hyperglycemic crisis, can continue to be diagnosed when a random (or casual) plasma glucose of ≥200 mg/dL (11.1 mmol/L) is found.[47] In the absence of classical diabetic symptoms, a test result diagnostic of diabetes (FPG or HbA1c) should be repeated to rule out laboratory error.[47]

Conclusion

In sexual medicine, the most important clinical actions for decision-making are not procedures based only on decision-tree testing algorithms or on shotgun medical or surgical prescriptions, but are instead the generation and evaluation of appropriate diagnostic hypotheses that can improve not only the sexual problem but also overall health. Because the majority of drugs employed in sexual medicine are agonists or antagonists of hormone receptors, and endocrinopathies affect a consistent proportion of subjects seeking medical care for ED (in our experience up to 70% of subjects consulting for ED have at least one of the conditions depicted in Figure 10.1), identifying endocrine disorders underlying the sexual problem is mandatory. In addition, quite often, correcting the endocrine disorder is a sufficient strategy to face the sexual problem. For example, successful treatment of obesity could reverse the hypogonadal state,[39] or treating hyperthyroidism can improve premature ejaculation.[19,31]

For all the aforementioned considerations, we strongly suggest that physicians who are experts in sexual medicine perform at least the following clinical procedures in all ED patients:

1 Breast and genital inspection and measurement of testis volume (Prader orchidometer), along with digito-rectal examination of the prostate and recording of blood pressure and waistline.
2 Collect a fasting morning blood sample for: total and HDL cholesterol, HbA1c, glucose, triglycerides, hematocrit/hemoglobin, TSH, PSA, LH, FSH, PRL, SHBG, and, obviously, total testosterone. The first four analytes are aimed at identifying metabolic derangements that are often comorbid with ED. The last seven analytes are useful in determining the existence and the nature of an eventual endocrinopathy, including hypogonadism. In addition, blood count and PSA are useful not only to corroborate the diagnosis, but also as a baseline value to monitor the efficacy of an eventual T supplementation.

References

1 Bhasin S, Cunningham GR, Hayes FJ, et al., Task Force, Endocrine Society. Testosterone therapy in men with androgen deficiency syndromes: an Endocrine Society clinical practice guideline. *J Clin Endocrinol Metab* 2010;95:2536–59.
2 Wang C, Nieschlag E, Swerdloff R, et al. Investigation, treatment and monitoring of late-onset hypogonadism in males: ISA, ISSAM, EAU, EAA and ASA recommendations. *Eur J Endocrinol* 2008;159:507–14.
3 Corona G, Rastrelli G, Vignozzi L, et al. Emerging medication for the treatment of male hypogonadism. *Expert Opin Emerg Drugs* 2012;17:239–59.
4 Corona G, Rastrelli G, Vignozzi L, et al. How to recognize late-onset hypogonadism in men with sexual dysfunction. *Asian J Androl* 2012;14:251–9.
5 Isidori AM, Buvat J, Corona G, et al. A critical analysis of the role of testosterone in erectile function: from pathophysiology to treatment – a systematic review. *Eur Urol* 2014;65:99–112.
6 Corona G, Rastrelli G, Maggi M. Diagnosis and treatment of late-onset hypogonadism: Systematic review and meta-analysis of TRT outcomes. *Best Pract Res Clin Endocrinol Metab* 2013;27:557–79.

7 Corona G, Rastrelli G, Morelli A, et al. Hypogonadism and metabolic syndrome. *J Endocrinol Invest* 2011;34:557–67.
8 Wu FC, Tajar A, Beynon JM, et al. Identification of late-onset hypogonadism in middle-aged and elderly men. *N Engl J Med* 2010;363:123–35.
9 Tajar A, Forti G, O'Neill TW, et al. Characteristics of secondary, primary, and compensated hypogonadism in aging men: evidence from the European Male Ageing Study. *J Clin Endocrinol Metab* 2010;95:1810–18.
10 Buvat J, Maggi M, Guay A, et al. Testosterone deficiency in men: systematic review and standard operating procedures for diagnosis and treatment. *J Sex Med.* 2013;10:245–84.
11 Rastrelli G, Corona G, Bandini E, et al. Investigation on psychological symptoms improves ANDROTEST accuracy in predicting hypogonadism in subjects with sexual dysfunction. *Int J Impot Res* 2013;25:34–9.
12 Rastrelli G, Corona G, Lotti F, et al. Relationship of testis size and LH levels with incidence of major adverse cardiovascular events in older men with sexual dysfunction. *J Sex Med* 2013;10:2761–73.
13 Maseroli E, Rastrelli G, Corona G, et al. Gynecomastia in subjects with sexual dysfunction. *J Endocrinol Invest* 2014;37:525–32.
14 Ghanem HM, Salonia A, Martin-Morales A. Standard operating procedures: physical examination and laboratory testing for men with erectile dysfunction. *J Sex Med* 2013;10:108–10.
15 Rastrelli G, Corona G, Vignozzi L, et al. Serum PSA as a predictor of testosterone deficiency. *J Sex Med* 2013;10: 2518–28.
16 Huhtaniemi IT, Tajar A, Lee DM, et al. Comparison of serum testosterone and estradiol measurements in 3174 European men using platform immunoassay and mass spectrometry; relevance for the diagnostics in aging men. *Eur J Endocrinol* 2012;166:983–91.
17 Corona G, Boddi V, Lotti F, et al. The relationship of testosterone to prostate-specific antigen in men with sexual dysfunction. *J Sex Med* 2010;7(1 Pt 1):284–92.
18 Morgentaler A, Traish AM. Shifting the paradigm of testosterone and prostate cancer: the saturation model and the limits of androgen-dependent growth. *Eur Urol* 2009;55:310–21.
19 Maggi M, Buvat J, Corona G, et al. Hormonal causes of male sexual dysfunctions and their management (hyperprolactinemia, thyroid disorders, GH disorders, DHEA). *J Sex Med* 2013;10:661–77.
20 Corona G, Mannucci E, Fisher AD, et al. Effect of hyperprolactinemia in male patients consulting for sexual dysfunction. *J Sex Med* 2007;4:1485–93.
21 Corona G, Rastrelli G, Ricca V, et al. Risk factors associated with primary and secondary reduced libido in male patients with sexual dysfunction. *J Sex Med* 2013;10:1074–89.
22 Buvat J, Lemaire A. Endocrine screening in 1,022 men with erectile dysfunction: clinical significance and cost-effective strategy. *J Urol* 1997;158:1764–7.
23 Buvat J. Hyperprolactinemia and sexual function in men: a short review. *Int J Impot Res* 2003;15:373–7.
24 Corona G, Mannucci E, Jannini EA, et al. Hypoprolactinemia: a new clinical syndrome in patients with sexual dysfunction. *J Sex Med* 2009;6:1457–66.
25 Corona G, Wu FCW, Rastrelli G, et al.. Low prolactin is associated with sexual dysfunction and psychological or metabolic disturbances in middle aged and elderly men: the European Male Aging Study (EMAS). *J Sex Med* 2014;11:240–53.
26 Drago F, Lissandrello CO. The "low-dose" concept and the paradoxical effects of prolactin on grooming and sexual behavior. *Eur J Pharmacol* 2000;405:131–7.
27 Gettler LT, McDade TW, Feranil AB, et al. Prolactin, fatherhood, and reproductive behavior in human males. *Am J Phys Anthropol* 2012;148:362–70.
28 Melmed S, Casanueva FF, Hoffman AR, et al. Diagnosis and treatment of hyperprolactinemia: an Endocrine Society clinical practice guideline. *J Clin Endocrinol Metab* 2011;96:273–88.
29 Corona G, Wu FCW, Forti G, et al. Thyroid hormones and male sexual function. *Int J Androl* 2012;35:668–79.
30 Carosa E, Di Sante S, Rossi S, et al. Ontogenetic profile of the expression of thyroid hormone receptors in rat and human corpora cavernosa of the penis. *J Sex Med* 2010;7(4 Pt 1):1381–90.
31 Carani C, Isidori AM, Granata A, et al. Multicenter study on the prevalence of sexual symptoms in male hypo- and hyperthyroid patients. *J Clin Endocrinol Metab* 2005;90:6472–9.
32 Corona G, Jannini EA, Lotti F, et al. Premature and delayed ejaculation: two ends of a single continuum influenced by hormonal milieu. *Int J Androl* 2011;34:41–8.
33 Corona G, Jannini EA, Vignozzi L, et al. The hormonal control of ejaculation. *Nat Rev Urol* 2012;9:508–19.
34 Helfand M, Crapo LM. Testing for suspected thyroid disease. In: Sox HC (ed.), *Common Diagnostic Tests.* Philadelphia: American College of Physicians, 1990.
35 Granata A, Tirabassi G, Pugni V, et al. Sexual dysfunctions in men affected by autoimmune Addison's disease before and after short-term gluco- and mineralocorticoid replacement therapy. *J Sex Med* 2013;10:2036–43.
36 Corona G, Rastrelli G, Giagulli V, et al. Dehydroepiandrosterone supplementation in elderly men: a meta-analysis study of placebo controlled trials. *J Clin Endocrinol Metab* 2013;98:3615–26.
37 Corona G, Rastrelli G, Filippi S, et al. Erectile dysfunction and central obesity: an Italian perspective. *Asian J Androl* 2014;16:581–91.
38 Corona G, Mannucci E, Lotti F, et al. Pulse pressure, an index of arterial stiffness, is associated with androgen deficiency and impaired penile blood flow in men with ED. *J Sex Med* 2009;6:285–93.
39 Corona G, Rastrelli G, Monami M, et al. Body weight loss reverts obesity-associated hypogonadotropic hypogonadism: a systematic review and meta-analysis. *Eur J Endocrinol* 2013;168:829–43.

40 Vignozzi L, Filippi S, Comeglio P, et al. Nonalcoholic steatohepatitis as a novel player in metabolic syndrome-induced erectile dysfunction: an experimental study in the rabbit. *Mol Cel Endocrinol* 2014;384:143–54.

41 Corona G, Giorda CB, Cucinotta D, et al., The SUBITO-DE study group. The SUBITO-DE study: Sexual dysfunction in newly diagnosed Type 2 diabetes male patients. *J Endocrinol Invest* 2013;36:864–8.

42 Yamada T, Hara K, Umematsu H, et al. Erectile dysfunction and cardiovascular events in diabetic men: a meta-analysis of observational studies. *PLoS One* 2012;7:e43673.

43 Corona G, Fagioli G, Mannucci E, et al. Penile doppler ultrasound in patients with erectile dysfunction (ED): role of peak systolic velocity measured in the flaccid state in predicting arteriogenic ED and silent coronary artery disease. *J Sex Med* 2008;5:2623–34.

44 Corona G, Rastrelli G, Silverii A, et al. The identification of pre-diabetes condition with ARIC algorithm, predicts long-term CV events in patients with erectile dysfunction. *J Sex Med* 2013;10:1114–23.

45 Corona G, Rastrelli G, Balercia G, et al. Hormonal associations and sexual dysfunctions in male patients with impaired fasting glucose: a cross-sectional and longitudinal study. *J Sex Med* 2012;9:1669–80.

46 Hatzimouratidis K, Amar E, Eardley I, et al. Guidelines on male sexual dysfunction: erectile dysfunction and premature ejaculation. *Eur Urol* 2010;57:804–14.

47 American Diabetes Association. Diagnosis and classification of diabetes mellitus. *Diab Care* 2014;37:S81–S90.

CHAPTER 11

Duplex ultrasonography and its role in the assessment of male sexual dysfunction

Conrad von Stempel and Miles Walkden
University College Hospital, London, UK

Introduction

Ultrasound of the penis is an adjunct to physical examination in the investigation of penile disease. It is a relatively non-invasive two-part test assessing the penis in both the flaccid and erect states. It can demonstrate penile structure, vasculature, pathological plaques, and anatomical variants. With the addition of Doppler spectral tracing it becomes a dynamic tool to assess penile vascular physiology, both venous and arterial. Measurement of peak blood flow in both the flaccid state and sequentially during an evolving erection demonstrates whether the penile vessels and corpora have normal compliance and physiological response.

Uses of penile Doppler

Penile Doppler was first formally described in 1985 by Lue,[1] who used a 4.5 MHz linear probe to quantify blood flow in the deep and dorsal penile arteries pre- and post-intracorporal pharmacostimulation.

Penile Doppler has a role in the investigation of a number of diseases, primarily erectile dysfunction, whilst it also has a role in the management of priapism and penile trauma, and in presurgical assessment for patients undergoing urethral and reconstructive surgery.

Erectile dysfunction

Penile Doppler is described in the European Association of Urology Guidelines as a second-line, specialist investigation indicated after thorough history, examination, and biochemistry and endocrine blood tests. It is most frequently carried out in assessing men with primary ED who have failed oral phosphodiesterase inhibitor therapy.[2]

If during the ultrasound examination the patient achieves and maintains a normal erection with pharmacostimulant injection, and Doppler examination reveals normal vascular physiology, further more invasive investigations of vasculogenic causes of ED are unnecessary. This in turn can guide andrology doctors to refer patients for a psychological opinion.[3,4]

Severe ED is more common in men with heart disease and in those with known classical risk factors: smoking, hypertension, hypercholesterolemia, and diabetes. Furthermore, men with ED and no prior diagnosis of cardiovascular disease have a risk ratio of 1.5 for all cardiovascular diseases including stroke, heart disease, and peripheral vascular disease when compared to patients without ED.[5] Vasculogenic ED was also demonstrated in a cohort of men who went on to develop angina and subsequent proven ischemic heart disease.[6] This has led ED to be described as a biomarker for cardiovascular disease. It is therefore now suggested that if penile Doppler demonstrates arterial insufficiency, specifically a reduced peak systolic velocity in at-risk patients with no previous history of heart disease, they should be referred for cardiovascular investigation.[7,8]

Priapism

Penile Doppler is not part of the routine management of acute priapism although it is the primary imaging investigation for differentiating between ischemic and non-ischemic priapism.[9] In addition, measuring peak systolic

Male Sexual Dysfunction: A Clinical Guide, First Edition. Edited by Suks Minhas and John Mulhall.

flow pre- and post-intervention such as corporal aspiration and shunt insertion can help guide management choices such as early penile implant insertion versus conservative treatment.[10]

Penile ultrasonographic anatomy

The nomenclature for the parts of the penis can sometimes be confusing, and varied terms are quoted in the literature. In particular two common terms are the "base" and "root" of the penis. For the sake of clarity in this chapter, the penoscrotal junction is taken to mean the base and the crura the root.

The penis is made up of three cylinders of tissue, namely the two corpora cavernosa and the corpus spongiosum. On ultrasound in the transverse plane the corpora cavernosa can be identified as heterogeneous circular structures surrounded by a thin echogenic layer of tunica with a bright midline septum separating them. The thickness of the tunica and therefore possible plaques can only be assessed in the tumescent state. The corpus spongiosum is visualized as a separate slightly brighter oval structure ventral to the cavernosa within which the hypoechoic urethra is sometimes seen.

The cavernosal arteries can be identified, even in the flaccid state, as tubular structures deep within the corporal tissues, the walls of which are hyperechoic giving a tram-track appearance. These are more readily visible when color Doppler is applied.

Penile vascular anatomy is extremely variable. The penis is supplied on each side by a common penile artery, which normally arises from the internal pudendal artery, which itself is a branch of the anterior division of the internal iliac artery.

The common penile artery normally has three branches: the bulbar, dorsal penile, and cavernosal arteries. It is the cavernosal arteries that are the most important in erection as they supply blood to the cavernosal sinusoids. They normally enter their respective corpora cavernosa at the level of the crura, and it is these vessels that should be used to measure blood flow. Perforators between the dorsal and cavernosal arteries are seen in around 20% of patients, whilst accessory cavernosal arteries are seen in around 60% of men.[11] These accessory cavernosal arteries tend to enter the corpora on the dorsal surface at the level of the penoscrotal junction. They can sometimes be the main supply and should always be looked for if the peak systolic velocity (PSV) in the crural cavernosal artery is low.

Cavernosal arterial blood enters branching helicine arteries, which supply the sinusoids with blood. The sinusoidal venules drain their blood into the subtunical venous plexus, which then drains via emissary veins that pierce the tunica albuginea surrounding the corpora. Emissary veins drain dorsally to the deep dorsal, laterally to the circumflex, and ventrally to the periurethral veins.

Beginning at the coronal sulcus, the prominent deep dorsal vein is the main venous drainage of the glans penis, the corpus spongiosum, and the distal two-thirds of the corpora cavernosa. It is this vein that is interrogated during Doppler if a venous leak is suspected from the arterial trace.

Standard operating technique

Pre-test

The investigator should take a brief history from the patient to determine whether they can ever achieve a normal erection and whether the patient has noticed a curve or wasting deformity in the erect penis. In addition a brief drug and past medical history should be sought to ensure there is no contraindication, absolute or relative, to intracavernosal injection, such as anticoagulant use, history of priapism, or condition predisposing to priapism such as sickle-cell disease, myeloma, or leukemia.

This information guides targeted ultrasound to look for plaques or cavernosal fibrosis and determines the dose of intracavernosal drug administered. Patients often have experience of intracavernosal injection, either in the andrology clinic or self-injection. In our practice a patient who achieves near normal erections may require as little as 5 μg of alprostadil, whilst those with severe ED will require significantly higher doses.

Several intracavernosal therapies are available; however, the most commonly used monotherapy is a single or split dose of 5–40 μg aprostadil into the left or right cavernosal corpus, which is effective in approximately three-quarters of men with ED.[12] Some centers describe using intracorporal phentolamine in cases where high forward end-diastolic flow but normal peak systolic velocities are recorded and the patient fails to maintain an erection. Phentolamine is an alpha-adrenergic antagonist that inhibits the sympathetic drive. High sympathetic drive in the context of a very anxious patient can lead to the recording of falsely low peak systolic velocities and increased end-diastolic flows, and the latter may be falsely interpreted as evidence of venous leak.[13]

A single combination injection with a mixture of phentolamine and alprostadil with or without papaverine (a non-selective phosphodiesterase inhibitor) is also available. There is evidence that a combination single injection can have greater efficacy over a monotherapy, but this is not readily available in the UK.[14]

Oral therapy has been used. However, the onset time of sildenafil is up to 90 minutes and, given the busy unpredictable nature of ultrasound clinics, the faster, more predictable injection is preferred. In addition a large proportion of the patients referred for penile Doppler have failed or have had inadequate responses to oral therapy.[15]

Other techniques have been advocated including use of audiovisual sexual media, vibrotactile devices, and manual self-stimulation.[16] When combined with intracavernosal injection, manual self-stimulation has been shown to achieve a higher rate of more rigid erections, providing a better representation of the patient's erections outside of the clinical environment.[17]

Before starting scanning, the investigator, or accompanying urologist, should explain that the test will involve scanning the underside of the penis and in between the legs for up to 30 minutes, initially in the flaccid state and then during erection.

The need for intracorporal injection and the risk of priapism should be carefully explained. The risk of priapism is usually quoted at around 1%. The patient should be made aware that he can try and alleviate the erection by ejaculation, cold water exposure, or exercise with the caveat that if this does not work within 3 hours of the injection they should return to hospital for possible intervention. Intervention normally takes the form of corporal aspiration with a 19-G needle and occasionally intracavernosal injection of phenylephrine, administered if aspiration fails.[2]

The patient should receive a physical information sheet, which documents the dose administered, site and time of injection, and where to present in case of complications post-examination.

Lastly, the investigator should explain that the aim of the test is to assess the erectile tissues and the changes in blood flow to the penis during erection. The vascular physiology of erection can be simplified when explaining to patients with the analogy of a filling bath: "In order to fill with water, the taps need to be fully on (cavernosal arteries) and the plug in place (venous outflow occlusion as the sinusoids engorge)."

The patient should be naked from the waist down and lying supine with their legs slightly apart to allow scanning of the crura. The initial examination should be made using high resolution B-mode (gray scale) on the flaccid penis. Historically the dorsal surface was scanned with a low-frequency (5–8 MHz) transducer. Today, with the advent of higher resolution transducers, the authors recommend ventral scanning for a number of reasons:

1 It is imperative to sample the most proximal, widest point on any vessel to record a representative flow reading. There is a steep negative gradient in the peak systolic flow of the cavernosal artery proximally to distally, as the helicine branches arise and the vessel tapers.
2 Arterial sampling at the crus allows accurate repeated sampling compared to the rather arbitrary "level of the penoscrotal junction" used in some papers.
3 At this site the vessel is least likely to be deformed by pressure exerted by the probe.[18,19]
4 Maximum Doppler signal is received from blood flowing in a vessel at 0° to the transducer (optimum angle of insonation), and a wide range of peak systolic velocities can be erroneously recorded from the same vessel if measured at different angles of insonation.[20] At the level of the crus as the cavernosal arteries pierce through the tunica, an optimum angle of insonation can be achieved, negating the need for excessive angle correction, which reduces the accuracy of recording.[21]

The cavernosal arteries have variable anatomy with multiple accessory vessels. These accessory vessels are sometimes but not always the dominant supply. It is therefore imperative that measurements are taken from both the crura and penoscrotal junction (where these accessory vessels are best seen) so that an erroneously low reading is not recorded (Figure 11.1).

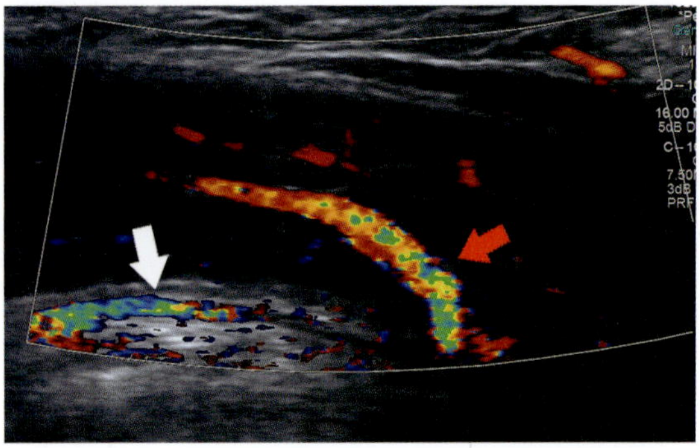

Figure 11.1 Longitudinal image of the penis at the level of the penoscrotal junction (evident by the slight dorsal curvature of the penis) showing an accessory cavernosal artery that, in this patient, forms the dominant supply to the penis (red arrow). This was discovered after abnormally low values for peak systolic velocity (PSV) were seen at the level of the crura in the setting of a normal erection, illustrating the importance of looking for accessory vessels. Also visible (white arrow) is the dorsal artery, which lies outside of the tunica.

How to scan

Scan the penis initially in the flaccid state. With the probe longitudinally and slightly obliqued, line the transducer up along each crus in turn. Identify where each cavernosal artery enters the crus. This will be the reference point to measure flow in subsequent time points. It is good practice to measure the peak systolic flow in each cavernosal artery.

In 2008 Corona et al. suggested that measurements of peak systolic velocity in the cavernosal arteries of less than 13 cm/s in the flaccid penis predict arterial insufficiency on dynamic scanning in 80% of cases from a cohort of over 1000 middle-aged men (45–65 years old). Mancini et al., 8 years previously, demonstrated that a PSV of greater than 12.5 cm/s in the flaccid penis predicted a normal PSV and normal arterial flow acceleration in the tumescent penis in over 90% of their cohort of over 100 participants. In our practice we regularly record a PSV of greater than 25 cm/s in the flaccid state, and further studies are needed to evaluate the correlation between blood flow in the flaccid and erect state.[22,23]

Next, with the transducer transverse and starting at the glans, sweep proximally along the shaft looking carefully for any calcified tunical plaques. Focal irregularities in the tunica and waisting can be better seen in the erect penis. At the penoscrotal junction scan from

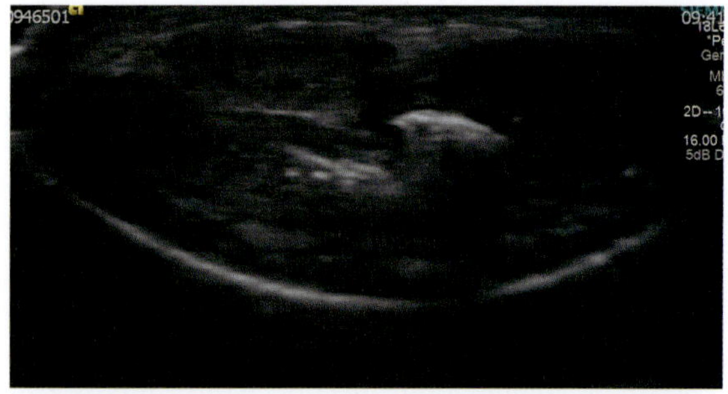

(a)

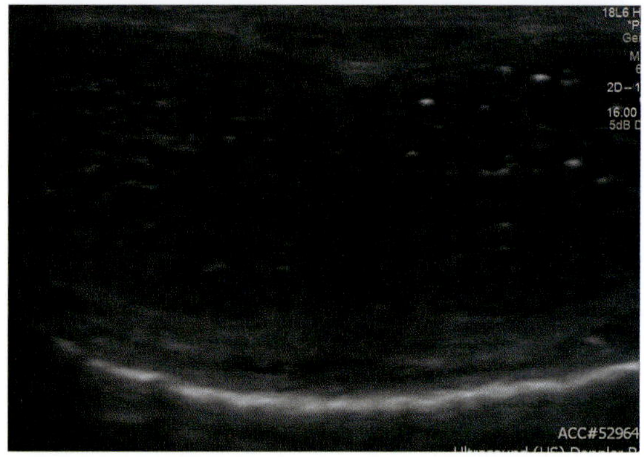

(b)

Figure 11.2 a) Axial image of the flaccid penis at the midshaft level immediately following intracorporal injection of alprostadil showing increased echogenic material within the corporal tissue close to the ventral tunica. This should not be confused with calcified plaque, and reinforces the importance of scanning preinjection. **b)** Axial image of the same patient at the same level 15 minutes later demonstrating almost complete dispersal of the drug (scattered echogenic foci in the left corpus are all that remain).

the undersurface of the scrotum at the penoscrotal junction proximally following each crus to its insertion.

In the assessment of ED and in planning penile surgery, the pharmacostimulation should then be administered. As the tunical septum is semipermeable, the drug can cross the midline into the contralateral corpus. The exception to this is in extrophy patients where the crura are completely separate and require individual injection.

It is important to ultrasound the injection site (a stream of echogenic bubbles can be identified in the corporal tissue), as incorrect placement will reduce the efficacy of the dose and can lead to the misdiagnosis of arterial insufficiency (Figure 11.2).

Formal Doppler interrogation of the cavernosal arteries consists of sequential sampling in a fixed location on the cavernosal artery on each side. There is no consensus in the literature as to when to commence arterial flow measurements, and there is a slight trade-off between continuous scanning, which can be awkward for the patient, and interval scanning, which can potentially miss the highest peak systolic velocity.

Sampling in each cavernosal artery should begin 2 minutes after injection. It is then reasonable to scan at 5-minute intervals until full rigidity with either a diastolic flow of less than 5 cm/s or reverse flow is achieved, or for up to a maximum of 30 minutes if there is a limited response.[22,24,25]

The peak systolic velocity normally is reached after 5–6 minutes but in approximately a quarter of patients who will respond to alprostadil there can be a substantial lag, necessitating scanning up to 30 minutes after injection

Acute priapism

In cases of acute priapism, the same systematic approach should be taken to ultrasound, with the exception of omitting the pharmacostimulation injection. The ultrasound report should document the state of tumescence, duration of priapism, and any prior interventions. Flow within the cavernosal arteries as well as the appearance of the cavernosal tissues should be assessed.

Findings

B-mode ultrasound

B-mode (gray-scale) ultrasound is normal in the vast majority of patients with erectile dysfunction. It can, however, demonstrate the stigmata of Peyronie's disease: plaques, penile wasting, and corporal fibrosis. Ultrasound is less sensitive than MRI in demonstrating early plaque formation but, in contrast, ultrasound readily shows calcification within plaques, something MRI cannot reliably do.[26,27] This impacts on the management of Peyronie's disease as calcium deposition is a hallmark of chronicity. It has been suggested that in patients with particularly large plaques and/or cavernosal fibrosis there is an increased incidence of arterial insufficiency and veno-occlusive failure.[28]

Cavernosal fibrosis can be identified as coarsened, usually hyperechoic, heterogeneous regions within the corpora, often accompanied by reduced blood flow on color Doppler. This can be seen in both subacute and chronic priapism as well as Peyronie's disease (Figure 11.3).

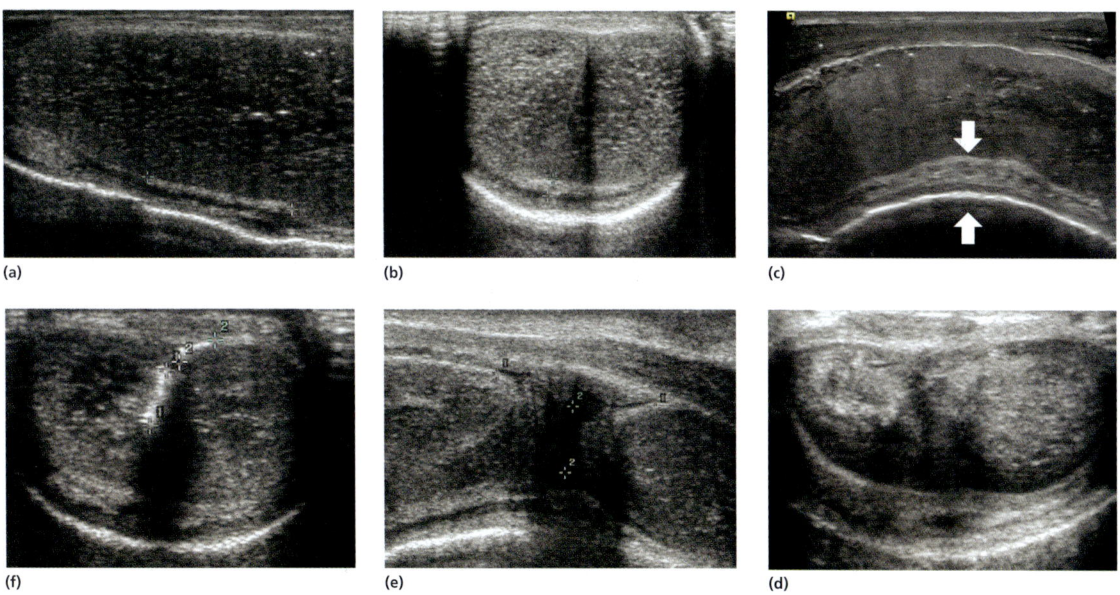

Figure 11.3 **a-f Clockwise from top left. a)** Longitudinal and **b)** axial: B-mode ultrasound of the distal penis showing a classical appearing non-calcified plaque on the dorsal tunical surface that appears as a focus of thickening (defined by the calipers). **c)** Longitudinal view of the midshaft showing a dorsal curvature cause by a non-calcified plaque (defined by arrows). **d)** Axial view of the midshaft demonstrating fibrosis of the right corpus cavernosum as shown by the reduced caliber compared to the left and the focus of increased echogenicity. **e)** Longitudinal view of the midshaft showing marked wasting of the corpus caused by a combination of tunica plaque and intracorporal fibrosis. **f)** Axial ultrasound of the midshaft showing two adjacent calcified plaques with post-acoustic shadowing involving the ventral tunica and septum (defined by calipers 1 and 2).

Vascular findings in the normal penis and in ED

In the unstimulated penis, there is high tone in the sinusoidal smooth muscle allowing limited inflow. With initiation of erection, parasympathetic drive via the pudendal nerves floods the sinusoids with nitric oxide. This quickly reduces the vascular resistance and results in rapid filling of the sinusoids. As the sinusoids engorge they compress their exiting venules creating a high arterial inflow, low venous outflow system. As the intracorporal pressure rises and it nears the systolic blood pressure, the inflow pressure plateaus then begins to drop.

The phases of a normal erection can be quantified with spectral tracing of the Doppler signal of the cavernosal arteries (Figure 11.4).

Historically the most useful parameters in assessment of ED are the peak systolic velocity (PSV), end-diastolic velocity (EDV), and resistive index (RI).[29] Modern approaches have included measurements of flow in the dorsal vein and the caliber change and undulation of cavernosal arteries.

Flow above 35 cm/s in the cavernosal arteries is widely accepted as equating to normal arterial flow, whereas flow of less than 25 cm/s is suggestive of arterial insufficiency with a sensitivity of 100% and specificity

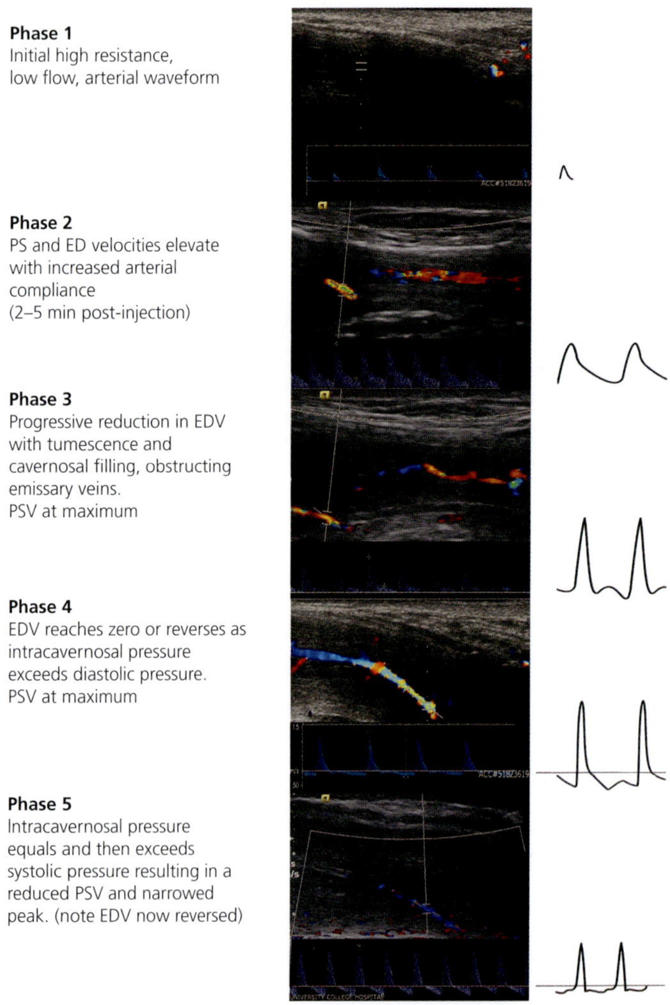

Figure 11.4 Waveforms. ED, end diastole; EDV, end-diastolic velocity; PS, peak systole; PSV, peak systolic velocity.

of 95%.[30] Intermediate values, between 25 and 35 cm/s, are not specific.[31]

A potential pitfall with these cut-off values is that they were calculated by Doppler correlation with arteriographic findings where the investigators identified overt stenosis. Vasculogenic ED is more likely due to a systemic, age-related process of endothelial dysfunction in the small helicine and cavernosal vessels, which is not factored into the current cut-off values.[32,33] An age-matched algorithm has been suggested, which multiplies age and PSV by a coefficient and promises to detect earlier stages of vascular insufficiency compared to current parameters; however, this has yet to be further evaluated.[34]

The peak systolic values should be compared between the cavernosal artery on each side as at a given time-point a discrepancy of more than 20% is suggestive of arterial insufficiency.[35] It is important, however, to identify any accessory vessels so as not to overdiagnose a deficient cavernosal artery on one side.

End-diastolic velocity is an indirect measure of intracorporal compliance and effective venous occlusion. As the pressure increases in the cavernosal sinusoids and equals diastolic pressure, the curve changes morphology and EDV steadily decreases and eventually equals zero. End-diastolic reversal can be seen as the intracavernosal pressure exceeds diastolic pressure. Lack of progression of EDV reduction with sequential scanning during erection is suggestive of veno-occlusive dysfunction[36] (Figure 11.5).

An EDV exceeding 5 cm/s is indicative of veno-occlusive dysfunction (VOD), although this is a normal finding in the early phases of erection.[37] Continuous high flow in the dorsal penile veins and any other venous shunting can be assessed, which in combination with an increased EDV may help in the diagnosis of VOD.[25] In the presence of arterial insufficiency, EDV cannot be reliably used to detect VOD. In the anxious patient, as previously mentioned, sympathetic drive can lead to increased diastolic flow incorrectly suggesting VOD.

It has been suggested that a RI of less than 0.75, a function of both PSV and EDV calculated as $RI = (PSV - EDV)/PSV$, can predict veno-occlusive disease in 95% of cases.[38] Other measurable variables that have been postulated as predictors of vasculogenic ED include degree of cavernosal artery tortuosity.[39] The caliber of cavernosal arteries is not thought to be a reliable variable as elasticity of vessels changes with remodeling and atherosclerosis with age, and there is a poor correlation between diameter change and rigidity.[25]

Vascular findings in priapism

In ischemic priapism with low flow in the cavernosal arteries, spectral trace reveals both a low PSV and low or absent EDV. These cases can be managed by immediate penile implantation, which preserves penile length and reduces complications of implant placement.[10]

There is an interesting subgroup of men with ischemic priapism who demonstrate high cavernosal artery PSV (up to 2 m/s in some cases) but importantly have a negative EDV indicating high resistance, and therefore negligible corporal perfusion. These cases need to be distinguished from high flow priapism (a non-ischemic pathology), and it is the end-diastolic velocity that is key to this difference.[40]

In non-ischemic priapism there is a low-resistance flow pattern with an elevated PSV and high EDV. Ultrasound demonstrates fistulae as areas of turbulent flow on color Doppler. Penile Doppler has an excellent sensitivity for A-V fistulae approaching 100%.[41] In these cases referral for internal pudendal artery angiography with selective catheterization and embolization is the gold-standard treatment[42–44] (Figure 11.6).

The advent of oral therapies has significantly improved the treatment of ED, and the vast majority of patients respond to such treatments and require no further investigation.[45] The role of penile Doppler in ED is therefore limited to patients who have failed a trial of oral therapy, and to a select group of mainly young men for whom a possible traumatic or congenital vascular abnormality is suspected.

There are, however, a number of problems with the test. The first and most important is that we rely on data obtained 20 years ago, performed using old ultrasound equipment on non-age-matched patients, for our cut-off values for abnormal and normal flow. We accept that a PSV of just above 35 cm/s in a 65-year-old man is probably within a normal range but for a younger man it would be logical that a normal value would be significantly higher. Age-matched normograms are required in order to more accurately diagnose arterial insufficiency.

The second problem is the artificial nature of the test with the likely sympathetic overlay no doubt seen in a large proportion of men. This has an effect on the veno-occlusive mechanism, and therefore the diagnosis of

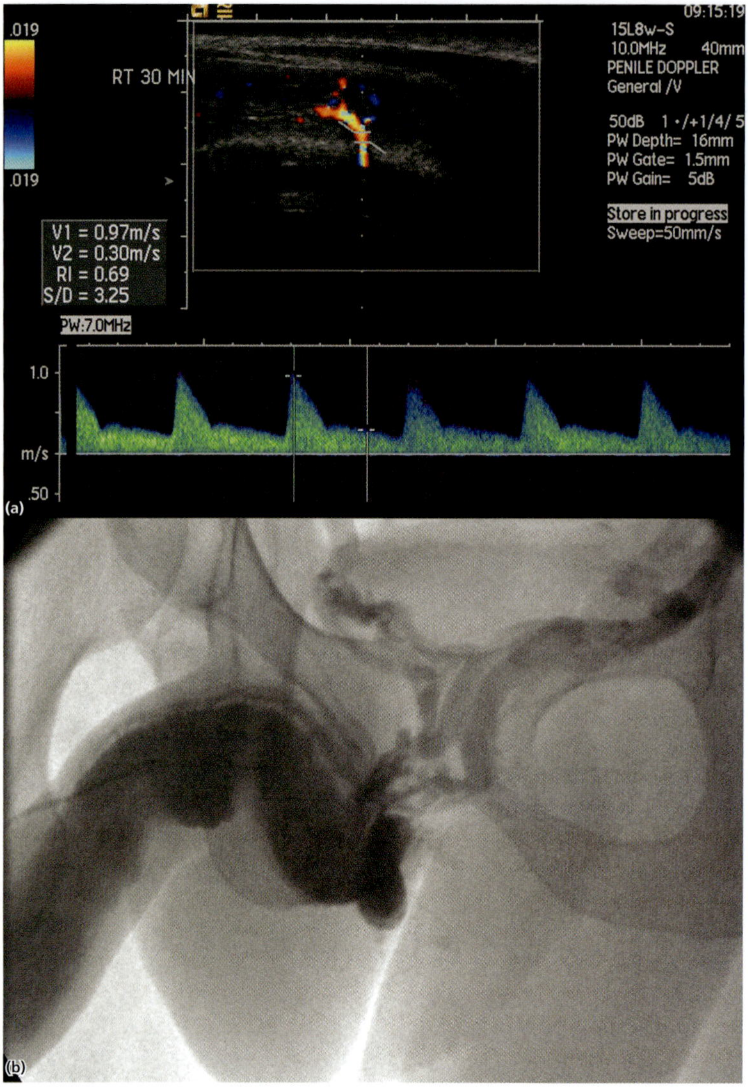

Figure 11.5 **a)** Longitudinal view of the cavernosal artery 30 minutes post-injection of alprostadil showing a normal peak systolic velocity (97 cm/s) but with sustained, high end-diastolic velocity of 30 cm/s (low resistance) suggestive of veno-occlusive dysfunction. The patient had 70% tumescence. **b)** Cavernosography in the same patient revealed early filling of the periprostatic plexus and pelvic veins consistent with a venous leak.

VOD on Doppler should be made with caution. In addition VOD cannot be identified in the presence of arterial insufficiency.

Lastly the result of any test should affect management of the patient. In the case of both arterial insufficiency and VOD no particularly successful treatment is currently available.

Arterial insufficiency in a subgroup of young men who have ED secondary to a traumatic arterial lesion may be treated by revascularization. Epigastric to dorsal penile artery anastomosis surgery is associated with the best results but is very complex surgery not recommended for routine use in patients with atherosclerosis. Furthermore, vein resection surgery for veno-occlusive disease has poor results and is no longer advised.[2,46,47]

In the older patient no routine treatments are offered but endovascular treatment options such as drug eluting stents are currently being assessed.[48] It may well be that

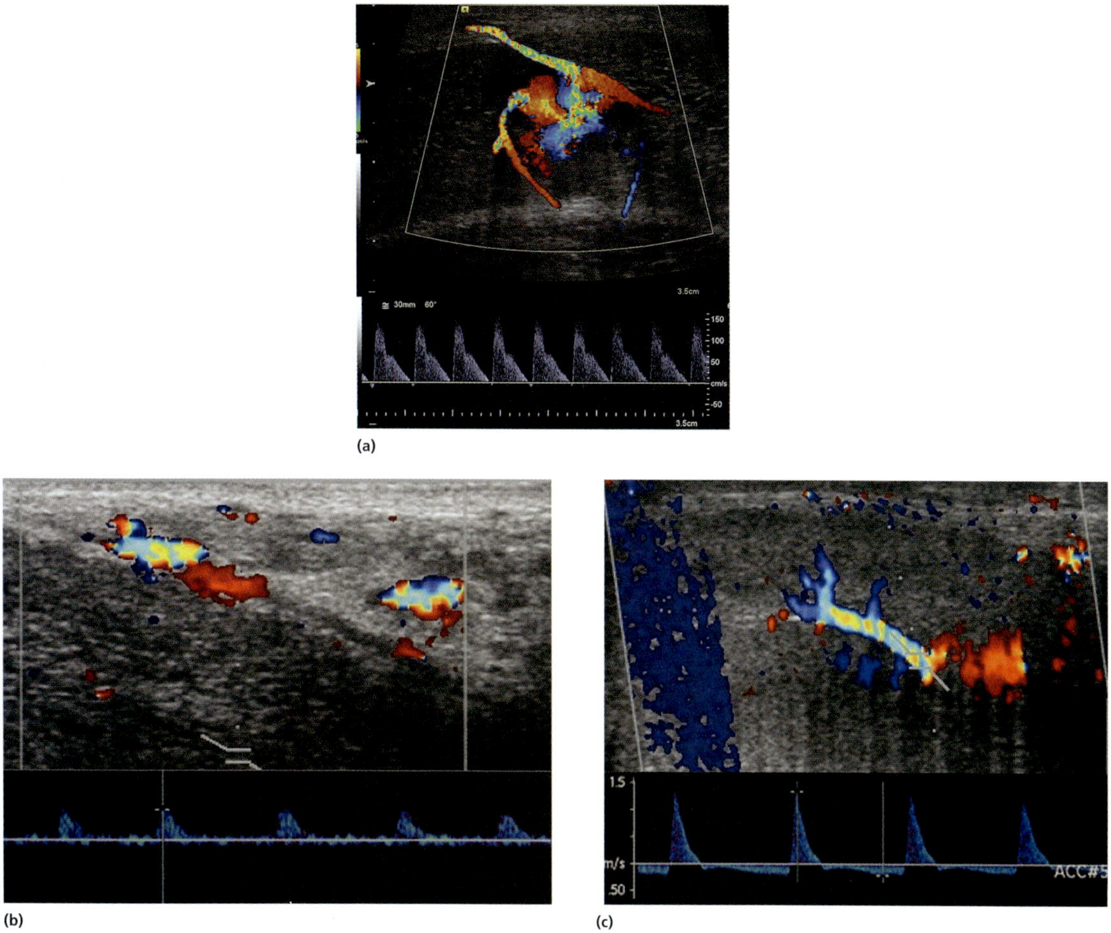

Figure 11.6 **a)** Longitudinal view of the penis at the penoscrotal junction showing a large fistula between the main cavernosal artery and the venous sinusoids as demonstrated by a focal area of turbulent flow in the corporal substance. Spectral trace shows both high peak systolic and high end-diastolic velocities consistent with a low resistance pattern seen in non-ischemic priapism. **b)** Longitudinal view at the level of the penoscrotal junction demonstrating the classically described ischemic waveform, which is low flow and high resistance. The calipers are positioned over the main cavernosal artery. The expanded corpora indicate tumescence, and the heterogeneity suggests early fibrosis. **c)** Longitudinal view of the penis in a second patient with ischemic priapism. This demonstrates very high peak systolic velocity (1.5 m/s) but crucially there is reversed flow in diastole, which clearly distinguishes it from both the high-flow, low-resistance waveform in image **a** (non-ischemic priapism) and image **b** (classical ischemic priapism).

the underlying problem is at the helicine endothelial level rather than stenosis in the larger proximal arteries.

Doppler in priapism is very useful and probably significantly under-used currently due to lack of evidence and research. There is no question it can differentiate between ischemic and non-ischemic priapism. The authors also postulate that it can be used to guide treatment of ischemic priapism. Two different waveforms have been noted, which are probably just different ends of the spectrum of evolution of the priapism. The first and most commonly described is a low-flow high-resistance waveform that likely indicates severe ischemia with little chance of reversal. The second is a high-flow high-resistance waveform (with reverse flow in diastole). This flow is similar to that seen in a normal erection and likely represents the early/less severe form of ischemia.

Penile Doppler is an excellent modality for assessing the vascular physiological response in erection. It also allows probably the best spatial resolution of the penile structures of any imaging modality.

References

1 Lue TF, Hricak H, Marich KW, Tanagho EA. Vasculogenic impotence evaluated by high-resolution ultrasonography and pulsed Doppler spectrum analysis. *Radiology* 1985;155:777–81.

2 Wespes E, Eardley I, Giuliano D, et al. Guidelines on male sexual dysfunction : Erectile dysfunction and premature ejaculation. European Association of Urology, 2013.

3 Meuleman EJ, Diemont WL. Investigation of erectile dysfunction. Diagnostic testing for vascular factors in erectile dysfunction. *Urol Clin North Am* 1995;22(4):803–19.

4 Patel DV, Halls J, Patel U. Investigation of erectile dysfunction. *Br J Radiol* 2012;85 (Special Issue 1):S69–78. doi:10.1259/bjr/20361140.

5 Banks E, Joshy G, Abhayaratna WP, et al. Erectile dysfunction severity as a risk marker for cardiovascular disease hospitalisation and all-cause mortality: a prospective cohort study. *PLoS Med* 2013;10(1):e1001372. doi:10.1371/journal.pmed.1001372.

6 Montorsi F, Briganti A, Salonia A, et al. Erectile dysfunction prevalence, time of onset and association with risk factors in 300 consecutive patients with acute chest pain and angiographically documented coronary artery disease. *Eur Urol* 2003;44:360–5.

7 Kawanishi Y, Lee KS, Kimura K, et al. Screening of ischemic heart disease with cavernous artery blood flow in erectile dysfunctional patients. *Int J Impot Res* 2001;13:100–3.

8 El-Sakka AI, Morsy AM. Screening for ischemic heart disease in patients with erectile dysfunction: Role of penile doppler ultrasonography. *Urology* 2004;64:346–50.

9 Montague D, Jarow J, Broderick GA, et al. American Urological Association guideline on the management of priapism. *J Urol* 2003;170:1318–24.

10 Ralph DJ, Borley NC, Allen C, et al. The use of high-resolution magnetic resonance imaging in the management of patients presenting with priapism. *BJU Int* 2010;106(11):1714–8.

11 Bookstein JJ, Lang EV. Penile magnification pharmacoarteriography: Details of intrapenile arterial anatomy. *Am J Roentgenol* 1987;148(5):883–8.

12 Linet OI, Ogrinc FG. Efficacy and safety of intracavernosal alprostadil in men with erectile dysfunction. The Alprostadil Study Group. *N Engl J Med* 1996;334(14):873–7.

13 Gontero P, Sriprasad S, Wilkins CJ, Donaldson N, Muir GH, Sidhu PS. Phentolamine re-dosing during penile dynamic colour Doppler ultrasound: A practical method to abolish a false diagnosis of venous leakage in patients with erectile dysfunction. *Br J Radiol* 2004;77:922–6.

14 Bechara A, Casabé A, Chéliz G, Romano S, Rey H, Fredotovich N. Comparative study of papaverine plus phentolamine versus prostaglandin E1 in erectile dysfunction. *J Urol* 1997;157(6):2132–4.

15 Arslan D, Esen AA, Secil M, et al. A new method for the evaluation of erectile dysfunction: sildenafil plus Doppler ultrasonography. *J Urol* 2001;66(1):181–4.

16 Incrocci L, Hop WC, Slob AK. Visual erotic and vibrotactile stimulation and intracavernous injection in screening men with erectile dysfunction: a 3 year experience with 406 cases. *Int J Impot Res* 1996;8:227–32.

17 Donatucci CF, Lue TF. The combined intracavernous injection and stimulation test: diagnostic accuracy. *J Urol* 1992;148:61–2.

18 Kim SH, Paick JS, Lee SE, et al. Doppler sonography of deep cavernosal artery of the penis: variation of peak systolic velocity according to sampling location. *J Ultrasound Med* 1994;13:591–4.

19 Halls J, Bydawell G, Patel U. Erectile dysfunction: The role of penile Doppler ultrasound in diagnosis. *Abdom Imaging* 2009;34(6):712–25.

20 Speel TGW, van Langen H, Wijkstra H, Meuleman EJH. Penile duplex pharmaco-ultrasonography revisited: revalidation of the parameters of the cavernous arterial response. *J Urol* 2003;169(1):216–20.

21 Kawanishi Y, Kimura K, Naroda T, et al. Evaluation of cavernous artery by color Doppler ultrasonography: Significance of ultrasonic beam angle. *Japanese J Urol* 1995;86:1142–9.

22 Corona G, Fagioli G, Mannucci E, et al. Penile doppler ultrasound in patients with erectile dysfunction (ED): Role of peak systolic velocity measured in the flaccid state in predicting arteriogenic ED and silent coronary artery disease. *J Sex Med* 2008;5:2623–34.

23 Mancini M, Bartolini M, Maggi M, Innocenti P, Villari N, Forti G. Duplex ultrasound evaluation of cavernosal peak systolic velocity and waveform acceleration in the penile flaccid state: clinical significance in the assessment of the arterial supply in patients with erectile dysfunction. *Int J Androl* 2000;23:199–204.

24 Sikka S, Hellstrom W, Brock G, Morales A. Standardization of vascular assessment of erectile dysfunction. *J Sex Med* 2013;10:120–9.

25 Wilkins CJ, Sriprasad S, Sidhu PS. Colour Doppler ultrasound of the penis. *Clin Radiol* 2003;58(7):514–23.

26 Fornara P, Gerbershagen HP. Ultrasound in patients affected with Peyronie's disease. *World J Urol* 2004;22(5):365–7.

27 Hauck EW, Hackstein N, Vosshenrich R, et al. Diagnostic value of magnetic resonance imaging in Peyronie's disease – a comparison both with palpation and ultrasound in the evaluation of plaque formation. *Eur Urol* 2003;43:293–9; discussion 299–300.

28 Chung E, De Young L, Brock GB. Penile duplex ultrasonography in men with Peyronie's disease: is it veno-occlusive dysfunction or poor cavernosal arterial inflow that contributes to erectile dysfunction? *J Sex Med* 2011;8(12):3446–51.

29 Broderick GA, Arger P. Duplex Doppler ultrasonography: Noninvasive assessment of penile anatomy and function. *Semin Roentgenol* 1993;XXVIII(1):43–56.

30 Benson CB, Aruny JE, Vickers MA. Correlation of duplex sonography with arteriography in patients with erectile dysfunction. *Am J Roentgenol* 1993;160:71–3.

31 Patel U, Amin Z, Friedman E, Vale J, Kirby R, Lees W. Colour flow and spectral Doppler imaging after papaverine-induced penile erection in 220 impotent men: repeated sampling, velocity asymmetry and vascular anomalies. *Clin Radiol* 1993;48:18–24.

32 Bocchio M, Desideri G, Scarpelli P, et al. Endothelial cell activation in men with erectile dysfunction without cardiovascular risk factors and overt vascular damage. *J Urol* 2004;171(4):1601–4.

33 Brunner H, Cockcroft JR, Deanfield J, et al. Endothelial function and dysfunction.Part II: Association with cardiovascular risk factors and diseases. A statement by the Working Group on Endothelins and Endothelial Factors of the European Society of Hypertension. *J Hypertens* 2005;23:233–46.

34 Caretta N, Palego P, Roverato A, Selice R, Ferlin A, Foresta C. Age-matched cavernous peak systolic velocity: a highly sensitive parameter in the diagnosis of arteriogenic erectile dysfunction. *Int J Impot Res* 2006;18(3):306–10.

35 Aversa A, Sarteschi LM. The role of penile color-duplex ultrasound for the evaluation of erectile dysfunction. *J Sex Med* 2007;4(5):1437–47.

36 Schwartz AN, Lowe M, Berger RE, Wang KY, Mack LA, Richardson ML. Assessment of normal and abnormal erectile function: color Doppler flow sonography versus conventional techniques. *Radiology* 1991;180(1):105–9.

37 Collins JP, Lewandowski BJ. Experience with intracorporeal injection of papaverine and duplex ultrasound scanning for assessment of arteriogenic impotence. *Br J Urol* 1987;59:84–8.

38 Naroda T, Yamanaka M, Matsushita K, et al. Clinical studies for venogenic impotence with color Doppler ultrasonography: Evaluation of resistance index of the cavernous artery. *Japanese J Urol* 1996;87:1231–5.

39 Yildirim D, Bozkurt IH, Gurses B, Cirakoglu A. A new parameter in the diagnosis of vascular erectile dysfunction with penile Doppler ultrasound: Cavernous artery ondulation index. *Eur Rev Med Pharmacol Sci* 2013;17(10):1382–8.

40 Halls JE, Patel DV, Walkden M, Patel U. Priapism: Pathophysiology and the role of the radiologist. *Br J Radiol* 2014. doi:10.1259/bjr/62360925.

41 Bastuba MD, Saenz de Tejada I, Dinlenc CZ, Sarazen A, Krane RJ, Goldstein I. Arterial priapism: diagnosis, treatment and long-term followup. *J Urol* 1994;151:1231–7.

42 Salonia A, Eardley I, Giuliano F, et al. European Association of Urology guidelines on priapism. *Eur Urol* 2014;65:480–9.

43 Walker TG, Grant PW, Goldstein I, Krane RJ, Greenfield AJ. "High-flow" priapism: treatment with superselective transcatheter embolization. *Radiology* 1990;174:1053–4.

44 Kang BC, Lee DY, Byun JY, et al. Post-traumatic arterial priapism: colour Doppler examination and superselective arterial embolization. *Clin Radiol* 1998;53:830–4.

45 Goldstein I, Lue T, Padma-Nathan H. Sildenafil Study Group. Oral sildenafil in the treatment of erectile dysfunction. *N Engl J Med* 1998;339(1):59.

46 Wespes E, Wildschutz T, Roumeguere T, Schulman CC. The place of surgery for vascular impotence in the third millennium. *J Urol* 2003;170(4 Pt 1):1284–6.

47 Siroky MB, Azadzoi KM. Vasculogenic erectile dysfunction: newer therapeutic strategies. *J Urol* 2003;170(2 Pt 2):S24–9; discussion S29–30.

48 Rogers JH, Goldstein I, Kandzari DE, et al. Zotarolimus-eluting peripheral stents for the treatment of erectile dysfunction in subjects with suboptimal response to phosphodiesterase-5 inhibitors. *J Am Coll Cardiol* 2012;60:2618–27.

CHAPTER 12

MRI in men with sexual dysfunction

Alex Kirkham
University College Hospital, London, UK

Introduction

Because most of the penis is readily examined both clinically and with ultrasound, MRI has a limited role compared to these simple and less expensive tests. Nevertheless, there are areas in which the combination of excellent soft tissue contrast and moderate resolution (with a carefully set up protocol) means that MRI is a useful – and in some cases first-line – investigation.

The one area in which MRI is of very limited utility is in the diagnosis of simple erectile dysfunction: ultrasound with pharmacological stimulation provides information about blood flow,[1] and is used together with the clinical response to stimulation and measurement of nocturnal penile tumescence. In cases where angiography is required, MRI is some way from providing adequate resolution of the internal pudendal vessels and their branches, though it can be used to identify men with "polyvascular" disease.[2]

We will therefore address four main areas in this chapter: (i) the diagnosis of penile fracture, which if missed can cause significant erectile dysfunction; (ii) the imaging of fibrosis and in particular Peyronie's disease; (iii) the imaging of priapism; and (iv) the utility of MRI in the problematic penile implant. Before addressing each of these subjects we will address the protocols used for scanning, and normal radiological anatomy.

Scanning protocol and radiological anatomy

Pharmacological stimulation

Prostaglandin E_1 (PGE_1; alprostadil) is routinely used to produce tumescence for the scan, as it greatly improves views of the whole penis. As well as improving spatial resolution and the contrast between tumescent corpora and their fibrous surroundings, it also aids positioning in the anatomical plane.

The risk of priapism with alprostadil is low in erectile dysfunction,[3] but it may be higher in men with normal erectile function – occurring in 1 out of 10 in one small series.[4] We err towards low doses (5 µg in young men with normal function, 10 µg in most, and 20 µg in men with established erectile dysfunction and previous exposure to alprostadil) because the aim is to achieve distension of the corpora for the scan rather than full tumescence. The treatment of any resulting priapism is covered elsewhere and is likely to be successful if initiated less than 4 h after injection.[5]

Positioning

Interpretation is greatly aided by positioning the penis in the midline. We let it lie on the lower abdominal wall: the disadvantage of some respiratory movement (usually small) is outweighed by a relatively fixed position throughout the scan. Tape may be used to secure, but it

Male Sexual Dysfunction: A Clinical Guide, First Edition. Edited by Suks Minhas and John Mulhall.

is sometimes better just to use some small bolsters on either side of the midline, as pressure on the corpus spongiosum easily compresses it and obscures fibrosis or urethral pathology within it.

Sequences (Table 12.1)

The mainstay of imaging the penis is high-resolution (in-plane resolution 0.7–1 mm), thin-slice (ideally 3 mm) T2-weighted images in three orthogonal planes. An adequate signal-to-noise ratio can be achieved using these parameters on all modern 1.5 T machines, and they may be exceeded at 3 T.

On T2-weighted sequences the corpus spongiosum (including the glans) and the corpora cavernosa are of high T2 signal (although there may be layering effects in tumescence giving areas of subtly different signal).[6] They are surrounded by a low T2 signal band, thickest around the corpora cavernosa, consisting of an inner layer of tunica albuginea and an outer layer of Buck's fascia. In some patients these two layers can be distinguished separately, particularly at the dorsum where the deep dorsal vein runs between them, but in general the distinction is hard to make.[6] The superficial dorsal vein is usually well seen, and lies superficial to Buck's fascia. The intracavernosal septum is low in T2 signal and usually shows characteristic "corrugations" (Figure 12.1).

The ischiocavernosus and bulbocavernosus muscles are particularly well seen on coronal images as low T2 structures. The urethra is usually seen as a subtly low signal slit, and foci of urethral thickening are seen at moderately high resolution (though considerably less than on ultrasound). Arteries are seen as low signal flow voids on T2, and the cavernosal arteries are usually easily distinguished (with the arterial anatomy variable and more than one artery commonly seen on each side[7,8]).

It is probably best to spend time preparing the patient (and in particular ensuring tumescence) instead of performing a large number of sequences, and in many cases (Peyronie's, the assessment of tumors, and some cases of fracture) the T2 images in three orthogonal planes suffice. Other sequences are useful in specific scenarios, as follows:

- T1 sequences: There are two scenarios in which T1 sequences (without enhancement) are likely to be useful. The first is thrombosis of the dorsal vein (Mondor's disease), where the vessel may be of conspicuously high signal (and some groups have gone on to use MR angiographic sequences to detect a filling defect[9]). The second is fracture, where T1 sequences may demonstrate hemorrhage, and in some rare cases reveal a fracture defect not seen on T2.[10]
- Contrast: While the vessels are visible on T2 sequences, enhancement is necessary to assess their patency, and is particularly useful in priapism. The normal corpora cavernosa enhance from proximal to distal, and from around the cavernosal arteries to peripherally. We perform T1 spin echo sequences in one plane (usually coronal), followed by dynamic gradient echo sequences in another, with a 30 s time resolution for at least 2 minutes. In priapism it is important to wait long enough for slow but intact perfusion to opacify the corpora cavernosa to assess likely tissue viability: at least 5 minutes after injection, and ideally 10 minutes, when we perform a spin echo sequence with exactly the same parameters as pre-contrast. The use of enhancement in Peyronie's and to assess penile implants is more speculative and will be discussed in the relevant sections; it is probably not useful in penile fracture (though this is debated[10,11]).

Table 12.1 Common MR sequences used in imaging the penis.

Sequence	Indication	In-plane resolution	Slice thickness
T2 spin echo Ax, cor, sag	Routine	0.7–0.9 mm	3 mm
STIR[a]	Infections (including implants)	1 mm	4 mm
T1	Fracture, priapism	0.8–1 mm	3 mm
T1 post-contrast	Priapism	0.8–1 mm	3 mm
Dynamic enhancement	Priapism; use in penile fracture, Peyronie's disease, and infected implants is debated	<1–1.2 mm, time resolution <30 s	3 mm

[a] STIR, short tau inversion recovery.

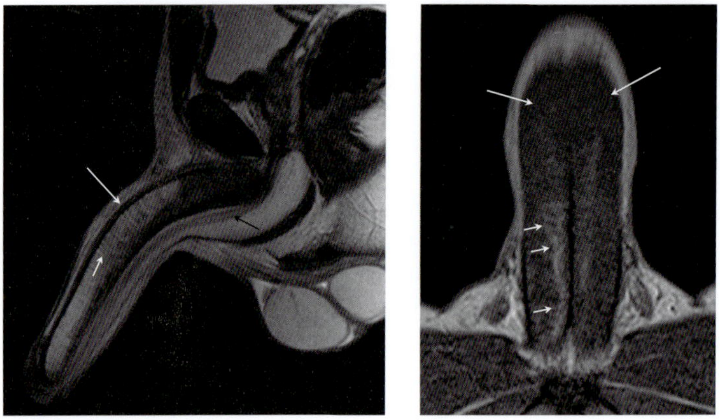

(a) (b)

Figure 12.1 **a)** T2 sagittal and **b)** T1 post-contrast images in a man with low-flow priapism. Note in **a)** the normal corrugations (short white arrow) and the normal urethra (black arrow). Also, Buck's fascia (long white arrow) is seen as a slightly higher signal layer than the adjacent (deeper) tunica albuginea. The T2 image shows low signal in the corpus cavernosum proximally, and high signal distally, but this does not correlate with the degree of infarction. For this, the post-contrast image **b)** obtained at 8 min is necessary: it shows generally no enhancement in the corpora cavernosa (long arrows), except around the proximal cavernosal arteries (short white arrows). The patient went on to have a penile implant the same week, with a good functional outcome.

- STIR/T2 fat saturated sequences: These show edema well, and may be useful for detecting inflammation (in particular when inflammation of an implant is suspected), although it can be difficult to distinguish low-level inflammation from normal postoperative appearances.

Penile fracture

Penile fracture is defined as a traumatic breach of the tunica albuginea, usually occurring with trauma to the tumescent penis,[12] and associated with the sensation of a "crack" and rapid detumescence with bruising.

In some cases, the defect of a penile fracture is palpable, but often it is obscured by bruising and hemorrhage (in particular because the majority of fractures are proximal).[13] For this reason, when there is clinical suspicion of a fracture, surgical exploration is usually performed with a relatively extensive (in some cases "degloving") approach, to locate the fracture or confidently exclude it.[14,15] This operation may result in significant morbidity,[16] but is worthwhile because conservative treatment almost certainly results in a higher rate of long-term sexual dysfunction.[17,18] Imaging would ideally (i) detect fracture with high sensitivity (and could therefore be used to rule it out in equivocal cases), and (ii) be used to plan the surgical approach and render the operation as minimally invasive as possible.

The first studies for fracture used cavernosography,[19] which has been superseded (it is not sufficiently accurate and is painful compared to the alternatives), and then ultrasound. The latter does diagnose the majority of fractures, and has the advantage that marking of the fracture site is straightforward.[20] However, there are limited data (in particular one small study of four patients) suggesting that MRI is more sensitive:[21] although ultrasound is of high spatial resolution, the heterogeneous tissue signal after a fracture can make it challenging to define the tunica albuginea. On MRI the margins of the low-signal tunica are usually better seen, even in the presence of edema and hematoma, and in one study MRI identified the fracture in all 13 patients in whom it was confirmed at operation.[22] Some groups advocate routine use of T1 sequences (in one small study identifying several fractures missed on T2[10]), and it adds little to the scan time, so should probably be used routinely. Whether intravenous contrast is necessary is more contentious; some reports suggest that it may help to define the margins of the defect, and others that there may be an early contrast blush after an acute fracture,[10] but the extra information is unlikely to alter the diagnosis and routine use of contrast is not currently justified by the data.

MRI may also be useful in making the diagnosis of other pathologies that mimic fracture. With intracavernosal hematoma,[16,22] the identification of a focus of altered signal within the corpus cavernosum (sometimes better seen after contrast administration) with an intact tunica allows conservative management (the symptoms are normally self-limiting). Similarly, MRI after rupture of a superficial vein (which is a common mimic of fracture[13]) shows hematoma but an intact tunica, and resolves without consequences.[23]

It is important to examine the corpus spongiosum, because fracture is associated with a urethral injury in around one-quarter of patients.[10] In some patients the MRI strongly suggests a urethral injury, but with the clinical finding of blood at the meatus, contrast urethrography remains the definitive (and simplest) investigation.[13]

The approach to suspected fracture should first involve examination: if the defect is palpable imaging is deemed unnecessary. Next, ultrasound if convincingly positive (some studies have shown false positives, and the technique is undoubtedly operator-dependent, so equivocal findings are probably not reliable) allows marking of the defect and is sufficient. However, in equivocal cases MRI is currently the most accurate imaging modality and a diagnostic scan can be obtained in 15–20minutes.

Priapism

The distinction between high-flow priapism (perfused corpora, often without pain, and sometimes post-traumatic) and low-flow (painful ischemia of the tumescent penis) can usually be made clinically and with the aid of blood gases. This is covered in detail in Chapter 20.

In most cases ultrasound is the primary radiological investigation. In high-flow priapism it is an excellent tool for the identification of high-volume, low-resistance, often chaotic flow characteristic of a pseudoaneurysm.[24] Such findings will often prompt conservative management or angiography and embolization. MRI in most cases shows some characteristic findings:

- a heterogeneous focus of signal void from high flow in the pseudoaneurysm, and sometimes prominent feeding arteries or draining veins;
- an early blush of enhancement on the dynamic images.[25,26]

Neither is as definitive as the Doppler ultrasound finding, however: in particular, the interpretation of cavernosal enhancement on early images can be challenging.

In low flow, ultrasound may give some indication of the degree of corporal blood flow. However, as in the case of most soft tissue tumors, Doppler is not sensitive enough to assess perfusion, and in particular the absence of visible flow is (i) operator-dependent, and (ii) does not imply that the tissue is not viable. In addition, ultrasound findings can be difficult to interpret in states that have elements of low and high flow: in particular, sickle-cell disease and after successful shunting for low-flow priapism.

MRI is probably the best tool we have for determining degree of infarction of the penis in low-flow priapism[27] (see Figure 12.1). It is important to perform both dynamic sequences to assess the vessels, and a delayed (we use a spin echo sequence, but gradient echo would suffice) sequence by at least 5 minutes (and ideally also 10 minutes) to assess corporal enhancement. The degree of infarction correlates well with both the blood gas and ultrasound findings, and in one paper non-enhancement on MRI predicted non-viable smooth muscle at histology in 10/10 patients.[27] In addition, all five patients with generally enhancing corpora cavernosa regained erectile function.[27] The result is important because it may affect management: there is good evidence that complete or almost complete non-enhancement after attempts at shunting has a poor functional outcome, and that early (acute) placement of a prosthesis may be optimal, before fibrosis has started to occur.[28]

MRI also demonstrates the much rarer unilateral or partial thrombosis,[29] and in cases of malignant priapism is usually diagnostic, with an irregular texture to the corpora on T2, and often peripheral (rather than periarterial) or distal early enhancement.[25]

Fibrosis and Peyronie's disease

Peyronie's plaques usually occur in the dependent part of the penis, and most are palpable.[30] For imaging (both ultrasound and MRI), stimulation with prostaglandin is extremely useful, stretching the tunica and distending the corpora cavernosa. The added benefit is that any resulting deformity can be documented and the images used for surgical planning.

On ultrasound Peyronie's plaques in the tunica are seen as areas of thickening, and if calcified are hyperechoic, with shadowing. Intracavernosal plaques are usually seen as irregular echogenic, non-shadowing foci, though it is important to emphasize that scattered thin strands across the distal half of each corpus cavernosum are a common, normal finding on both ultrasound and MRI.

On MRI fibrosis is low signal on both T1 and T2 sequences, and plaques (including those that are calcified) appear as foci of low signal thickening in the tunica and low signal in the corpora cavernosa. Calcification is almost impossible to delineate on MRI because it creates a signal void similar to fibrosis.[30] Scanning in three orthogonal planes with the penis well positioned allows assessment of angulation and of variations in caliber (which are common[31]).

One study has compared ultrasound and MRI for the assessment of palpable plaques, and found that (i) MRI detected a few more (58/93 vs 52/93) palpable plaques than ultrasound, and (ii) MRI detected eight plaques that were too proximal to be detected by ultrasound. On the other hand, ultrasound identified calcification in 14 plaques that could not be specifically identified on MRI.[30]

One final benefit of MRI may be in the assessment of enhancement. Many urologists would not operate on patients who have symptoms of active disease (in particular pain) because ongoing fibrosis formation and deformity can prejudice the surgical outcome.[32] An attractive hypothesis is that if Peyronie's disease represents an abnormal response to minor injuries, then the inflammatory component of active disease might be seen as enhancement on MRI (between 9%[32] and 35%[33] of plaques are associated with early enhancement). For now, however, this hypothesis remains unproven, and it is interesting that in a recent series *none* of the eight patients who had pain showed any plaque enhancement.[32]

A degree of fibrosis at the site of injury is to be expected after penile fracture (and indeed around 90% of patients have a palpable "nodule" at the site postoperatively[18]), and there are other causes of intracavernosal fibrosis – in particular priapism and regular use of intracavernosal agents, though this is debated.[34] In all of these cases ultrasound may suffice but is probably not definitive: fibrosis appears echogenic within the corpora in ultrasound, but the soft tissue contrast is better on MRI, and scanning in three planes provides a more reproducible assessment of deformity (both angulation and change in caliber). We use MRI routinely in this context.

Penile implants

All current inflatable penile implants are safe in 1.5 T machines. Two malleable prostheses (OmniPhase and DuraPhase: Dacomed, Minneapolis, MN) show significant deflection of their metal components in 1.5 T magnets and should not be scanned.

The fluid within inflatable prostheses means that they are well delineated on T2 and STIR sequences. We scan with the implant inflated where possible, and take particular care in positioning: it is easy to produce artefactual "kinking" at the base of the pendulous part with over-zealous taping to the abdominal wall, and we usually use just bolsters on each side.

Several causes of malfunctioning penile implant can be difficult to diagnose clinically, but are well seen on MRI:

- crossover (two inflatable parts lying in one corpus cavernosum for part of their length) (Figure 12.2);
- kinking from overlong cavernosal components (relatively common, a potent cause of pain and often hard to diagnose clinically[35]);
- aneurysmal dilatation;[36]
- distal flaccidity from too short components.

These are all well demonstrated. In one study of 14 patients with a painful prosthesis, all showed an abnormality on MRI but in only five was the cause apparent clinically.[35] Too short a prosthesis needs to be distinguished from the "floppy glans" or supersonic transformer deformity,[37] which is best diagnosed clinically or with ultrasound, when the movement of the different soft tissue structures can be assessed dynamically.

Fluid around the prosthesis can have several causes. In the immediate postoperative period it is common to have either hematoma or a little serous fluid, which may persist for several months (with some moderate surrounding edema on STIR sequences also common). Prosthesis infection is fairly uncommon (1–5% of virgin implants, though higher for revisions[38]) but can occur within weeks, and also causes periprosthetic fluid and edema, seen in particular on STIR sequences.[39] The difference between the benign early reactive changes and infection is one of degree, and there are no published data on the performance of MRI in this context compared to clinical and biochemical findings. We suspect that in cases where the infection is advanced enough to cause definitive findings on MRI it will be apparent clinically too. Finally, rupture of the prosthesis

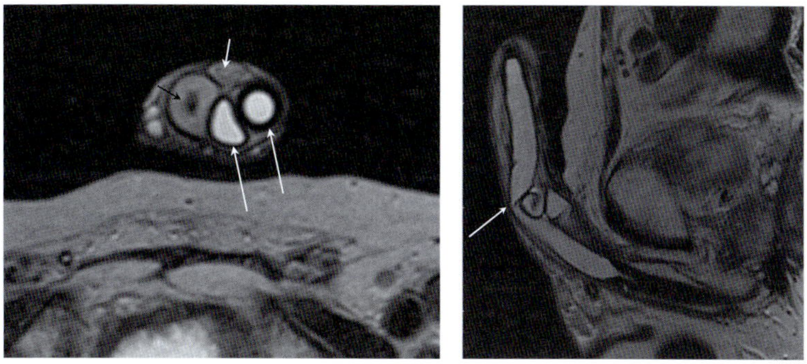

(a) (b)

Figure 12.2 **a)** T2 axial and **b)** sagittal images of a penile implant. **a)** This shows the two cavernosal components (long white arrows) lying in the left corpus cavernosum (true crossover). Note the periarterial post-priapism fibrosis in the right corpus cavernosum (black arrow) and the normal urethra (short white arrow). The sagittal image in **b)** shows a "kink" at the point where the right cavernosal component crosses over to the left (long white arrow).

can lead to the finding of fluid outside it, persisting particularly if a fibrous capsule has developed. The key in this scenario is the finding of a partially or completely deflated reservoir balloon.

Other conditions

The role of MRI in penile cancer is debated, and is outside the remit of this chapter, but there are several review articles summarizing the data.[40,41] In patients with congenital abnormalities, MRI can be very useful (with or without alprostadil) for delineating the size and anatomical relationships of the corpora.

References

1 Sikka SC, Hellstrom WJ, Brock G, Morales AM. Standardization of vascular assessment of erectile dysfunction: standard operating procedures for duplex ultrasound. *J Sex Med* 2013;10(1):120–9. [Review]

2 Vlachopoulos C, Terentes-Printzios D, Stefanadis C. How to identify subjects with poly-vascular disease? *Curr Vasc Pharmacol*. 2012;10(6):728–30. [Review]

3 Linet OI, Neff LL. Intracavernous prostaglandin E1 in erectile dysfunction. *Clin Invest* 1994;72(2):139–49. [Review]

4 Scardino E, Villa G, Bonomo G, et al. Magnetic resonance imaging combined with artificial erection for local staging of penile cancer. *Urology* 2004;63(6):1158–62.

5 Muruve N, Hosking DH. Intracorporeal phenylephrine in the treatment of priapism. *J Urol* 1996;155(1):141–3.

6 Kirkham AP, Illing RO, Minhas S, Allen C. MR imaging of nonmalignant penile lesions. *Radiographics* 2008;28(3): 837–53. [Review]

7 Martínez-Piñeiro L, Julve E, Martínez-Piñeiro JA. Topographical anatomy of the penile arteries. *Brit J Urol* 1997;80(3):463–7.

8 Bookstein JJ, Lang EV. Penile magnification pharmacoarteriography: details of intrapenile arterial anatomy. *AJR Am J Roentgenol* 1987;148(5):883–8.

9 Boscolo-Berto R, Iafrate M, Casarrubea G, Ficarra V. Magnetic resonance angiography findings of penile Mondor's disease. *J Magn Reson Imaging* 2009;30(2):407–10.

10 Uder M, Gohl D, Takahashi M, et al. MRI of penile fracture: diagnosis and therapeutic follow-up. *Eur Radiol* 2002;12(1):113–20.

11 Choi MH, Kim B, Ryu JA, Lee SW, Lee KS. MR imaging of acute penile fracture. *Radiographics* 2000;20:1397–405.

12 Kramer AC. Penile fracture seems more likely during sex under stressful situations. *J Sex Med* 2011;8(12):3414–7.

13 Koifman L, Barros R, Junior RA, Cavalcanti AG, Favorito LA. Penile fracture: diagnosis, treatment and outcomes of 150 patients. *Urology* 2010;76(6):1488–92.

14 Kamdar C, Mooppan UMM, Kim H, Gulmi FA. Penile fracture: preoperative evaluation and surgical technique for optimal patient outcome. *BJU Int* 2008;102(11): 1640–4.

15 Yapanoglu T, Aksoy Y, Adanur S, Kabadayi B, Ozturk G, Ozbey I. Seventeen years' experience of penile fracture: conservative vs. surgical treatment. *J Sex Med* 2009;6(7): 2058–63.

16 Abolyosr A, Moneim AEA, Abdelatif AM, Abdalla MA, Imam HM. The management of penile fracture based on clinical and magnetic resonance imaging findings. *BJU Int* 2005;96(3):373–7.

17 Fergany AF, Angermeier KW, Montague DK. Review of Cleveland Clinic experience with penile fracture. *Urology* 1999;54(2):352–5.

18 Zargooshi J. Sexual function and tunica albuginea wound healing following penile fracture: An 18-year follow-up study of 352 patients from Kermanshah, Iran. *J Sex Med* 2009;6(4):1141–50.

19 Grosman H, Gray RR, St Louis EL, Casey R, Keresteci AG, Elliott DS. The role of corpus cavernosography in acute "fracture" of the penis. *Radiology* 1982;144(4):787–8.

20 Dierks PR, Hawkins H. Sonography and penile trauma. *J Ultras Med* 1983;2(9):417–9.

21 Fedel M, Venz S, Andreessen R, Sudhoff F, Loening SA. The value of magnetic resonance imaging in the diagnosis of suspected penile fracture with atypical clinical findings. *J Urol* 1996;155(6):1924–7.

22 Abolyosr A, Moneim A, Abdelatif A, Abdalla M, Imam H. The management of penile fracture based on clinical and magnetic resonance imaging findings. *BJU Int* 2005;96(3): 373–7.

23 Nehru-Babu M, Hendry D, Ai-Saffar N. Rupture of the dorsal vein mimicking fracture of the penis. *BJU Int* 1999;84(1):179–80.

24 Bertolotto M, Quaia E, Mucelli FP, Ciampalini S, Forgács B, Gattuccio I. Color Doppler imaging of posttraumatic priapism before and after selective embolization. *Radiographics* 2003;23(2):495–503.

25 Kirkham APS, Illing RO, Minhas S, Minhas S, Allen C. MR imaging of nonmalignant penile lesions. *Radiographics* 2008;28(3):837–53.

26 Eracleous E, Kondou M, Aristidou K, et al. Use of Doppler ultrasound and 3-dimensional contrast-enhanced MR angiography in the diagnosis and follow-up of post-traumatic high-flow priapism in a child. *Pediatr Radiol* 2000;30(4):265–7.

27 Ralph DJ, Borley NC, Allen C, et al. The use of high-resolution magnetic resonance imaging in the management of patients presenting with priapism. *BJU Int* 2010;106(11): 1714–8.

28 Rees RW, Kalsi J, Minhas S, Peters J, Kell P, Ralph DJ. The management of low-flow priapism with the immediate insertion of a penile prosthesis. *BJU Int* 2002;90(9):893–7.

29 Asbach P, Oelrich B, Haase O, Lenk SV, Loening SA. Acute partial segmental thrombosis of the corpus cavernosum: imaging findings on ultrasound, computed tomography, and magnetic resonance imaging. *Clin Imag* 2008;32(5):400–2.

30 Hauck E. Diagnostic value of magnetic resonance imaging in Peyronie's disease – a comparison both with palpation and ultrasound in the evaluation of plaque formation. *Eur Urol* 2003;43(3):293–300.

31 Levine LA, Lenting EL. A surgical algorithm for the treatment of Peyronie's disease. *J Urol* 1997;158(6):2149–52.

32 Hauck EW, Weidner W. François de la Peyronie and the disease named after him. *Lancet* 2001;357(9273): 2049–51.

33 Helweg G, Judmaier W, Buchberger W, et al. Peyronie's disease: MR findings in 28 patients. *AJR Am J Roentgenol* 1992;158(6):1261–4.

34 Tal R, Mulhall JP. Intracavernosal injections and fibrosis: myth or reality? *BJU Int* 2008;102(5):525–6.

35 Moncada I, Hernández C, Jara J, et al. Buckling of cylinders may cause prolonged penile pain after prosthesis implantation: a case control study using magnetic resonance imaging of the penis. *J Urol* 1998;160(1):67–71.

36 Kirkham A. MRI of the penis. *Brit J Radiol* 2012;85 (Spec. No 1):S86–93.

37 Mulhall JP, Kim FJ. Reconstructing penile supersonic transporter (SST) deformity using glanulopexy (glans fixation). *Urology* 2001;57(6):1160–2.

38 Carson C. Diagnosis, treatment and prevention of penile prosthesis infection. *Int J Impot Res* 2003;15:S139–S46.

39 Moncada I, Jara J, Cabello R, Monzo J, Hernandez C. Radiological assessment of penile prosthesis: the role of magnetic resonance imaging. *World J Urol* 2004;22(5): 371–7.

40 Kirkham APS. Radiological imaging in penile cancer. In: Muneer A, Arya A, Horenblas S (eds), *Textbook of Penile Cancer*. London: Springer, 2012; pp. 69–102.

41 Kochhar R, Taylor B, Sangar V. Imaging in primary penile cancer: current status and future directions. *Eur Radiol* 2009;6:1–12.

CHAPTER 13

The metabolic syndrome and ED

Mark Paulos and Martin Miner

Brown University, Providence, RI, USA

Introduction

Erectile dysfunction (ED), defined as the inability to maintain and achieve an erection sufficient for satisfactory intercourse, has a high prevalence and incidence worldwide.[1] A systematic review of epidemiological evidence undertaken in 2002 showed a clear increase in prevalence with advancing age, with rates for men younger than 40 years ranging from approximately 2% to 9%, compared with 18% to 86% for those older than 80 years.[2] Although not life-threatening, it may be a precursor or marker of more serious conditions, particularly coronary artery disease (CAD). Inman et al.[3] have shown that when ED occurs in younger men, it is associated with a marked increase in the risk of future cardiac events, and that overall ED may be associated with an approximately 80% higher risk of subsequent CAD.

Sexual function is a complex, multifactorial process. The development of ED is attributable to both psychogenic factors and physiological alterations in neural, vascular, hormonal, and metabolic perturbations, all mediated through endothelial and smooth muscle dysfunction. While this cascade of metabolic parameters can lead to early endothelial dysfunction and, eventually, late cardiovascular events, this chapter will focus on the metabolic investigation of erectile dysfunction. Specifically, we will illustrate from our practice a clinical case and the value of the metabolic workup of the ED patient and the evolving concept of "cardiometabolic risk."

Cardiometabolic risk entails the risk of developing any of the following: type 2 diabetes (T2DM), cardiovascular disease (CVD), or metabolic syndrome (MetS). The assessment of cardiometabolic risk uses traditional risk factors such as smoking, high low-density-lipoprotein cholesterol (LDL-C), hypertension, and elevated serum glucose as well as emerging risk factors closely related to abdominal obesity, especially intra-abdominal or visceral obesity. The relationship between traditional cardiovascular risk factors (hypercholesterolemia, hypertension, and smoking) and the occurrence of cardiovascular events is well understood. Our increasing understanding of the pathophysiology of cardiovascular disease is now defining the value of a range of new cardiovascular risk factors. Risk stratification requires measurement tools of CVD risk that must be valid in the general male population, and measurement tests or biomarkers that help predict cardiac risk.[4] ED should become part of this CVD risk assessment.

Traditional models of cardiovascular risk such as Framingham Risk Score (FRS) are weighted toward age, and 80% of men aged 40–59 will have a low 10- year risk.[5] Incorporating some assessment of lifetime risk has been proposed as an added step to evaluate cardiovascular risk in this younger middle-aged population, in which those with ED, as noted by Inman, are at particularly elevated cardiovascular risk.[3]

New data have emerged to justify a new version, though controversial, to better target lipid management therapies for the reduction of cardiovascular events in the adult population.[6] New guidelines have attempted to address the shortcomings of older risk models. ED guidelines such as Princeton III[7] have attempted to utilize evidence-based evaluation to further stratify men for cardiovascular (CVS) risk following the utilization of keen history taking and traditional risk models to establish the presence of predominantly vasculogenic ED and the volume of subclinical atherosclerotic burden, which are markers for subsequent CVS events of myocardial infarction (MI) and cerebrovascular accident (CVA) in men.[8]

Male Sexual Dysfunction: A Clinical Guide, First Edition. Edited by Suks Minhas and John Mulhall.

Box 13.1 TS: A 44-year-old male with 20-year history of ED.

TS is a 44-year-old male who presented to the Men's Health Center with a longstanding history of erectile dysfunction (ED). He is married and is a broker attorney for a large investment firm. In this global recession, he is under enormous work stress. He had consulted a urologist 10 years prior, and underwent nocturnal penile tumescence testing, which was normal. He was thought to have "psychogenic" ED. He was treated with the first-line oral therapies: sildenafil, vardenafil, and tadalafil but with limited success.

In fact, he noted increasing unresponsiveness to these medications over time, achieving penetration in less than 40% of attempts. Upon further questioning, his ED appeared in his mid-20s, and affected multiple domains of his sexual function. His complaints included decreased firmness of erection, and an inability to sustain his erections often leading to an inability to complete intercourse. His desire was good, and he and his wife adapted their sexual intimacy to include genital intimacy without penetration. Yet, Mr S felt there should be more that could be done to help him both understand the cause of his ED, and improve his sexual functioning.

His past medical history was unremarkable: no allergies; no medications; no chronic diseases. His life habits too revealed little in the way of cause: no history of cigarettes or marijuana use; rare alcohol intake. He walked 30–45 minutes each day, used a functional weight trainer for an anaerobic workout for 1 hour 2–3 days each week, and though his diet included beef 2–3 times per week, it was generally "low fat" and of moderate calories.

His family history was positive for premature heart disease: his father suffered a myocardial infarction (MI) at age 57 and succumbed to leukemia at 58. His paternal uncle had a fatal MI at age 52. His mother was alive and well at age 70 without any chronic diseases.

On physical exam his blood pressure was 118/74 mmHg sitting, and 112/70 mmHg supine. Pulse was 74 beats/minute and regular. Height was 5 feet 11 inches, weight 211 pounds, abdominal girth 37 inches, and a BMI of 29.4. He had no systemic evidence of vascular disease. There were no arteriolar venous nicking or soft exudate on fundoscopic exam. Heart exam revealed no murmurs; pulses were all intact without auscultated bruits. Genitourinary exam revealed a normal phallus without plaque and normal testes.

Mr S's laboratories revealed: serum fasting glucose of 116 mg/dL; total cholesterol of 178 mg/dL; triglycerides of 80 mg/dL; HDL-C of 37 mg/dL; and LDL-C cholesterol of 125 ng/dL. Total Chol/HDL ratio was 4.81, suggestive of moderate risk.[9] Total testosterone: 616 ng/dL (normal 300–1000); bioavailable testosterone: 248 ng/dL (normal: 40–49 years: 95–350); sex-hormone binding globulin (SHBG): 32 nmol/L. High-sensitivity C-reactive protein (hs CRP): 3.2 mg/L.

Mr S's case raises several questions:

- Is a history of ED a harbinger for future cardiovascular risk? This is especially of concern given Mr S's family history of premature cardiovascular disease on the male side.
- Are there cost-effective, sensitive, and specific metabolic tests that might indicate increased cardiovascular risk?
- Will these tests delineate treatment based on identification of obstructive coronary artery disease (CAD) and atherosclerotic burden and thereby lower future CVS risk and improve erectile function?

The metabolic syndrome: a cluster of findings increasing the risk of type 2 DM and CVD: its relationship to ED

Metabolic syndrome (MetS) is a complex disorder with high socioeconomic cost that is considered a worldwide epidemic. MetS is defined by a cluster of interconnected factors that directly increase the risk of coronary heart disease (CHD), other forms of cardiovascular atherosclerotic diseases (CVD), and type 2 DM. Its main components are dyslipidemia – elevated triglycerides and apolipoprotein B (apoB)-containing lipoproteins, and low high-density lipoproteins (HDL) – hypertension, and deregulated glucose homeostasis, while abdominal obesity and/or insulin resistance (IR) have gained increasing attention as the core manifestations of the syndrome. Recently, other abnormalities such as chronic proinflammatory and prothrombotic states, non-alcoholic fatty liver disease, and sleep apnea have been added to the syndrome, making its definition even more complex. Besides the many components and clinical implications of MetS, there is still no universally accepted pathogenic mechanism or clearly defined diagnostic criteria. Furthermore, there is still debate as to whether this entity represents a specific syndrome or is a surrogate of combined risk factors that put the individual at particular risk.[10]

The most current definition incorporates the International Diabetes Federation (IDF) and American Heart Association/National Heart, Lung and Blood Institute (AHA/NHLBI) definitions and requires a patient to have any three of the following five conditions:[11]

- Elevated waist circumference (ethnicity specific values, e.g., European males >102 cm (40 in) and females >89 cm (35 in)).
- Triglycerides >150 nmol/L.
- HDL-cholesterol <1.03 mmol/L (<40 mg/dL).
- BP >135/85 mmHg.
- Fasting glucose >5.6 mmol/L (>100 mg/dL).

ED has been linked to multiple selected aspects of the metabolic syndrome, including type 2 diabetes mellitus,[12,13] increased fasting blood glucose,[14,15] arteriosclerotic disease manifestations,[16–18] hypertension,[13,14,19,20] and obesity,[13–15] and to the metabolic syndrome as defined by different health organizations.[14,15,20,21] Moreover, Bal et al.[15] noted that the risk of ED increased in line with the number of MetS factors exhibited by a patient. Several interrelated mechanisms may explain the observed relationship between the MetS and ED. One obvious mechanism could be a low testosterone level, which has been shown to be associated with moderate and severe ED,[22] possibly via a mechanism of diminished NO synthesis.[23] This hypothesis was supported by a report that testosterone treatment increases cavernosal expression of NO synthetase mRNA in rats.[24] In this way, hypogonadism as a manifestation of the MetS could result in diminished NO synthesis and subsequent ED. Another mechanism is peripheral arterial insufficiency due to an atherosclerotic disease. The presence of arterial vasculogenic ED is associated with ischemic heart disease in men over 40 years old in several studies.[25] Furthermore, men with ED are twice as likely to have sustained a myocardial infarction compared with men without ED, and the risk becomes more pronounced with increasing age.[26] Increasing alpha-adrenergic activity has been linked to several established aspects of the MetS, and is an attractive potential mechanism that could explain the link between the MetS and ED. Evidence supporting this mechanism has come from a study demonstrating that patients with non-organic ED have significantly higher sympathetic activity than those without ($p<0.05$).[27] This mechanism has been supported by studies that have concluded that treatment with alpha-receptor antagonists, doxazosin[28] and alfuzosin,[29,30] may improve sexual function including ED. This mechanism is also attractive because it explains the link between ED and lower urinary tract symptoms (LUTS), which was confirmed by the Multinational Survey of the Aging Male (MSAM7) study.[32] This study included more than 14,000 men, aged 50–80 years, representative of the population of six European countries and the United States.[31]

A fourth mechanism explaining the link between the MetS and ED involves increased activation of the Rho/Rhokinase pathway, acting downstream of norepinephrine and endothelin1 receptors. Diabetes and hypertension have been linked to increased activity in this pathway.[28] Increased activity in the Rho/Rho-kinase pathway results in the inhibition of smooth muscle and subsequent smooth muscle contraction.[33] Although this mechanism has not been specifically demonstrated in erectile tissue, it adds to the body of evidence suggesting that ED is also an expression of the MetS and could arise via this mechanism.[34]

There are several hypotheses concerning the mechanism linking the metabolic syndrome and male hypogonadism. Obesity, especially visceral obesity, is an established aspect of the metabolic syndrome. Activity of aromatase, an adipose enzyme that is involved in the irreversible conversion of testosterone into estradiol,[35] is higher in men who are obese and, consequently, they tend to have a decreased testosterone level and increased estradiol level.[35,36] Thus, the MetS provides an endocrine mechanism to explain the development of hypogonadotropic hypogonadism, as it is believed that the effect of estradiol on gonadotropin suppression is more potent than that of testosterone.[37] The findings of Zumoff and colleagues,[38] who treated six obese men with oral testolactone (an aromatase inhibitor), support this conclusion. After 6 weeks, men treated with testolactone had higher levels of testosterone and luteinizing hormone (LH) and decreased levels of estrogen compared with their baseline levels.[38]

The hypothalamic-pituitary-adrenal (HPA) axis provides yet another mechanism that could explain the link between the metabolic syndrome and hypogonadism. The HPA axis has been shown to be overactive in subjects suffering from the metabolic syndrome,[39] and it is well established that cortisol inhibits the reproductive axis at several levels, including secretion of gonadotropin-releasing hormone (GnRH) and LH and also at the level of the testes themselves.[40] This emerging link between the metabolic syndrome and male hypogonadism via increased aromatase activity, hypogonadotropic hypogonadism, and increased activity of the HPA axis seems to suggest that male hypogonadism is also a urological aspect of the metabolic syndrome.

Novel biomarkers (metabolic and imaging) to clarify CVS risk in the ED patient

By definition, cardiac biomarkers are measurement tests that help predict cardiac risk.[41] They include traditional measurements of cardiovascular risk: the lipid panel; blood sugar; and blood pressure. They can include anthropomorphic measurements such as waist circumference (WC), body mass index (BMI), and other measures of visceral obesity. They can include imaging studies such as coronary artery calcification (CAC) as measured by electron-beam computed tomography or computed tomography or carotid intima-media thickness (CIMT) or carotid plaque. They can be surrogate measures of endothelial function such as peripheral arterial tonometry, or serum asymmetric dimethylarginine (ADMA). They can be surrogate measures of arterial inflammation: highly sensitive C-reactive protein (hsCRP), tumor necrosis factor α (TNF-α), adipokines, or interleukin-6 (IL-6). They can measure insulin resistance and include fasting serum insulin, Homeostatic Model Assessment of Insulin Resistance (HOMA-IR), fasting glucose, or glycated hemoglobin A1c (HbA1C). Lastly, they might include the measurement of the extremely atherogenic level of small, dense LDL particles (LDL-P) or apolipoprotein B (apo-B) as measured by nuclear magnetic resonance.

Therefore, a range of important novel risk factors or biomarkers for cardiovascular disease are associated with the MetS, although not yet included within its definition. Most have yet to be validated for efficacy and cost-effective screening in both the asymptomatic or symptomatic ED patient. These include the above noted chronic, low-grade inflammation, and disturbances in the secretion of bioactive substances from adipocytes ("adipokines"),[42,43] hsCRP, apo-B, and vitamin D levels.

The cardiovascular risk factors associated with the MetS, whether included within its diagnostic criteria or not, contribute to the progression of atherosclerotic cardiometabolic disease. Current diagnostic and therapeutic approaches do not adequately address these factors, and further clarification of the utility of these biomarkers in the ED patient is required.

We examine a few non-traditional markers and evaluate the quality of the evidence for their value as potential markers for cardiometabolic disease and, thereby, in the ED patient. These have been graded according to the recommendations of the Centre for Evidence-Based medicine (www.cebm.net). Levels of evidence have been determined by consensus of the authors following review of the present literature.

Waist circumference (intra-abdominal adiposity) (IAA) in men with ED: level of evidence = 1a

Intra-abdominal adiposity (IAA) drives the progression of multiple risk factors directly, through the secretion of excess free fatty acids and inflammatory adipokines, and decreased secretion of adiponectin. The important contributions of IAA to dyslipidemia and insulin resistance provide an indirect, though clinically important, link to the genesis and progression of atherosclerosis and cardiovascular disease.[44–46] Presence of excess IAA is an important determinant of cardiometabolic risk. IAA is associated with insulin resistance, hyperglycemia, dyslipidemia, hypertension, and prothrombotic/proinflammatory states. Excess IAA typically is accompanied by elevated levels of C-reactive protein and free fatty acids (FFAs), as well as decreased levels of adiponectin. Abdominal obesity has been shown to be associated with the inflammation cascade, with adipose tissue expressing a number of inflammatory cytokines. Inflammation is now believed to play a role in the development of atherosclerosis and type 2 DM. Elevated levels of CRP are considered to be predictive of cardiovascular disease and insulin resistance.[46,47]

These components help to explain why excess abdominal adiposity is considered to be a great threat to cardiovascular and metabolic health. Abdominal obesity is associated with multiple cardiometabolic risk factors, including dyslipidemia,[48] elevated blood glucose,[49] and inflammation[41] – all factors leading to the development of CVD and DM in male ED patients. DM is, after age, the greatest risk factor for ED.[2] Patients with DM were three times more likely to develop ED than those who did not have DM.[50,51] The prevalence for ED in these patients was as high as 75%.[52–54] The Cologne Male Survey noted a four-fold increase in ED in men with DM as compared to the general population.[55] In the

Health Professionals Follow-up Study, which involved greater than 30,000 subjects, Bacon et al.[56] found the duration of DM to be strongly associated with the incidence of ED. Rhoden et al.[57] found that higher glycated hemoglobin levels in patients with DM were significantly associated with more severe ED ($p<0.05$). The risk of ED in men with DM is also significantly associated with other diabetic complications such as diabetic neuropathy ($p<0.05$).[58]

Adipocytes generate inflammatory cytokines, and patients with obesity and T2DM tend to have a higher inflammatory profile. Inflammatory markers, such as IL-6,[59,60] TNF-α,[59] or hsCRP,[47] are elevated and have been associated with impaired endothelial function, cardiovascular events, and ED.[60,61]

Testosterone levels and cardiometabolic risk: level of evidence = 2a

Hypogonadism is a common condition in men – especially older men – that can affect both health status and quality of life. Mulligan et al.[62] examined the prevalence rates and odds ratios for selected comorbidities associated with low testosterone levels in 2162 primary care patients. They observed that the odds ratios of having low testosterone levels (hypogonadism is both the presence of low levels and clinical signs and symptoms) were increased in the presence of certain risk factors. The odds ratios for the presence of hypogonadism (the odds of having hypogonadism if one has this risk factor versus not having the risk factor) were 2.38 for obesity, 2.09 for diabetes, 1.84 for hypertension, and 1.47 for hyperlipidemia.[62]

Research to date strongly and consistently shows testosterone replacement therapy (TRT), at least over the short term (up to ~3 years), has positive effects on body composition – decreasing fat mass, and increasing muscle mass – which in turn can reduce the risk for MetS and T2DM.[63] Evidence is moderately consistent for TRT improving bone mineral density. Research to date also is strong in showing that TRT has positive effects on various aspects of sexual function, though the specific effects differ from study to study. Most studies to date showed that TRT increased sexual awareness and arousal, erectile function, and the frequency of spontaneous erections, but was less consistent in enhancing actual sexual behavior and performance.[64] It is beyond the scope of this chapter to address the conflicting issues regarding testosterone and CVS events and mortality. One can simply say that studies thus far, both positive and negative, are cross-sectional and, hence, inconclusive. Yet, the authors feel it is vital to screen all men with ED for testosterone deficiency, and thereby perhaps gain a sense of a man's overall health and stress. This is especially true in those men with a history of inadequate response to prior phosphodiesterase type 5 (PDE5) inhibitors.[65]

CAC potential role in ED management: level of evidence = 1b

Coronary artery calcium (CAC) scores are better than carotid intima media thickness (CIMT), as shown in a cohort of 44,052 asymptomatic patients referred for cardiovascular risk stratification. All-cause mortality rates (MRs) were calculated after stratifying by age groups and CAC score.[66] Another aim was to determine if CAC scoring is independently predictive of mortality in young adults and in the elderly population, and if a young person with high CAC has a higher mortality risk than an older person with lower CAC. Indeed, the value of CAC for predicting mortality extends to both elderly patients and those less than 45 years old. Elderly persons with no CAC have a lower MR than younger persons with high CAC.[66]

In another Multi-Ethnic Study of Atherosclerosis (MESA) subanalysis, Detrano et al.[67] collected data on risk factors and performed coronary calcium scoring in an ethnically diverse population without cardiovascular disease at entry who were followed for a median of 3.8 years. They found that the adjusted risk of a CVD event was increased by a factor of 7.73 among participants with a CAC score of 101 to 300 compared to those individuals with no coronary calcium.[67] This risk increased to 9.67 among those with CAC scores exceeding 300.[67] They noted that CAC scores are a strong predictor of incident CHD and provide predictive value beyond the standard Framingham risk data, regardless of race or ethnicity.

Thus, we propose the use of CAC scoring in men with ED deemed at intermediate risk of CAD according to the Framingham Risk Stratification or in patients with low ACC/AHA risk but who might fall outside the present grading criteria.[8] The absence of CAC is conclusive of minimal to no risk of Atherosclerotic Cardiovascular Disease (ASCVD) in the following 10 years. The presence of CAC may help guide the clinician regarding appropriate primary prevention therapy and certainly is one of the strongest discriminatory tests for the intermediate-risk patient in CVD risk stratification.

The role for peripheral arterial tonometry (PAT) assessment, asymmetric dimethylarginine (ADMA) as markers of endothelial cell function in men with ED: level of evidence = 2a

Because endothelial dysfunction is considered the first step toward the generation of atherosclerotic plaque[68] and can be found in patients with cardiovascular risk factors,[69,70] the use of flow-mediated vasodilation (FMD) has long had a role in the evaluation of the pathology of erectile dysfunction. Indeed, Kaiser et al.[71] studied 30 men with ED and no other clinical cardiovascular disease, and compared them with 27 age-matched controls without ED. The ED group had penile vascular disease present on Doppler ultrasound testing (mean peak systolic flow of 28 cm/s ± 3), an IIEF-5 score of 12.9 versus 22.3 (p=0.000,001) with a cut-off value for ED <21. While no significant differences were noted in fasting lipids, glucose, homocysteine, and CAC scores in the two groups, there was a significant difference in brachial artery flow-mediated vasodilation studies, thereby illustrating the idea that ED appears to occur before the development of overt structural or functional systemic vascular disease, and that abnormalities in the penile cavernosal nitric oxide/cyclic GMP vasodilator system may result in ED as an early clinical manifestation of vascular disease.[72]

This led to the theory that endothelial dysfunction is believed to be the common initiator of ED and other atherosclerotic diseases. The importance of this study cannot be understated. Men with ED but no other clinical cardiovascular disease were found to have reduced flow-mediated vasodilation in the brachial artery in response to sublingual nitroglycerine, indicating endothelial dysfunction and abnormal smooth muscle relaxation. Evidence is accumulating that endothelial dysfunction is an early functional change thought to precede ASCVD changes in the cerebrovascular, coronary, and peripheral circulations.[72]

Obesity is associated with increased activation of the renin-angiotensin system, which in turn leads to vasoconstriction and impaired endothelial function.[73] DM is associated with higher levels of asymmetric dimethylarginine (ADMA).[74] ADMA is an endogenous analog of L-arginine that competitively inhibits nitric oxide synthase (NOS).[75] Elevated plasma ADMA levels signify impaired endothelial cell function[74,75] and predict cardiovascular events.[76–80] A strong link of ADMA to CAD and ED has been reported.[81]

Endothelial dysfunction is characterized by a reduction in endogenous nitric oxide activity, which may be attributed to an elevation in ADMA levels.[82] Thus, it may be speculated that the elevation of endogenous ADMA may be associated with the systemic manifestations of endothelial dysfunction in patients with cardiovascular risk factors and ED.[83]

Vitamin D and cardiovascular health: level of evidence = 2b

Vitamin D is known to have a well-defined role in bone and calcium metabolism, but it has also been implicated as a factor in cardiovascular health. Vitamin D deficiency, defined by the American Endocrine Society as less than 20 ng/mL, of blood affects nearly 50% of the world's population.[84] It has been observed that the incidence of cardiovascular disease increases with increasing distance from the Equator, and correlation with vitamin D deficiency has been proposed as a mechanism.[85] Both the Framingham Offspring Study and the Health Professionals Follow-up Study showed an approximately doubled risk for cardiovascular events in vitamin D-deficient subjects.[86,87] Analysis of retrospectively collected data from 27,686 patients in the Intermountain Heart Collaborative Study Group (IHC) demonstrated that vitamin D levels were highly associated with coronary artery disease and myocardial infarction.[88] In the Multi-Ethnic Study of Atherosclerosis, lower 25 Hydroxyvitamin D concentration was associated with an increased risk for incident coronary artery calcification, a measure of coronary atherosclerosis.[89]

Study of the effects of the vitamin D receptor (VDR) has revealed potential mechanisms for the effects of vitamin D on vascular health. Vitamin D receptors are present in all of the key mediators of atherosclerosis including endothelial cells, vascular smooth muscle cells, and immune cells.[90] Vascular cell growth, migration, and differentiation along with immune response modulation and cytokine expression are tied to activation of the VDR. Vitamin D is also directly involved in the systemic inflammatory response contributing to atherosclerosis.[90] Although interventional studies have not yet shown benefits of vitamin D supplementation in risk reduction, it is clearly evolving as an important marker of risk.

Box 13.2 The follow-up visit of Mr TS.

Mr TS returned to the Center and underwent further studies. A reactive hyperemic index ratio (RHI) evaluation revealed a result of 2.08, suggestive of fair endothelial function. ADMA returned elevated at 0.55 (suggestive of impairment of endothelial function), in the 5th quintile, with a 95% reference range of 0.26–0.67. LDL particle number (LDL-P) was elevated at 1655 nmol/L (optimal <1000) with small LDL-P of 1220 nmol/L (optimal <600), and LDL particle size was 20.4 nm (consistent with the increased risk of small particle pattern B). Repeat LDL-C was 141 mg/dL, HDL-C 33 mg/dL, TG 46 mg/dL, and total cholesterol of 183 mg/dL. A penile Doppler ultrasound study was normal with the left cavernosal arterial systolic velocity of 36.17 cm/s and right cavernosal velocity of 41.93 cm/s, at 60% tumescence following injection with 0.2 mL of a standard tri-mix (papaverine; phentolamine; alprostadil). Repeat hsCRP remained elevated at 4.0 mg/L.

With use of the 2013 ASCVD Risk Estimator, published jointly by the American College of Cardiology (ACC) and the American Heart Association (AHA) to help healthcare providers and patients estimate 10-year and lifetime risks for atherosclerotic cardiovascular disease (ASCVD) using the Pooled Cohort Equations and lifetime risk prediction tools, his 10-year ASCVD risk is 1.9% and 1.0% with optimal risk factors. His lifetime ASCVD risk is 5.0% calculated and 5.0% with optimal risk factors.

His recommendation is not to be in the statin group given a 10-year ASCVD risk <5%, with the following caveat: in individuals for whom after quantitative risk assessment a risk-based treatment decision is uncertain, additional factors may be considered to inform treatment decision-making. These factors may include: primary LDL-C ≥160 mg/dL or other evidence of genetic hyperlipidemias; family history of premature ASCVD with onset <55 years of age in a first-degree male relative or <65 years of age in a first-degree female relative; high-sensitivity C-reactive protein ≥2 mg/L; CAC score ≥300 Agatston units or ≥75 percentile for age, sex, and ethnicity; ankle-brachial index <0.9, or elevated lifetime risk of ASCVD. Additional factors may be identified in the future. (IIb C)

Given Mr TS's repeat laboratories and tests, how might we stratify his cardiovascular risk and make recommendations?

While it is true that Mr TS's penile Doppler studies suggest good penile arterial flow, and that some of his ED may be psychogenic or related to performance anxiety, his elevated hsCRP on two occasions and his elevated LDL-P number are reflective of a greater atherogenic risk, and given his low HDL-C and his family history of premature MI, one could make a case for implementing statin therapy, based on the JUPITER and Inman studies discussed above. In reality, Mr TS has agreed to a 3-month trial of a strict Mediterranean diet and a repeat of his laboratory parameters, a greater commitment to exercise, and psychological counseling with his wife with our clinical psychologist who specializes in sexual therapy.

Most importantly, the use of these novel biomarkers and surrogates begs the question whether this discovery of Mr TS's dyslipidemia is a cause for his ED, and whether modification of his dyslipidemia can improve both his ED and lessen his overall CVD risk? The honest answer is that we do not have clarification of this at present. There remains a disconnect between imaging surrogates and outcomes.

From the above evidence and our experience, we propose the following metabolic investigation of men with ED, including anthropomorphic and vital sign measurements:

- 2013 ASCVD Risk Estimator
- Waist circumference measured at the umbilicus
- Blood pressure/heart rate
- Fasting insulin and glucose levels
- Baseline renal function (BUN/creatinine)
- Fasting lipid profile
- Morning total testosterone level
- hsCRP
- Vitamin D3 (OH)
- If any doubt with use of the 2013 ASCVD Risk Estimator, then CT calcium scoring may clarify risk and treatment options.

The use of biomarkers to define risk

When we examine the use of biomarkers, we must distinguish between screening to define a population at risk that we are not currently treating, or reducing surrogate endpoints (e.g., MI, acute coronary syndrome, stroke). These questions, together with the issue posed by Thompson:[86] "Could erectile dysfunction serve as a surrogate measure of treatment efficacy in preventive interventions for cardiac disease?"[91] can only be answered by further studies of cardiovascular disease prevention strategies in men with largely vasculogenic ED. Men with ED with or without CVS risk factors, should be considered an "intermediate" risk group for future cardiovascular events. It is this group of men, particularly under the age of 60 years, who may benefit from utilization of some of these surrogate markers of cardiometabolic risk in a cost-effective manner to stratify them for subsequent aggressive treatment of preventative cardiovascular risk factors. These men, many of whom may be missed by the traditional Framingham risk criteria, may find the risk elaborated with prudent use of these biomarkers or imaging studies. Only further studies of men with vasculogenic ED and preventative measures will provide evidence as to which of the surrogate markers are impactful and efficacious in the delineation of such risk.

Conclusion

The metabolic investigation of erectile dysfunction involves primarily the investigation of metabolic sequelae of visceral adiposity leading to type 2 DM or CVD. This is known as cardiometabolic risk. Older models of cardiovascular risk assessment (FRS) have generally underestimated risk in younger and middle-aged populations. The authors of the new risk models make adjustments for this and introduce the idea of balancing 10-year risk with lifetime risk to aid in decision-making in younger adults. Whether it is lifetime risk or ED that is used to enhance 10-year risk assessment, the concept is the same: to discern those who have started down the path of inflammation, endothelial dysfunction, and vulnerable plaque formation, and thereby intervene somewhere upstream from the first ASCVD event. Lifetime risk may be something abstract to most patients, and current evidence does not support its use to guide pharmacotherapy. The value is to motivate therapeutic lifestyle changes. ED is something tangible. It affects mental health and quality of life. Young and middle-aged male patients with ED are likely to make changes that will have an immediate impact on both their CVS risk and overall sexual function.

References

1 Hatsimouratidis K, Amar E, Eardley I, et al. Guidelines on male sexual dysfunction and premature ejaculation. *Eur Urol* 2010;57:804–14.

2 Prins J, Blanker MH, Bohnen AM, et al. Prevalence of erectile dysfunction: a systematic review of population-based studies. *Int J Impot Res* 2002;14:422–32.

3 Inman BA, St Sauver JL, Jacobson DJ, et al. A population-based, longitudinal study of erectile dysfunction and future coronary artery disease. *Mayo Clin Proc* 2009;84:108–13.

4 Marma AK, Berry JD, Ning H, et al. Distribution of 10-year and lifetime predicted risks for cardiovascular disease in US adults: findings from the National Health and Nutrition Examination Survey 2003 to 2006. *Circ Cardiovasc Qual Outcomes* 2010;3:8–14.

5 Dhaliwal SS, Welborn TA. Central obesity and multivariable cardiovascular risk as assessed by the Framingham prediction scores. *Am J Cardiol* 2009;103:1403–7.

6 Stone NJ, Robinson J, Lichtenstein AH, et al. 2013 ACC/AHA guideline on the treatment of blood cholesterol to reduce atherosclerotic cardiovascular risk in adults. *J Am Coll Cardiol* 2013. doi: 10.1161/01.cir.0000437738.63853.7a.

7 Nehra A, Jackson G, Miner M, et al. The Princeton III Consensus Recommendations for the Management of Erectile Dysfunction and Cardiovascular Disease. *Mayo Clin Proc* 2012;87(8):766–78.

8 Miner M, Nehra A, Jackson G, et al. All men with vasculogenic ED require a cardiovascular workup. *Am J Med* 2014; 127:174–82.

9 Castelli WP, Abbott RD, McNamara PM. Summary estimates of cholesterol used to predict coronary heart disease. *Circulation* 1983;67(4):730–4.

10 Kassi E, Pervanidou P, Kaltsas G, et al. Metabolic syndrome: definitions and controversies. *BMC Med* 2011;9:48–61.

11 Alberti KG, Eckel RH, Grundy SM, et al. International Diabetes Task Force on Epidemiology and Prevention, National Heart, Lung and Blood Institute, American Heart Association, World Heart Federation, International Atherosclerosis Society, International Association for the Study of Obesity: harmonizing the metabolic syndrome: a joint interim statement of the International Diabetes Task Force on Epidemiology and Prevention; National Heart, Lung, and Blood Institute; American Heart Association; World Heart Federation; International Atherosclerosis Society; and International Association for the Study of Obesity. *Circulation* 2009;120:1640–5.

12 Aslan, Y, Sezgin T, Tuncel A, Tekdogan UY, Guler S, Atan A. Is type 2 diabetes mellitus a cause of severe erectile dysfunction in patients with metabolic syndrome. *Urology* 2009;74:561–5.

13 Saigal CS, Wessels H, Pace J, Schonlau M, Wilt TJ. Predictors and prevalence of erectile dysfunction in a racially diverse population. *Arch Intern Med* 2006;166:207–12.

14 Demir T. Prevalence of erectile dysfunction in patients with metabolic syndrome. *Int J Urol* 2006;13:385–8.

15 Bal K, Oder M, Sahin AS, et al. Prevalence of metabolic syndrome and its association with erectile dysfunction among urologic patients: metabolic backgrounds of erectile dysfunction. *Urology* 2007;69:356–60.

16 El-Sakka AI, Morsy AM. Screening for ischemic heart disease in patients with erectile dysfunction: role of penile Doppler ultrasonography. *Urology* 2004;64:346–50.

17 El-Sakka AI, Morsy AM, Fagih BI, Nassar, AH. Coronary artery risk factors in patients with erectile dysfunction. *J Urol* 2004;172: 251–4.

18 Jackson G. Sexual response in cardiovascular disease. *J Sex Res* 2009;46:233–6.

19 Al-Hunayan A, Al-Mutar M, Kehind EO, Thalib L, Al-Ghorory M. The prevalence and predictors of erectile dysfunction in men with newly diagnosed type 2 diabetes mellitus. *BJU Int* 2007;99:130–4.

20 Tomada N, Tomada I, Botelho F, Cruz F, Vendeira P. Are all metabolic syndrome components responsible for penile hemodynamics impairment in patients with erectile dysfunction? The role of body fat mass assessment. *J Sex Med* 2011;8:831–9.

21 Kupelian V, Shabsig R, Araujo AB, O'Donell, AB, McKinlay JB. Erectile dysfunction as a predictor of the metabolic syndrome in aging men: results from the Massachusetts Male Aging Study. *J Urol* 2006;176:222–6.

22 Corona G. Mannucci E, Ricca V, et al. The age-related decline of testosterone is associated with different specific symptoms and signs in patients with sexual dysfunction. *Int J Androl* 2009;32:720–8.

23 Gorbachinsky I, Akpinar H, Assimos, DG. Metabolic syndrome and urologic diseases. *Rev Urol* 2010;12:157–80.

24 Reilly, CM, Zamorano P, Stopper VS, Mills TM. Androgenic regulation of NO availability in rat penile erection. *J Androl* 1997;18:110–15.

25 Shamloul R, Ghanem HM, Salem A, et al. Correlation between penile duplex findings and stress electrocardiography in men with erectile dysfunction. *Int J Impot Res* 2004;16:235–7.

26 Chen CJ, Kuo TB, Tseng YJ, Yang CC. Combined cardiac sympathetic excitation and vagal impairment in patients with non-organic erectile dysfunction. *Clin Neurophysiol* 2009;120:348–52.

27 Kirby RS, O'Leary M P, Carson C. Efficacy of extended-release doxazosin and doxazosin standard in patients with concomitant benign prostatic hyperplasia and sexual dysfunction. *BJU Int* 2005;95:103–9.

28 De Rose AF, Carmignani G, Corbu C, et al. Observational multicentric trial performed with doxazosin: evaluation of sexual effects on patients with diagnosed benign prostatic hyperplasia. *Urol Int* 2002;68:95–8.

29 Liguori G, Trombetta C, Di Giorgi G, et al. Efficacy of combined oral therapy with tadalafil and alfuzosin: an integrated approach to management of patients with lower urinary tract symptoms and erectile dysfunction. Preliminary report. *J Sex Med* 2009;6:544–52.

30 Kaplan SA, Gonzeles RR, Te AE. Combination of alfuzosin and sildenafil is superior to monotherapy in treating lower urinary tract symptoms and erectile dysfunction. *Eur Urol* 2007;51:1717–23.

31 Rosen R, Altwein J, Boyle P, et al. Lower urinary tract symptoms and male sexual dysfunction: the multinational survey of the aging male (MSAM-7). *Eur Urol* 2003;44:637–49.

32 McVary KT. Lower urinary tract symptoms and sexual dysfunction: epidemiology and pathophysiology. *BJU Int* 2006;97(Suppl. 2):23–8.

33 Faris JE, Smith MR. Metabolic sequelae associated with androgen deprivation therapy for prostate cancer. *Curr Opin Endocrinol Diabetes Obes* 2010;17:240–6.

34 Hammarsten J, Peeker R. Urologic aspects of the metabolic syndrome. *Nat Rev Urol* 2011;8:483–94.

35 Cohen PG Obesity in men: the hypogonadal-estrogen receptor relationship and its effect on glucose homeostasis. *Med Hypotheses* 2008;70:358–60.

36 Vermeulen A, Kaufman JM, Deslypere JP, Thomas G. Attenuated luteinizing hormone (LH) pulse amplitude but normal pulse frequency, and its relation to plasma androgens in hypogonadism of obese men. *J Clin Endocrinol Metab* 1993;76:1140–6.

37 Cohen PG. The role of estradiol in the maintenance of secondary hypogonadism in males in erectile dysfunction. *Med Hypotheses* 1998;50:331–3.

38 Zumoff B, Miller LK, Strain GW. Reversal of the hypogonadotropic hypogonadism of obese men by administration of the aromatase inhibitor testolactone. *Metabolism* 1993; 52:1126–8.

39 Rosmond R, Dallman MF, Björntorp P. Stress-related cortisol secretion in men: relationships with abdominal obesity and endocrine, metabolic and hemodynamic abnormalities. *J Clin Endocrinol Metab* 1998;83:1853–9.

40 Chrousos GP. Stressors, stress, and neuroendocrine integration of the adaptive response. The 1997 Hans Selye Memorial Lecture. *Ann NY Acad Sci* 1998;851:311–35.

41 Billups KL, Kaiser DR, Kelly AS, et al. Relation of C-reactive protein and other cardiovascular risk factors to penile vascular disease in men with erectile dysfunction. *Int J Impot Res* 2003;15:231–6.

42 Gelfand EV, Cannon CP. Rimonabant: a cannabinoid receptor type 1 blocker for management of multiple cardiometabolic risk factors. *JACC* 2006;47(10);1919–26.

43 Vasudevan AR, Ballantyne CM. Cardiometabolic risk assessment: an approach to the prevention of cardiovascular disease and diabetes mellitus. *Clin Conerstone* 2005; 7(2–3):7–16.

44 Rathmann W, Haastert B, Herder C, et al. Differential association of adiponectin with cardiovascular risk markers in men and women? The KORA survey 2000. *Int J Obes* 2007;31:770–6.

45 Yamauchi T, Kamon J, Minokoshi Y, et al. Adiponectin stimulates glucose utilization and fatty-acid oxidation by activating AMP-activated protein kinase. *Nat Med* 2002;8: 1288–95.

46 Snijder MB, Heine RJ, Seidell JC, et al. Associations of adiponectin levels with incident impaired glucose metabolism

and type 2 diabetes in older men and women. The Hoorn study. *Diabetes Care* 2006;29:2498–503.

47 Silvestro A, Brevetti G, Schiano V, et al. Adhesion molecules and cardiovascular risk in peripheral arterial disease. Soluble vascular cell adhesion molecule-1 improves risk stratification. *Thromb Haemost* 2005;93:559–63.

48 Nikoobakht M, Nasseh H, Pourkasmaee M. The relationship between lipid profile and erectile dysfunction. *Int J Impot Res* 2005;17:523–6.

49 Burke JP, Jacobson DJ, McGree ME, et al. Diabetes and sexual dysfunction: Results from the Olmsted County Study of urinary symptoms and health status among men. *J Urol* 2007;177:1438–42.

50 Ponholzer A, Temml C, Mock K, et al. Prevalence and risk factors for erectile dysfunction in 2869 men using a validated questionnaire. *Eur Urol* 2005;47:80–5.

51 Saigal CS, Wessels H, Pace J, et al. for the Urologic Diseases in America Project. Predictors and prevalence of erectile dysfunction in a racially diverse population. *Arch Intern Med* 2006;166:207–12.

52 Fonseca V, Jawa A. Endothelial and erectile dysfunction, diabetes mellitus, and the metabolic syndrome: Common pathways and treatments? *Am J Cardiol* 2005;96:13M–18M.

53 Vinik A, Richardson D. Erectile dysfunction in diabetes. *Diabetes Rev* 1998;6:16–33.

54 Fedele D, Coscelli C, Santeusanio F, et al. for the Gruppo Italiano Studio Deficit Erecttile nei Diabetici. Erectile dysfunction in diabetic subjects in Italy. *Diabetes Care* 1998; 21:1973–7.

55 Braun M, Wassmer G, Klotz T, et al. Epidemiology of erectile dysfunction: Results of the 'Cologne Male Survey.' *Int J Impot Res* 2000;12:305–11.

56 Bacon CG, Hu FB, Giovannucci E, et al. Association and type and duration of diabetes with erectile dysfunction in a large cohort of men. *Diabetes Care* 2002;25:1458–63.

57 Rhoden EL, Ribeiro EP, Riedner CE, et al. Glycosylated hemoglobin levels and the severity of erectile function in diabetic men. *BJU Int* 2005;95:615–17.

58 Gazzaruso C, Pujia A, Solerte SB, et al. Erectile dysfunction and angiographic extent of coronary artery disease in type II diabetic patients. *Int J Impot Res* 2006;18:311–15.

59 Naya M, Tsukamoto T, Morita K, et al. Plasma interleukin-6 and tumor necrosis factor-alpha can predict coronary endothelial dysfunction in hypertensive patients. *Hypertens Res* 2007;30:541–8.

60 Vlachopoulos C, Aznaouridis K, Ioakeimidis N, et al. Unfavourable endothelial and inflammatory state in erectile dysfunction patients with or without coronary artery disease. *Eur Heart J* 2006;27:2640–48.

61 Giugliano F, Esposito K, Di Palo C, et al. Erectile dysfunction associates with endothelial dysfunction and raised proinflammatory cytokine levels in obese men. *J Endocrinol Invest* 2004;27:665–9.

62 Mulligan T, Frick MF, Zuraw QC, et al. Prevalence of hypogonadism in males at least 45 years: the HIM study. *Int J Clin Pract* 2006;60:762–9.

63 Buvat J, Maggi M, Guay A, Octavio Torres L. Testosterone deficiency in men: systematic review and standard operating procedures for diagnosis and treatment. *J Sex Med* 2013; 10:245–84.

64 Miner M, Canty D, Shabsigh R. Testosterone replacement therapy in hypogonadal men: assessing benefits, risks, and best practices. *Postgrad Med* 2008;120(3):130–52.

65 Shabsigh R, Kaufman JM, Steidle C, Padma-Nathan H. Randomized study of testosterone gel as adjunctive therapy to sildenafil in hypogonadal men with erectile dysfunction who do not respond to sildenafil alone. *J Urol* 2004;172(2): 658–63.

66 Tota-Maharaj R, Blaha MJ. Coronary artery calcium for the prediction of mortality in young adults <45 years old and elderly adults >75 years old. *Eur Heart J* 2012;33:2955–62.

67 Detrano R, Guerci AD, Carr JJ, et al. Coronary calcium as a predictor of coronary events in four racial or ethnic groups. *N Engl J Med* 2008;358:1336–45.

68 Cooke JP. The endothelium: A new target for therapy. *Vasc Med* 2000;5:49–53.

69 Lekakis J, Papamichael C, Vemmos C, et al. Effects of acute cigarette smoking on endothelium-dependent arterial dilatation in normal subjects. *Am J Cardiol* 1998;81:1225–8.

70 Higashi Y, Sasaki S, Nakagawa K, et al. Effect of obesity on endothelium-dependent, nitric oxide-mediated vasodilation in normotensive individuals and patients with essential hypertension. *Am J Hypertens* 2001;14:1038–45.

71 Kaiser DR, Billups KL, Bank AL, et al. Impaired brachial artery endothelium-dependent and -independent vasodilation in men with erectile dysfunction and no other clinical cardiovascular disease. *J Am Coll Cardiol* 2004;43:179–84.

72 Shabsigh R. Correlation between erectile dysfunction and metabolic syndrome. In: Sadovsky R (ed.), *Heart of the Matter: Erectile Dysfunction as an Early Sign of Vasculopathy.* Livingston, NJ: CogniMed Inc., 2005; pp. 14–21.

73 Segura J, Ruilope LM. Obesity, essential hypertension and rennin-angiotensin system. *Public Health Nutr* 2007; 10:1151–5.

74 Yamagishi S, Ueda S, Nakamura K, et al. Role of asymmetric dimethylarginine (ADMA) in diabetic vascular complications. *Curr Pharm Des* 2008;25:2613–8.

75 Palmer RM, Ferrige AG, Moncada S. Nitric oxide release accounts for the biological activity of endothelium-derived relaxing factor. *Nature* 1987;327:524–6.

76 Juonala M, Viikari J, Alfthan G, et al. Brachial artery flow-mediated dilation and asymmetrical dimethylarginine in the cardiovascular risk in young Finns study. *Circulation* 2007; 116:1367–73.

77 Ardigo D, Stuehlinger M, Franzini L, et al. ADMA is independently related to flow-mediated vasodilation in

subjects at low cardiovascular risk. *Eur J Clinic Invest* 2007; 37:263–9.

78 Valkonen V, Paiva H, Salonen J, et al. Risk of acute coronary events and serum concentration of asymmetric dimethylarginine. *Lancet* 2001;358:2127–8.

79 Mittermayer F, Krzyzanowska K, Exner M, et al. Asymmetric dimethylarginine predicts major adverse cardiovascular events in patients with advanced peripheral artery disease. *Arterioscler Thromb Vasc Biol* 2006;26:2536–40.

80 Schnabel R, Blankenberg S, Lubos E, et al. Asymmetric dimethylarginine and the risk of cardiovascular events and death in patients with coronary artery disease: Results from the AtheroGene Study. *Circ Res* 2005;97:e53–e59.

81 Maas R, Wenske S, Zabel M, et al. Elevation of asymmetric dimethylarginine (ADMA) and coronary artery disease in men with erectile dysfunction. *Euro Urol* 2005;48:1004–11.

82 Cooke JP. Does ADMA cause endothelial dysfunction? *Arterioscler Thromb Vasc Biol* 2000;20: 2032–7.

83 Kielstein JT, Impraim B, Simmel S, et al. Cardiovascular effects of systemic nitric oxide synthase inhibition with ADMA in humans. *Circulation* 2004;109:172–177.

84 Hollick MF, Binkley NC, Heike BA, et al. Evaluation, treatment, and prevention of vitamin D deficiency: an Endocrine Society Clinical Practice Guideline. *J Clin Endocrinol Metab* 2011;96:1911–30.

85 Judd S, Tangpricha V. Vitamin D deficiency and risk for cardiovascular disease. *Lancet* 1989;1:613.

86 Wallis D, Penckofer S, Sizemore G. The "sunshine deficit" and cardiovascular disease. *Circulation* 2008;118:1476–85.

87 Kuhn T, Kaaks R. Plasma 25-hydroxyvitamin D and its genetic determinants in relation to incident myocardial infarction and stroke in the European Prospective Investigation into Cancer and Nutrition (EPIC)-Germany Study. *Arch Int Med* 2008;168:1174–80.

88 Mullie P, Autier P. Relation of vitamin D deficiency to cardiovascular disease. *Am J Cardiol* 2010;106:963–8.

89 de Boer, I, Kestenbaum B, Shoben A, Michos E, Sarnak M, Siscovick D. 25-Hydroxyvitamin D levels inversely associate with risk for developing coronary artery calcification. *J Am Soc Nephrol* 2009;20:1805–12.

90 Danik J, Manson J. Vitamin D and cardiovascular disease. *Curr Treat Options Cardiovasc Med* 2012;14:414–24.

91 Thompson IM, Tamgen CM, Goodman PJ, Probstfield JL, Moinpour CM, Coltman CA. Erectile dysfunction and subsequent cardiovascular disease. *JAMA* 2005;294: 2296–3002.

CHAPTER 14

Psychological assessment of patients with ED

Catherine Benedict and Christian J. Nelson

Memorial Sloan Kettering Cancer Center, New York, USA

Introduction

It is well established that both physical and psychosocial factors can contribute to the etiology of erectile dysfunction (ED) and that psychogenic components of ED are often present regardless of original etiology. Pre-existing distress and psychological reactions to ED can significantly exacerbate even mild cases of organic disorder and impede treatment compliance and success. The majority of men with ED are ashamed of their condition. Emotional reaction to ED may also include reduced confidence and performance anxiety, loss of masculine identity and self-esteem, ED "bother," and depressive symptoms.[1–3] Men who experience ED may avoid sexual contact because of anxiety that a sexual attempt will ultimately end in failure.[4,5] This avoidance may lead to fewer sexual encounters, loss of intimacy, and emotional distancing with one's partner.[6–10] Over time, sexual problems may erode the quality of intimate relationships and general relationship functioning. Despite the fact that men with all degrees of ED experience some distress, many men do not speak with their doctors about their ED, or only do so when symptoms are severe. A growing body of literature suggests that underdiagnosed and untreated psychosocial factors contributing to ED result in early treatment termination and failure.[11,12] A thorough assessment of biopsychosocial etiological factors and the psychological and behavioral responses to ED is required to develop a comprehensive treatment plan and address potential barriers to treatment success. This chapter will review the psychosocial impact of ED and clinical assessment strategies to obtain relevant information for the treatment of ED.

Psychosocial impact of ED

Anxiety and depression

It is quite common that men with ED have comorbid symptoms of depression and/or anxiety.[13–17] Depressive and anxiety symptoms may have etiological significance or may be in reaction to ED symptoms.[18] In one study of 120 men presenting to a sexuality clinic, 33% had a major current psychiatric disorder, with major depression being the most common.[19] Of note, only about one-third of these men were identified by their urologist as having a mental disorder.[19] In another study of 103 men with ED, 63% had a detectable psychiatric diagnosis, including 25% with depressive disorders, 12% with anxiety disorders, and 7% with depression-anxiety comorbidity.[20]

Anxiety often plays a role in the development and maintenance of ED. Fears of inadequacy may coexist with fears of performance to cause erectile problems. Other fears that contribute to the development of sexual anxieties include excessive need to please partners and demands for performance on the part of the partner.[21] Erectile problems, in turn, may also heighten sexual anxieties due to increased concerns about erectile response and durability leading up to and during sexual encounters.[17] This heightened focus on performance and feeling self-conscious are cognitive distractions that exacerbate problems with arousal and performance.[22,23] Men who are unable to become aroused due to sexual anxieties and experience erectile problems as a result will have greater fears leading up to the next sexual encounter, increasing the likelihood of failure, and reinforcing the pressure to perform during successive encounters. All the while, sexual confidence and esteem

Male Sexual Dysfunction: A Clinical Guide, First Edition. Edited by Suks Minhas and John Mulhall.

are further and further damaged. This results in a vicious cycle of failure and escalating performance anxiety.[17] Ultimately, the anticipation of failure may cause a man to start to avoid sex all together, which may also encompass other aspects of intimacy in his relationship.

Anxiety may also overlap with depression in men with ED. With or without symptoms of anxiety, depression is among the most common comorbid problems in patients with ED.[16,24] The association between ED and depression is bidirectional, in which the two conditions reinforce each other in a "downward spiral."[25] One of the diagnostic criteria of depression is loss of interest in pleasurable activities, including sex. ED, along with loss of libido and orgasm problems, is among the most common sexual complaints among depressed men.[26] The association between ED and depression has been demonstrated in three large, well-designed, population-based studies of aging men in the United States, Finland, Brazil, Japan, and Malaysia.[14,15,27] Data from the Massachusetts Male Aging Study (MMAS) confirm that men (aged 40–70 years) with clinically significant depressive symptoms are nearly two times more likely to report ED compared to their non-depressed peers, controlling for important sociodemographic and medical factors.[25] ED is associated with a higher incidence of depressive symptoms independent of age, marital status, and comorbid medical conditions.[13] Men with depression and ED have lower libido than men with ED alone and are less likely to discuss their ED with their partners.[13,20]

Partner and relationship difficulties

Psychological distress stemming from ED may come from internal expectations and values such as long-held beliefs about manhood and sexual self-concept, or from partner and relationship factors. These may include perceptions of partner expectations regarding sexual ability, level of intimacy in the relationship, and communication around sexual difficulties. Men often feel uncomfortable sharing their feelings about their erectile problems with their partners.[3,28] They may feel shameful and try to conceal their ED, causing further reason to avoid physical closeness and more general intimacy with their partner.[29–31] This can have broad implications for the general functioning of the relationship, cause emotional distancing, increase men's sense of social isolation, and exacerbate psychological distress.

Partners may also want to hold back or avoid discussions regarding sexual changes to "protect" patients from increased distress (i.e., protective buffering). This has been consistently shown among couples coping with ED and the sexual sequelae after treatment for prostate cancer.[28,32] Couples that avoid discussing changes in their sexual relationship have more difficulty adjusting to sexual difficulties and are also more likely to experience more general problems in their relationship. They are less likely to engage in sexual problem-solving, modify sexual practices to accommodate the sexual changes in the relationship, and to explore new ways to maintain sexual satisfaction. For example, among couples coping with ED after prostate cancer, couples' engagement in constructive communication about the sexual changes in their relationship is associated with intercourse satisfaction and overall marital adjustment.[33] Conversely, non-communication regarding sexual changes is associated with increased distress in both partners, emotional distancing and marital tension, reduced likelihood of initiating sexual interactions, and lowered relationship intimacy.[28,33]

Both partners are impacted by the changes that ED may have on their relationship and must adjust to those changes individually and as a couple. Regret and feelings of loss are reported by both men and their partners in the face of sexual dysfunction.[34] Partner and relationship factors are important considerations in assessing men's reactions to ED and the impact ED may have on their psychological well-being and quality of life.

Avoidance

Given the psychological consequences of ED, it is not surprising that many men have difficulty accepting their condition and delay pursuing treatment. Most men place an extremely high value on sexual functioning, and often view the ability to have erections as the core of what it means to be a man. In many ways, ED may be perceived as a threat to a man's identity and sense of self. Men often make excuses for their ED hoping it will improve and often feel shame or embarrassment in pursuing treatments. In fact, research has indicated that as many as 69% of men deny their ED, and the median time to pursue treatment for ED is 2 years.[35] Although the embarrassment related to ED may be mitigated in men whose ED is caused by an alternative medical condition or treatment (e.g., prostate cancer, certain prescription medications), many men still delay seeking treatment hoping their ED will improve spontaneously. Only 50% of men who report an interest in ED treatment actually pursue it.[36] Additionally, a growing body of literature is showing that compliance with ED treatments is poor. Disappointment, shame, and relationship strain may impact men's ability to commit to and sustain the use of medications for ED. Data indicate that 50–80% of men discontinue use of medical interventions (i.e., pills, injections, vacuum devices) for ED within a year.[37,38] Phosphodiesterase type 5 inhibitors (PDE5Is) are used to treat about 90% of men who seek ED treatment; however, despite being a safe and effective treatment, dropout rates are estimated to be 30–50%.[39–41] Although men may discontinue ED treatment for a number of reasons, those who develop a pattern of avoidance may be particularly prone to poor adherence. Avoidance may lead to chronic forms of ED and further prolong or exacerbate the negative effects of ED on emotional and relational well-being.

Psychological assessment of patients with ED

It is important that clinicians treating men with ED take a thorough history to gather information on potential organic as well as psychogenic components of erectile problems. As reviewed, the psychological manifestation of ED often goes beyond mere performance anxiety and may have significant implications for patients' level of distress and well-being, sexual and intimate relationships, and broader psychosocial functioning. The assessment of ED should therefore identify any psychological (patients' and their partners') and interpersonal factors that may be contributing to ED etiology as well as potential sources of resistance, non-adherence, or treatment dropout. Gathering this information will help the clinician to identify potential barriers to treatment, which can then be addressed early to optimize pharmaceutical treatment and restoration of sexual health. The initial history will likely be the most comprehensive part of the psychological assessment. However, follow-up care should involve ongoing assessment of psychological and behavioral responses to treatment. Treatment is improved by adding components of sexual therapy to pharmaceutical treatment and addressing the various psychosocial obstacles that may lead to early dropout.[42] It is also suggested that clinicians assess patients' (and their partners') expectations for treatment and provide pre-treatment education if needed.[30] Using a biopsychosocial model, clinicians should discuss the ways in which biological, psychological, relational, and contextual factors contribute to the onset and maintenance of erectile problems. Rather than focusing solely on ED symptoms, clinicians should address the impact of ED and treatment on the broader sexual experience for men and their partners. This should be based on a shared understanding of realistic expectations for the course of treatment.

It is important to note that these discussions can be difficult for both patients and clinicians. Although some patients may be relieved by the opportunity to discuss their sexual difficulties, others may feel uncomfortable, embarrassed, or anxious.[31] Clinicians should be conscious of not having their questions appear threatening. A discussion may be initiated with a general statement and non-threatening question, such as:

- It is very common for men to experience changes in their sexual functioning (particularly if there is a relevant medical condition such as diabetes). Men may notice that they are starting to have problems maintaining an erection during sex or that the quality of their erections has changed. Is this something that bothers you and would you like to talk about it?

Alternatively, patients may complete a brief questionnaire to assess erectile and sexual problems, such as those reviewed at the end of the chapter. Completing a questionnaire introduces the subject and may make it easier for patients to acknowledge the problem and share information with the clinician without the pressure of a face-to-face conversation or feeling put on the spot.[31] This may also normalize symptomatology, help to organize a man's thoughts regarding his erectile functioning, and introduce appropriate language to use when later speaking with the clinician.

Likewise, clinicians who are inexperienced in taking a sexual history or treating ED may feel ill-prepared to ask specific and intimate questions regarding patients' sex lives. Nonetheless, it is important for clinicians to portray a confident, non-judgmental, and empathetic demeanor to make patients feel comfortable and open to sharing their story.[12] Using a direct approach and specific screening questions to guide patients and elicit necessary information is often helpful. The interview should always be conducted within the bounds of patients' comfort level and with sensitivity to patients' anxieties or reticence. Maintaining a positive therapeutic alliance is the most important aspect of the assessment. The goal is to build a therapeutic relationship based on clear communication and mutual respect.

Depending on whether patients are single or coupled, the format for evaluation and treatment may vary. Most patients will be seen alone; however, if time permits, the clinician may want to ask partners to accompany patients and encourage their participation. This allows partners to provide their perspective and also gives clinicians the opportunity to evaluate couples' interactions. This can provide valuable information regarding relationship functioning and couples' expectations for treatment. However, partner involvement should never be forced and the clinician should defer to the patient's preference. Again, maintaining rapport and building a trusting therapeutic relationship is most important. Men who are in a new relationship or in a relationship that does not feel safe to discuss such topics would most likely be better off seeing the clinician alone. Patients may have a multitude of personal and interpersonal reasons for their preference to either see the clinician alone or as a couple and, at least at first, this should be respected. As treatment progresses and a trusting therapeutic alliance has been established, the clinician may encourage a patient to overcome his initial resistance to including his partner, if there is an important reason to do so. If this is the case, the clinician should first have a good understanding of the patient's initial reasons for not wanting to include his partner to ensure that it would be a safe and beneficial addition to treatment.

Background information and sex history

The assessment of ED will naturally begin with a clear and detailed description of the patient's sexual symptoms and a thorough medical history to determine whether illness or medication is the cause of symptoms. A sex history should be used to obtain information related to potential organic and psychogenic factors connected to erectile problems, and should be a comprehensive assessment of a patient's overall sexual health and relationships.[12] The objective of this evaluation is to identify any predisposing, precipitating, and maintaining factors related to the etiology of ED.[43] This information will give insight into potential psychosocial factors related to ED to be further evaluated as the assessment goes on or later in treatment. An integrated medical and psychosocial history will also provide context to understand the patient's experience of ED within his broader sexual experience and life.[12] From a biopsychosocial approach, Althof and colleagues[44] recommend a comprehensive initial evaluation that not only examines the patient's or couple's sexual history, but also includes current sexual practices, relationship quality and history, emotional or psychological health, and any relevant contextual factors (e.g., young children, financial concerns, cultural beliefs). Similarly, Perelman[12] highlights the importance of taking a thorough assessment of patients' psychological and relational well-being as it relates to sexual experiences and current problems. This includes assessment of proximal ("immediate") and longstanding ("remote") causes of ED.[12] Proximal factors include current cognitions, emotions, and behaviors that maintain sexual problems, whereas longstanding factors refer to more remote causes (predisposing and/or precipitating events).[12] Critical information may be obtained from assessing a patient's developmental history for influences on current sexual functioning (such as sexual or physical abuse).[44] The background and sexual history evaluation should include any previous treatments the patient has sought and outcomes of treatment. Were they successful? Why or why not? This information may give insight into treatment avoidance and barriers to treatment success.

Focused questions may be used to quickly identify potential etiological factors related to ED, which can then be followed up with more probing questions and asking patients to elaborate. Clinicians may ask patients to describe a recent sexual experience, which may readily identify immediate and remote causes of ED such as insufficient stimulation, fatigue, or relationship distress.[12] It is also helpful to ask patients about their beliefs regarding the cause of sexual changes and experience of ED, psychological reactions to ED, and expectations for treatment. This may elicit critical pieces of information that can be used to inform the treatment plan or give insight into potential barriers to compliance. Addressing any factors that could lead to early dropout as early as possible is of course optimal. For example, identifying unrealistic expectations for what treatment will entail and addressing relevant concerns will increase the likelihood of treatment success. Follow-up clinical visits should include constant re-evaluations of any problematic factors identified in the initial visit and monitoring response to treatment with those factors in mind. Problematic factors that are not easily resolved may signal the need to refer the patient to additional services or support such as sex therapy or counseling.

Importantly, a patient may not spontaneously provide information pertaining to the psychological experience of ED or other relational and contextual factors that may turn out to be important. Patients may not perceive such information to be relevant, may be unable to identify or articulate emotional reactions, or may avoid certain topics out of embarrassment or shame.[44] Specific and direct questions can be used to elicit information if the patient is reluctant to spontaneously provide relevant information.

Assessing for ED-related anxiety and depression

Assessment of a patient's psychological function in relation to ED will overlap and be integrated into the sexual history. Depending on the role of the clinician, the extent to which sexual anxieties and depression are evaluated may vary. Urologists, for example, do not usually pursue in-depth assessment of ED-related anxiety or depression, though sex therapists will. Nevertheless, as stated prior, it is important for any treating clinician to have at least a cursory understanding of the roles anxiety and depression are currently playing in maintaining ED. Which psychological factors are leading to distracted thoughts during sexual encounters and either implicitly or explicitly affecting sexual arousal? Likewise, what psychological factors are relevant to treatment compliance and success? Although some clinicians will be interested in obtaining a full history of the predisposing factors that led to the critical anxiety or depressive symptoms causing ED, it is only critical to know and understand the current psychological obstacles that are maintaining the dysfunctional process.[12] Much of this information may be obtained through questions used during the sexual history described above. If not, clinicians should use more pointed questions or standardized assessment tools (described at the end of this chapter).

Negative cognitions related to ED will likely underlie any anxiety or depressive symptomatology that is observed. Assessment of these negative cognitions surrounding ED must be included in the sexual history and psychological assessment. Clinicians should specifically ask patients to describe the thoughts and emotions that occur before, during, and after sexual activity if not spontaneously provided.[12] Clinicians may consider the following questions:

- Does the patient worry about his sexual performance before he is even in the sexual situation?
- Does he engage in negative self-evaluation during or after the sexual experience?
- Do these negative thoughts affect his overall self-concept and esteem in other areas of functioning?
- Do negative thoughts occur with regularity or in particular situations?

It is important to understand psychological processes that are distracting, reduce arousal, and maintain problematic behaviors that affect later sexual experiences. All of these factors may contribute to a cycle of increasing performance anxiety and failure or to a pattern of avoidance. Clinicians should assess whether patients are avoiding sexual activity as a way to cope with distressing or anxiety-provoking thoughts and situations.

Other personality factors may contribute to sexual difficulties, such as fragile self-esteem, fear of being negatively evaluated by others, and higher levels of interpersonal sensitivity.[45] Problematic interpersonal sensitivity (being "too sensitive") is characterized by a chronic tendency to perceive and elicit criticism from others and perceptions of rejection.[46] The clinician will likely pick up on these characteristics as the therapeutic relationship grows without using specific questions. It is beyond the scope of ED treatment to try to change longstanding problematic personality traits, but it is helpful if the clinician is aware of these factors as treatment progresses. If problematic behaviors are causing the patient significant distress or dysfunction in multiple areas of his life, the clinician should make a referral for more general psychological assessment and support.

Assessing for partner and relationship difficulties

Treatment for ED must include an understanding of a patient's sexual relationship(s). Clinicians should ask questions to explore how couples have communicated and coped with sexual changes thus far, and be aware of both partners' expectations for ED treatment and recovery. Questions should assess partners' initial reactions to ED and current feelings.[44] The assessment may be guided by the following questions:

- How does the partner feel about the patient's ED and ED treatment?
- Is the partner upset, angry, or relieved?

- How did the couple try to cope with changes in their sexual relationship initially? Were they successful? Why or why not?

Assessment of these factors will help identify barriers to sexual rehabilitation and may help guide treatment strategies and/or signal a need for referral to additional supportive resources such as couples counseling. Partners often want to be helpful and supportive during this process but may be unsure of how best to be involved and supportive. The degree to which men perceive their partners as being (un)supportive will likely correlate with the degree of distress patients experience related to ED and/or adherence to ED treatment.

Clinicians may want to invite partners to attend a clinical visit to share their perspectives. Partners may be able to provide additional information and important insight about the couples' sexual relationship and relationship dynamics.[44] When partners are present, providers should encourage both patients and partners to ask questions and also to communicate any reservations, concerns, or fears. Supportive partners may be allies for both patients and clinicians to facilitate ED treatment adherence and successful intervention.[44] Alternatively, clinicians may observe unsupportive behaviors or destructive interactions within a couple that can inform the treatment plan. Minor problems may be due to misunderstandings or misinformation and can easily be addressed through education and helpful suggestions by the clinician. Alternatively, the couple may be referred to couples' counseling if relationship problems are more systemic. Importantly, single patients may also benefit from feeling open to discuss their concerns regarding how ED treatment may impact sexual experiences with potential future partners and dating. Both single and partnered men may have fears of rejection or negative reactions from partners. Providing an opportunity for men to discuss their fears can provide insight into patients' expectations, anticipatory anxiety using ED treatments during sexual experiences, or other potential barriers to adherence. The mere opportunity to voice such concerns may be beneficial to patients.

Clinicians should also determine the nature of partners' sexual function:

- Does the partner suffer from low desire, genital pain, or other sexual problem?
- Does the partner miss sexual intimacy?
- Is the partner interested in or motivated to improve their sexual relationship?

This information may identify potential barriers to treatment success and inform the treatment plan. Clinicians may consider educating couples about the use of lubrication, non-penetrative sexual activity, and alternative ways of maintaining intimacy. Couples are better able to adjust to sexual changes in their relationships when there is open, positive communication of mutual respect. Some couples choose to accept the changes caused by ED and are satisfied with non-penetrative sexual activity and alternative ways of maintaining intimacy. However, those couples seeking treatment are motivated to address ED and hoping for recovery. The clinician should encourage couples to discuss their concerns as they progress through treatment and engage in joint problem-solving to adjust to treatments and have satisfying sexual experiences for both partners.

General psychopathology

All patients who present with erectile difficulties should be screened for distress.[12,44] As reviewed, sexual dysfunction may result from depression and anxiety disorders. These should be considered particularly for men with acquired or situational ED.[12] Importantly, the clinician should at least gather enough information to determine whether psychiatric symptoms are the cause or result of the ED.[12] This should be done in a way that does not interfere with rapport.

Depression may be evaluated by asking patients to describe their mood, sleep, appetite, energy, concentration, and outlook on the future. If depressive symptoms are endorsed, the severity of depression should be clarified. Any indication of major depression should be followed by an evaluation of the patient's suicide risk. Again, the clinician should determine whether depression (or antidepressant medications) is causing ED or whether ED is causing depression. Obtaining information on any prior depressive episodes or family history of depression may help clarify these relations. To do this, standardized questionnaires may be useful. Two common questionnaires are the Patient Health Questionnaire-9 (PHQ-9)[47,48] and the Beck Depression Inventory-II.[49] The PHQ-9 is a nine-item measure that was developed specifically for the medical office to screen, diagnose, monitor, and measure the severity of depression in patients. It may be completed by the patient, or by the clinician interviewing the patient. The Beck Depression Inventory is

Table 14.1 Scales that measure anxiety and distress.

Measure of psychological function	Abbreviation	Number of items	Description
Beck Anxiety Inventory[52]	BAI	21	Measures the physiological and cognitive symptoms of anxiety. Discriminates between anxious and non-anxious diagnostic groups and may be used as a screening tool
Beck Depression Inventory II[49]	BDI	21	The most widely used instrument for detecting depression. Measures the intensity of depression in clinical and normal patients including an item that assesses suicidal ideation
Brief Symptoms Inventory – Depression and Anxiety subscales[54]	BSI	6	Designed to measure the psychological function of psychiatric, medical, and normal individuals. The scale includes Depression and Anxiety subscales (6 items each)
Center for Epidemiologic Studies Depression Scale[55]	CESD	20	Measures symptoms that make up diagnostic criteria of a major depressive episode. Designed to be a screening test for depression and depressive disorder
General Anxiety Disorder Questionnaire[51]	GAD	7	Brief screening and assessment tool to measure symptoms of anxiety
Patient Health Questionnaire[47]	PHQ-9	9	Designed to screen, diagnose, monitor, and measure the severity of depression including the presence and duration of suicidal ideation

one of the most widely used measures of depression severity. It is a 21-item measure that can also be used by clinicians as a depression screening tool. Alternatively, Chochinov and colleagues demonstrated that simply asking a patient "Are you depressed?" was at least as effective as using a questionnaire to assess depression.[50]

Anxiety disorders should also be evaluated as a standard part of the assessment. Situational anxiety such as performance anxiety should be distinguished from other anxiety disorders. The assessment of situational or performance anxiety should be assessed first, as stated above; this type of anxiety is frequently present in men with ED. Generalized anxiety disorder may be evaluated by determining whether patients experience shortness of breath, racing heart, decreased concentration, nervousness or agitation, sleep disturbances, and excessive or unrealistic fears. The Generalized Anxiety Disorder 7-item (GAD-7) scale was developed for use in primary care clinics and may be used as a screening tool to determine whether a more extensive assessment is indicated.[51] The Beck Anxiety Inventory may be used to screen and assess the severity of anxiety.[52] It measures both the physiological and cognitive symptoms of anxiety. Additional measures of depression and anxiety are reviewed in Table 14.1.

Making referrals

It is beyond the scope of clinicians treating ED to address longstanding psychopathology or disordered personality traits, though assessment of these factors will give insight into potential psychological and interpersonal causes of ED. Nevertheless, collecting at least cursory information on general levels of distress and mental health history may provide insight into patients' propensity for psychological difficulties, typical coping styles (adaptive vs maladaptive), and effective coping strategies that have been useful in the past and can be encouraged again (e.g., counseling or support groups).

The clinician must determine whether the patient's psychological functioning will permit a focused approach to ED treatment, whether adjunct medical or psychosocial therapy should be started with ED treatment, or whether ED treatment should be postponed until the patient's emotional distress is under control or other conflicting stressors resolve.[12] A mental health counselor or sex therapist may be able to help address underlying psychosocial factors related to sexual difficulties, support the ED treatment plan, and promote good compliance. Of note, patients who believe their ED is purely a medical problem or who fail to recognize their psychological difficulties may object to seeing a mental health counselor at first. This should be normalized and the relation between ED and relevant psychosocial factors should be briefly explained using examples from the patient's own personal and sexual history.

Questionnaires

Self-administered questionnaires and symptom scales may be valuable adjuncts to the assessment of the psychological assessment of ED. Table 14.1 lists some of the most common scales that assess anxiety and depression. A thorough assessment of published scales on male sexual dysfunction has been made by Rosen and Nelson.[53]

References

1 Zaider T, Manne S, Nelson C, Mulhall J, Kissane D. Loss of masculine identity, marital affection, and sexual bother in men with localized prostate cancer. *J Sex Med* 2012;9(10):2724–32.

2 Nelson CJ, Deveci S, Stasi J, Scardino PT, Mulhall JP. Sexual bother following radical prostatectomy. *J Sex Med* 2010;7:129–35.

3 Steidle CP, Stecher VJ, Pace C, Tseng LJ. Correlation of improved erectile function and rate of successful intercourse with improved emotional well-being assessed with the Self-Esteem And Relationship questionnaire in men treated with sildenafil for erectile dysfunction and stratified by age. *Curr Med Res Opin* 2006;22(5):939–48.

4 Hedon F. Anxiety and erectile dysfunction: a global approach to ED enhances results and quality of life. *Int J Impot Res* 2003;15(Suppl 2):S16–9.

5 Graham JW, Hofer SM, Donaldson SI, MacKinnon DP, Schafer JL. Analysis with missing data in prevention research. In: Bryant KJ, Windle MT, West SG (eds), *The Science of Prevention: Methodological Advances from Alcohol and Substance Abuse Research*, 1st edn. Washington, DC: American Psychological Association, 1997; pp. 325–66.

6 Carroll JL, Bagley DH. Evaluation of sexual satisfaction in partners of men experiencing erectile failure. *J Sex Marital Ther* 1990;16(2):70–8.

7 Chevret M, Jaudinot E, Sullivan K, Marrel A, De Gendre AS. Impact of erectile dysfunction (ED) on sexual life of female partners: assessment with the Index of Sexual Life (ISL) questionnaire. *J Sex Marital Ther* 2004;30(3):157–72.

8 Muller MJ, Ruof J, Graf-Morgenstern M, Porst H, Benkert O. Quality of partnership in patients with erectile dysfunction after sildenafil treatment. *Pharmacopsychiatry* 2001;34(3):91–5.

9 Riley A, Riley E. Behavioural and clinical findings in couples where the man presents with erectile disorder: a retrospective study. *Int J Clin Pract* 2000;54(4):220–4.

10 Nelson CJ. The impact of male sexual dysfunction on the female partner. *Curr Sex Health Rep* 2006;3:37–41.

11 Althof SE. Sexual therapy in the age of pharmacotherapy. *Annu Rev Sex Res* 2006;17(1):116–31.

12 Perelman MA. Psychosocial evaluation and combination treatment of men with erectile dysfunction. *Urol Clin North Am* 2005;32(4):431–45.

13 Shabsigh R, Klein LT, Seidman S, Kaplan SA, Lehrhoff BJ, Ritter JS. Increased incidence of depressive symptoms in men with erectile dysfunction. *Urology* 1998;52(5):848–52.

14 Araujo AB, Durante R, Feldman HA, Goldstein I, McKinlay JB. The relationship between depressive symptoms and male erectile dysfunction: cross-sectional results from the Massachusetts Male Aging Study. *Psychosom Med* 1998;60(4):458–65.

15 Shiri RR, Koskimäki JJ, Tammela TLTLJ, Häkkinen JJ, Auvinen AA, Hakama MM. Bidirectional relationship between depression and erectile dysfunction. *J Urol* 2007;177(2):669–73.

16 Perelman MA. Erectile dysfunction and depression: screening and treatment. *Urol Clin North Am* 2011;38(2):125–39.

17 Hedon F. Anxiety and erectile dysfunction: a global approach to ED enhances results and quality of life. *Int J Impot Res* 2003;15(Suppl 2):S16–9.

18 Rosen RC. Psychogenic erectile dysfunction. Classification and management. *Urol Clin North Am* 2001;28(2):269–78.

19 Lee IC, Surridge D, Morales A, Heaton JP. The prevalence and influence of significant psychiatric abnormalities in men undergoing comprehensive management of organic erectile dysfunction. *Int J Impot Res* 2000;12(1):47–51.

20 Mallis D, Moysidis K, Nakopoulou E, Papaharitou S, Hatzimouratidis K, Hatzichristou D. Psychiatric morbidity is frequently undetected in patients with erectile dysfunction. *J Urol* 2005;174(5):1913–6.

21 Barlow DH. Causes of sexual dysfunction: The role of anxiety and cognitive interference. *J Consult Clin Psych* 1986;54(2):140–8.

22 Hale VE, Strassberg DS. The role of anxiety on sexual arousal. *Arch Sex Behav* 1990;19(6):569–81.

23 Beck JG, Barlow DH. The effects of anxiety and attentional focus on sexual responding – II: Cognitive and affective patterns in erectile dysfunction. *Behav Res Ther* 1986;24(1):19–26.

24 Makhlouf A, Kparker A, Niederberger CS. Depression and erectile dysfunction. *Urol Clin North Am* 2007;34(4):565–74, vii.

25 Araujo AB, Durante R, Feldman HA, Goldstein I, McKinlay JB. The relationship between depressive symptoms and male erectile dysfunction: cross-sectional results from the Massachusetts Male Aging Study. *Psychosom Med* 1998;60(4):458–65.

26 Kennedy SH, Eisfeld BS, Dickens SE, Bacchiochi JR, Bagby RM. Antidepressant-induced sexual dysfunction during treatment with moclobemide, paroxetine, sertraline, and venlafaxine. *J Clin Psychiat* 2000;61(4):276–81.

27 Nicolosi A, Moreira ED Jr, Villa M, Glasser DB. A population study of the association between sexual function, sexual satisfaction and depressive symptoms in men. *J Affect Disorders* 2004;82(2):235–43.
28 Boehmer U, Clark JA. Communication about prostate cancer between men and their wives. *J Fam Pract* 2001;50(3):226–31.
29 Dean J, de Boer BJ, Graziottin A, Hatzichristou D, Heaton J, Tailor A. Partner satisfaction and successful treatment outcomes for men with erectile dysfunction (ED). *Eur Urol Suppl* 2006;5(13):779–85.
30 Dean J, de Boer BJ, Graziottin A, Hatzichristou D, Heaton J, Tailor A. Psychological, social, and behavioural benefits for men following effective erectile dysfunction (ED) treatment: Men who enjoy better sex experience improved psychological well-being. *Eur Urol Suppl* 2006;5(13):773–8.
31 Dean J, de Boer BJ, Graziottin A, Hatzichristou D, Heaton J, Tailor A. Effective erectile dysfunction (ED) treatment enables men to enjoy better sex: The importance of erection hardness, psychological well-being, and partner satisfaction. *Eur Urol Suppl* 2006;5(13):761–6.
32 Wittmann D, Northouse L, Crossley H, et al. A pilot study of potential pre-operative barriers to couples' sexual recovery after radical prostatectomy for prostate cancer. *J Sex Marital Ther* 2015;41:155–68.
33 Badr H, Taylor CL. Sexual dysfunction and spousal communication in couples coping with prostate cancer. *Psycho-oncology* 2009;18(7):735–46.
34 Resendes LA, McCorkle R. Spousal responses to prostate cancer: an integrative review. *Cancer Invest* 2006;24(2): 192–8.
35 de Boer BJ, Bots ML, Nijeholt AA, Moors JP, Verheij TJ. The prevalence of bother, acceptance, and need for help in men with erectile dysfunction. *J Sex Med* 2005;2(3):445–50.
36 Salonia A, Abdollah F, Gallina A, et al. Does educational status affect a patient's behavior toward erectile dysfunction? *J Sex Med* 2008;5(8):1941–8.
37 Schover LR, Fouladi RT, Warneke CL, et al. Defining sexual outcomes after treatment for localized prostate carcinoma. *Cancer* 2002;95(8):1773–85 [see comment].
38 Sundaram CP, Thomas W, Pryor LE, Sidi AA, Billups K, Pryor JL. Long-term follow-up of patients receiving injection therapy for erectile dysfunction. *Urology* 1997;49(6):932–5.
39 Huang SA, Lie JD. Phosphodiesterase-5 (PDE5) inhibitors in the management of erectile dysfunction. *P&T* 2013;38(7):407–19.
40 Jiann BP, Yu CC, Su CC, Tsai JY. Compliance of sildenafil treatment for erectile dysfunction and factors affecting it. *Int J Impot Res* 2006;18(2):146–9.
41 Klotz T, Mathers M, Klotz R, Sommer F. Why do patients with erectile dysfunction abandon effective therapy with sildenafil (Viagra)? *Int J Impot Res* 2005;17(1):2–4.
42 Perelman MA. Sex coaching for physicians: combination treatment for patient and partner. *Int J Impot Res* 2003;15(Suppl. 5):S67–S74.
43 McCabe M, Althof SE, Assalian P, et al. Psychological and interpersonal dimensions of sexual function and dysfunction. *J Sex Med* 2010;7(1 Pt 2):327–36.
44 Althof SE, Needle RB. Psychological factors associated with male sexual dysfunction: screening and treatment for the urologist. *Urol Clin North Am* 2011;38(2):141–6.
45 Molton IR, Siegel SD, Penedo FJ, et al. Promoting recovery of sexual functioning after radical prostatectomy with group-based stress management: the role of interpersonal sensitivity. *J Psychosom Res* 2008;64(5):527–36.
46 Stern BL, Kim Y, Trull TJ, Scarpa A, Pilkonis P. Inventory of Interpersonal Problems Personality Disorder scales: operating characteristics and confirmatory factor analysis in nonclinical samples. *J Pers Assess* 2000;74(3):459–71.
47 Kroenke K, Spitzer RL, Williams JB. The PHQ-9: validity of a brief depression severity measure. *J Gen Intern Med* 2001;16(9):606–13.
48 Williams JW Jr, Noel PH, Cordes JA, Ramirez G, Pignone M. Is this patient clinically depressed? *JAMA* 2002;287(9):1160–70.
49 Beck AT, Steer RA, Brown GK. *Manual for the Beck Depression Inventory-II*. San Antonio, TX: Psychological Corporation, 1996.
50 Chochinov HM, Wilson KG, Enns M, Lander S. "Are you depressed?" Screening for depression in the terminally ill. *Am J Psychiatry* 1997;154(5):674–6.
51 Spitzer RL, Kroenke K, Williams JB, Lowe B. A brief measure for assessing generalized anxiety disorder: the GAD-7. *Arch Intern Med* 2006;166(10):1092–7.
52 Steer RA, Beck AT. Beck Anxiety Inventory. In: Wood CPZRJ (ed.), *Evaluating Stress: A Book of Resources*. Lanham, MD: Scarecrow Education, 1997; pp. 23–40.
53 Rosen R, Nelson C. Validated questionnaires in male sexual function assessment. In: Mulhall JP, Incrocci L, Goldstein I, Rosen R (eds), *Cancer and Sexual Health*. Current Clinical Urology series. Humana Press, 2011; pp. 339–49.
54 Derogatis LR. *Brief Symptom Inventory (BSI): Administration, Scoring, and Procedures Manual*, 3rd edn. Minneapolis, MN: NCS Pearson, 1992.
55 Eaton WW, Smith C, Ybarra M, Muntaner C, Tien A. *Center for Epidemiologic Studies Depression Scale: Review and Revision (CESD and CESD-R). The use of psychological testing for treatment planning and outcomes assessment: Vol. 3: Instruments for adults*, 3rd edn. Mahwah, NJ: Lawrence Erlbaum Associates, 2004; pp. 363–77.

CHAPTER 15

Nocturnal penile tumescence study

Chi-Ying Li[1], Stephen Larsen[1], and Tet Yap[2]

[1] *University College Hospital London, London, UK*

[2] *St George's Hospital, London, UK*

Introduction

Nocturnal penile tumescence (NPT) is spontaneous penile tumescence occurring during sleep, and typically associated with rapid eye movement (REM) sleep.

The exact physiological mechanism underlying NPT is not known, but various mechanisms have been hypothesized. These include centrally mediated mechanisms whereby reduction of inhibitory supraspinal control of the spinal pathways during REM sleep (including the noradrenergic neurons of the locus ceruleus, which are inhibitory to penile erection) results in increased NPT.[1]

During REM sleep NPT has been hypothesized to be due to modulation from the lateral preoptic area of the forebrain, which coordinates the spinal erectile mechanism mediated by descending excitation from the paraventricular nucleus and the removal of descending inhibition, as demonstrated by lesion experiments in the lateral preoptic area in the forebrain.[2]

Clinical studies have also pointed to the role of spinal regulation, in showing that the isolated thoracic cord is less effective than the isolated cervical cord in maintaining NPT. Furthermore, despite the presence of NPT, psychogenic or reflexogenic erectile function in spinal cord injured men is significantly impaired.[3]

In contrast to our knowledge of the physiological processes underlying erection at the peripheral level, the physiological process of NPT and its association with REM sleep is relatively unknown.

NPT monitoring was first documented in the 1940 in infants,[4] and subsequently Karacan et al.[5] demonstrated that 80% of NPT occurred during REM sleep. The total NPT peaks at the age of puberty, when tumescence may occur as much as 20% of the total sleep time.

Initially NPT studies were conducted by psychologists to study sleep and dreams; subsequently, NPT has been used to differentiate psychogenic causes of erectile dysfunction (ED) from organic ED.

Indications for NPT monitoring include:[6]

1 Suspected psychogenic ED and to differentiate from organic ED.
2 Non-response to ED treatment therapy, with or without planned subsequent surgical intervention.
3 Excluding causes of ED.
4 Medicolegal.
5 Measurement of drug effects in clinical trials.
6 Suspected sleep disorders.

Investigation

In its classic form, NPT study consists of a nocturnal monitoring device that measures the number of tumescence episodes during sleep, duration of each erection, penile circumference change, and maximal penile rigidity.[7]

NPT has been measured by a variety of methods,[8] including:

1 Stamp test (Barry et al. 1980).
2 Snap gauges (Diedrich et al. 1992).
3 Sleep laboratory nocturnal penile tumescence and rigidity (NPTR).
4 RigiScan® (Endocare Inc., Irvine, CA).
5 NPT electrobioimpedence volumetric assessment (NEVA™; American Medical Systems, Minnetonka, MN; which has now been acquired by Boston Scientific.).

Stamp test

The postage stamp test is a low-cost, simple screening test that can be carried out in the home. Postage

Male Sexual Dysfunction: A Clinical Guide, First Edition. Edited by Suks Minhas and John Mulhall.

stamp(s) are wrapped around the flaccid penis and pasted or fastened at bedtime. If the stamps are found broken in the morning, presumptions are made that nocturnal erection(s) have taken place, whereas lack of such a finding suggests the absence of NPT and thus the cause of ED is presumed to be organic.

The drawback of the stamp test is that it has limited diagnostic value as it only indicates the probable ability to obtain nocturnal erection without any further information on number of episodes, duration of each episode, penile circumference change, or rigidity.

Snap gauges

A similar concept in NPT monitoring is the snap-gauge band. This consists of pre-set snap-gauges with different release-force constants applied around the penile shaft. The ability of the nocturnal tumescence to break the band measures not only the ability to have nocturnal tumescence but also the force/rigidity of the erection.

Previous studies using the snap-gauge band tested simultaneously with recording of nocturnal penile tumescence measuring penile rigidity has demonstrated that the snap-gauge band is relatively reliable and inexpensive compared to the RigiScan® Plus and has a role as a screening device in evaluation of ED.[9,10]

Sleep laboratory nocturnal penile tumescence and rigidity

Traditionally studies of NPT were conducted by psychologists to study sleep/dreams disorders. NPT was measured in conjunction with electroencephalography, electrooculography, and electromyography (EMG) with nasal air flow and oxygen saturation to confirm that patients were in the REM sleep phase. Sleep movement patterns were also monitored as periodic limb movement disorders are associated with abnormal NPT.

The patient is awakened during maximal tumescence and the erection is quantified with measurement of penile axial rigidity using a device applied to the tip of the penis. A buckling resistance of 500 g is considered the minimum force required for vaginal penetration, while a buckling resistance of 1500 g is considered complete rigidity.

Clinicians using NPT studies to differentiate psychogenic from organic ED in a sleep laboratory have used mercury strain gauges to measure NPT. These have a reported accuracy of 85–90%, and measure penile expansion but not rigidity. This can be overcome by direct visual inspection with subsequent measurement of buckling force/axial rigidity.

This method of direct visual monitoring together with NPT study and EEG confirmation of REM sleep is considered the most accurate but also the most expensive method of evaluating NPT.

RigiScan®

RigiScan® was introduced in 1985 as the first apparatus to provide automated NPT measurement. It consists of a small portable recording device that is able to collect data for three nights, for a maximum duration of 10 hours each night. It has the advantage of being performed at home when sleep is more likely to be normal, thus reducing the risks of false-positive NPT tests frequently associated with the laboratory-based NPT studies, where normal sleep may be difficult under an artificial laboratory environment.

The device consists of two loops, one placed at the base of the penis whilst the other is placed at the coronal sulcus. The loops are constricted, thus measuring penile circumference and radial rigidity at both the base and the tip (coronal sulcus).

A measurement is taken for 15–20 minutes with the patient awake to establish the individual's baseline; subsequently the penile rigidity is registered every 3 minutes by constricting the loops, applying a radial compression of 2.8 N. If the base detects a circumference increase of more than 10 mm, sampling is increased to every 30 seconds.

The device combines the measurement of: (i) number of erection episodes; (ii) duration of each event; (iii) penile circumference changes; and (iv) maximal radial penile rigidity.

The range of normal parameters includes:

- Between 3–6[11] and 4–5 erectile episodes per night.[12]
- Duration on average from 10 minutes[13] to 10–15 minutes per erection episode,[11] to a duration of more than 30 minutes in total.[12]
- An increase in circumference of >3 cm at the base and >2 cm at the tip/coronal sulcus.[12]
- A maximum rigidity of >70% at both base and tip/coronal sulcus[12] or rigidity of >60% at the tip/corona sulcus.[13] Rigidity of >70% represents a normal non-buckling erection and a rigidity of <40% represents a flaccid penis.
- Recorded on at least two consecutive nights.[13]

Previous studies have questioned the use of radial rigidity as opposed to axial rigidity as a measurement for erectile function,[14] and the validity of using radial rigidity of greater than 60% as a cut-off of normal. Other study[15] has confirmed that radial rigidity measured by RigiScan® correlated well with axial rigidity. However, when radial rigidity exceeded 60% of maximum, there was a poor correlation between radial and axial rigidity. The RigiScan® failed to discriminate axial rigidities of between 450 and 900g of buckling force, and since traditionally an axial rigidity of 500–550g is considered adequate for vaginal penetration, the RigiScan® may not be able to detect mild abnormalities in erectile function. Therefore using a cut-off of radial rigidity in excess of 60% of maximum should be interpreted cautiously.

Previous studies[16] have found considerable variations in individual responses over three nights in healthy volunteers without a history of ED. Therefore a nomogram has been developed to allow rapid computerized comparison of NPT study results. This utilizes the principle of "area under the curve" measurements,[17] expressed as tumescence activity units (TAU) and radial activity units (RAU). An example of a normal NPT trace is shown in (Figure 15.1) and an abnormal trace is shown in (Figure 15.2).

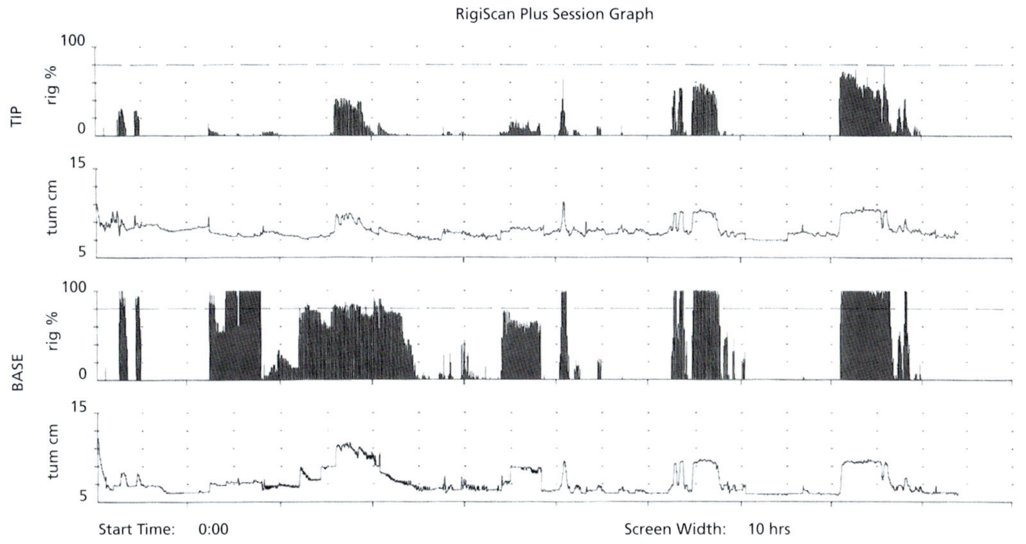

Figure 15.1 A normal NPT trace.

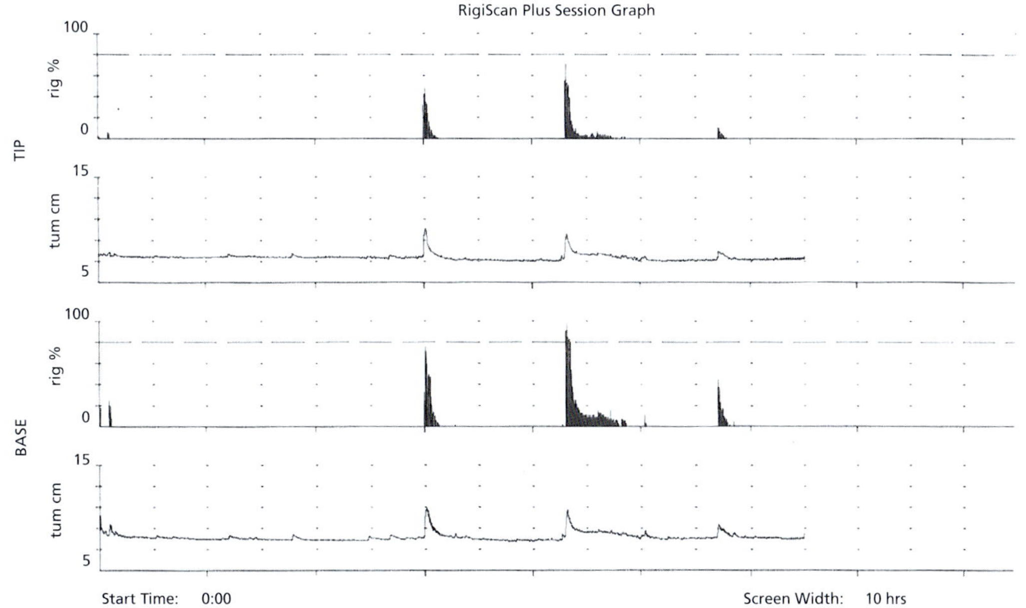

Figure 15.2 An abnormal NPT trace.

NPT electrobioimpedence volumetric assessment (NEVA™)

The newest addition to NPT testing is NEVA™. This measures electrobioimpedance to assess volumetric changes in the penis during NPT. A small recording device is attached to the patient's thigh and three small electrode pads are applied to the hip, the base of the penis, and the glans penis.

An undetectable alternating current is sent from the glans electrode to the hip ground. The penile base electrode measures impedance and changes in penile length: the impedance decreases as the cross-sectional area of the penis increases with nocturnal tumescence.[18]

This has been used to measure parameters of NPT including: (i) number of erection episodes; (ii) duration of each episode; and (iii) changes in penile length and blood volume in both healthy volunteers and patients with ED. The mean volume change in 10 controls was 213%/14.4 mL.

The NEVA™ system can be used to document NPT, but the relationship between volume changes and rigidity needs to be further quantified, although previous study using an erectometer has demonstrated close correlation between penile circumference changes and rigidity.[19]

Conclusion

The main advantage of NPT study is its utility in distinguishing psychogenic from organic ED. The presence of NPT indicates that the neurovascular axis is functionally intact and that the cause of ED is most likely psychogenic. The main disadvantage of NPT studies is their cost, as they are ideally performed with a RigiScan® in a specially equipped sleep laboratory with trained observers.

Due to diagnostic uncertainties associated with various NPT tests, NPT testing is not recommended as a routine part of ED evaluation. Nevertheless, NPT assessment remains the single best non-invasive method to differentiate between organic and psychogenic ED.

References

1 Bancroft J. The endocrinology of sexual arousal. *J Endocrinol* 2005;186;411–27.

2 Mann K, Sohn M. Spontaneous nocturnal erection – physiology and clinical application. *Somnologie* 2005:9;119–26.

3 Suh DD, Yang CC, Clowers DE. Nocturnal penile tumescence and effects of complete spinal cord injury: possible physiologic mechanisms. *Urology* 2003;61(1):184–9.

4 Halverson HM. Genital and sphincter behaviour of the male infant. *J Gen Psycho* 1940;56(1):95–136.

5 Karacan I, Goodenough DR, Shapiro A, Starker S. Erection cycle during sleep in relation to dream anxiety. *Arch Gen Psychiatry* 1966;15(2):183–9.

6 Heaton JP, Morales A. Facts and controversies on the application of penile tumescence and rigidity; recording for erectile dysfunction. In Hellstrom WJG (ed.), *Male Infertility and Sexual Dysfunction*. New York: Springer-Verlag, 1997; pp. 579–92.

7 Kessler WO. Nocturnal penile tumescence. *Urol Clin North Am* 1988;15(1):81–6.

8 Lue, TF and Broderick, GA. (2007). Campbell-Walsh Urology. 9th Edition. Saunders Elsevier. Wein, Alan J. Kavoussi, Louis R. Novick, Andrew C. Partin, Alan W. Peters, Craig A. Ch 22. P763–764.

9 Ek A, Bradley WE, Krane RJ. Nocturnal penile rigidity measured by the snap-gauge band. *J Urol* 1983;129(5):964–6.

10 Mizuno I, Fuse H, Fujiuchi Y. Snap-gauge band compared to RigiScan Plus in a nocturnal penile tumescence study for evaluation of erectile dysfunction. *Urol Int* 2003;71(1):96–9.

11 Levine LA, Lenting EL. Use of nocturnal penile tumescence and rigidity in the evaluation of male erectile dysfunction. *Urol Clin North Am* 1995;22(4):775–88.

12 Cilurzo P, Canale D, Turchi P, Giorgi PM, Menchini Fabris GF. The RigiScan System in the diagnosis of male sexual impotence. *Arch Ital Urol Nefrol Androl* 1992;64 (Suppl 2):81–5.

13 Hatzichristou DG, Hatzimouratidis K, Ioannides E, Yannakoyorgos K, Dimitriadis G, Kalinderis A. Nocturnal penile tumescence and rigidity monitoring in young potent volunteers: reproducibility, evaluation criteria and the effect of sexual intercourse. *J Urol* 1998;159(6):1921-6.

14 Udelson D, Park K, Sadeghi-Nejad H, Salimpour P, Krane RJ, Goldstein I. Axial penile buckling forces vs Rigiscan radial rigidity as a function of intracavernosal pressure: why Rigiscan does not predict functional erections in individual patients. *Int J Impot Res* 1999;11(6):327–37; discusion 337–9.

15 Allen RP, Smolev JK, Engel RM, Brendler CB. Comparison of RigiScan and formal nocturnal penile tumescence testing in the evaluation of erectile rigidity. *J Urol* 1993;149(5 Pt 2): 1265–8.

16 Levine LA, Carroll RA. Nocturnal penile tumescence and rigidity in men without complaints of erectile dysfunction using a new quantitative analysis software. *J Urol* 1994;152(4):1103–7.

17 Burris AS, Banks SM, Sherins RJ. Quantitative assessment of nocturnal penile tumescence and rigidity in normal men using a home monitor. *J Androl* 1989;10(6):492–7.

18 Knoll LD, Abrams JH. Nocturnal electrobioimpedance volumetric assessment of patients with erectile dysfunction. *Urology* 1999;53(6):1200–4.

19 Suzuki K, Sato Y, Horita H, et al. The correlation between penile tumescence measured by the erectometer and penile rigidity by the RigiScan. *Int J Urol* 2001;8(11):594–8.

CHAPTER 16

Psychosexual therapy for male sexual dysfunction

Angela Gregory
Nottingham University Hospital, Nottingham, UK

Introduction

It was not until the 1960s that the pioneering work of Dr William Masters and Dr Virginia Johnson began to expand our knowledge and understanding of human sexual functioning. In laboratory conditions they observed, monitored, and assessed individuals and couples engaging in sexual activity. Their research formed the basis of a model of human sexual response that is still widely accepted today.[1] This model identified four distinct phases and described the physiological changes that occurred in each phase. They believed that sexual difficulties occurred due to breaks in the sexual response cycle, and designed a treatment approach called "sensate focus" to address them.[2] At the time, problems with sexual function were widely believed to be psychological in nature, and perhaps the most frequently used and widely adopted diagnostic criteria for a range of sexual disorders can be found in the *Diagnostic and Statistical Manual of Mental Disorders* (DSM-5).[3]

Beliefs and assumptions about the etiology of erectile dysfunction (ED) dramatically changed with the approval of Viagra (sildenafil) on March 27th, 1998, followed by Cialis (tadalafil) and Levitra (vardenafil) in 2003. As well as enhancing the sexual performance of millions of men around the world, the impact on the pharmaceutical industry and the medical research generated by the launch of these drugs was equally dramatic. This research provided a wealth of knowledge about comorbid conditions such as diabetes and established the link between erectile dysfunction and cardiovascular disease. Whilst the era of the phosphodiesterase type 5 inhibitors (PDE5i) revolutionized the sex lives of men and their partners, some have argued that it also medicalized sexual functioning and led to the psychological/behavioral/interpersonal and contextual aspects of sexual function being ignored.[4] More recently, however, there has been increasing acknowledgment of the multi-faceted nature of erectile dysfunction including the importance of the couple relationship in the success of treatment interventions. As Masters and Johnson stated, "there is no such thing as an uninvolved partner in a relationship where sexual dysfunction exists."[2]

Psychosexual therapy

Sex therapy today is a specialized form of psychotherapy that draws on an array of technical interventions known to effectively treat male sexual dysfunction.[5] It comprises cognitive/behavioral interventions, systems/couple interventions, and sometimes psychodynamic/psychoanalytic interventions. For men with erectile dysfunction, psychotherapeutic approaches combined with oral medication may provide the most comprehensive and promising treatment, regardless of etiology.[6]

A predominantly behavioral sex therapy program comprises of:[7]

- Assessment/history taking (treatment goal)
- Education
- Formulation
- Treatment.

Male Sexual Dysfunction: A Clinical Guide, First Edition. Edited by Suks Minhas and John Mulhall.

Assessment/history

The main focus of assessment/history taking is to identify whether a sexual difficulty is lifelong or acquired, generalized or situational. It focuses on highlighting the relevant predisposing, precipitating ("triggering events"), and maintaining factors. *Predisposing* factors relate to any negative experiences during childhood or teenage years that could make a person vulnerable to developing a sexual difficulty in later life. *Precipitating* factors, or "triggering events," are related to what was happening at the time sexual problems began apparent, for example, redundancy, bereavement, divorce, commencing medication, surgery, or illness. It is important to ask patients what they first noticed, how the sexual problem developed, and the context in which it is experienced. Identifying current *maintaining* factors helps explain why problems persist long after the original *precipitating* event. Asking specific and detailed questions can highlight *maintaining* factors relatively easily and can be employed in a variety of clinical settings. For example, a common *maintaining* factor for men with erectile dysfunction is avoidance of sexual intimacy, which if identified, can be addressed during treatment. It should be noted, however, that in some complex cases therapy or counseling may need to focus on the *predisposing* or *precipitating* events, if emotional issues related to these remain current. Examples could be childhood sexual abuse or bereavement.

Masturbation

Research suggests that many people masturbate, yet its role is often neglected by researchers and healthcare professionals alike.[8,9] Of all the sexual practices it remains one that few enquire about or discuss.[10] Over 20 years ago Perelman reported that in his clinical experience masturbatory frequency and technique were often implicated in difficulties with male sexual desire, erection, and ejaculation and that specific details about masturbation provide a wealth of diagnostic information.[11]

Erectile dysfunction

Questions about masturbation can identify whether a man's ED is situational which helps to diagnose whether it is primarily psychogenic in nature. Accessibility to online hard core pornography can result in high-frequency masturbation and negatively impact on a man's ability to become sufficiently aroused during partnered sex. Some men also masturbate in an attempt to "test out" their erectile responses, paying little attention to feelings of sexual desire or arousal thus leading to further failure.

Premature ejaculation

Asking about masturbatory technique can help identify if a man has learned any control of his arousal during self-stimulation. Questions about speed of stimulation, privacy, and pornography use can help identify factors potentially creating heightened physiological and psychological responses that could "trigger" early ejaculation and highlight whether a masturbatory retraining program would be beneficial. The focus of retraining is to help gain more control of arousal with an emphasis on physiological relaxation and changes to the type and nature of the stimulation. Whether this approach is appropriate due to cultural or religious reasons needs to be established.

Delayed ejaculation

If a man experiences problems with ejaculation during partnered sex, it is essential to find out about his ability to ejaculate during masturbation. If there are no issues with self-stimulation then questions relating to frequency and pornography use need to be asked. Highly arousing material and/or vigorous stimulation can result in a man finding it difficult to achieve similar arousal/stimulation during partnered sex. Asking about masturbatory technique can also identify an idiosyncratic style that includes very specific stimulation or a physical position unlikely to be experienced during sexual intercourse, thus making it difficult to achieve sufficient levels of sexual arousal to facilitate orgasm and ejaculation. Such detail can provide valuable information for inclusion into a masturbatory retraining program.

Relationship

Questions should focus on current levels of affection and intimate or sexual activity. These identify issues of avoidance and provide clarification for the appropriateness of treatment suggestions given to a couple in the form of homework assignments. Those who have experienced long periods of intimate or sexual abstinence generally require more psychological/pharmacological input to re-establish a satisfying sexual relationship, which can takes weeks or even months in some cases.[6]

Exploration of a couple's general relationship can establish whether there is significant relational distress that could impede behavioral and/or pharmacological treatment, and can highlight whether a couple need to access relationship counseling.

Negative behaviors

Negative behaviors can arise as a consequence of sexual difficulties. Common behaviors include apologizing during sexual activity, arguments as the result of failure, avoidance of any intimate or sexual activity, "testing out" erectile responses, and rushing or avoiding foreplay due to the fear that an erectile response will be short lived, which can in turn "trigger" a secondary problem with premature ejaculation (PE). In general, negative behaviors lead to further failure and dissatisfaction, increase performance anxiety, and create relationship distress. Negative behaviors will often contribute to the *maintenance* of sexual difficulties, and explaining their role provides the rationale for behavior change.

Previous treatments

Questions about any previous treatments, psychological or pharmacological, are important. If PDE5 inhibitors have been prescribed, then detailed questions should be asked about which medications were tried, at what dose, how many were taken, the context in which they were used, and what response was achieved. The answers will highlight what needs to be addressed to optimize future success. A lack of education, inadequate dosing, insufficient medication, negative side effects, unrealistic expectations, performance anxiety, or partner's response are some of the many for reasons for failure. In the current climate of the UK's National Health Service (NHS), where cost is often the paramount consideration, the cheapest PDE5i is commonly prescribed. However, several sponsored and non-sponsored studies have investigated whether patient/couples prefer one drug over another once they have been offered the opportunity to try them all over a reasonably long period. A recent literature review (2000–2010) of patients' preference studies concluded 52–65% preferred tadalafil compared to vardenafil (12–20%) and sildenafil (8–30%). The reasons for the preference were mainly due to the longer duration of action and increased spontaneity.[12] Spontaneity reduces performance anxiety as the patient can take a tablet well ahead of any hoped for, expected, or planned sexual activity. Therefore it is essential that patient preference should be taken into consideration.

Medical history

Sexual dysfunction is often multi-factorial therefore it is necessary to identify all *maintaining* factors including organic causes and prescribed medications. As ED and coronary artery disease (CAD) frequently coexist, ED may be an early warning sign for occult CAD, giving a window of opportunity for CAD risk reduction of 2–5 years.[13] There is evidence that regular physical activity and weight loss can significantly improve erectile function, improve the efficacy of PDE5 inhibitors and reduce the risk of cardiovascular diseases/events.[13]

Context

Contextual factors can contribute to or help *maintain* sexual difficulties; examples such as work-related stress, disability, financial worries, shift work, or caring for family members may be relevant. Assessing the impact these have on the individual/couple is important, especially in relation to the quality time a couple have to spend together.

Goal setting

Discussing the goal of treatment allows the therapist to ensure that the outcome the patient expects is realistic and achievable, it also identifies what treatment interventions are necessary and the level of time and motivation required from the individual or couple.

Education

Education is an essential aspect of sex therapy as it helps patients understand how the body works, normalizes some of their experiences, especially around age-/disease-related changes, and highlights possible reasons for unsuccessful pharmacological treatment. It also provides an opportunity to explain the role of performance anxiety, common in both organic and psychogenic erectile dysfunction. Performance anxiety is the fear of future sexual failure based on previous failures; it interferes with sexual arousal, distracts from sensual feelings, undermines sexual self-confidence, and ultimately contributes to sexual avoidance.[14]

Myths and assumptions about sexual performance are perhaps the most negative influences on male satisfaction.[15] Identifying and challenging these myths is an important aspect of the therapy process because it provides an opportunity for discussion about "normal" sexual functioning. Over the past few years there has been an explosion of online hard core pornography that is influencing and educating people about what is "normal" and creating a cultural context to which they aspire and judge themselves against. This presents serious challenges for healthcare professionals and therapists alike.

In the author's opinion providing education as part of the assessment process can sometimes prevent the need for more formal therapy as described below.

Formulation

This has four main purposes:

1. It provides the rationale for the treatment approach.
2. It should provide the couple or individual with further understanding of their sexual difficulties.
3. It can encourage a sense of optimism about the outcome of treatment.
4. It enables the therapist to check that the information obtained during the assessment has been correctly understood.

Treatments

Sensate focus

This is perhaps the most widely known behavioral treatment for sexual dysfunction. It provides:

- A structured approach that allows a couple to rebuild their intimate and sexual relationship gradually, which is important when a couple have not been intimate or sexual for some time.
- Specific techniques for a couple or individual to deal with particular problems.

Depending on the outcome of the assessment process and identification of *maintaining* factors, couples are given specific relaxing/sensual and/or erotic/sexual suggestions to be carried out at home on a regular basis. They are usually asked to abstain from sexual intercourse as this reduces the inhibitory role of performance anxiety and maximizes relaxation and arousal. Ideally therapy should be flexible and creative, giving couples a choice over what they want to do or feel comfortable with. With established couples, finding out what they did together before the onset of the sexual problem is a good way of ensuring that homework suggestions are appropriate for them. With individuals who are in a relationship but whose partner cannot attend, then they should be asked to discuss this approach with their partner.

The rationale for suggesting sensate focus is that behaviors that elicit positive emotions and feelings are likely to be continued and repeated, whilst behaviors that evoke negative emotions and feelings are likely to be avoided.

Erectile dysfunction: case examples using sex therapy techniques

According to DSM-5 Erectile Dysfunction is defined as "the persistent or recurrent inability to achieve and/or maintain an erection sufficient for satisfactory sexual activity that has persisted for at least 6 months, experienced 75%–100% of the time and caused significant distress."[3]

Psychogenic erectile dysfunction

This is a physical problem that is emotional or psychological in origin; performance anxiety related to the "fear of failure" and a loss of sexual self-confidence is the most common cause. Performance anxiety leads to what is described as "spectatoring." This means that during sexual contact the man's focus is on mentally monitoring his performance (or lack of) rather than on pleasure and sexual cues, this detracts attention from the pleasurable aspects of sexual activity, making it difficult to achieve and maintain arousal. From a physiological perspective, anxiety or stress can stimulate the production of norepinephrine/epinephrine, which has an inhibitory impact on sexual arousal.[6]

Case study: The use of psychosexual therapy for a man presenting with psychogenic erectile dysfunction (Box 16.1)

Assessment identified:

Predisposing factors: Lost his erection when he first attempted sexual intercourse aged 16 years. His partner told everyone about it via Facebook; he felt humiliated and ashamed and as a result he stopped socializing and avoided sexual relationships.

Precipitating factors: At 19 years he met his new girlfriend; he couldn't get an erection for sexual intercourse but he had no problems with masturbation. He felt the medication his GP prescribed did not make any difference to his erections but admitted he only tried it on two occasions.

Maintaining factors: Performance anxiety, loss of sexual confidence, his girlfriend gets upset because she

Box 16.1 Case study: James 19 years

- New relationship of 3 months.
- Difficulties gaining and maintaining an erection for sexual intercourse but no difficulties with masturbation.
- Worried his relationship will end because of his erection problem.
- His GP prescribed 4 × sildenafil 50 mg.
- As treatment was unsuccessful his GP referred him to an NHS Psychosexual Clinic.

James said he felt humiliated by his first failure at 16 years and that it prevented him from having another sexual relationship until he met his current girlfriend. He was afraid she would leave him, was constantly worried about his lack of erections, and said he often avoided attempting sexual intercourse. He went to see his GP, who had reassured him that his ED was psychological and prescribed a PDE5i. When the medication didn't work, he felt "useless" and worried there was something seriously wrong. His girlfriend was invited to attend with him but James felt she would be "too embarrassed." His goal was to have successful sexual intercourse.

thinks he doesn't find her attractive, generalized anxiety, masturbatory frequency (four times per day) often with pornography for added arousal.

Preliminary diagnosis: Situational Psychogenic Erectile Dysfunction

Treatment

The nature of psychogenic ED, and the role of performance anxiety and inhibitory function of norepinephrine/epinephrine was discussed, as was the potentially negative impact of his masturbatory and pornography habit. The treatment plan (Box 16.2) was negotiated and a follow-up appointment arranged for 4 weeks hence.

When he returned to the clinic James had not used pornography for 4 weeks although he had masturbated on two occasions. He was getting good erectile responses with his girlfriend but was still very anxious about attempting sexual intercourse. He was prescribed tadalafil 20 mg × 8 as its longer half-life would allow for spontaneity and frequency, both of which were important for James. At his appointment 4 weeks later he was enjoying regular sexual intercourse both with and without medication. He was given a further prescription and a review appointment was booked. The overall aim

Box 16.2 "A Man with a Plan" (4 weeks)

- Discuss plan with his girlfriend.
- Sensate focus – No attempt at sexual intercourse but kissing, cuddling, mutual masturbation, and oral sex included.
- Abstain from masturbation and pornography use.
- Pelvic floor exercises.
- Lubricant.

was to reduce the need for medication as his sexual confidence grew and the role of performance anxiety diminished.

Organic erectile dysfunction

Sex therapy can be useful for men with organic erectile dysfunction if psychological/behavioral/relationship or contextual factors are helping to *maintain* the sexual dysfunction and negatively impact on the success of PDE5 inhibitor treatment. In the case below, diabetes is *likely* to be the primary *maintaining* factor; however, other factors may explain why treatment with PDE5 inhibitors failed, and addressing these during therapy could optimize efficacy.

Case study: Example of the use of psychosexual therapy for a man presenting with organic erectile dysfunction (Box 16.3)

Many men do not try sufficient medication before they cease using it and what they require is better education in order to manage their expectations, encourage partner involvement, and improve the sensual/sexual context. McCullough et al. showed that about one-third of patients need to try at least six to eight doses before they can more accurately assess their response.[16] Similarly the NHS Diabetes Factsheet 33 recommends that men with diabetes should be treated for 3 months or daily dosing for 2 months at maximum dose before being deemed non-responders.[17] This case study also highlights the importance of enquiring about a partner's sexual experience. In women, dyspareunia can be related to a lack of arousal, reduced lubrication, infrequent sexual intercourse, and pelvic floor hypertonicity. However, the most frequent cause in post-menopausal women is vaginal atrophy, which can be treated with local estrogen preparations.[18] For post-menopausal women who are unsuited for local estrogen treatment,

Box 16.3 Case study: Simon 54 years and Kim 49 years

- Diagnosed diabetic 5 years ago.
- CAD risk assessment carried out by GP.
- Simvastatin 20 mg.
- BP 140/80.
- Testosterone 16 nmol/L.
- Unsuccessfully treated with sildenafil, tadalafil, and vardenafil.
- Married for 30 years
- Referred from Urology to an NHS Psychosexual Clinic.

Simon and his wife had not had successful sexual intercourse for 4 years. Kim said he avoided being intimate with her even though she had told him that what she missed most was kissing and cuddling. His GP prescribed sildenafil 50 mg; he tried one tablet, didn't tell Kim, and attempted intercourse without any prior discussion or foreplay. She experienced dyspareunia (painful intercourse) and he lost his erection. He subsequently tried tadalafil 20 mg × 2 with the same results and described himself as a "total failure." His GP had then prescribed him vardenafil 20 mg but he admitted he had yet to try it.

a non-hormonal vaginal moisturizer like Hyalofemme® or Replens™ should be suggested. These products help rehydrate the vagina and can be used alongside lubricant. Silicone/oil-based lubricants such as Sylk, Yes, and TLC make penetration easier and more comfortable.

Assessment identified:

Predisposing factors: Nothing highlighted at initial assessment.

Precipitating factors: Diabetes and medication effects.

Maintaining factors: Diabetes, medication, performance anxiety, loss of sexual confidence, avoidance of intimacy/sexual activity, his masturbatory habit (frequently "testing" out his erectile responses), his wife's experience of dyspareunia during previous attempts at penetration.

Preliminary diagnosis: Secondary Mixed Erectile Dysfunction

Treatment

A treatment plan (Box 16.4) was negotiated and a follow-up appointment arranged for 4 weeks hence.

When they returned to the clinic Simon was getting very good erectile responses during sexual intimacy, he was also experiencing a return of morning erections and

Box 16.4 "A Man with a Plan" (4 weeks).

- Sensate focus – Re-establish intimacy, lots of kissing, cuddling, and touching. But no attempt at sexual intercourse.
- Medication × 2 per week or daily dosing.
- General exercise advice.
- Pelvic floor exercises
- Self-hypnosis CD for confidence.
- Lubricant/vaginal moisturizer discussed with Kim, and medical assessment suggested.

Kim was feeling much happier. It was decided that they would continue with the plan (Box 16.4) for another 4 weeks, but if Simon was feeling sexually confident they would attempt intercourse prior to their next appointment. However, a discussion also took place regarding a strategy for dealing with ED should it recur – that is, they would continue to be loving and intimate with each other and not revert to previous negative behaviors.

These case studies highlight the importance of patient motivation, and a good quality relationship where both partners desire a satisfying sexual life with no barriers preventing them from making use of medical interventions. Men/couples with complex maintaining factors or health issues may require more in-depth psychotherapeutic interventions than the ones described above.

Pelvic floor exercises in treating sexual dysfunction

Pelvic floor exercises were taught in both of the case scenarios, and in the author's clinic this is routine procedure. The four functions of the male pelvic floor are:

- Support abdominal contents
- Maintain urinary/fecal continence
- Allow elimination of urine and feces
- Important role in sexual activity.

Among the multiple factors involved in the presence of sexual dysfunction, the pelvic floor appears to have an important influence, although its exact role is unclear.[19] Contractions of the ischiocavernosus muscles produce an increase in the intracavernous pressure and influence penile rigidity. Rhythmic contractions of the bulbocavernosus muscle propel the semen down the urethra resulting in ejaculation.[20] In a small randomized study carried out by Dorey et al., evidence showed that pelvic floor muscle exercises were significantly effective for some men with erectile dysfunction.[21] Pelvic floor exercises have also been reported in the treatment of premature ejaculation. La Pera and Nicestro published their findings that 61% of patients with PE reported that they were better able to control the ejaculatory reflex after 15–20 sessions of pelvic floor rehabilitation.[22]

Ejaculatory dysfunction

After erectile dysfunction the most common male sexual dysfunction is premature ejaculation, although delayed ejaculation is also common in the author's clinical setting. Medical and therapeutic interventions exist, but there is no first-line treatment for either type of ejaculatory dysfunction, and men should be assessed and treated on a case-by-case basis.

Premature (early) ejaculation (PE)

DSM-5 defines this as "ejaculation which occurs prior to or within one minute of vaginal penetration and an inability to delay ejaculation that has persisted for at least 6 months, occurs 75%–100% of the time and causes significant distress."[3] The International Society for Sexual Medicine 2010 also includes the addition of "avoidance of sexual intimacy" in their definition of premature ejaculation.[23]

Currently a number of selective serotonin reuptake inhibitors (SSRIs) are used off-label in long-term daily dosing regimens to treat PE.[24] In the author's experience the results are variable, with some men experiencing significant improvement whilst others experience little or no improvement and/or unpleasant side effects. In 2013, Priligy (dapoxetine), an SSRI with a short half-life, was licensed specifically to treat PE. In terms of topical treatments a mixture of prilocaine and lidocaine has also been shown to improve ejaculatory latency and control.[25] Pharmacological treatment options should be discussed with patients and considered in conjunction with sex therapy; as there is a general consensus that the latter offers additional benefits for patients with PE.[26] The checklist in Table 16.1 can be useful for identifying some common *maintaining* factors for PE and indicates which behavioral/psychological interventions may be of benefit.

An individualized masturbatory retraining program that takes into account specific details gained during assessment can be suggested. Breathing and pelvic floor relaxation techniques should be taught as these can help men learn more conscious control over their feelings of sexual arousal and excitement.[27]

A masturbatory retraining program for men with PE includes varying physiological and psychological stimulation using a variety of techniques, useful for learning control of sexual arousal during self-stimulation. Once learnt, such techniques can then be applied to controlling arousal during partnered sex.[27] Due to cultural or religious reasons this intervention may not be acceptable or appropriate for some men.

Delayed ejaculation (DE)

The DSM-V defines this as "a marked difficulty or inability to achieve desired ejaculation despite the presence of adequate desire, arousal, and stimulation." The difficulty needs to occur 75–100% of the time, for a period of at least 6 months and cause significant distress.[3] The checklist in Table 16.2 highlights many of the

Table 16.1 Checklist for assessment of premature ejaculation (PE).

Maintaining factors for PE	Behavioral/psychological interventions
Frequency of sexual intercourse	Explore reasons why? Increase frequency? Sensate focus
Pornography use	Reduce or abstain
Masturbatory technique	Masturbatory retraining program
Glans hypersensitivity	Lidocaine, regular massage of glans
Lack of experience and sexual skills	Masturbatory program, sensate focus, time
PE is secondary to erectile dysfunction (ED)	Treatment for ED should be initiated, relaxation techniques, sensate focus
Relationship distress	Couple counseling, sensate focus
Generalized anxiety	Cognitive behavioral therapy (CBT), self-hypnosis, relaxation techniques, yoga, exercise
Withdrawal from opiates	Education and time before considering any of the above

Table 16.2 Checklist for assessment of delayed ejaculation (DE).

Maintaining factors for DE	Behavioral/psychological interventions
Excessive masturbation/pornography use	Reduce or abstain
Idiosyncratic masturbatory style	Masturbatory retraining program
Never masturbated to orgasm/ejaculation	Masturbation program focusing on arousal
Lack of relaxation – "Trying too hard"	General relaxation techniques, sensate focus
Lack of arousal – "Trying too hard"	Experimentation with arousal, stimulation techniques, sensate focus
Consciously/unconsciously slowing down or stopping arousing stimulus during masturbation or sexual intercourse	Speed up stimulation
Problems with retracting foreskin	Encourage movement during self-stimulation, regularly massage foreskin back during washing using water-based emollient or lubricant. If psychological response is phobic avoidance then CBT desensitization may be necessary
Overly focused on a partner's sexual pleasure	Education, explore ways of increasing the man's arousal during sexual intimacy, direct penile stimulation, sensate focus
Psychological factors (fear of pregnancy, guilt, religious/cultural beliefs)	Psychotherapy, counseling, sensate focus
Medication (SSRIs)	Education about medication effects and techniques for increasing arousal, follow-up after reducing or ceasing medication
Alcohol	Reduce or abstain

maintaining factors associated with DE and identifies some possible treatment interventions.

Men who find it difficult to retract their foreskin during masturbation or penetration require a clinical assessment, and those with primary delayed (or absent) ejaculation in all situations should be investigated to exclude any organic causes. However, the most common presentation in the author's clinical practice are men who can orgasm and ejaculate during masturbation but not during partner sex. In such cases, masturbatory frequency, pornography use, or an idiosyncratic masturbatory style are often significant *maintaining* factors. If an idiosyncratic masturbatory style is identified then a masturbatory retraining program can be initiated, which incorporates a position and stimulation that more closely reflects penetration. Retraining takes time and needs to be carried out regularly to challenge the well-established conditioning nature of the previous stimulus. Again, however, this would not be an option for men who do not wish to engage in self-stimulation for cultural or religious reasons, for instance. Other men with DE get into the habit of "trying too hard" to ejaculate during intercourse, which negatively impacts on both relaxation and arousal and establishes a pattern of performance anxiety with similar inhibitory effects to those experienced by men with ED. Clear boundaries about stopping penetration before it becomes "hard work" or uncomfortable for the partner should be discussed, and advice about using manual stimulation to achieve ejaculation inside the vagina could be suggested. The latter is especially important for couples who would like to conceive.

PLISSIT: a sexuality assessment and intervention tool

The goal of healthcare provision is to maintain, restore, or improve a patient's quality of life, and sexual function should be a routine part of that clinical service mandate.[28] Annon's model (Figure 16.1) is a framework for assessing and managing patients with sexual difficulties and provides a structure that can be adapted for use in a range of clinical specialities.[29] It recognizes that different levels of psychological/behavioral and medical interventions are required, and identifies that early intervention may prevent many patients needing more specialist help. In the author's opinion prescribed medical treatments could be included at any level, provided there is time available for an assessment and patient education.

PLISSIT is an acronym for the following:

P: *Permission*. This level is the least complex. Discussing potential sexual changes as a result of illness, disease, medication, cancer, or surgery, gives the patient

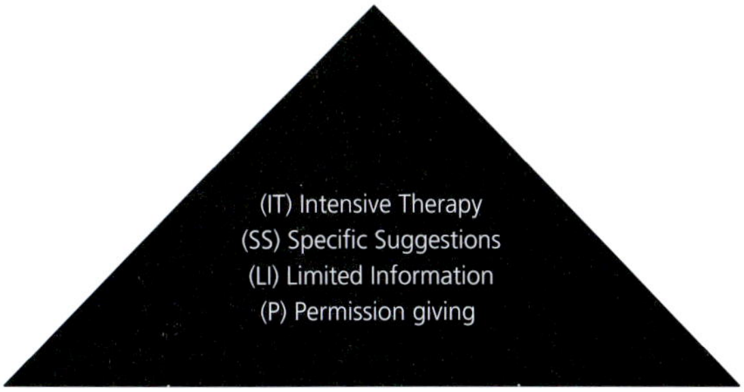

Figure 16.1 Annon's PLISSIT model.

permission to discuss any concerns, and simple reassurance can often be enough. If due to illness or surgery patients are finding sex difficult then *permission* can be given to experiment with new forms of sexual expression, to try different sexual positions, or even, if appropriate, to abstain from sexual activity.

LI: *Limited Information*. Giving limited information provides patients with specific facts directly related to their area of concern. This may relate to how their age, ill-health and/or treatment can affect their sexual abilities, and include basic facts about normal sexual response, and challenge myths and unrealistic expectations about the norms of sexual functioning. Websites could be recommended to enhance the patient's knowledge and understanding.

SS: *Specific Suggestions*. This level of intervention involves providing suggestions that directly address the specific problem presented by the patient. Sexual difficulties with a sudden onset and/or short duration are the most responsive to this form of brief treatment and could include many of the suggestions already mentioned in this chapter, such as lubrication, masturbatory retraining, and pelvic floor exercises. General ideas for rebuilding intimacy such as sitting together watching a film or having breakfast in bed sound simple but can be effective in re-establishing a more intimate relationship. Showering or bathing together can be a non-threatening way of touching each other again if there have been longer periods of sexual abstinence. For couples that have very little quality time together "Staying in Dates" and "Going out Dates" can be discussed. Some people have limited financial resources or young children so it is important for any suggestions to be realistic and affordable. Once specific suggestions have been made a follow-up appointment is necessary to identify the outcome of these suggestions.

IT: *Intensive Therapy*. This final level of intervention is the most complex and is used when a patient's sexual problem has not been resolved by the other three levels. It involves highly individualized therapy that is more involved, takes more time, and should only be undertaken by a suitably trained therapist. If there is no local NHS provision, information about sex therapy and how to access private therapists can be found on the College of Sexual and Relationship Therapy website (www.cosrt.org.uk).

Conclusion

The long-term impact of sexual dysfunction can be devastating for both the individual and their partner; for many men it will rob them of everything they value most, their self-respect, sexual confidence, and the most intimate part of their relationship. Therefore helping men maintain or restore their sexual functioning is not a lifestyle issue but a quality of life issue, and healthcare professionals have a major role in providing an opportunity for early discussion and treatment of sexual difficulties.

References

1 Masters WH, Johnson VE. *Human Sexual Response*. London: Churchill, 1966.
2 Masters WH, Johnson VE. *Human Sexual Inadequacy*. London: Churchill, 1970.
3 American Psychiatric Association. *Diagnostic and Statistical Manual of Mental Disorders*, 5th edn. Arlington, VA: American Psychiatric Press, 2013.
4 Tiefer L. *Sex is Not a Natural Act & Other Essays*. Colorado: Westview Press, 1995.
5 Althof S. What's new in sex therapy? *J Sex Med* 2010;7(1):5–13.
6 Kirana PS, Porst H. Erectile dysfunction. In: Kirana PS, Tripoldi R, Reisman Y, Porst H (eds), *The EFS & ESSM Syllabus of Clinical Sexology*. Amsterdam: Medix, 2013; pp. 596–635.
7 Hawton K. *Sex Therapy A Practical Guide*. Oxford: Oxford University Press, 1993.
8 Laumann EO, Gagnon JH, Michael RT, Michaels S. *The Social Organization of Sexuality*. Chicago: University of Chicago Press, 1994.
9 Gerressu M, Mercer CH, Graham CA, Wellings K, Johnson AM. Prevalence of masturbation and associated factors in a British National Probability Survey. *Arch Sex Behav* 2008;37(2):266–78.

10 Lipsith J, McCann D, Goldmeier D. Male psychogenic sexual dysfunction: the role of masturbation. *J Sex Relat Ther* 2003;18(4):447–71.

11 Perelman MA. Masturbation revisited. *Contemp Urol* 1994;6:67–80

12 Porst H. Erectile dysfunction (ED). In: Porst H, Reisman Y (eds), *The ESSM Syllabus of Sexual Medicine*. Amsterdam: Medix, 2012; pp. 433–533.

13 Jackson G, Boon N, Eardley I, et al. Erectile dysfunction and coronary artery disease prediction: evidence based guidance and consensus. *Int J Clin Pract* 2010;64(7):848–57.

14 Tripodi F, Silvagg C, Simonelli C. Psychology of sexual response. In: Porst H, Reisman Y (eds), *The ESSM Syllabus of Sexual Medicine*. Amsterdam: Medix, 2012; pp. 83–139.

15 Zilbergeld B. *The New Male Sexuality*. New York: Bantam, 1999.

16 McCullough AR, Barada JH, Fawzy A, Guay AT, Hatzichristou D. Achieving treatment optimization with sildenafil citrate in patients with erectile dysfunction. *Urology* 2002;60 (Suppl. 2):28–38.

17 NHS Diabetes Factsheet 33. Diabetes and erectile dysfunction: 'ED is a marker of ill health'. NHS, 2011.

18 Lev-Sagie A, Nyirjesy P. Noninfectious vaginitis. In: Goldstein A, Pukhall C, Goldstein I (eds), *Female Sexual Pain Disorders*. Chichester: Wiley Blackwell, 2009; pp. 105–11.

19 Rosenbaum TY. Pelvic floor involvement in male and female sexual dysfunction and the role of pelvic floor rehabilitation in treatment: a literature review. *J Sex Med* 2007;4:4–13.

20 Dorey G. Male pelvic floor: History and update. *Urol Nurs* 2005;25(4):277–84.

21 Dorey G, Speakman M, Feneley R, Swinkels A, Dunn C, Ewings P. Randomised controlled trial of pelvic floor muscle exercises and manometric biofeedback for erectile dysfunction. *Brit J Gen Pract* 2004;54:819–25.

22 La Pera G. Nicastro A. A new treatment for premature ejaculation: The rehabilitation of the pelvic floor. *J Sex Marital Ther* 1996;22:22–6.

23 Althof SE, Abdo CH, Dean J, et al. International Society for Sexual Medicine's guidelines for the diagnosis and treatment of premature ejaculation. *J Sex Med* 2010;7:2947–69.

24 McCarty EJ, Dinsmore WW. Dapoxetine: an evidence-based review of its effectiveness in treatment of premature ejaculation. *Core Evid* 2012;7:1–14.

25 Dinsmore WW, Wyllie MG. PSD502 improves ejaculatory latency, control and sexual satisfaction when applied topically 5 mins before intercourse in men with premature ejaculation: results of a phase II, multicentre, double blind, placebo-controlled study. *BJU Int* 2009;103:940–9.

26 Althof S. Integrated and combined therapy. In: Kirana PS, Tripoldi F, Reisman Y, Porst H (eds), *The EFS & ESSM Syllabus of Clinical Sexology*. Amsterdam: Medix, 2013; pp. 516–27.

27 Metz E, McCarthy W. *Coping with Premature Ejaculation*. New Harbinger Publications, 2003.

28 Stevenson R, Elliott S. Sexual disorders with comorbid psychiatric or physical illness. In: Balon R. Segraves RT (eds), *Clinical Manual of Sexual Disorders*, 1st edn. New York: American Psychiatric Publishing, 2009.

29 Annon JS. The PLISSIT model: a proposed conceptual scheme for the behavioural treatment of sexual problems. *J Sex Educ Ther* 1976;2:1–15.

CHAPTER 17

Treatment of premature ejaculation and ejaculatory disorders

Michael Kirby
The Prostate Centre, London, UK

Introduction

Premature ejaculation (PE) is an important topic because of the high prevalence and the stress that it causes to both sufferer and partner alike. Other ejaculatory disorders include delayed ejaculation, painful ejaculation and post-orgasmic pain, anejaculation, and retrograde ejaculation.

The first report on PE was in 1887, which was a practical treatise on impotence and sterility and allied disorders of the male sexual organs by S. Gross.[1] Rapid ejaculation is the most common form of male sexual dysfunction, sometimes referred to as ejaculation praecox. The sexual response cycle consists of four different stages: desire, arousal, orgasm, and resolution. In men, the fourth stage of orgasm is usually coincident with ejaculation, and it is disruption of this fourth stage of orgasm that is described as ejaculatory dysfunction.

Definition of premature ejaculation

Many definitions have been proposed for PE, and this has caused problems with understanding the prevalence and epidemiology of the condition. In 1980, the American Psychiatric Association[2] defined the condition as "Ejaculation occurs before the individual wishes because of recurrent and persistent absence of reasonable voluntary control of ejaculation and orgasm during sexual activity." Over subsequent years the definition was revised several times and finally adopted by DSM-IV-TR in 2000[3] as:

- The persistent or recurrent ejaculation with minimal sexual stimulation before, on or shortly after penetration and before the person wishes it. The clinician must take into account the factors that affect the duration of the excitement phase, such as age, novelty of the sexual partner or situation and recent frequency of sexual activity.
- The disturbance causes marked distress or interpersonal difficulty.
- Premature ejaculation is not due exclusively to the direct effects of a substance (e.g., withdrawal from opioids).

This definition has been used as the starting point for most epidemiological studies on PE over the last 10 years.

The International Society for Sexual Medicine (ISSM) produced an evidence-based definition of PE in 2008,[4] describing lifelong PE as:

- A male sexual dysfunction characterised by ejaculation that always or nearly always occurs prior to, or within about 1 minute of, vaginal penetration.
- The inability to delay ejaculation on all, or nearly all, vaginal penetrations.
- Negative personal consequences such as distress, bother, frustration, and/or the avoidance of sexual intimacy.

The 60 second rule is not absolute, since many men will seek treatment for lifelong PE with intravaginal ejaculation latency times (IELT) of up to 2 minutes. Factors to bear in mind are the duration of the excitement phase, age, novelty of the sexual partner, the situation, and the frequency of sexual activity.

Waldinger and co-workers described the IELT in 1994, and it was defined as the time between intravaginal entry and the beginning of intravaginal ejaculation.[5] The stopwatch technique was used by the female partner to measure ejaculation latency time during intercourse in a 4-week period.[6,7] One would think that this would interfere with normal sexual function and be

Male Sexual Dysfunction: A Clinical Guide, First Edition. Edited by Suks Minhas and John Mulhall.

quite intrusive on the relationship, but in research studies, patients do not appear to object to the use of a stopwatch.[8,9]

Defining PE as lifelong or acquired was proposed by Godpodinoff in 1989.[10] The 2010 ISSM guideline for the diagnosis and treatment of PE allows the proposed criteria for lifelong and acquired PE.[11] There are two other important PE syndromes in men who consult with concerns about premature ejaculation.[12–14] It is important to understand these differences in order to tailor advice and treatment (see Table 17.1).

We therefore have four PE syndromes:[15]

- Lifelong PE (LPE)
- Acquired PE (APE)
- Natural variable PE (NVPE)
- Premature-like ejaculatory dysfunction (PLED).

In men with lifelong PE, the ejaculation occurs in most cases within 30–60 seconds (80%) or between 1 and 2 minutes (20%). This occurs from about the first sexual encounter and with nearly every woman with whom sexual intercourse has taken place. Ejaculation occurs too early in nearly every episode of sexual intercourse and remains rapid throughout the lifetime of the subject, suggesting a neurobiological/genetic cause.[15]

In acquired PE, the IELT is short (less than 2 minutes). This syndrome occurs at some point in a man's life and follows normal ejaculation experiences previously. It may develop suddenly or gradually and result from urological or thyroid dysfunctions, or psychological or relationship problems.[15]

In natural variable PE, the ejaculation time may be short or normal. Early ejaculations are inconsistent and irregular. However, the ability to delay ejaculation may be diminished or lacking, giving the impression of reduced control of ejaculation. Psychological support is first-line treatment in these men.[15]

Premature-like ejaculatory dysfunction has been described when the IELT is in the normal range or may even be of longer duration. There is a subjective perception of consistent or inconsistent fast ejaculation. The ability to delay ejaculation may be reduced or absent, and there may be imagined early ejaculation or lack of control of ejaculation. The preoccupation with ejaculation may be accounted for by a psychiatric disorder.[15]

These definitions are helpful from a clinical point of view, because they require different approaches to management.

The prospect that underlying genetic differences may account for PE in certain men is intriguing. There was in 1998 a report of a high PE prevalence among first-degree male relatives of Dutch men with lifelong PE, with an IELT of less than a minute. This generated a hypothesis of a genetic cause for lifelong PE, suggesting a neurobiological cause rather than a psychological one.[6,16] There is, of course, biological plausibility for this explanation.

These first reports were subsequently supported by studies based in Finland. One study by Jern et al. identified male twins between the ages of 33 and 43 years, of whom 91 were identical and 110 complete twin pairs.

Table 17.1 Summary of the symptoms of the four premature ejaculation (PE) syndromes used in the classification of men with complaints of PE.[15]

Lifelong PE (LPE)	Acquired PE (APE)	Natural variable PE (NVPE)	Premature-like ejaculatory dysfunction (PLED)
Most cases (80%) occur within 30–60 seconds, fewer (20%) within 1–2 minutes	Intravaginal ejaculation latency time (IELT) is short (<2 minutes)	Ejaculation time may be short/normal	IELT is normal/longer
Starts from about the first sexual encounter	PE occurs at some point in their life	Early ejaculations are inconsistent and irregular	Subjective perception of inconsistent/ consistent rapid ejaculation
Occurs with almost every woman	Normal ejaculation experienced previously	Ability to delay ejaculation may be diminished/lacking	Ability to delay ejaculation may be diminished/lacking
Occurs too early in almost every intercourse	Onset gradual or sudden	Impression of reduced control of ejaculation	Imagined PE or lack of control of ejaculation
Remains rapid throughout lifetime (neurobiological/ genetic cause)	May result from urological/thyroid dysfunctions or psychological/ relationship problems	Psychotherapy should be considered first-line	Preoccupation not better accounted for by another mental disorder

Results showed a moderate genetic influence (28%) for PE but not on delayed ejaculation.[17]

Further evidence came from another study by Jern et al., where they investigated a large number of male twins ($n = 3946$, mean age 29.9 years) and their siblings. Again, a significant moderate genetic effect was found for PE (28%), but there was no clear-cut familial effect for delayed ejaculation.[18]

There are some common features of men with lifelong PE in both the serotonin-transporter-gene-linked polymorphic region (5-HTTLPR) and the dopamine transporter protein (DAT).[19,20]

When erectile dysfunction (ED) occurs in conjunction with PE it can lead to performance anxiety, and fear of losing the erection can contribute to early ejaculation.[21] It is therefore important to enquire about erectile difficulties in men presenting with PE.

Epidemiology and etiology of premature ejaculation

With varying definitions of PE, it is difficult to evaluate the various prevalence studies. Many studies have been conducted, reporting conflicting results, especially in the primary care setting, with prevalence rates varying between 2 and 31%.[22,23] Nathan reanalysed 22 general population sex surveys to assess the prevalence and distribution of psychosexual dysfunctions as defined by the third edition of the *Diagnostic and Statistical Manual of Mental Disorders* (DSM-III). The prevalence of premature ejaculation was in the order of 35%.[24] Other general population prevalence estimates have reported rates from 4% to 39%, although most estimates fell between 22% and 38%.[25–27]

In the trials that used the DSM-IV-TR (DSM-IV Text Revision) definition, PE has been recognized as the most common male sexual dysfunction, with a prevalence of 20–30%.[28–30] McMahon et al. evaluated 4997 men in the Asia-Pacific countries, of whom two-thirds were younger than 46 years. Self-reported PE was in fact more prevalent than self-reported ED, 13% versus 8%.[31]

There are, of course, physiological, medical, and psychological causes for PE. There has been speculation that the prolongation of intercourse may be a learnt response, since it has been observed how brief intercourse is in animals, particularly under conditions where the animal may be forced to fight or flee from danger.[32] Clearly, lifelong PE is unlikely to have a psychological cause, but the psychological effect is severe and needs to be dealt with.

Studies involving self-stimulation have demonstrated that premature ejaculators continue to reach orgasm in about half the time of those without the problem, and self-reported anxiety was very prominent.[33,34]

Endocrine abnormalities seem unlikely to be involved in the etiology of this problem, but can occur.[35] Neurological disorders commonly cause ejaculatory problems. Interruption of the long spinal tracts between the cortex and the sacral cord or the pelvic autonomic nerves interferes with genital engorgement, erections, ejaculation, and orgasm. Ejaculatory disorders are common in spinal cord injury patients. The absence of ejaculation causes fertility problems and, interestingly, congenital spinal anomalies such as spina bifida can also impair ejaculation. Some men with lifelong anejaculation have been found to have occult dysplasia of the lower spinal cord.[36]

Diabetes leads to ejaculatory problems. It may cause decreased volume of ejaculate or retrograde ejaculation. PE may be related to autonomic neuropathy and both central and peripheral neurotransmitters in diabetes.[37]

Cerebrovascular disease may lead to sexual problems, not only related to injury to the brain but also comorbidities, leading to poor libido, erectile difficulties, and difficulties with ejaculation.[38] The medial preoptic area of the hypothalamus is important for ejaculation due to its relationship with the serotonergic pathways of the nucleus paragigantocellularis (nPGi) in the pons.[6,39]

Penile hypersensitivity and a rapid bulbocavernosal reflex have been postulated as a cause for PE.[40] This hypothesis has been explored by Xin et al.[41,42] and although unproven, it is the basis for the use of topical anesthetics.

Treatment of premature ejaculation

The British Society for Sexual Medicine (BSSM) has produced a useful algorithm for the management of PE (http://www.bssm.org.uk/downloads/).

When developing a treatment plan for this troublesome disorder, it is essential to take a careful patient and partner history to establish the presenting complaint. The time taken to ejaculate after vaginal penetration is important and it is necessary to establish the perceived degree of ejaculatory control. Enquiry should be made about the degree of patient and partner distress caused by the ejaculatory problem. The onset and duration of PE should be established. Underlying psychological causes or problems should be explored, and past medical history and any other current complaints should be established.

A targeted physical examination may be appropriate at this stage, depending on the medical history. For lifelong PE, a physical examination is advisable, but in acquired PE it is mandatory. A genital examination may expose a phimosis or a short frenulum. An examination of the prostate should be performed if the history suggests the need to do so, and likewise bacterial cultures of the urine and/or semen. Evidence of any thyroid disease or neurological cause should be sought.

There are six important questions to help identify PE:

- Can you delay ejaculation before vaginal penetration?
- What is the time between penetration and ejaculation?
- Can you delay ejaculation?
- Do you and your partner feel bothered, annoyed, or frustrated by your PE?
- Is your PE affecting your relationship?
- Do you or your partner avoid sexual intercourse because of embarrassment?

It is also important to distinguish between ED and PE, and the following questions are useful:

- Is your erection hard enough to penetrate?
- Do you have difficulty in maintaining your erection until you ejaculate during intercourse?
- Do you ever rush intercourse to prevent loss of your erection?

Patients with PLED or NVPE often simply require reassurance and education. Sometimes behavioral therapy and psychotherapy may be necessary. When PE is secondary to ED or other sexual dysfunctions, the primary cause should be dealt with. Lifelong and acquired PE can be differentiated by enquiring when the patient first experienced PE and whether he has experienced PE since his first sexual experience on every, or almost every, attempt with every partner?

In APE, treatment initially should be behavioral therapy or psychotherapy followed by, or combined, with pharmacotherapy. In LPE, pharmacotherapy is almost always necessary but added benefit comes from the use of behavioral therapy or psychotherapy in combination. In APE, attempted gradual withdrawal of drug therapy may be appropriate in selected patients after 6–8 weeks (Table 17.2).

The treatment options for pharmacotherapy include oral therapies with a short half-life taken on demand, specifically suggesting a role in treating PE, for example, dapoxetine, which is the only oral licensed selective serotonin reuptake inhibitor (SSRI) medication for the treatment of PE. Off-label SSRIs and tricyclic antidepressant drugs have been used as daily treatments for PE, including paroxetine, sertraline, fluoxetine, citalopram, and clomipramine. The evidence base for using these drugs (off license) was extensively reviewed in the AUA guideline on The Pharmacologic Treatment of Premature Ejaculation 2003.[43]

Phosphodiesterase type 5 (PDE5) inhibitors used on demand as combination treatment with SSRIs can be helpful when PE coexists with ED.[44] Tramadol, an opiate derivative usually used as an analgesic, has also been shown to have efficacy for the treatment of PE and is particularly useful when PE coexists with a need for analgesia.[45] Topical therapies include currently off-label lidocaine/prilocaine.[46]

Behavioral and psychological therapies have been incorporated for a number of years, and studies suggest that combination therapy, as opposed to medication alone, can produce some positive outcomes.[47]

SSRIs when used as daily dosing, produce a therapeutic benefit after 1–2 weeks. A meta-analysis of published data suggests that paroxetine is the most effective, increasing IELT approximately 8.8-fold over baseline.[49] Daily dosing allows for a more spontaneous sexual experience but is, of course, more likely to produce side effects. Side effects observed using daily dosing of paroxetine, sertraline, and fluoxetine were drowsiness (0–13%), nausea (3–22%), dizziness (3–12%), dry mouth (4–19%), ED (4–6%), and anejaculation (3–22%).[50] Concerns have been raised about sperm DNA fragmentation with daily dosing of paroxetine,[51] and currently the advice is to avoid daily dosing with SSRIs in couples wishing to achieve pregnancy. The same advice applies to duloxetine[52] and escitalopram,[53] which have been shown to be effective in treating PE. However, escitalopram has been shown to cause significant decreases in sperm concentration, motility, and morphology when compared with the baseline semen measures.[54]

Dapoxetine is a short-acting SSRI developed principally for the treatment of PE and can be used on demand when taken a few hours before the expected sexual encounter, thereby reducing the possibility of side effects. It is the first drug to be licensed for this

Table 17.2 Treatment options for the management of premature ejaculation (PE).

Treatment	Comment
Sexual/behavioral therapy	• Limited or low efficacy as monotherapy, particularly in LPE • Improves success of PE medications if used in combination
Topical analgesics (lidocaine/prilocaine)	• Good efficacy but risk of over-application and vaginal transfer causing numbness
SSRIs (dapoxetine, paroxetine 10–40 mg, sertraline 50–200 mg, fluoxetine 20–40 mg, citalopram 20–40 mg)	• On-demand dapoxetine has proven efficacy with a 3–4-fold increase in IELT. Common side effects include headache, dizziness, nausea, and diarrhea • Daily dosing with paroxetine provides good efficacy rates, with upto 8-fold increase in IELT. On-demand dosing provides little or no efficacy. Common side effects include yawning, fatigue, perspiration, nausea, diarrhea, ED, and absent ejaculation. Has fertility issues
Tricyclic antidepressants (clomipramine 12.5–50 mg)	• Daily and on-demand dosing have proven efficacy with a 4–6-fold increase in IELT • Common side effects include dizziness, fatigue, nausea, dry mouth, ED
PDE5 inhibitors	• Efficacy not well established in pure PE • Good efficacy in PE + ED either alone or as combination therapy
Tramadol 12 mg, 5–50 mg	• Limited data report a 6-fold increase in IELT • Common side effects include dyspepsia and somnolence • High potential for addiction
Alpha1-adrenoreceptor agonists (tamsulosin, silodosin, terazosin)	• Very limited data report success rates of upto 50% • High potential for anejaculation
Combination therapies (PDE5 inhibitor + dapoxetine/off-label SSRI or topical lidocaine/prilocaine)	• Superior efficacy reported with PDE5 inhibitor + SSRI vs either as monotherapy • Superior efficacy reported with PDE5 inhibitor + topical lidocaine/prilocaine vs either as monotherapy
Management of PE-related risk factors (hyperthyroidism and bacterial prostatitis)	• PE improves with normalization of thyroid hormones or antibiotic treatment of bacterial prostatitis

Adapted from Kirana et al.[48]

indication. A review by Hutchinson et al. concluded that dapoxetine is well tolerated as an on-demand therapy and with continual dosing, but there are few data regarding long-term adverse events. There were reports in the development program that there were rare vasovagal-mediated syncopal events, but there were no other associated significant cardiovascular adverse events.[55] With a starting dose of 30 mg, clinicians have not found this to be an issue at the current time.

Tramadol is used widely as an analgesic and has been shown to be effective in the management of PE. A meta-analysis identified five trials involving 715 patients,[56] and the authors concluded that tramadol may be effective in PE treatment, especially when patients have failed therapies similar to the chronic use of SSRIs. It is not licensed for this indication and addiction to this drug needs to be borne in mind, as well as the side-effect profile, and hence it should only be used as a last resort in difficult patients.

If there is ED as well as PE, treatment of the ED with a PDE5 inhibitor should be prescribed first, followed by secondary PE treatment after 2–3 months if needed. Regarding the combination of PDE5 inhibitors and dapoxetine, pharmacokinetic studies have shown that adding sildenafil or tadalafil to dapoxetine does not alter the pharmacokinetics of either drug.[57]

Topical anesthetics are useful in some patients. They contain lidocaine or a combination of lidocaine and prilocaine in a spray, ointment, or cream preparation. They are sometimes used within condoms and sold as over-the-counter (OTC) products. The role of these agents in PE has been reviewed by Wylie and Powell, who concluded that they could be an acceptable first-line option. However, they are not licensed for this indication and can cause numbness of the glans and penile skin, and there may also be some transvaginal absorption and numbness if the medication is not removed prior to coitus. The creams and gels need to be applied 10–20 minutes before sexual intercourse.[58]

Recently a new lidocaine-prilocaine-containing spray (TEMPE/Fortacin) has been investigated,[58] which only needs to be applied 5 minutes before sexual intercourse.

It has been shown to increase the IELT from a baseline of 0.58 minutes to 3.17 minutes during 3 months of double-blind treatment. There was a 3.3-fold delay in ejaculation compared to placebo ($p<0.001$), and this formulation has been approved by the EMA.

Anejaculation

Anejaculation is the complete absence of antegrade or retrograde ejaculation. It is caused by failure of emission of semen from the prostate and seminal ducts into the urethra.[59] Anejaculation is usually associated with a normal orgasmic sensation. Occasionally, for example in incomplete spinal cord injuries, this sensation may be altered or decreased. True anejaculation is caused by central or peripheral nervous system dysfunctions or the effect of drugs. Neural causes include spinal cord injury, cauda equina lesions, multiple sclerosis, Parkinson's disease, autonomic neuropathy (juvenile diabetes), retroperitoneal lymphadenectomy, aortoiliac surgery, and colorectal surgery. Drug-related anejaculation is associated with the use of antihypertensives, antidepressants, antipsychotics, and alcoho.[60]

Sexual dysfunction after radical prostatectomy occurs commonly. It is well understood that concomitant surgical removal of the seminal vesicles along with the prostate produces a "dry" orgasm and that most men retain the ability to achieve a sexual climax.

In anejaculation it is possible to evoke the ejaculation reflex with penile vibratory stimulation.[61] Assisted reproductive technologies have improved so much over the last few years that infertility issues can usually be solved.

Delayed ejaculation

Delayed or retarded ejaculation is much less common. It is important to determine whether it is lifelong or acquired, and whether it is generalized or situational. Prevalence is less than 3%.[62] There may be anatomical or congenital causes. Other causes include neurogenic, infective, endocrine, and drugs that interfere with either the central control of ejaculation or the nerves that supply the reproductive organs. There are also psychological causes that need to be taken into consideration (Table 17.3).

The British Association of Sexual Health and HIV (BASHH) Special Interest Group for Sexual Dysfunction has provided some helpful recommendations for the management of retarded ejaculation.[63] A variety of drugs have been used to facilitate SSRI-induced retarded ejaculation by either central dopaminergic or antiserotonergic effects[63] (Table 17.4).

Table 17.3 Causes of retarded ejaculation.[63]

Physiological	Reduced penile sensitivity
	Slower bulbocavernosal reflexes
	Idiosyncratic genital stimulation
Congenital	Müllerian duct cyst
	Wolffian duct abnormality
	Prune belly syndrome
Anatomical	Transurethral resection of prostate (TURP)
	Bladder neck incision
Neurological	Spinal cord injury
	Diabetic neuropathy
	Radical prostatectomy
	Proctocolectomy
	Bilateral sympathectomy
	Abdominal aortic aneurysmectomy
	Para-aortic lymphadenectomy
Endocrine	Hypogonadism
	Hypothyroidism
	Diabetes
Drugs	Alpha blockers
	Beta blockers
	Adrenergic neuron blockers
	Antipsychotics
	Tricyclic antidepressants
	Atypical antidepressants (e.g. trazodone)
	Benzodiazepines
	Opiates
	SSRIs
	Thiazides
	Monoamine oxidase inhibitors
	Naproxen
	Baclofen
	Alcohol
Psychological	Psychosocial

Table 17.4 Adjunctive pharmacotherapy for SSRI-induced retarded ejaculation.[64]

Drug	As required	Daily
Amantadine	100–400 mg (for 2 days before coitus)	75–100 mg b.d. or t.d.s.
Bupropion	75–150 mg	75 mg b.d. or t.d.s.
Buspirone	15–60 mg	5–15 mg b.d.
Cyproheptadine	4–12 mg	On demand
Yohimbine	5–10 mg	5 mg t.d.s.

It is important to identify a treatable organic cause if it is present or withdraw a drug if it is known to impair ejaculatory dysfunction. Following this, the mainstay of treatment would be by psychotherapy, but drug therapy can be tried on an individual basis.

Retrograde ejaculation

Antegrade ejaculation requires a closed bladder neck and proximal urethra, and when this mechanism fails related to anatomical, neurological, pharmacological, or idiopathic factors, ejaculation occurs into the bladder.[65] Retrograde ejaculation can be confirmed on examination of a urine sample post-ejaculation to look for spermatozoa.[66] It is common after transurethral resection of the prostate (TURP) procedures.

As with anejaculation, it is important to determine the cause and remove any offending drugs from the treatment list. Medical treatments are based on increasing the sympathetic tone of the bladder neck or decreasing the parasympathetic activity using drugs such as ephedrine or imipramine.[65,66]

Assisted reproductive technologies have improved so much over the last few years that infertility issues can usually be solved. Urinary sperm retrieval aims to obtain sufficient viable sperm from the post-ejaculatory urine for insemination, in vitro fertilization (IVF), or intracytoplasmic sperm injection (ICSI).[67] In urinary sperm retrieval, a post-ejaculatory urine specimen is obtained either by voiding or catheterization, usually after alkalinization of the urine using oral sodium bicarbonate or by increasing oral fluid intake to dilute the urine.

Painful ejaculation

Painful ejaculation may occur in relation to benign prostatic hypertropthy (BPH), infection, or inflammation from acute prostatitis, chronic prostatitis, or chronic pelvic pain syndrome. It is also described in patients following radical prostatectomy. The incidence of post-orgasmic pain is 1–9.7%.[68] Occasionally, seminal vesicle inflammation or seminal vesicle calculi can cause problems, together with ejaculatory duct obstruction.[69–72] The cause should be thoroughly investigated. Theories as to the etiology include those referring to abnormal bladder neck closure and pudendal neuropathy. The treatment options include: self-care; a perineal hyperprotection program; and medication with the alpha blocker, topiramate. Surgical procedures that include removing a section of the sacrotuberous ligament, neurolysis of the pudendal nerve, or removing a section of the sacrospinous ligament have also been tried.[68]

Men with BPH and painful ejaculation tend to have more severe lower urinary tract symptoms (LUTS), report greater bother, and have a higher prevalence of ED and reduced ejaculation than men with LUTS only.[73]

Where a cause is found, dealing with the underlying problem can be helpful, but sometimes no etiological factor can be found.

References

1 Gross S. *Practical Treatise on Impotence, Sterility and Allied Disorders of the Male Sexual Organs*. Edinburg: YL Pentland, 1887.

2 American Psychiatric Association. *Diagnostic and Statistical Manual of Mental Disorders*, 3rd edn (DSM-III). Washington, DC: American Psychiatric Association, 1980.

3 American Psychiatric Association. *Diagnostic and Statistical Manual of Mental Disorders*, 4th edn, Text Revision (DSM-IV-TR). Washington, DC: American Psychiatric Association, 2000.

4 McMahon CG, Althof SE, Waldinger MD, et al. An evidence-based definition of lifelong premature ejaculation: Report of the International Society for Sexual Medicine (ISSM) Ad Hoc Committee for the definition of premature ejaculation. *J Sex Med* 2008;5:1590–606.

5 Waldinger MD, Hengeveld MW, Zwinderman AH. Paroxetine treatment of premature ejaculation: a double-blind, randomized, placebo-controlled study. *Am J Psychiatry* 1994;151:1377–9.

6 Waldinger MD. The neurobiological approach to premature ejaculation. *J Urol* 2002;168:2359–67.

7 Waldinger MD, Hengeveld MW, Zwinderman AH, et al. Effect of SSRI antidepressants on ejaculation: a double-blind, randomized, placebo-controlled study with fluoxetine, fluvoxamine, paroxetine, and sertraline. *J Clin Psychopharmacol* 1998;18:274–81.

8 Althof SE. Evidence based assessment of rapid ejaculation. *Int J Impot Res* 1998;10: (Suppl. 2):S74–S76; discussion S77–S79.

9 Althof SE. Pharmacologic treatment of rapid ejaculation. *Psychiatr Clin North Am* 1995;18:85–94.

10 Godpodinoff ML. Premature ejaculation: clinical subgroups and etiology. *J Sex Marital Ther* 1989;15:130–4.

11 Althof SE, Abdo CH, Dean J, et al. International Society for Sexual Medicine's guidelines for the diagnosis and treatment of premature ejaculation. *J Sex Med* 2010;7:2947–69.

12 Waldinger MD, Schweitzer DH. Changing paradigms from a historical DSM-III and DSM-IV view towards an evidence-based definition of premature ejaculation. Part I – validity of DSM-IV-TR. *J Sex Med* 2006;3:682–92.

13 Waldinger MD, Schweitzer DH. Changing paradigms from a historical DSM-III and DSM-IV view towards an evidence-based definition of premature ejaculation. Part II – proposals for DSM-V and ICD-11. *J Sex Med* 2006;3:693–705.
14 Waldinger MD. Recent advances in the classification, neurobiology and treatment of premature ejaculation. *Adv Psychosom Med* 2008;29:50–69.
15 Masters WH, Johnson VE. *Human Sexual Inadequacy*. Boston, MA: Little & Brown, 1970. In: Serefoglu EC, Saitz TR. New insights on premature ejaculation: a review of definition, classification, prevalence and treatment. *Asian J Androl* 2012;14:822–9.
16 Waldinger M, Rietschel M, Nothen N, et al. Familial occurrence of primary premature ejaculation. *Psychiatr Genet* 1998;8:37–40.
17 Jern P, Santtila P, Witting K, et al. Premature and delayed ejaculation: Genetic and environmental effects in a population-based sample of Finnish twins. *J Sex Med* 2007;4:1739–49.
18 Jern P, Santtila P, Johansson A, et al. Evidence for a genetic etiology to ejaculatory dysfunction. *Int J Impot Res* 2009;21: 62–7.
19 Janssen PKC, Bakker SC, Réthelyi J, et al. Serotonin transporter promoter region (5-HTTLPR) polymorphism is associated with the intravaginal ejaculation latency in Dutch men with lifelong premature ejaculation. *J Sex Med* 2009;6:276–84.
20 Santtila P, Jern P, Westberg L, et al. The dopamine transporter gene (DAT) polymorphism is associated with premature ejaculation. *J Sex Med* 2010;7:1538–46.
21 Corona G, Petrone L, Mannucci E, et al. Psycho-biological correlates of rapid ejaculation in patients attending an andrologic unit for sexual dysfunctions. *Eur Urol* 2004;46:615–22.
22 Nirenberg TD, Wincze JP, Bansal S, et al. Volunteer bias in a study of male alcoholic's sexual behaviour. *Arch Sex Behav* 1991;20:371–9.
23 Read S, King M, Watson J. Sexual dysfunction in primary medical care: prevalence, characteristics and detection by the general practitioner. *J Public Health Med* 1007;19: 387–91.
24 Nathan SG. The epidemiology of the DSM-III psychosexual dysfunctions. *J Sex Marital Ther* 1986;12:267–81.
25 Reading AE, Wiest WM. An analysis of self-reported sexual behaviour in a sample of normal males. *Arch Sex Behav* 1984;13:69–83.
26 Spector IP, Carey MP. Incidence and prevalence of the sexual dysfunctions: a critical review of the empirical literature. *Arch Sex Behav* 1990;19:389–408.
27 Grenier G, Byers ES. Rapid ejaculation: a review of conceptual, etiological and treatment issues. *Arch Sex Behav* 1995;24:447–72.
28 Laumann EO, Paik A, Rosen RC. Sexual dysfunction in the United States: prevalence and predictors. *JAMA* 1999;281: 537–44.
29 Laumann EO, Nicolosi A, Glasser DB, et al. Sexual problems among women and men aged 40–80 y: prevalence and correlates identified in the Global Study of Sexual Attitudes and Behaviours. *Int J Impot Res* 2005;17:39–57.
30 Porst H, Montorsi F, Rosen RC, et al. The Premature Ejaculation Prevalence and Attitudes (PEPA) survey: prevalence, comorbidities and professional help-seeking. *Eur Urol* 2007;51:816–23; discussion 824.
31 McMahon CG, Lee G, Park JK, et al. Premature ejaculation and erectile dysfunction prevalence and attitudes in the Asia-Pacific region. *J Sex Med* 2012;9:454–65.
32 Hong J. Survival of the fastest: on the origins of premature ejaculation. *J Sex Res* 1984;20:109–12.
33 Strassberg DS, Kelly MP, Carroll C, et al. The psychophysiological nature of premature ejaculation. *Arch Sex Behav* 1987;16:327–36.
34 Strassberg DS, Mahoney JM, Schaugaard M, et al. The role of anxiety in premature ejaculation: a psychophysiological model. *Arch Sex Behav* 1990;19:251–7.
35 Pirke KM, Kockott G, Aldenhoff J, et al. Pituitary gonadal system function in patients with erectile impotence and premature ejaculation. *Arch Sex Behav* 1979;8:41–8.
36 Lundberg PO, Ertekin C, Ghezzi A, et al. Neurosexology. Guidelines for Neurologists European Federation of Neurological Societies Task Force on Neurosexology. *Eur J Neurol* 2001;8:2–24.
37 El-Sakka AI. Premature ejaculation in non-insulin-dependent diabetic patients. *Int J Androl* 2003;26:329–34.
38 Pistoia F, Govoni S, Boselli C. Sex after stroke: a CNS only dysfunction? *Pharmacol Res* 2006;54:11–8.
39 McLean PD. Brain mechanisms of primal sexual functions and related behaviour. In: Gessa GL, Sandler M (eds), *Sexual Behaviour: Pharmacology and Biochemistry*. New York: Raven Press, 1975.
40 Fanciullaci FCG, Beretta G, Zanillo A. Cortical evoked potentials in subjects with true premature ejaculation. *Andrologia* 1988;20:326–30.
41 Xin ZC, Chung WS, Choi YD, et al. Penile sensitivity in patients with primary premature ejaculation. *J Urol* 1996;156:979–81.
42 Xin ZC, Choi YD, Rha KH, et al. Somatosensory evoked potentials in patients with primary premature ejaculation. *J Urol* 1997;158:451–5.
43 Montague DK, Jarow J, Broderick GA et al. AUA guideline on the pharmacologic management of premature ejaculation. 2003. Available at: https://www.auanet.org/common/pdf/education/clinical-guidance/Premature-Ejaculation.pdf (Accessed April 2016).
44 Wang WF, Minhas S, Ralph DJ. Phosphodiesterase 5 inhibitors in the treatment of premature ejaculation. *Int J Androl* 2006;29:503–9.
45 Safarinejad MR, Hosseini SY. Safety and efficacy of tramadol in the treatment of premature ejaculation: a double-blind, placebo-controlled, fixed-dose, randomized study. *J Clin Psychopharmacol* 2006;26:27–31.

46 Wyllie MG, Powell JA. The role of local anaesthetics in premature ejaculation. *BJU Int* 2012;110(11 Pt C):E943–8.

47 Fruhauf S, Gerger H, Schmidt HM, et al. Efficacy of psychological interventions for sexual dysfunction: a systematic review and meta-analysis. *Arch Sex Behav* 2013;42:915–33.

48 Kirana PS, Tripodi F, Reisman Y, Porst H (eds). *The EFS and ESSM Syllabus of Clinical Sexology*. Amsterdam: Medix Publishers, 2013.

49 Waldinger MD. Towards evidence-based drug treatment research on premature ejaculation: a critical evaluation of methodology. *Int J Impot Res* 2003;15:309–13.

50 Monague DK, Jarow J, Broderick GA, et al. AUA guideline on the pharmacologic management of premature ejaculation. *J Urol* 2004;172:290–4.

51 Tanrikut C, Feldman AS, Altemus M, et al. Adverse effect of paroxetine on sperm. *Fertil Steril* 2010;94:1021–6.

52 Athanasios Z, Polyanthi P, George K. The efficacy of duloxetine in the treatment of premature ejaculation. *Int Urol Nephrol* 2007;39:115–8.

53 Safarinejad MRMD. Safety and efficacy of escitalopram in the treatment of premature ejaculation: a double-blind, placebo-controlled, fixed-dose, randomized study. *J Clin Psychopharmacol* 2007;27:444–50.

54 Koyuncu H, Serefoglu EC, Yencilek E, et al. Citalopram treatment for premature ejaculation has a negative effect on semen parameters. *Int J Impot Res* 2011;23:257–61.

55 Hutchinson K, Cruickshank K, Wyclie K. A benefit-risk assessment of dapoxetine in the treatment of premature ejaculation. *Drug Saf* 2012;35:359–72.

56 Yang L, Qian S, Liu H, et al. Role of tramadol in premature ejaculation: a systematic review and meta-analaysis. *Urol Int* 2013;91:197–205.

57 Dresser MJ, Kang D, Staehr P, et al. Pharmacokinetics of dapoxetine, a new treatment for premature ejaculation: Impact of age and effects of a high-fat meal. *J Clin Pharmacol* 2006;46:1023–9.

58 Wyllie MG, Powell JA. The role of local anaesthetics in premature ejaculation. *BJU Int* 2012;110:E943–48.

59 Buvat J. Glossaire. Les pertubations de l'éjaculation. In: Buvat J, Jouannet P (eds), *L'éjaculation et ses pertubations*. Lyon-Villeurbanne : SIMEP, 1983, p. 9.

60 Wang R, Monga M, Hellstrom WJ. Ejaculatory dysfunction. In: Comhaire FH (ed), *Male Infertility: Clinical Investigation. Cause Evaluation and Treatment*. London: Chapman & Hall, 1996; pp. 205–21.

61 Brindley GS. Reflex ejaculation under vibratory stimulation in paraplegic men. *Paraplegia* 1981;19:299–302.

62 Perelman MA. Delayed ejaculation. *J Sex Med* 2013;10: 1189–90.

63 Richardson D, Goldmeier D. Recommendations for the management of retarded ejaculation: BASHH Special Interest Group for Sexual Dysfunction. *Int J STD AIDS* 2006;17:7–13.

64 McMahon CG, Abdo C, Incrocci L, et al. Disorders of orgasm and ejaculation in men. *J Sex Med* 2004;1:58–64.

65 Ralph DJ, Wylie KR. Ejaculatory disorders and sexual function. *BJU Int* 2005;95:1181–6.

66 Colpi G, Weidner W, Jungwirth A, et al. EAU guidelines on ejaculatory dysfunction. *Eur Urol* 2004;46:555–8.

67 Jefferys A, Siassakos D, Wardle P. The management of retrograde ejaculation: A systematic review and update. *Fertil Steril* 2012;97(2):306–12.

68 Ilie CP, Mischianu DL, Pemberton RJ. Painful ejaculation. *BJU Int* 2007;99:1335–9.

69 Weintraub MP. De Mouy E, Hellstrom WJ. Newer modalities in the diagnosis and treatment of ejaculatory duct obstruction. *J Urol* 1993;150:1150–4.

70 Corriere JN Jr. Painful ejaculation due to seminal vesicle calculi. *J Urol* 1997;157:626.

71 Kochakarn W, Leenanupunth C, Muangman V, et al. Ejaculatory duct obstruction in the infertile male: experience of 7 cases at Ramathibodi Hospital. *J Med Assoc Thai* 2001;84:1148–52.

72 Nickel JC, Elhilai M, Vallancien G. Benign prostatic hyperplasia (BPH) and prostatitis: prevalence of painful ejaculation in men with clinical BPH. *BJU Int* 2005;95: 571–4.

73 Osen R, ALtwein J, Boyle P, et al. Lower urinary tract symptoms and male sexual dysfunction: the multinational survey of the aging male (MSAM-7). *Eur Urol* 2003;44:637–49.

CHAPTER 18

Erectile dysfunction and infertility

Vikram Soni, Alexander W. Pastuszak, and Mohit Khera
Baylor College of Medicine, Houston, TX, USA

Infertility and sexual dysfunction in men, specifically erectile dysfunction (ED), are distinct entities that share a complex and interdependent relationship with one another. This chapter discusses the similarities and differences between the etiologies and treatments for each condition, and highlights the potential impact infertility may have on male sexual function. It is important to consider these as linked entities during evaluation of affected men, and to structure treatment approaches while considering the numerous and varied causes of both ED and male infertility, given the close relationship between the two conditions.

Approximately 60–75% of couples conceive within 6 months of initiating unprotected sexual intercourse, with 90% conceiving within one year.[1,2] Based on these data, infertility is defined as an inability to conceive after at least 12 months of regular, unprotected intercourse. Approximately 15% of couples have fertility difficulties, with a male factor implicated in up to 50% of these cases.[3] Extrapolated further, these data suggest that close to 8% of all men of reproductive age will seek medical treatment for infertility at some point in their lives.[4] Clearly, these numbers are not insignificant. Fortunately the treatment of both male and female infertility has dramatically improved over the past three decades with the advent of assisted reproductive technologies (ART), including in vitro fertilization (IVF) and intracytoplasmic sperm injection (ICSI). These treatment methods have offered the ability to bypass many of the most vexing causes of male infertility, but also come at a substantial cost: an estimated $1.8 billion dollars was spent on ART in the United States in the year 2000 alone.[5] According to a recent industry analysis, ART now results in more than 50,000 babies per year in the United States via more than 140,000 IVF procedures, a number that has nearly tripled since 1999. There are more than 450 infertility clinics, over 100 sperm banks, an unknown number of egg donors, and more than 1700 reproductive specialists competing for a slice of a very lucrative business – the infertility services sector has swelled to an estimated US$4 billion dollar industry.[6]

However, these approaches often do not take into consideration the fundamental causes of male infertility, which are increasingly known to be genetic in nature, leading to an increased risk of genetic disease in the offspring as well as an increased risk of masking significant medical pathology in the male partner.[7,8] The causes of male infertility are numerous and include a variety of congenital and acquired disorders (Table 18.1). Inherent to an inability to father a child naturally is the inability to have an erection sufficient for penetration and duration of sexual intercourse, and men with ED may have difficulties with fertility as a result, not only due to their inability to achieve vaginal penetration, but also potentially due to dysregulation of the hypothalamic-pituitary-gonadal (HPG) axis, which may result from hormonal imbalance, leading to both infertility and ED.

Erectile dysfunction is defined as an inability to achieve or maintain an erection sufficient for satisfactory sexual intercourse.[9] ED is estimated to affect 30 million men in the United States and has a 10–20% worldwide prevalence rate.[10,11] Despite a growing understanding of the pathophysiology of ED and persistent improvements in treatment modalities, ED prevalence rates continue to rise, and approximately 322 million men are expected to have ED by 2025, a large increase from 152 million men in 1995.[12] Furthermore, the prevalence of ED increases with age and coincides with numerous chronic health

Male Sexual Dysfunction: A Clinical Guide, First Edition. Edited by Suks Minhas and John Mulhall.

Table 18.1 Causes and distribution of male infertility.

Hypothalamic-pituitary disorders (1–2%)	
Congenital disorders	• Congenital GnRH deficiency (Kallmann syndrome) • Hemochromatosis • Multi-organ genetic disorders (Prader–Willi syndrome, Laurence–Moon–Biedl syndrome, familial cerebellar ataxia)
Acquired disorders	• Pituitary and hypothalamic tumors (macroadenoma, craniopharyngioma) • Infiltrative disorders (sarcoidosis, histiocytosis, tuberculosis, fungal infections) • Trauma, post-surgery, post-irradiation • Vascular (infarction, aneurysm) • Hormonal (hyperprolactinemia, androgen excess, estrogen excess, cortisol excess) • Drugs (opioids and psychotropic medications, GnRH agonists or antagonists)
Systemic disorders	• Chronic illnesses • Nutritional deficiencies • Obesity
Primary gonadal disorders (30–40%)	
Congenital disorders	• Klinefelter's syndrome (XXY) and its variants (XXY/XY; XXXY) • Cryptorchidism • Myotonic dystrophy • Functional prepubertal castrate syndrome (congenital anorchia) • Varicocele • Androgen insensitivity syndromes • 5α-reductase deficiency • Y chromosome deletions
Acquired disorders	• Varicocele • Viral orchitis (mumps, echovirus, arbovirus) • Granulomatous orchitis (leprosy, tuberculosis) • Epididymo-orchitis (gonorrhea, chlamydia) • Drugs (e.g., alkylating agents, alcohol, marijuana, antiandrogens, ketoconazole, spironolactone, H2 receptor antagonists) • Ionizing radiation • Environmental toxins (e.g., dibromochloropropane, carbon disulfide, cadmium, lead, mercury, environmental estrogens and phytoestrogens) • Hyperthermia • Immunologic disorders, including polyglandular autoimmune disease • Trauma • Torsion • Castration • Systemic illness (e.g., renal failure, hepatic cirrhosis, cancer, sickle-cell disease, amyloidosis, vasculitis, celiac disease)
Disorders of sperm transport (10–20%)	
• Epididymal dysfunction (drugs, infection) • Abnormalities of the vas deferens (congenital absence, Young's syndrome, infection, vasectomy) • Ejaculatory dysfunction (spinal cord disease, autonomic dysfunction, premature ejaculation)	
Idiopathic male infertility (40–50%)	

conditions, including type II diabetes, cardiovascular disease, depression, dyslipidemia, hypertension, benign prostatic hypertrophy, lower urinary tract symptoms, and hypogonadism. Given the world's aging population and the increasing prevalence of the aforementioned comorbidities it is likely that the prevalence of ED will continue to increase.[13–18] As with infertility, ED also places a substantial economic burden on both patients and society. Between 1994 and 2000, expenditures for the management of ED, excluding the cost of pharmaceuticals, almost doubled from US$185 million to US$330 million.[19,20] This increase in spending on ED treatment may represent an increased societal acceptance of ED as a treatable condition and a corresponding increase in self-reporting and acceptance of treatment on behalf of the male population.[20] With regards to incidence, a recent study found that during the period 1995–2000 the incidence of ED increased from 5% to 6.5% but has since stabilized at approximately 5% per year.[21] However, as the prevalence of the above comorbidities continues to rise, we can expect the economic burden of ED to correspondingly increase.

Taken separately, infertility and ED have been well studied, and treatment strategies for these two conditions have dramatically improved over the past two decades, coinciding with the development of ICSI in 1992 and the approval of phosphodiesterase-5 (PDE5) inhibitors in 1998. As the relationship between male infertility and ED becomes clearer, it is apparent that these conditions are inextricably linked. Evaluation and treatment of the infertile male may influence erectile function, and conversely, ED can impact a man's fertility. Given this relationship, the clinician should consider both conditions when developing a management plan for affected men. In this chapter we provide a discussion of the similarities and differences between ED and male infertility – in terms of etiology and treatment – as well as the potential impact a diagnosis of infertility may have on male erectile function. Our goal is to provide clinicians and healthcare providers with a clearer understanding of the emerging links between ED and male factor infertility.

Differences and common links between male infertility and erectile dysfunction

Numerous causes of ED and male infertility have been identified to date, though it is clear that not all etiologies are known for either condition. The causes of ED are frequently multifactorial, comprising a mix of organic and psychogenic factors[22] (Table 18.2). Many of the disorders in Table 18.2 are chronic and systemic in nature, leading to damage of multiple tissue types, including vascular and nervous tissues, and often leading to effects on endocrine signaling. Together, the effects of these system-wide insults may result in ED.[23–25] Fortunately, the disease processes contributing to ED can often be identified, and in some cases risk modification by way of smoking cessation, increased exercise, weight control, diet optimization, and modification of activities leading to penile and perineal trauma, have been shown to significantly improve erectile function.[26–33] In cases where ED may be attributed to the effects of medications, drug substitution, dosage adjustment, drug holidays, or drug cessation may restore sexual function in some men.[22,34,35] If further treatment of ED symptoms is required, a multi-modal therapeutic plan incorporating medications, lifestyle modification, and surgery may be implemented. Many treatment modalities for ED, including oral therapy via PDE5 inhibitors, intracavernous injections, and intraurethral suppositories containing vasoactive medications; vacuum erection devices and penile prostheses; or revascularization surgery, have been extensively studied and efficacy rates clearly established.[36–42] This is helpful in giving both patients and clinicians a clear understanding of the benefits and risks of each therapeutic option.

Although many causes of male infertility are known (see Table 18.1), 40–50% of causes remain unidentified, despite significant improvements in our diagnostic armamentarium and the use of new technologies in diagnosis.[43–45] Without establishing a cause for a man's fertility difficulties, it is not possible to develop a targeted treatment plan. As a result, empiric pharmacotherapy is frequently utilized in affected men after limited laboratory evaluation of the HPG axis. Empiric therapies include gonadotropin-releasing hormone (GnRH)-, follicle-stimulating hormone (FSH)-, and luteinizing hormone (LH)-modulating drugs, anti-estrogens (clomiphene citrate, tamoxifen citrate), aromatase inhibitors (testolactone, anastrozole), and antioxidants such as L-carnitine, α-tocopherol, ascorbic acid, and retinoids. Unfortunately, large-scale, randomized, placebo-controlled studies in infertile men of most of the above agents are lacking, and smaller studies have produced conflicting results as to the efficacy of these treatments.[46–59] Assisted reproduction has become an increasingly popular treatment option for couples in whom a cause of infertility is not established or other therapies have failed. Intrauterine insemination (IUI) may be used to achieve conception in the setting of male subfertility, with a recent meta-analysis finding that couples were three times more likely to achieve a pregnancy through IUI when compared with timed intercourse.[60] Successful fertilization rates using ICSI have been reported to be 70–80%, with corresponding pregnancy rates of up to 45%.[61] What is frequently overlooked in both men and women with fertility difficulties is the possibility of a transmissible genetic lesion that may

Table 18.2 Classification of causes of erectile dysfunction.

Organic	
Vasculogenic	• Atherosclerosis • Hypertension • Hypercholesterolemia • Diabetes mellitus • Pelvic/perineal trauma or irradiation • Smoking • Peyronie's disease • Venous shunts (may be acquired after penile surgery)
Neurogenic	• Stroke • Parkinson's disease • Alzheimer's disease • Encephalitis • Temporal lobe epilepsy • Spinal cord injury or associated CNS disorder (disk herniation, tumor, spina bifida, multiple sclerosis) • Pelvic trauma or surgery • Diabetic neuropathy
Endocrinological	• Hypogonadism • Hyperprolactinemia • Hyper- and hypothyroidism
Drug-induced	• Antihypertensives (diuretics, non-selective β-adrenergic blockers, spironolactone) • Antipsychotics (clozapine, risperidone, haloperidol) • Antidepressants (tricyclic antidepressants, monoamine oxidase inhibitors, selective serotonin reuptake inhibitors) • Lithium • Anxiolotics (benzodiazepines); newer anxiolytics (bupropion, buspirone) not associated with sexual side effects • Antiandrogens (LHRH agonists, finasteride, dutasteride) • Alcohol abuse
Psychogenic	
Generalized	• Primary lack of sexual arousability • Age-related decline in sexual arousability
Situational	• Performance anxiety • Depression • Partner-related (lack of arousability, partner conflict)

affect the couple's offspring. Recent data indicate that 10–30% of male infertility is genetic in origin,[62] yet testing for genetic lesions is rarely performed, in part due to a lack of clinically available assays to test for a broad range of genetic defects.

Despite the differences between many of the etiologies and treatments of ED and male factor infertility, numerous common links exist between the two conditions, and having an awareness of these is crucial to a thorough workup of patients presenting with these conditions.

Any condition that interferes with signaling through the HPG axis can potentially result in both male infertility as well as ED.[63,64] Disorders resulting in testosterone (T) deficiency are common causes of both conditions, as androgens influence the development of the male reproductive tract and affect libido and sexual behavior.[65] A study conducted in the Boston area reported a 5.6% prevalence of symptomatic androgen deficiency (hypogonadism) in men between 30 and 79 years old. Of symptomatic men, ED was reported as the primary symptom in 16% of cases.[66] Hypogonadism is generally diagnosed via serum total T levels ≤300 ng/dL on two consecutive blood samples, as well as the presence of hypogonadal symptoms, including fatigue, decreased energy and libido, ED, insomnia, and increased fat mass, and may contribute to both ED and infertility.[64,66–71] Of the various forms of T deficiency, hypogonadotropic hypogonadism (HH) is the most common and best described.[64] HH may be subdivided into congenital, acquired, or idiopathic etiologies. Congenital causes of HH include Kallmann syndrome

(KS), Prader–Willi and Laurence–Moon–Biedl syndromes, and hereditary hemochromatosis, with KS being the most common of these.[64,72,73] In cases of HH, T secretion from Leydig cells is diminished, which may result in both ED and infertility.[74] Furthermore, in cases of HH, a decline in FSH production leads to impaired spermatogenesis.

Hypogonadotropic hypogonadism may also be acquired secondary to hyperprolactinemia, defined as a serum prolactin of ≥20 ng/mL.[64] Excessive prolactin suppresses GnRH release, impairs binding of LH to receptors on Leydig cells, and may decrease ejaculate volumes, culminating in both infertility and ED.[75,76] Hyperprolactinemia is most commonly caused by a prolactin-secreting pituitary adenoma, but may also be secondary to conditions that interfere with the secretion of dopamine, which inhibits prolactin release. Lesions that inhibit dopamine secretion include tumors of the hypothalamus, infiltrative diseases such as sarcoidosis that damage dopamine-secreting cells in the central nervous system, or damage to the hypothalamic-pituitary stalk following trauma or surgery. Numerous drugs, including the antipsychotics risperidone and haloperidol, gastric motility agents such as metoclopramide and domperidone, and antihypertensive medications including methyldopa and verapamil, can also cause hyperprolactinemia and consequently HH.[77]

Thyroid disease has also been implicated in ED and male factor infertility. Both hyper- and hypothyroidism are known to affect steroid hormone metabolism and sperm quality and have been associated with subfertility.[78–80] Hyperthyroidism in particular has been shown to be associated with ED, whereas hypothyroidism has been postulated to primarily affect sexual desire and ejaculatory function.[81,82]

Iatrogenic causes of both male infertility and ED have also been reported. Surgical procedures that violate the retroperitoneum may result in obstruction of the vas deferens or ejaculatory ducts, or cause damage to the nerves involved in penile erection, seminal emission, and ejaculation.[83] Bilateral retroperitoneal lymphadenectomy can result in sympathetic nerve injury leading to anejaculation or retrograde ejaculation, having a clear impact on male fertility, and may also lead to ED.[84,85] Radical prostatectomy and radical cystoprostatectomy also carry with them a risk of ED from neurovascular injury and infertility due to transection of the vas deferens, removal of the seminal vesicles, and injury to nerves involved in ejaculation and erection, as above.[83] Hormonal therapies for metastatic prostate carcinoma impact both male fertility and erectile function, given that these medications reduce serum testosterone levels.[86] An improved understanding of the neuroanatomy of the pelvis has resulted in modification of surgical techniques to lower the incidence of iatrogenically induced sexual dysfunction.[87] Indeed, nerve-sparing techniques during radical prostatectomy have decreased the incidence of ED from 43–100% to 30–50% following radical prostatectomy, and to less than 10% (from 15–100%) after radical rectal surgery.[87–92] Similarly, use of nerve-sparing techniques during radical cystectomy has been shown to improve postoperative quality of life and sexual function, with preservation of erectile function in 62%, 47%, 43%, and 20% of men between the ages of 40–49, 50–59, 60–69, and 70–79 years old, respectively.[93]

Other medications are also known to negatively impact both male fertility and sexual function. Spironolactone, a non-selective mineralocorticoid receptor antagonist, blocks both the epithelial and non-epithelial actions of aldosterone. With its moderate affinity for both progesterone and androgen receptors, spironolactone use carries with it a risk of sexual side effects, including ED, and through inhibition of testosterone production, infertility.[94,95] A variety of psychotherapeutic medications have also been shown to affect erectile function and fertility. Antidepressant medications, including selective serotonin reuptake inhibitors (SSRIs), monoamine oxidase inhibitors (MAOIs), and tricyclic antidepressants (TCAs), may lead to both ED and ejaculatory dysfunction.[96–98] Antipsychotics such as phenothiazines and the mood-stabilizer lithium, owing to their anti-β-adrenergic, anticholinergic, and/or anti-dopaminergic effects within the CNS, may also disrupt the HPG axis, leading to ejaculatory and erectile dysfunction, and reduction in libido.[99,100] 5α-Reductase inhibitors (5ARIs), including finasteride and dutasteride, often used in the treatment of benign prostatic hypertrophy, have also been associated with a reduction in semen volume, ejaculatory disturbances, and ED.[101] In addition, 5ARI usage has been associated with reduced libido, and several studies have reported this effect in up to 5% of subjects. In some cases, persistent loss of libido even after discontinuation of the drug has been reported.[102–106]

Although many of the above medications reduce serum androgen levels, the use of exogenous androgens may also affect male fertility. Exogenous androgen supplementation can impair spermatogenesis by suppressing GnRH secretion, and exogenous androgens can induce azoospermia, which may last 6 months or longer and in some cases be irreversible following cessation of androgen administration.[59] While T therapy may be part of an appropriate treatment approach to the hypogonadal patient, its use should be limited in men desiring fertility, and alternative treatments, including anti-estrogens and GnRH receptor blockers, should be considered instead. Alternatively, recent studies indicate that judicious use of exogenous androgen concomitantly with medications that stimulate testicular testosterone production, including human chorionic gonadotropin (hCG) and FSH, may preserve semen parameters in hypogonadal men.[107,108]

It should be noted that the links between male factor infertility and ED discussed above, and summarized in Table 18.3, do not represent the most common causes of infertility and/or ED. Though pathologies common to both male infertility and ED exist, most causes of both male infertility and ED are independent of one

Table 18.3 Etiologies common to male infertility and erectile dysfunction (ED).

Category	Disorders	Mechanism of dysfunction
Endocrinological	*Congenital hypogonadotropic hypogonadism (HH)*	In all cases gonadotropin deficiency results in T deficiency, impaired spermatogenesis, and sexual dysfunction (loss of libido, ED in some cases)
	Kallmann's syndrome	
	Prader–Willi	
	Gonadotropin subunit mutation	
	DAX1 mutation	
	GPR54 mutation	
	Leptin or leptin receptor mutation	
	Hyperprolactinemia	Excess prolactin inhibits GnRH secretion, leading to HH
	Pituitary adenoma	
	Hypothalamic tumors (i.e., craniopharyngiomas)	
	Section of hypothalamic-pituitary stalk	
	Antipsychotics (phenothiazines, haloperidol, pimozide, risperidone, molindone, olanzapine)	
	Antidepressants (clomipramine, desipramine)	
	Gastrointestinal drugs (cimetidine, metoclopramide)	
	Antihypertensives (methyldopa, reserpine, verapamil)	
	Hyper-/hypothyroidism	Both impair steroid metabolism, lower sperm quality, and are associated with ED
Infiltrative disease	Sarcoidosis	Deposition and accumulation of compounds in hypothalamus or pituitary damages GnRH-, LH-, or FSH-secreting cells leading to HH
	Langerhans cell histiocytosis	
	Hemochromatosis	
Drug-induced	*Suppression of gonadotropins*	Suppression of gonadotropins leads to HH, ED, ejaculatory dysfunction, or orgasmic dysfunction plus infertility via CNS activity
	Exogenous gonadal steroids	
	Glucocorticoids	
	Opiates	
	GnRH analogs	
	Psychotropic medication (SSRIs, MAOIs, TCAs)	
	Antiandrogens (spironolactone, 5α-reductase inhibitors)	Suppress production of T/DHT
Iatrogenic	Radical prostatectomy	All pose risk of neurovascular injury and obstruction of sperm transport. Newer techniques have reduced incidence of such injuries
	Radical cystectomy	
	Bilateral pelvic lymphadenectomy	

DHT, dihydrotestosterone; FSH, follicle-stimulating hormone; GnRH, gonadotropin-releasing hormone; LH, luteinizing hormone; MAOI, monoamine oxidase inhibitor; SSRI, selective serotonin reuptake inhibitor; T, testosterone; TCA, tricyclic antidepressant.

another (see Tables 18.1 and 18.2). However, there is also a psychological relationship between an infertility diagnosis and ED that may pose interesting challenges to patients, their partners, and the clinicians treating them. This relationship is explored in the following section.

The impact of infertility on erectile dysfunction

Achieving a sense of sexual compatibility is integral to most intimate relationships, and in many of these relationships, one or both partners report a strong desire for a child.[109] While society's expectations of procreation may influence sexual behavior, at least to some degree, a feeling of sexual togetherness is important to overall sexual health and relationship stability. Thus, sexual satisfaction and the desire to have children are interrelated, and it therefore seems intuitive that a diagnosis of infertility, which can heighten anxiety and increase stress levels, may be associated with an increased incidence of male sexual dysfunction.

A diagnosis of male factor infertility is associated with a loss of self-esteem, increased anxiety, and overall diminished feelings of self-worth in the male partner.[110] Shindel et al., in a study of 121 infertile couples, found that male subjects reported significantly lower scores on the Mental Health subscale of the Short Form 36 (SF-36) questionnaire, a validated instrument for assessing one's perception of physical health, than the general population, indicating a poorer perception of their mental health. Furthermore, 11% and 12% of men in this study reported moderate and severe depressive symptoms, respectively, as assessed by the Center for Epidemiologic Studies Depression Scale (CES-D) questionnaire, a validated tool for assessment of depressive symptoms. The same study found that while mean erectile function domain (EFD) scores of the International Index of Erectile Function (IIEF) questionnaire were above the cut-off value for a diagnosis of ED, 22% of men had EFD scores of less than 26 and of these, 18% and 4% had mild and moderate ED, respectively.[111] Monga et al. similarly found that infertile men had significantly lower total and intercourse satisfaction scores on the IIEF compared with controls, and Jain et al. found, in a survey of 175 infertile couples in India, that premature ejaculation, erectile dysfunction, decreased libido, and orgasmic failure were reported by 66%, 15%, 11%, and 8% of male partners, respectively.[112,113]

The stress induced by both the diagnosis and treatment of infertility may result in increased male sexual dysfunction and reduced sexual activity among infertile men.[114] When the male factor is identified as the sole cause of infertility in a couple, men experience greater distress and sexual dysfunction than when a female or mixed etiology is responsible.[115] Furthermore, the prevalence of ED, determined by a score of less than 22 on the Sexual Health Inventory in Men (SHIM) questionnaire, and the frequency of hypogonadal symptoms, determined by a positive finding on the Androgen Deficiency in the Aging Male (ADAM) questionnaire, were both significantly higher among infertile men compared with men with proven fertility. The investigators further postulated that, due to the relatively young age and overall good health of the subjects in this study, as well as the lack of correlation between ED, hypogonadal symptoms, and serum T levels, both ED and hypogonadal symptoms were "likely multifactorial and probably largely due to psychogenic factors" related to infertility.[116] Given these associations, it is not surprising to find that a link exists between depression, anxiety, and stress, and reduced sexual frequency, desire, and overall sexuality, particularly in men who already have diminished fertility.[117–120] Given that corporal smooth muscle contraction, and therefore detumescence, is mediated in part by noradrenaline (norepinephrine), ED in this setting may be due to increased noradrenaline production in response to the stress associated with an infertility diagnosis.

Diagnostic tests performed as a result of a standard infertility workup may also exacerbate difficulties with sexual function in men. Semen analysis, generally the first diagnostic test of an infertility workup, frequently requires the patient to provide a semen sample in the clinic and under time constraints. Under these circumstances, transient ED and ejaculatory difficulties may be experienced by the male patient.[121] In addition, the identification of abnormal semen parameters on the first semen analysis can also lead to erectile and orgasmic difficulties. Saleh et al. observed that 11% of men undergoing infertility evaluation experienced problems with erection or orgasm after detection of an abnormality in their first semen analysis.[122]

Some clinics may try to ameliorate difficulties in obtaining a semen sample by offering patients the option to collect samples at home and bring them to the clinic within 1 hour. However, even in this scenario the potential for transient ED arises owing to the "forced" nature of sexual activity. Many couples are also advised to schedule sexual intercourse around the period of female ovulation, which may diminish the spontaneity of the sexual act and result in performance anxiety, ED, and ejaculatory dysfunction.[123] Owing to the "calculated" nature of the resulting sexual intercourse, many men have reported avoiding sex outside of this time frame and a decline in libido has been reported in almost 10% of men after fertility evaluation.[120,124]

It is important to note that the results of these studies do not necessarily establish a causal relationship between infertility and ED, and our aim here is not to make such a claim. Rather, the data show that an association between the two very well might exist, and that the initial diagnosis and workup of infertility can have a substantial impact on male sexuality. In addition, outside influences and social pressures related to successful reproduction may also have marked effects upon male psychosexual function, and may ultimately lead to sexual dysfunction.[125] As such, it is important for the clinician to be aware of these associations and take proactive measures to counsel and treat these patients accordingly.

Overview of the evaluation of erectile dysfunction

The modern management of ED has been marked by a drive to establish evidence-based best practices that are both standardized and proceed in a step-wise, goal-orientated fashion. The current philosophy behind the management and treatment of ED revolves around a "patient-centered, goal-directed" approach, originally described by Lue.[126,127] The foundations of this paradigm stress the importance of pursuing ED management and treatment in a methodical, evidence-based manner, beginning with a thorough medical, sexual, and psychosocial history followed by a focused physical examination and pertinent laboratory testing (Figure 18.1).[128] The clinician is then encouraged to present treatment options to the patient or couple in a manner that is sensitive to the cultural, ethnic, and religious factors that may influence the patient's preferred treatment path.[129] The goal of this approach is to allow the patient or couple to make an informed decision regarding treatment that is consistent with their view of sexual fulfillment.[130,131] Since its initial description, this model has been further buoyed by a series of internationally accepted consensus meetings, chief among these being a series of reports generated from the International Consultations on Sexual Medicine (ICSM).[132,133]

A step-wise approach to the management and treatment of ED begins with the understanding that, unlike a variety of disease processes, a diagnosis of ED commonly hinges upon the subjective complaint(s) of the patient. Extensive diagnostic testing and objective data gathering are not necessarily required to initiate ED treatment, although such data may be helpful in guiding treatment in particular cases.[134] Regardless, an essential first step in ED management is a comprehensive sexual, medical, and psychosocial history.[135–137]

Given the association between ED and several chronic medical conditions and adverse lifestyle habits (e.g., diabetes, cardiovascular disease (CVD), hypertension, prostate disease, obesity, sedentary lifestyle, cigarette smoking), the medical history of the ED patient should focus on elucidating the existence and extent of these underlying conditions.[13–18,138] The third Princeton Consensus Guidelines Panel, acknowledging the frequent coexistence of ED and CVD, recommended that all men presenting with ED should undergo an initial cardiac assessment with stratification of their cardiac risk, regardless of the presence or absence of overt cardiac symptoms.[139] This algorithm places ED patients into three categories – low, medium, or high cardiac risk – and guides management based upon this stratification (Figure 18.2). A complete medical history would also include an assessment of the known organic causes of ED, such as neurological disease, hypogonadism, thyroid disorders, pelvic trauma, medication usage, and so forth. These known organic causes of ED have been described previously and are presented in Table 18.2.

The sexual and psychosocial history of the ED patient is also of vital importance in framing the patient's overall sexual well-being and confirming the diagnosis.[140] This includes establishing the duration and severity of erectile dysfunction, as well as assessing the entirety of the male sexual response cycle (i.e., libido, ejaculation, and orgasm). Partner sexual function and the patient's relationship satisfaction (both past and present relationships) are also important in establishing the broader picture of the patient's overall sexual health. Inquiring

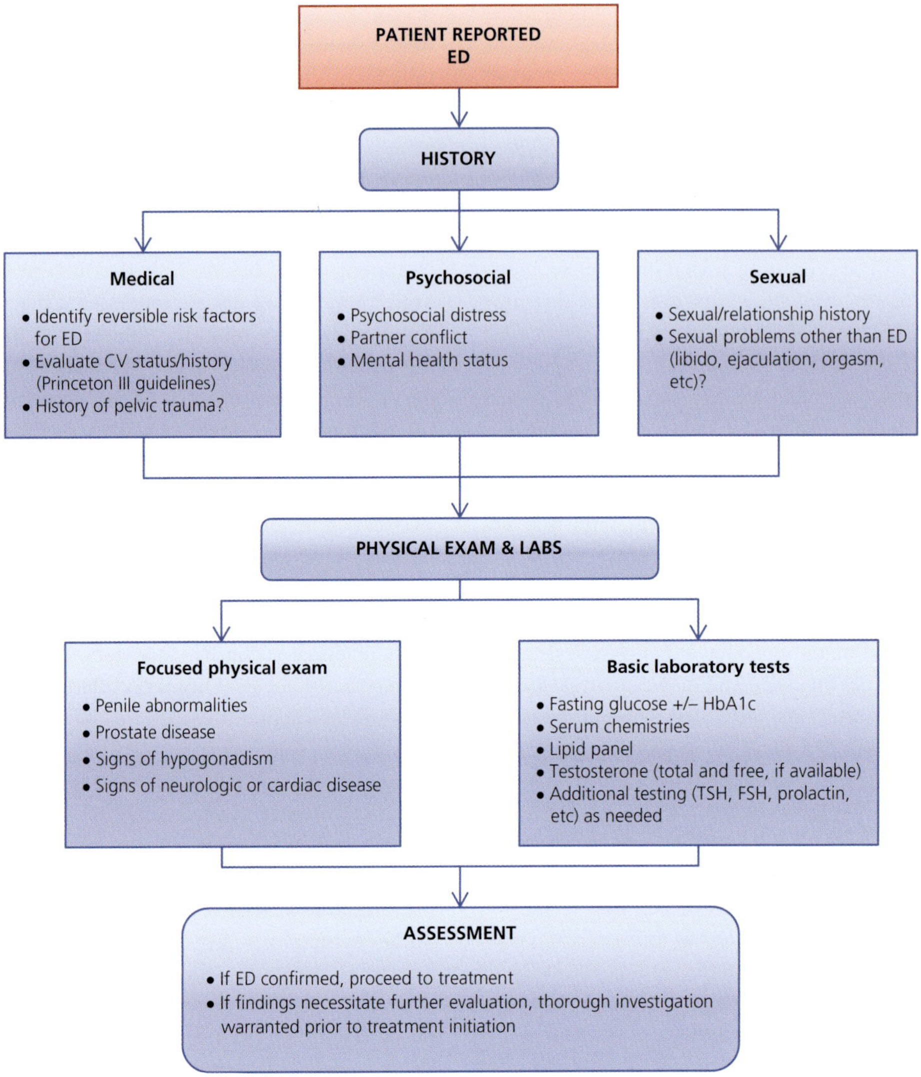

Figure 18.1 Algorithm for the diagnostic evaluation of erectile dysfunction (ED).

about potential sources of anxiety, depression, or relationship distress may serve to reveal emotional or environmental stressors that might contribute to, or exacerbate, ED.[141] There are several validated, self-administered ED questionnaires, such as the IIEF and SHIM, and these may provide useful information to supplement the history. The IIEF, mentioned previously, consists of 15 questions addressing five domains of sexual function – erectile function, orgasmic function, sexual desire, intercourse satisfaction, and overall satisfaction. The SHIM, a five-item questionnaire adapted from the IIEF, focuses specifically on erectile function and serves as a useful, brief, and easily administered ED screening tool. Information gleaned from patient responses to questionnaires may help stratify patients based on ED severity and can aid the clinician in establishing a clearer understanding of the patient's sexual health status.[10,142]

A focused physical exam is also highly recommended and should include an assessment of the cardiovascular, neurological, and genital systems.[129] A finding of elevated blood pressure or reduced peripheral pulses,

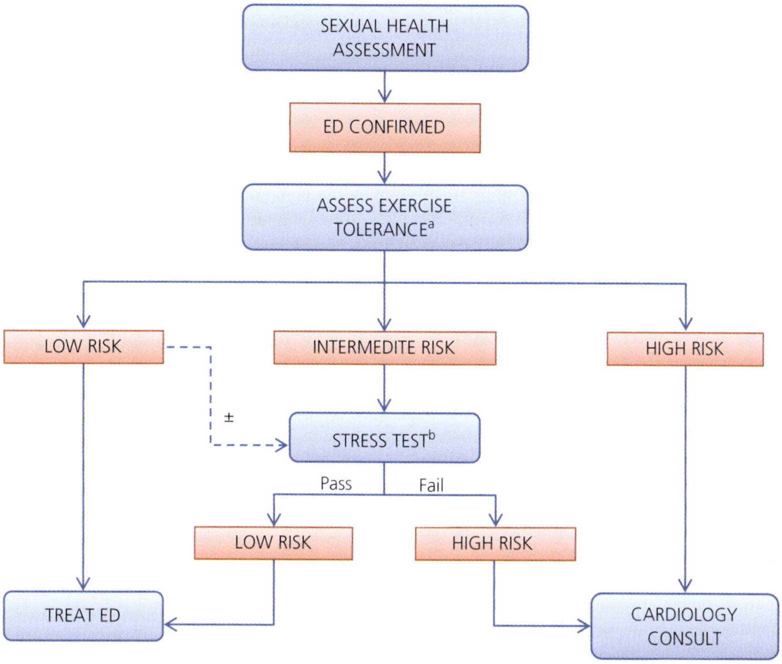

Figure 18.2 Princeton III Consensus Panel recommendations for management of erectile dysfunction (ED) in cardiovascular disease (CVD). [a]Sexual activity is equivalent to walking one mile on flat surface in 20 minutes or briskly climbing two flights of stairs in 10 seconds. [b]Sexual activity is equivalent to four minutes of the Bruce treadmill protocol. Low-risk patients are those able to perform exercise of moderate intensity without symptoms. This group also includes patients with a history of successful revascularization, asymptomatic controlled hypertension, mild valvular dysfunction, and left ventricular dysfunction (New York Heart Association (NYHA) class I and II). High-risk patients are those with moderate to severe cardiac symptoms, including unstable angina pectoris, uncontrolled hypertension, congestive heart failure (NYHA class IV), recent myocardial infarction (MI; <2 weeks), high-risk arrhythmia, severe cardiomyopathy, and moderate to severe valve disease.Source: Kostis et al. (2005).[139] Reproduced with permission of Elsevier.

for example, may reveal undiagnosed cardiovascular disease concomitant with the patient's ED.[23,143] The absence of secondary sex characteristics or presence of a distinctive body habitus might point to an underlying endocrine disorder or congenital abnormality (e.g., Klinefelter's or Kallmann syndrome). An evaluation of the genital system may uncover evidence of pelvic trauma, penile deformity (Peyronie's disease), or testicular abnormality, while findings of an abnormal neurological exam may suggest the presence of a peripheral neuropathy portending a diagnosis of diabetes mellitus. Given that the etiology of ED is often multifactorial, physical exam findings alone might not pinpoint a specific cause. Rather, the physical exam may help corroborate aspects of the history, provide direction to subsequent diagnostic testing and laboratory work, and in some cases, uncover undiagnosed comorbidities.[133,137]

The choice of laboratory testing should be equally focused and flow from the information obtained from the history and physical examination. Recommended laboratory tests for the evaluation of ED include serum chemistries, fasting glucose, HbA1c, complete blood count, lipid profile, and serum total testosterone (Figure 18.1).[128] In select cases, additional testing may be ordered at the clinician's discretion if particular etiologies, such as hypogonadism, thyroid disease, hyperprolactinemia, or others are suspected.[66,71,128,133,144–146]

Treatment considerations for erectile dysfunction

Once a diagnosis of ED has been established appropriate treatment may commence (Figure 18.3). Given the association between ED and comorbid health conditions

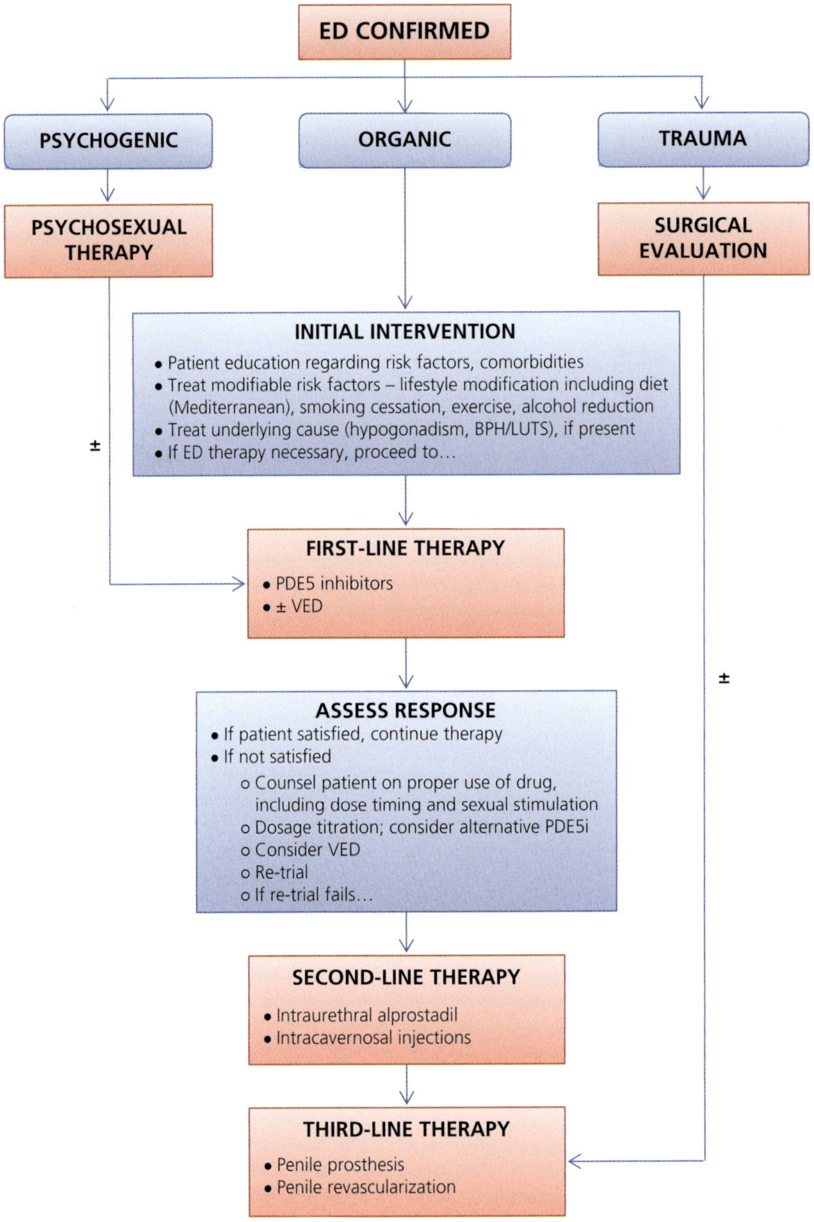

Figure 18.3 Treatment algorithm for management of erectile dysfunction (ED). BPH, benign prostatic hyperplasia; LUTS, lower urinary tract symptoms; PDE5i,phosphodiesterase type 5 inhibitor; VED, vacuum erection device.

such as diabetes, hypertension, and cardiovascular disease it is logical to presume that lifestyle modification might play a role in optimization of overall sexual health. Several reports have suggested such a beneficial effect. For example, smoking cessation, weight reduction, increased exercise, and adoption of a healthy diet have all been shown to provide a beneficial effect on erectile function.[26,28,32,147–149] However, few data exist evaluating the effects of lifestyle modification on ED, and reports often differ on the efficacy of lifestyle changes and reversal of ED symptoms.[30,31] However, it is advisable to counsel patients on the importance of adopting healthy lifestyle habits to improve sexual health, notwithstanding the need for pharmacotherapy or medical interventions.[150,151]

Given their relative convenience, simplicity, and ease of use, oral pharmacotherapy in the form of PDE5 inhibitors (PDE5is) represent a first-line treatment option for ED.[150] Currently, three oral PDE5is comprise the mainstay of oral ED therapies: sildenafil, vardenafil, and tadalafil. Each of these oral agents blocks phosphodiesterase-5 from degrading cGMP, the penultimate downstream mediator of corporal smooth muscle relaxation that mediates erection. All three PDE5is have similar efficacy and tolerability, although subtle differences between these three agents exist. However, superiority of one agent over the others has not been established, mostly owing to lack of comparative, head-to-head clinical trials.[36] While sildenafil and vardenafil exhibit similar half-lives of 3–5 hours, tadalafil possesses a half-life of approximately 18 hours, which has led to a daily dosing protocol for tadalafil, and it may be a useful alternative for patients in select cases.[152] All three medications interact to some degree with α-adrenergic receptor blockers, such as those used to treat hypertension and lower urinary tract symptoms (LUTS). Vardenafil is contraindicated in all patients taking alpha blockers, and both sildenafil (50 mg and 100 mg doses) and tadalafil should be administered with caution to such patients. All three PDE5is are absolutely contraindicated in patients taking any form of nitrate medication.[150]

Overall, PDE5is are effective, with successful sexual intercourse rates of approximately 70%. However, these medications are not effective or sufficient in all patients.[36] In the event a patient fails a trial of PDE5is, the best next step is to reassess the therapeutic plan. Several modifiable factors influence the success or failure of PDE5i therapy. For example, the timing of medication use is important. PDE5is should be taken on demand approximately 1 hour before initiating sexual activity. This interval allows sufficient time for achievement of peak serum concentrations and peak efficacy. In addition, achieving an erection sufficient for intercourse also depends on the presence of adequate sexual stimulation. PDE5is inhibit degradation of nitric oxide (NO) by cGMP, but NO release is dependent on sexual stimulation and arousal. Insufficient stimulation may therefore result in suboptimal NO levels and diminished PDE5i efficacy. PDE5i efficacy may be also be limited by high fat intake, and reduction of fat intake proximal to drug usage may improve PDE5i efficacy. The patient should also be aware that up to 10 attempts with PDE5i may be necessary to achieve satisfactory erections, although high first-use response rates can occur.[36,153–156] If treatment failure persists despite appropriate medication usage, the clinician may consider second-line options.

Second-line therapy for the treatment of ED consists of intracavernous injectable (ICI) agents or intraurethral suppositories.[157] Alprostadil, a synthetic formulation of the potent vasodilator prostaglandin E_1 (PGE_1), is available as an intraurethral suppository, which is inserted through the urethral meatus to the distal urethra, from where the drug is absorbed through the urethral mucosa and into the corpora cavernosa, stimulating erection. Up to 56% of men will engage in intercourse to completion in two of three attempts using intraurethral alprostadil (IUA).[158] However, other studies have shown lower success rates and a lack of consistency in treatment response.[159,160] Clinicians must take care to present realistic expectations to patients in light of the variable data on outcomes with IUA. Of note, the efficacy of IUA may be supplemented with the use of an adjustable penile constriction band designed to prevent medication migration out of the corpora. PDE5is may also serve as an adjunct to patients using IUA, with combination therapy with PDE5is having improved efficacy compared with IUA alone.[161–163] The most common adverse events associated with IUA are penile or urethral pain, seen in upwards of 50% of cases. Headache, dizziness, or minor bleeding are also associated with IUA usage, but at much lower rates (between 1 and 10%).[164]

Intracavernosal injection of vasoactive agents represents the most effective non-surgical treatment for ED, and is successful in otherwise normal men with ED as well as difficult-to-treat subgroups of men with ED, including those with diabetes, cardiovascular disease, and other chronic illnesses.[164–166] As the name suggests, ICI involves the direct injection of vasodilatory drug into the corpora cavernosa. Alprostadil, papaverine, and phentolamine are the three agents regularly used in clinical practice, and they may be administered either as single agent or in combination. Success rates of up to 70–90% have been reported with ICI, depending on the combination of agents used.[167–173] Possible side effects of ICI include pain at the injection site, penile pain with erection, penile fibrosis, and priapism.[165,172] However, these side effects may be mitigated by using combination rather than monotherapy.[171] ICI is contraindicated in patients with a history of psychiatric disorder or mental instability, risk of priapism, coagulopathy, or cardiovascular disease, or in those deemed unable to administer self-injections (e.g., poor manual dexterity, morbid obesity).

A brief note regarding vacuum erection devices (VEDs) is also warranted in this discussion. These may be used as first-line ED therapy or as an adjunct to first- or second-line therapies.[173] VEDs are medical devices consisting of a cylindrical chamber into which the penis is inserted. Air is extracted from the chamber, creating negative pressure around the penis and drawing blood into the corpora, resulting in erection. An elastic constriction band is then placed around the base of the penis to prevent blood regress and the device is removed.[174,175] The constriction band should be left in place for no longer than 30 minutes, given the risk of cavernosal ischemia, and if the patient requires an erection lasting more than 30 minutes, the band must be released, detumesence achieved, and the procedure repeated.[176,177] Unlike medical therapies, VEDs do not activate or modulate a biochemical signaling pathway, and as such, do not produce a "physiologic" erection.[174,178] Nevertheless, they are effective in generating erections sufficient for intercourse 60–90% of the time. Unfortunately, patient satisfaction rates with VEDs are low overall, between 30 and 68%.[179–184] Complications associated with VEDs are relatively infrequent, tend to decrease with continued use of the device, and include penile pain, petechiae, bruising, and difficulty with ejaculation given the physical obstruction of ejaculate passage.[180,185]

If a patient fails oral, intraurethral, or injectable therapy, third-line treatment for ED involves surgical management via implantation of a penile prosthesis or, in select cases, penile revascularization surgery.[157,186,187] However, an in-depth discussion of the surgical management of ED is beyond the scope of this chapter.

Erectile dysfunction treatment for infertile men

In the setting of male infertility, the algorithm for ED management does not deviate greatly from Figure 18.3. However, the clinician should be aware that in the setting of male infertility, overall ED rates, as well as prevalence of psychogenic ED, may be higher than in the general population.[116,188] This interplay has been discussed above, and in such cases, psychosexual therapy might be a valuable treatment option.[189–191] Unfortunately, the necessary volume of evidence-based, well-controlled, and large-scale trials investigating the effectiveness of psychosexual therapy in ED treatment is lacking. That said, psychosexual therapy has shown benefit in men with ED, especially those who continued therapy for longer time intervals.[191] The dearth of evidence notwithstanding, consultation with a trained sexual therapist is an important treatment modality to consider in the infertile male, as integrated treatment plans combining psychosexual and medical therapy may aid the patient in achieving overall sexual well-being.[190,192]

The spectrum of ED treatments affects the male sexual response cycle, and may therefore negatively impact male fertility. The effect of PDE5is on male fertility and seminal parameters is discussed elsewhere in this text, although no apparent negative effects have been reported.

Studies investigating the effects of IUA on semen parameters have reported no adverse effects on sperm motility, viability, or membrane integrity.[193] In contrast, phentolamine and other α1-receptor antagonists may negatively impact sperm quality and ejaculatory function. Andrade et al. showed a dose-dependent reduction in sperm motility in men using phentolamine, while Kobayashi et al. observed loss of seminal emission in 15 healthy male volunteers while on silodosin, an α1-receptor antagonist.[194,195] The general association between α1-receptor antagonists, such as prazosin and phentolamine, and impaired ejaculation is also well established.[196,197] However, consensus data regarding the effect on male fertility of intracavernous phentolamine, specifically when delivered in combination with other ICI agents such as alprostadil and papaverine, has not been established.

As mentioned previously, VEDs may cause difficulty with ejaculation and trapping of ejaculate due to urethral compression in 12–30% of patients; this may pose a problem for men seeking treatment for both infertility and ED.[184]

Overall, the current evidence base examining the effects of ED therapies on infertility shows little detrimental effect on fertility apart from several specific drugs, supporting the use of most ED therapies in men with fertility concerns or difficulties.

Conclusion

Since the first successful delivery resulting from in vitro fertilization was reported in 1982, progress in the field of ART has been dramatic.[198] Consumer consumption and the increased availability of ART, and consequently the number of babies born via these technologies, have significantly increased in recent years. An area of particular excitement in this new age of reproductive healthcare is that of male factor infertility. Couples who previously would have no recourse other than donor insemination or adoption, due to the presence of a severe male factor or prior treatment failures, may now achieve pregnancies thanks to the breakthroughs in ART. One area of future investigation in this realm is that of the relationship between male infertility and ED. While recent work describes clear relationships between ED and male infertility on numerous levels, including causes and treatments, numerous etiologies of both conditions, as well as cause-specific treatments, remain to be elucidated.

Ultimately, the clear association between ED and male infertility highlights the need to consider these entities together when evaluating the infertile male or the male with erectile difficulties, and to target the evaluation and treatment approaches to afflicted men.

References

1 Tietze C, Guttmacher AF, Rubin S. Time required for conception in 1727 planned pregnancies. *Fertil Steril* 1950;1(4):338–46.

2 Spira A. Epidemiology of human reproduction. *Hum Reprod* 1986;1(2):111–5.

3 Thonneau P, Marchand S, Tallec A, et al. Incidence and main causes of infertility in a resident population (1,850,000) of three French regions (1988–1989). *Hum Reprod* 1991;6(6):811–6.

4 Martinez GM, Chandra A, Abma JC, Jones J, Mosher WD. Fertility, contraception, and fatherhood: Data on men and women from cycle 6 (2002) of the 2002 National Survey of Family Growth. *Vital Health Stat 23* 2006;(26)(26):1–142.

5 Meacham RB, Joyce GF, Wise M, Kparker A, Niederberger C, Urologic Diseases in America Project. Male infertility. *J Urol* 2007;177(6):2058–66.

6 Marketdata Enterprises I. U.S. fertility clinics & infertility services: An industry analysis. 2009. Available at: http://www.marketdataenterprises.com/wp-content/uploads/2014/01/Fertility%20Clinics%20PR%202013.pdf

7 Kolettis PN, Sabanegh ES. Significant medical pathology discovered during a male infertility evaluation. *J Urol* 2001;166(1):178–80.

8 Eisenberg ML, Park Y, Hollenbeck AR, Lipshultz LI, Schatzkin A, Pletcher MJ. Fatherhood and the risk of cardiovascular mortality in the NIH-AARP Diet and Health Study. *Hum Reprod* 2011;26(12):3479–85.

9 NIH consensus conference. impotence. NIH consensus development panel on impotence. *JAMA* 1993;270(1):83–90.

10 Rosen RC, Riley A, Wagner G, Osterloh IH, Kirkpatrick J, Mishra A. The international index of erectile function (IIEF): A multidimensional scale for assessment of erectile dysfunction. *Urology* 1997;49(6):822–30.

11 Derogatis LR, Burnett AL. The epidemiology of sexual dysfunctions. *J Sex Med* 2008;5(2):289–300.

12 Ayta IA, McKinlay JB, Krane RJ. The likely worldwide increase in erectile dysfunction between 1995 and 2025 and some possible policy consequences. *BJU Int* 1999;84(1):50–6.

13 Braun M, Wassmer G, Klotz T, Reifenrath B, Mathers M, Engelmann U. Epidemiology of erectile dysfunction: Results of the 'Cologne Male Survey'. *Int J Impot Res* 2000;12(6):305–11.

14 Nicolosi A, Laumann EO, Glasser DB, et al. Sexual behavior and sexual dysfunctions after age 40: The global study of sexual attitudes and behaviors. *Urology* 2004;64(5):991–7.

15 Rosen RC, Fisher WA, Eardley I, et al. The Multinational Men's Attitudes to Life Events and Sexuality (MALES) study: I. prevalence of erectile dysfunction and related health concerns in the general population. *Curr Med Res Opin* 2004;20(5):607–17.

16 Saigal CS, Wessells H, Pace J, Schonlau M, Wilt TJ, Urologic Diseases in America Project. Predictors and prevalence of erectile dysfunction in a racially diverse population. *Arch Intern Med* 2006;166(2):207–12.

17 Laumann EO, West S, Glasser D, Carson C, Rosen R, Kang JH. Prevalence and correlates of erectile dysfunction by race and ethnicity among men aged 40 or older in the United States: From the Male Attitudes Regarding Sexual Health Survey. *J Sex Med* 2007;4(1):57–65.

18 Selvin E, Burnett AL, Platz EA. Prevalence and risk factors for erectile dysfunction in the US. *Am J Med* 2007;120(2):151–7.

19 Litwin MS, Saigal CS, Yano EM, et al. Urologic Diseases in America Project: Analytical methods and principal findings. *J Urol* 2005;173(3):933–7.

20 Wessells H, Joyce GF, Wise M, Wilt TJ. Erectile dysfunction. *J Urol* 2007;177(5):1675–81.

21 Schouten BW, Bohnen AM, Groeneveld FP, Dohle GR, Thomas S, Bosch JL. Erectile dysfunction in the community: Trends over time in incidence, prevalence, GP consultation

and medication use – the Krimpen Study: Trends in ED. *J Sex Med* 2010;7(7):2547–53.

22 Ralph D, McNicholas T. UK management guidelines for erectile dysfunction. *BMJ* 2000;321(7259):499–503.

23 Seftel AD, Miner MM, Kloner RA, Althof SE. Office evaluation of male sexual dysfunction. *Urol Clin North Am* 2007;34(4):463–82, v.

24 Shabsigh R, Klein LT, Seidman S, Kaplan SA, Lehrhoff BJ, Ritter JS. Increased incidence of depressive symptoms in men with erectile dysfunction. *Urology* 1998;52(5):848–52.

25 Araujo AB, Durante R, Feldman HA, Goldstein I, McKinlay JB. The relationship between depressive symptoms and male erectile dysfunction: Cross-sectional results from the Massachusetts Male Aging Study. *Psychosom Med* 1998;60(4):458–65.

26 Mannino DM, Klevens RM, Flanders WD. Cigarette smoking: An independent risk factor for impotence? *Am J Epidemiol* 1994;140(11):1003–8.

27 Feldman HA, Johannes CB, Derby CA, et al. Erectile dysfunction and coronary risk factors: Prospective results from the Massachusetts Male Aging Study. *Prev Med* 2000; 30(4):328–38.

28 Bacon CG, Mittleman MA, Kawachi I, Giovannucci E, Glasser DB, Rimm EB. A prospective study of risk factors for erectile dysfunction. *J Urol* 2006;176(1):217–21.

29 Feldman HA, Goldstein I, Hatzichristou DG, Krane RJ, McKinlay JB. Impotence and its medical and psychosocial correlates: Results of the Massachusetts Male Aging Study. *J Urol* 1994;151(1):54–61.

30 Derby CA, Mohr BA, Goldstein I, Feldman HA, Johannes CB, McKinlay JB. Modifiable risk factors and erectile dysfunction: Can lifestyle changes modify risk? *Urology* 2000;56(2):302–6.

31 Esposito K, Giugliano F, Di Palo C, et al. Effect of lifestyle changes on erectile dysfunction in obese men: A randomized controlled trial. *JAMA* 2004;291(24):2978–84.

32 Esposito K, Ciotola M, Giugliano F, et al. Mediterranean diet improves erectile function in subjects with the metabolic syndrome. *Int J Impot Res* 2006;18(4):405–10.

33 Schrader SM, Breitenstein MJ, Lowe BD. Cutting off the nose to save the penis. *J Sex Med* 2008;5(8):1932–40.

34 Rosen RC, Lane RM, Menza M. Effects of SSRIs on sexual function: A critical review. *J Clin Psychopharmacol* 1999;19(1): 67–85.

35 Nurnberg HG, Gelenberg A, Hargreave TB, Harrison WM, Siegel RL, Smith MD. Efficacy of sildenafil citrate for the treatment of erectile dysfunction in men taking serotonin reuptake inhibitors. *Am J Psychiatry* 2001;158(11):1926–8.

36 Carson CC, Lue TF. Phosphodiesterase type 5 inhibitors for erectile dysfunction. *BJU Int* 2005;96(3):257–80.

37 Linet OI, Neff LL. Intracavernous prostaglandin E1 in erectile dysfunction. *Clin Investig* 1994;72(2):139–49.

38 Lakin MM, Montague DK, VanderBrug Medendorp S, Tesar L, Schover LR. Intracavernous injection therapy: Analysis of results and complications. *J Urol* 1990;143(6):1138–41.

39 Hellstrom WJ, Bennett AH, Gesundheit N, et al. A double-blind, placebo-controlled evaluation of the erectile response to transurethral alprostadil. *Urology* 1996;48(6):851–6.

40 Padma-Nathan H, Hellstrom WJ, Kaiser FE, et al. Treatment of men with erectile dysfunction with transurethral alprostadil. Medicated Urethral System for Erection (MUSE) study group. *N Engl J Med* 1997;336(1):1–7.

41 Guay AT, Perez JB, Velasquez E, Newton RA, Jacobson JP. Clinical experience with intraurethral alprostadil (MUSE) in the treatment of men with erectile dysfunction. A retrospective study. Medicated Urethral System for Erection. *Eur Urol* 2000;38(6):671–6.

42 Hellstrom WJ, Montague DK, Moncada I, et al. Implants, mechanical devices, and vascular surgery for erectile dysfunction. *J Sex Med* 2010;7(1 Pt 2):501–23.

43 Nagler HM. Varicocele. In: Lipshultz LI (ed.), *Infertility in the Male*. St Louis: Mosby Year Book, 1997; pp. 336–59.

44 Nieschlag E. Classification of andrological disorders. In: Nieschlag E, Behre H, Nieschlag S (eds), *Andrology: Male Reproductive Health and Dysfunction*, 2nd edn. Berlin: Springer-Verlag, 1997; pp. 83–7.

45 de Kretser D. Male infertility. *Lancet* 1997;349(9054): 787–90.

46 Badenoch DF, Waxman J, Boorman L, et al. Administration of a gonadotropin releasing hormone analogue in oligozoospermic infertile males. *Acta Endocrinol (Copenh)* 1988;117(2): 265–7.

47 Crottaz B, Senn A, Reymond MJ, Rey F, Germond M, Gomez F. Follicle-stimulating hormone bioactivity in idiopathic normogonadotropic oligoasthenozoospermia: Double-blind trial with gonadotropin-releasing hormone. *Fertil Steril* 1992;57(5):1034–43.

48 Attia AM, Al-Inany HG, Proctor ML. Gonadotrophins for idiopathic male factor subfertility. *Cochrane Database Syst Rev* 2006;8:CD005071. doi: 10.1002/14651858. CD005071.pub2.

49 Ashkenazi J, Bar-Hava I, Farhi J, et al. The role of purified follicle stimulating hormone therapy in the male partner before intracytoplasmic sperm injection. *Fertil Steril* 1999; 72(4):670–3.

50 Baccetti B, Piomboni P, Bruni E, et al. Effect of follicle-stimulating hormone on sperm quality and pregnancy rate. *Asian J Androl* 2004;6(2):133–7.

51 Micic S, Dotlic R. Evaluation of sperm parameters in clinical trial with clomiphene citrate of oligospermic men. *J Urol* 1985;133(2):221–2.

52 Liu PY, Handelsman DJ. The present and future state of hormonal treatment for male infertility. *Hum Reprod Update* 2003;9(1):9–23.

53 Pavlovich CP, King P, Goldstein M, Schlegel PN. Evidence of a treatable endocrinopathy in infertile men. *J Urol* 2001; 165(3):837–41.

54 Clark RV, Sherins RJ. Treatment of men with idiopathic oligozoospermic infertility using the aromatase inhibitor,

testolactone. results of a double-blinded, randomized, placebo-controlled trial with crossover. *J Androl* 1989;10(3):240–7.
55 Suleiman SA, Ali ME, Zaki ZM, el-Malik EM, Nasr MA. Lipid peroxidation and human sperm motility: Protective role of vitamin E. *J Androl* 1996;17(5):530–7.
56 Rolf C, Cooper TG, Yeung CH, Nieschlag E. Antioxidant treatment of patients with asthenozoospermia or moderate oligoasthenozoospermia with high-dose vitamin C and vitamin E: A randomized, placebo-controlled, double-blind study. *Hum Reprod* 1999;14(4):1028–33.
57 Keskes-Ammar L, Feki-Chakroun N, Rebai T, et al. Sperm oxidative stress and the effect of an oral vitamin E and selenium supplement on semen quality in infertile men. *Arch Androl* 2003;49(2):83–94.
58 Balercia G, Regoli F, Armeni T, Koverech A, Mantero F, Boscaro M. Placebo-controlled double-blind randomized trial on the use of L-carnitine, L-acetylcarnitine, or combined L-carnitine and L-acetylcarnitine in men with idiopathic asthenozoospermia. *Fertil Steril* 2005;84(3):662–71.
59 Sigman M, Glass S, Campagnone J, Pryor JL. Carnitine for the treatment of idiopathic asthenospermia: A randomized, double-blind, placebo-controlled trial. *Fertil Steril* 2006; 85(5):1409–14.
60 Cohlen BJ. Should we continue performing intrauterine inseminations in the year 2004? *Gynecol Obstet Invest* 2005; 59(1):3–13.
61 Palermo GD, Neri QV, Takeuchi T, Rosenwaks Z. ICSI: Where we have been and where we are going. *Semin Reprod Med* 2009;27(2):191–201.
62 Hwang K, Yatsenko AN, Jorgez CJ, et al. Mendelian genetics of male infertility. *Ann N Y Acad Sci* 2010;1214(1):E1–E17.
63 Lue TF. Erectile dysfunction. *N Engl J Med* 2000;342(24): 1802–13.
64 Hwang K, Walters RC, Lipshultz LI. Contemporary concepts in the evaluation and management of male infertility. *Nat Rev Urol* 2011;8(2):86–94.
65 Mulligan T, Schmitt B. Testosterone for erectile failure. *J Gen Intern Med* 1993;8(9):517–21.
66 Araujo AB, Esche GR, Kupelian V, et al. Prevalence of symptomatic androgen deficiency in men. *J Clin Endocrinol Metab* 2007;92(11):4241–7.
67 Diagnostic evaluation of the infertile male: A committee opinion. *Fertil Steril* 2012;98(2):294–301.
68 Slag MF, Morley JE, Elson MK, et al. Impotence in medical clinic outpatients. *JAMA* 1983;249(13):1736–40.
69 Spark RF, White RA, Connolly PB. Impotence is not always psychogenic. newer insights into hypothalamic-pituitary-gonadal dysfunction. *JAMA* 1980;243(8):750–5.
70 Buvat J, Lemaire A. Endocrine screening in 1,022 men with erectile dysfunction: Clinical significance and cost-effective strategy. *J Urol* 1997;158(5):1764–7.
71 Earle CM, Stuckey BG. Biochemical screening in the assessment of erectile dysfunction: What tests decide future therapy? *Urology* 2003;62(4):727–31.
72 Kelly TM, Edwards CQ, Meikle AW, Kushner JP. Hypogonadism in hemochromatosis: Reversal with iron depletion. *Ann Intern Med* 1984;101(5):629–32.
73 Walton C, Kelly WF, Laing I, Bu'lock DE. Endocrine abnormalities in idiopathic haemochromatosis. *Q J Med* 1983;52(205):99–110.
74 Schwanzel-Fukuda M, Bick D, Pfaff DW. Luteinizing hormone-releasing hormone (LHRH)-expressing cells do not migrate normally in an inherited hypogonadal (Kallmann) syndrome. *Brain Res Mol Brain Res* 1989;6(4):311–26.
75 Carter JN, Tyson JE, Tolis G, Van Vliet S, Faiman C, Friesen HG. Prolactin-screening tumors and hypogonadism in 22 men. *N Engl J Med* 1978;299(16):847–52.
76 Segal S, Yaffe H, Laufer N, Ben-David M. Male hyperprolactinemia: Effects on fertility. *Fertil Steril* 1979;32(5): 556–61.
77 Melmed S, Casanueva FF, Hoffman AR, et al. Diagnosis and treatment of hyperprolactinemia: An Endocrine Society clinical practice guideline. *J Clin Endocrinol Metab* 2011; 96(2):273–88.
78 Velazquez EM, Bellabarba Arata G. Effects of thyroid status on pituitary gonadotropin and testicular reserve in men. *Arch Androl* 1997;38(1):85–92.
79 Abalovich M, Levalle O, Hermes R, et al. Hypothalamic-pituitary-testicular axis and seminal parameters in hyperthyroid males. *Thyroid* 1999;9(9):857–63.
80 Krassas GE, Pontikides N, Deligianni V, Miras K. A prospective controlled study of the impact of hyperthyroidism on reproductive function in males. *J Clin Endocrinol Metab* 2002;87(8):3667–71.
81 Corona G, Wu FCW, Forti G, et al. Thyroid hormones and male sexual function. *Int J Androl* 2012;35(5):668–79.
82 Maggi M, Buvat J, Corona G, Guay A, Torres LO. Hormonal causes of male sexual dysfunctions and their management (hyperprolactinemia, thyroid disorders, GH disorders, and DHEA). *J Sex Med* 2013;10(3):661–77.
83 Hendry WF. Iatrogenic damage to male reproductive function. *J R Soc Med* 1995;88(10):579P–584P.
84 Kedia KR, Markland C, Fraley EE. Sexual function after high retroperitoneal lymphadenectomy. *Urol Clin North Am* 1977;4(3):523–8.
85 Nijman JM, Schraffordt Koops H, Oldhoff J, Kremer J, Sleijfer DT. Sexual function after surgery and combination chemotherapy in men with disseminated nonseminomatous testicular cancer. *J Surg Oncol* 1988;38(3):182–6.
86 Schover LR. Sexuality and fertility in urologic cancer patients. *Cancer* 1987;60(3 Suppl.):553–8.
87 Walsh PC, Donker PJ. Impotence following radical prostatectomy: Insight into etiology and prevention. *J Urol* 2002;167(2 Pt 2):1005–10.
88 Quinlan DM, Epstein JI, Carter BS, Walsh PC. Sexual function following radical prostatectomy: Influence of preservation of neurovascular bundles. *J Urol* 1991;145(5): 998–1002.

89 Borchers H, Brehmer B, Kirschner-Hermanns R, Reineke T, Tietze L, Jakse G. Erectile function after non-nerve-sparing radical prostatectomy: Fact or fiction? *Urol Int* 2006; 76(3):213–6.
90 Weinstein M, Roberts M. Sexual potency following surgery for rectal carcinoma. A follow-up of 44 patients. *Ann Surg* 1977;185(3):295–300.
91 Catalona WJ, Bigg SW. Nerve-sparing radical prostatectomy: Evaluation of results after 250 patients. *J Urol* 1990;143(3):538–43; discussion 544.
92 Liang JT, Lai HS, Lee PH, Chang KJ. Laparoscopic pelvic autonomic nerve-preserving surgery for sigmoid colon cancer. *Ann Surg Oncol* 2008;15(6):1609–16.
93 Schoenberg MP, Walsh PC, Breazeale DR, Marshall FF, Mostwin JL, Brendler CB. Local recurrence and survival following nerve sparing radical cystoprostatectomy for bladder cancer: 10-year follow-up. *J Urol* 1996;155(2):490–4.
94 Sica DA. Pharmacokinetics and pharmacodynamics of mineralocorticoid blocking agents and their effects on potassium homeostasis. *Heart Fail Rev* 2005;10(1):23–9.
95 Griffin JE, Wilson JD. Disorders of the testes and male reproductive tract. In: Wilson JD (ed.), *Williams Textbook of Endocrinology*, 10th edn. Philadelphia: Saunders, 2003; pp. 709–69.
96 Harrison WM, Rabkin JG, Ehrhardt AA, et al. Effects of antidepressant medication on sexual function: A controlled study. *J Clin Psychopharmacol* 1986;6(3):144–9.
97 Monteiro WO, Noshirvani HF, Marks IM, Lelliott PT. Anorgasmia from clomipramine in obsessive-compulsive disorder. A controlled trial. *Br J Psychiatry* 1987;151: 107–12.
98 Keltner NL, McAfee KM, Taylor CL. Mechanisms and treatments of SSRI-induced sexual dysfunction. *Perspect Psychiatr Care* 2002;38(3):111–16.
99 Sullivan G, Lukoff D. Sexual side effects of antipsychotic medication: Evaluation and interventions. *Hosp Community Psychiatry* 1990;41(11):1238–41.
100 Nudell DM, Monoski MM, Lipshultz LI. Common medications and drugs: How they affect male fertility. *Urol Clin North Am* 2002;29(4):965–73.
101 Giuliano F. Impact of medical treatments for benign prostatic hyperplasia on sexual function. *BJU Int* 2006;97 (Suppl. 2):34–8; discussion 44–5.
102 Traish AM, Hassani J, Guay AT, Zitzmann M, Hansen ML. Adverse side effects of 5alpha-reductase inhibitors therapy: Persistent diminished libido and erectile dysfunction and depression in a subset of patients. *J Sex Med* 2011;8(3):872–84.
103 Roehrborn CG, Siami P, Barkin J, et al. The effects of dutasteride, tamsulosin and combination therapy on lower urinary tract symptoms in men with benign prostatic hyperplasia and prostatic enlargement: 2-year results from the CombAT study. *J Urol* 2008;179(2):616–21; discussion 621.
104 Amory JK, Anawalt BD, Matsumoto AM, et al. The effect of 5alpha-reductase inhibition with dutasteride and finasteride on bone mineral density, serum lipoproteins, hemoglobin, prostate specific antigen and sexual function in healthy young men. *J Urol* 2008;179(6):2333–8.
105 AUA Practice Guidelines Committee. AUA guideline on management of benign prostatic hyperplasia (2003). Chapter 1: Diagnosis and treatment recommendations. *J Urol* 2003;170(2 Pt 1):530–47.
106 Marberger M, Roehrborn CG, Marks LS, Wilson T, Rittmaster RS. Relationship among serum testosterone, sexual function, and response to treatment in men receiving dutasteride for benign prostatic hyperplasia. *J Clin Endocrinol Metab* 2006;91(4):1323–8.
107 Hsieh TC, Pastuszak AW, Hwang K, Lipshultz LI. Concomitant intramuscular human chorionic gonadotropin preserves spermatogenesis in men undergoing testosterone replacement therapy. *J Urol* 2013;189(2): 647–50.
108 Zacharin M, Sabin MA, Nair VV, Dagabdhao P. Addition of recombinant follicle-stimulating hormone to human chorionic gonadotropin treatment in adolescents and young adults with hypogonadotropic hypogonadism promotes normal testicular growth and may promote early spermatogenesis. *Fertil Steril* 2012;98(4):836–42.
109 Wischmann T, Stammer H, Scherg H, Gerhard I, Verres R. Psychosocial characteristics of infertile couples: A study by the 'Heidelberg Fertility Consultation Service'. *Hum Reprod* 2001;16(8):1753–61.
110 Kedem P, Mikulincer M, Nathanson YE, Bartoov B. Psychological aspects of male infertility. *Br J Med Psychol* 1990;63(Pt 1)(Pt 1):73–80.
111 Shindel AW, Nelson CJ, Naughton CK, Ohebshalom M, Mulhall JP. Sexual function and quality of life in the male partner of infertile couples: Prevalence and correlates of dysfunction. *J Urol* 2008;179(3):1056–9.
112 Monga M, Alexandrescu B, Katz SE, Stein M, Ganiats T. Impact of infertility on quality of life, marital adjustment, and sexual function. *Urology* 2004;63(1):126–30.
113 Jain K, Radhakrishnan G, Agrawal P. Infertility and psychosexual disorders: Relationship in infertile couples. *Indian J Med Sci* 2000;54(1):1–7.
114 Benazon N, Wright J, Sabourin S. Stress, sexual satisfaction, and marital adjustment in infertile couples. *J Sex Marital Ther* 1992;18(4):273–84.
115 Slade P, Raval H, Buck P, Lieberman BE. A 3-year follow-up of emotional, marital and sexual functioning in couples who were infertile. *J Reprod Infant Psyc* 1992;10(4): 233–43.
116 O'Brien JH, Lazarou S, Deane L, Jarvi K, Zini A. Erectile dysfunction and andropause symptoms in infertile men. *J Urol* 2005;174(5):1932–4; discussion 1934.
117 Mahlstedt PP. The psychological component of infertility. *Fertil Steril* 1985;43(3):335–46.

118 Glover L, Gannon K, Sherr L, Abel PD. Psychological distress before and immediately after attendance at a male sub-fertility clinic. *J R Soc Med* 1994;87(8):448–9.

119 Keye WR Jr. Psychosexual responses to infertility. *Clin Obstet Gynecol* 1984;27(3):760–6.

120 Sigg C. Sexuality and sterility. *Ther Umsch* 1994;51(2): 115–9.

121 Gurkan L, Raynor MC, Hellstrom WJ. Sex and the infertile male. *Semin Reprod Med* 2009;27(2):186–90.

122 Saleh RA, Ranga GM, Raina R, Nelson DR, Agarwal A. Sexual dysfunction in men undergoing infertility evaluation: A cohort observational study. *Fertil Steril* 2003;79(4): 909–12.

123 Nachtigall RD, Becker G, Wozny M. The effects of gender-specific diagnosis on men's and women's response to infertility. *Fertil Steril* 1992;57(1):113–21.

124 Drake TS, Grunert GM. A cyclic pattern of sexual dysfunction in the infertility investigation. *Fertil Steril* 1979;32(5):542–5.

125 Burns LH. Psychiatric aspects of infertility and infertility treatments. *Psychiatr Clin North Am* 2007;30(4):689–716.

126 Lue TF. Impotence: A patient's goal-directed approach to treatment. *World J Urol* 1990;8(2):67–74.

127 Lue TF. A patient's goal-directed approach to erectile dysfunction and Peyronie's disease. *Can J Urol* 1995;2 (Suppl. 1):13–17.

128 Hatzichristou D, Rosen RC, Broderick G, et al. Clinical evaluation and management strategy for sexual dysfunction in men and women. *J Sex Med* 2004;1(1): 49–57.

129 Hatzichristou D, Rosen RC, Derogatis LR, et al. Recommendations for the clinical evaluation of men and women with sexual dysfunction. *J Sex Med* 2010;7(1 pt 2): 337–348.

130 Jarow JP, Nana-Sinkam P, Sabbagh M, Eskew A. Outcome analysis of goal directed therapy for impotence. *J Urol* 1996;155(5):1609–12.

131 Hanash KA. Comparative results of goal oriented therapy for erectile dysfunction. *J Urol* 1997;157(6):2135–8.

132 Lue TF, Giuliano F, Montorsi F, et al. Summary of the recommendations on sexual dysfunctions in men. *J Sex Med* 2004;1(1):6–23.

133 Montorsi F, Adaikan G, Becher E, et al. Summary of the recommendations on sexual dysfunctions in men. *J Sex Med* 2010;7(11):3572–88.

134 Lewis JM, Osbourne AL, O'Leary MP. Erectile dysfunction. *J Med Liban* 2004;52(4):213–6.

135 Nusbaum MR, Hamilton CD. The proactive sexual health history. *Am Fam Physician* 2002;66(9):1705–12.

136 Burnett AL. Erectile dysfunction: A practical approach for primary care. *Geriatrics* 1998;53(2):34.

137 Davis-Joseph B, Tiefer L, Melman A. Accuracy of the initial history and physical examination to establish the etiology of erectile dysfunction. *Urology* 1995;45(3):498–502.

138 Martin-Morales A, Sanchez-Cruz JJ, Saenz de Tejada I, Rodriguez-Vela L, Jimenez-Cruz JF, Burgos-Rodriguez R. Prevalence and independent risk factors for erectile dysfunction in Spain: Results of the Epidemiologia de la Disfuncion Erectil Masculina Study. *J Urol* 2001; 166(2):569–74; discussion 574–5.

139 Kostis JB, Jackson G, Rosen R, et al. Sexual dysfunction and cardiac risk (the Second Princeton Consensus Conference). *Am J Cardiol* 2005;96 (12, Suppl. 2):85–93.

140 Kingsberg SA. Taking a sexual history. *Obstet Gynecol Clin North Am* 2006;33(4):535–47.

141 Fisher WA, Eardley I, McCabe M, Sand M. Erectile dysfunction (ED) is a shared sexual concern of couples I: Couple conceptions of ED. *J Sex Med* 2009;6(10): 2746–60.

142 Rosen RC, Cappelleri JC, Smith MD, Lipsky J, Pena BM. Development and evaluation of an abridged, 5-item version of the International Index of Erectile Function (IIEF-5) as a diagnostic tool for erectile dysfunction. *Int J Impot Res* 1999;11(6):319–26.

143 Sun P, Swindle R. Are men with erectile dysfunction more likely to have hypertension than men without erectile dysfunction? A naturalistic national cohort study. *J Urol* 2005;174(1):244–8.

144 Zonszein J. Diagnosis and management of endocrine disorders of erectile dysfunction. *Urol Clin North Am* 1995;22(4):789–802.

145 Ghanem HM, Salonia A, Martin-Morales A. Physical examination and laboratory testing for men with ED. *J Sex Med* 2013;10(1):108–10.

146 Ghanem HM, Salonia A, Martin-Morales A. SOP: Physical examination and laboratory testing for men with erectile dysfunction. *J Sex Med* 2013;10(1):108–10.

147 Wing RR, Rosen RC, Fava JL, et al. Effects of weight loss intervention on erectile function in older men with type 2 diabetes in the look AHEAD trial. *J Sex Med* 2010;7(1 Pt 1): 156–65.

148 Lamina S, Okoye CG, Dagogo TT. Therapeutic effect of an interval exercise training program in the management of erectile dysfunction in hypertensive patients. *J Clin Hypertens (Greenwich)* 2009;11(3):125–9.

149 Gupta BP, Murad MH, Clifton MM, Prokop L, Nehra A, Kopecky SL. The effect of lifestyle modification and cardiovascular risk factor reduction on erectile dysfunction: A systematic review and meta-analysis. *Arch Intern Med* 2011;171(20):1797–803.

150 Montague DK, Jarow JP, Broderick GA, et al. Chapter 1: The management of erectile dysfunction: An AUA update. *J Urol* 2005;174(1):230–9.

151 Esposito K, Giugliano D. Lifestyle for erectile dysfunction: A good choice. *Arch Intern Med* 2012;172(3):295–6; author reply 296.

152 Shabsigh R, Donatucci C, Costabile R, et al. Reliability of efficacy in men with erectile dysfunction treated with

tadalafil once daily after initial success. *Int J Impot Res* 2010;22(1):1–8.

153 Montorsi F, Padma-Nathan H, Buvat J, et al. Earliest time to onset of action leading to successful intercourse with vardenafil determined in an at-home setting: A randomized, double-blind, placebo-controlled trial. *J Sex Med* 2004;1(2):168–178.

154 Padma-Nathan H, Stecher VJ, Sweeney M, Orazem J, Tseng LJ, Deriesthal H. Minimal time to successful intercourse after sildenafil citrate: Results of a randomized, double-blind, placebo-controlled trial. *Urology* 2003;62(3): 400–3.

155 Carson CC. Erectile dysfunction in the 21st century: Whom we can treat, whom we cannot treat and patient education. *Int J Impot Res* 2002;14 (Suppl. 1):S29–34.

156 Rajagopalan P, Mazzu A, Xia C, Dawkins R, Sundaresan P. Effect of high-fat breakfast and moderate-fat evening meal on the pharmacokinetics of vardenafil, an oral phosphodiesterase-5 inhibitor for the treatment of erectile dysfunction. *J Clin Pharmacol* 2003;43(3):260–7.

157 Wespes E, Amar E, Hatzichristou D, et al. EAU guidelines on erectile dysfunction: An update. *Eur Urol* 2006;49(5): 806–15.

158 Guay AT, Perez JB, Velasquez E, Newton RA, Jacobson JP. Clinical experience with intraurethral alprostadil (MUSE) in the treatment of men with erectile dysfunction. A retrospective study. medicated urethral system for erection. *Eur Urol* 2000;38(6):671–6.

159 Fulgham PF, Cochran JS, Denman JL, et al. Disappointing initial results with transurethral alprostadil for erectile dysfunction in a urology practice setting. *J Urol* 1998;160 (6 Pt 1):2041–6.

160 Mulhall JP, Jahoda AE, Ahmed A, Parker M. Analysis of the consistency of intraurethral prostaglandin E(1) (MUSE) during at-home use. *Urology* 2001;58(2):262–6.

161 Nehra A, Blute ML, Barrett DM, Moreland RB. Rationale for combination therapy of intraurethral prostaglandin E(1) and sildenafil in the salvage of erectile dysfunction patients desiring noninvasive therapy. *Int J Impot Res* 2002;14 (Suppl. 1):S38–42.

162 Mydlo JH, Volpe MA, MacChia RJ. Results from different patient populations using combined therapy with alprostadil and sildenafil: Predictors of satisfaction. *BJU Int* 2000;86(4):469–73.

163 Lewis RW. Intraurethral and topical agents. *Drugs Today (Barc)* 2000;36(2–3):113–9.

164 Costa P, Potempa AJ. Intraurethral alprostadil for erectile dysfunction: A review of the literature. *Drugs* 2012;72(17): 2243–54.

165 Linet OI, Ogrinc FG. Efficacy and safety of intracavernosal alprostadil in men with erectile dysfunction. The Alprostadil Study Group. *N Engl J Med* 1996;334(14):873–7.

166 Heaton JP, Lording D, Liu SN, et al. Intracavernosal alprostadil is effective for the treatment of erectile dysfunction in diabetic men. *Int J Impot Res* 2001;13(6): 317–21.

167 Sidi AA, Cameron JS, Duffy LM, Lange PH. Intracavernous drug-induced erections in the management of male erectile dysfunction: Experience with 100 patients. *J Urol* 1986;135(4):704–6.

168 Zorgniotti AW, Lefleur RS. Auto-injection of the corpus cavernosum with a vasoactive drug combination for vasculogenic impotence. *J Urol* 1985;133(1):39–41.

169 Robinette MA, Moffat MJ. Intracorporal injection of papaverine and phentolamine in the management of impotence. *Br J Urol* 1986;58(6):692–5.

170 Porst H. The rationale for prostaglandin E1 in erectile failure: A survey of worldwide experience. *J Urol* 1996; 155(3):802–15.

171 Bennett AH, Carpenter AJ, Barada JH. An improved vasoactive drug combination for a pharmacological erection program. *J Urol* 1991;146(6):1564–5.

172 Moemen MN, Hamed HA, Kamel II, Shamloul RM, Ghanem HM. Clinical and sonographic assessment of the side effects of intracavernous injection of vasoactive substances. *Int J Impot Res* 2004;16(2):143–5.

173 Hackett G, Kell P, Ralph D, et al. British Society for Sexual Medicine guidelines on the management of erectile dysfunction. *J Sex Med* 2008;5(8):1841–65.

174 Broderick GA, McGahan JP, Stone AR, White RD. The hemodynamics of vacuum constriction erections: Assessment by color Doppler ultrasound. *J Urol* 1992;147(1):57–61.

175 McMahon CG. Nonsurgical treatment of cavernosal venous leakage. *Urology* 1997;49(1):97–100.

176 Witherington R. Vacuum constriction device for management of erectile impotence. *J Urol* 1989;141(2): 320–2.

177 Sidi AA, Becher EF, Zhang G, Lewis JH. Patient acceptance of and satisfaction with an external negative pressure device for impotence. *J Urol* 1990;144(5):1154–6.

178 Nadig PW, Ware JC, Blumoff R. Noninvasive device to produce and maintain an erection-like state. *Urology* 1986;27(2):126–31.

179 Vrijhof HJ, Delaere KP. Vacuum constriction devices in erectile dysfunction: Acceptance and effectiveness in patients with impotence of organic or mixed aetiology. *Br J Urol* 1994;74(1):102–5.

180 Dutta TC, Eid JF. Vacuum constriction devices for erectile dysfunction: A long-term, prospective study of patients with mild, moderate, and severe dysfunction. *Urology* 1999;54(5):891–3.

181 Blackard CE, Borkon WD, Lima JS, Nelson J. Use of vacuum tumescence device for impotence secondary to venous leakage. *Urology* 1993;41(3):225–30.

182 Baltaci S, Aydos K, Kosar A, Anafarta K. Treating erectile dysfunction with a vacuum tumescence device: A retrospective analysis of acceptance and satisfaction. *Br J Urol* 1995;76(6):757–60.

183 Turner LA, Althof SE, Levine SB, et al. Treating erectile dysfunction with external vacuum devices: Impact upon sexual, psychological and marital functioning. *J Urol* 1990;144(1):79–82.

184 Turner LA, Althof SE, Levine SB, Bodner DR, Kursh ED, Resnick MI. External vacuum devices in the treatment of erectile dysfunction: A one-year study of sexual and psychosocial impact. *J Sex Marital Ther* 1991;17(2):81–93.

185 Cookson MS, Nadig PW. Long-term results with vacuum constriction device. *J Urol* 1993;149(2):290–4.

186 Montague DK, Angermeier KW. Penile prosthesis implantation. *Urol Clin North Am* 2001;28(2):355–61.

187 Montague DK, Angermeier KW. Contemporary aspects of penile prosthesis implantation. *Urol Int* 2003;70(2):141–6.

188 Lotti F, Corona G, Rastrelli G, Forti G, Jannini EA, Maggi M. Clinical correlates of erectile dysfunction and premature ejaculation in men with couple infertility. *J Sex Med* 2012;9(10):2698–707.

189 Rosen RC. Psychogenic erectile dysfunction. Classification and management. *Urol Clin North Am* 2001;28(2):269–78.

190 McCabe M, Althof SE, Assalian P, et al. Psychological and interpersonal dimensions of sexual function and dysfunction. *J Sex Med* 2010;7(1 Pt 2):327–36.

191 Wylie KR. Treatment outcome of brief couple therapy in psychogenic male erectile disorder. *Arch Sex Behav* 1997;26(5):527–45.

192 Hawton K. Integration of treatments for male erectile dysfunction. *Lancet* 1998;351(9095):7–8.

193 Hellstrom WJ, Wang R, Peterson CA, Varady JC, Gesundheit N, Sikka SC. Effects of alprostadil and prazosin on motility, viability and membrane integrity of human sperm. *J Urol* 1998;159(5):1559–62.

194 Kobayashi K, Masumori N, Hisasue S, et al. Inhibition of seminal emission is the main cause of anejaculation induced by a new highly selective alpha1A-blocker in normal volunteers. *J Sex Med* 2008;5(9):2185–90.

195 Andrade JR, Traboulsi A, Hussain A, Dubin NH. In vitro effects of sildenafil and phentolamine, drugs used for erectile dysfunction, on human sperm motility. *Am J Obstet Gynecol* 2000;182(5):1093–5.

196 Tillem SM, Mellinger BC. Azoospermia due to aperistalsis of the vas deferens: Successful treatment with pseudoephedrine. *Urology* 1999;53(2):417–9.

197 Smith JF, Walsh TJ, Turek PJ. Ejaculatory duct obstruction. *Urol Clin North Am* 2008;35(2):221–7, viii.

198 Jones HW Jr, Jones GS, Andrews MC, et al. The program for in vitro fertilization at Norfolk. *Fertil Steril* 1982;38(1):14–21.

CHAPTER 19

Drug therapy for erectile dysfunction

Francisco J. Garcia[1,2,3], Eric Chung[4], and Gerald Brock[2,3]

[1] *University of Western Ontario, London, ON, Canada*

[2] *St Joseph's Health Sciences Centre, London, ON, Canada*

[3] *Lawson Health Research Institute, London, ON, Canada*

[4] *Princess Alexandra Hospital, Brisbane, Queensland, Australia*

Effective drug therapy for erectile dysfunction (ED) is a relatively recent advance in management. Historically, ED was treated with a presumption that the major underlying abnormalities were psychological. As a result, the management of ED was under the care of psychologists and sex therapist in the early 20th century. Therapies typically were psychoanalysis, sex therapy, and hormonal manipulation. With a better understanding of the etiology of ED and the vascular anatomy of the penis, it became apparent that a significant proportion of men suffered from organic ED. Management shifted from a predominantly psychoanalytic approach, towards surgery. With increasing knowledge and research activity, local therapies such as intracavernosal injection (ICI) were introduced in the 1980s. Brindley most famously injected his own penis prior to the start of a presentation at a conference, and then demonstrated his erection to the audience at the presentation's conclusion.[1] These discoveries led to better understanding of erectile physiology and allowed for the regulatory approval of new agents and identification of novel targets for pro-erectile therapy by several different routes (oral, sublingual, buccal, topical, etc.). Today there is a surge of research being performed on maximizing existing approaches, developing new agents with enhanced tolerability and efficacy profiles. However, the ideal therapy of the future, one that would have the potential to permanently cure the patient's ED such that ongoing medical treatment would not be required, still remains to be discovered.

General approach to drug therapy

Medication effects

Prior to initiating new drug therapy for erectile dysfunction it is important to review existing medications and comorbidities, identifying all contributing factors to erectile dysfunction. In particular, when a patient complains of sexual symptoms after initiating a new medication, it is important to determine if the symptoms are related primarily to sexual drive, erectile dysfunction, or alterations in ejaculation. Our current understanding of normal erectile physiology makes it easy to understand how some medications can interact with erections. Older antihypertensives, such as methyldopa and reserpine, have a high incidence of sexual dysfunction due to their central suppressive effects. Thiazides also have an association with ED,[2] as does spironolactone, which may interfere with testosterone synthesis.[3,4] Specific alpha-1 blockade may, however, be protective of ED.[2] Interestingly, statin therapy may salvage hypercholesterolemic sildenafil non-responders,[5] but has also been shown to induce a primary hypogonadism.[6]

While it seems intuitive that cardiac specific diagnoses and medications may exacerbate erectile dysfunction, many other medications across a wide range of therapeutic fields can induce erectile dysfunction. Table 19.1 summarizes a sample of drugs from different classes with reported effects on erectile function.

Male Sexual Dysfunction: A Clinical Guide, First Edition. Edited by Suks Minhas and John Mulhall.

Table 19.1 Selection of drugs reported to cause erectile dysfunction as a side effect.

Class	Example
Gastrointestinal	Metoclopramide,[187] cimetidine[188,189]
Neuropsychoactive	Typical antipsychotics,[190] atypical antipsychotics,[191] cannabis,[192] ethanol,[193,194] antidepressants,[189] gabapentin[195]
Analgesics	Opioids,[196] celecoxib,[197] indometacin[198]
Antihypertensives	Clonidine,[189,199] reserpine,[200] spironolactone,[3,4,200] thiazides[2]
Antiandrogens	5-Alpha-reductase inhibitors (dutasteride, finasteride),[201,202] goserelin,[203] triptorelin,[204] leuprolide[205]
Anti-infectives	Ketoconazole,[189] protease inhibitors,[206] antivirals[207]

Testosterone replacement

Men with ED secondary to low testosterone will often require some degree of supplementation in order to regain their erectile capacity. The specifics of managing these endocrinopathies and the different formulations of testosterone are discussed elsewhere. However, a note should be made that in cases of phosphodiesterase-5 inhibitor (PDE5-inhibitor) failure with concomitant hypogonadism, testosterone replacement therapy may salvage the ability to respond and allow for a more robust response to PDE5 inhibitor therapy.[7,8]

Pharmacological therapies

The clinical efficacy of a drug for ED can be determined through a variety of methods. The simplest is a subjective assessment of efficacy by asking the patient "Has the treatment you have been taking over the past 4 weeks improved your erectile function? Yes/No"[9] In much of the early literature on erectile dysfunction this was considered the General Assessment Question (GAQ). While it does not give the investigators any information on rigidity, reliability, or intercourse success, it does provide a subjective assessment of the patient's perspective. During the initial studies on sildenafil, the International Index of Erectile Function (IIEF) was developed to quantify the efficacy of treatment.[10] This was a carefully constructed questionnaire of 15 questions, covering five domains including erectile function, orgasmic function, sexual desire, sexual satisfaction, and overall satisfaction. A couple of interesting points need to be addressed about the original IIEF questionnaire; +primarily that all men with anatomical abnormalities of the penis (e.g., Peyronie's disease) and men with a history of priapism were excluded from the development of the questionnaire. Additionally, almost 50% of those in the study had no organic component to their ED.[10] However, the questionnaire did demonstrate excellent test-retest, construct, and discriminatory validity, and has since become a "gold standard" for evaluation of the efficacy of erectogenic interventions. At 15 questions the tool was cumbersome at times, and many authors began reporting only on the erectile function domain (IIEF-EF), which consisted of questions 1–5 and 15. The final metamorphosis of the IIEF came when a desire to design a diagnostic tool for ED arose, and an abridged version of the IIEF was produced that was able to categorize men into five categories of severity of erectile dysfunction.[11] A final questionnaire is the Sexual Encounter Profile (SEP), which is a series of five yes/no questions that the patient fills out after each attempt at intercourse. Question 2 ("Were you able to insert your penis into your partner's vagina?") and Question 3 ("Did your erection last long enough for you to have successful intercourse?") are the most reported values from the questionnaire. In particular, SEP Question 3 (SEP3) is considered the most rigorous measure of clinical efficacy in ED trials.[9]

Oral phosphodiesterase-5 (PDE5) inhibitors

Like many major breakthroughs in medicine, the discovery of PDE5 inhibitors for management of ED was a happy accident. In an attempt to develop a new way to manage angina, the PDE5 enzyme was specifically targeted due to its exclusive catalytic activity on cyclic guanosine monophosphate (cGMP).[12] The hope for Pfizer was that finding an endogenous method of augmenting the response of NO would allow them to avoid the tachyphylaxis associated with exogenous administration of NO in the management of angina.[12] However, as the preclinical studies progressed, the efficacy for treatment of angina was not sufficient, and the short half-life necessitated a cumbersome three times a day administration. It was at this juncture that the side effect reported by many of the males in the study of increased penile erectile capacity, which had been ignored previously, was then exploited.[12] In 1994 the first studies looking into sildenafil's use as an erectogenic aid began, and these were reported in 1996.[13] This first study not only demonstrated the efficacy of PDE5 inhibition on erections, but also showed a favorable dose-response curve, demonstrated tolerability of the medication,[13] and exploited the short half-life by successfully demonstrating on-demand use.[14]

Some level of sexual stimulation or arousal is required to initiate the release of NO to activate soluble guanyl cyclase to create cGMP. PDE5 inhibitors inhibit the breakdown of cGMP thereby augmenting the original pro-erectile signal leading to a decrease in intracellular calcium and ultimately smooth muscle relaxation.[15] An important distinction is that the drug does not cause erections directly and still requires sexual stimulation and arousal in order to augment the pro-erectile signal.

Clinically relevant pharmacokinetics of the three most used PDE5 inhibitors (sildenafil, vardenafil, and tadalafil) involves an understanding of time to peak concentrations, half-life, PDE5 affinity, and cross-reactivity. These are summarized in Table 19.2. Notable points include the similar half-lives of sildenafil and vardenafil versus the prolonged half-life of tadalafil, which has obvious implications towards length of time one must wait before administering nitrates. Each agent has unique side effects or cautions, such as PDE6 crossover inhibition with sildenafil causing blue vision; more backaches and myalgias with tadalafil; and a caution against concomitant use of antiarrhythmics with vardenafil. There are also differences in the affinity of each agent to the PDE5 enzyme, which would explain why vardenafil seems to have a larger therapeutic window despite a similar half-life to sildenafil. These features may become important when discussing which agent to try first, and what to expect.

Despite the minor structural differences between the PDE5 inhibitors, all have demonstrated efficacy in multiple large multicenter trials. The Global Assessment Question (GAQ) is typically positive in approximately 80% of

Table 19.2 Characteristics of three major phosphodiesterase inhibitors.

	Sildenafil	**Vardenafil**	**Tadalafil**
Half-life (h)[a]	3.82 ± 0.84	3.94 ± 1.31	17.5
Earliest onset (min)[a]	14	11	16
>50% part response (min)[a]	20	25	30
Success (%) measured at time (h) [vs placebo (%)][a]	69 % at 1 h	78% at 4 h [vs 57%]	60.9% at 24 h ± 2 [vs 36.8%]
	81% at 4 h [vs 31%]	70% at >6 h [vs 24%]	64.1% at 36 h ± 2 [vs 41.8%]
	60% at 8 h	87% at 8 h [vs 57%]	
	31% at 12 h		
Dosage[a]	100 mg	20 mg	20 mg
PDE6 affinity/PDE5 affinity[b,c]	0.09	0.0053	0.04
Side effects:[d,e,f]			
• Headache	14.6%	15%	14%
• Flush	14.1%	11%	4%
• Dyspepsia	6.2%	4%	10%
• Back pain	0%	2%	6%
• Rhinitis	2.6%	9%	5%
• Color visual disturbances	5.2%	0%	0%

Data sources:

[a] Shabsigh et al.[208]

[b] Gbekor et al.[209]

[c] Blount et al.[210]

[d] Padma-Nathan et al. (sildenafil).[211]

[e] Reffelmann et al. (vardenafil).[212]

[f] Brock et al. (tadalafil).[17]

ED patients treated with any of the PDE5 inhibitors as compared to approximately 30% with placebo.[16–18] Similarly, the SEP3 is positive in approximately 65–75% of treated patients, as compared to 30% with placebo. However, when the same agents are used in special populations they do not perform as well as with a mixed cohort. In particular, men with diabetes report GAQ and SEP3 positively approximately 50–70% of the time if treated with a PDE5 inhibitor as compared to 10–30% with placebo.[19–21] Additionally, tadalafil and vardenafil have been tried in a post-prostatectomy nerve spare situation and demonstrate positive GAQ and SEP3 on 60% and 40%, as compared to 15–20% and 10–20% with placebo.[22,23] While efficacy is obviously present, these unique populations do not have a response similar to the mixed cohort, and it should be discussed when initiating therapy. While some literature suggests that up to 80% of couples may be successful with the first dose,[24] other reports suggest that it takes approximately 3–8 attempts to maximize therapy.[25] However, despite the ease of administration, high efficacy, and easy tolerability, discontinuation rates are still around 45–78% after 6–24 months. Reasons for discontinuation are:

- efficacy below expectations (42%)
- cost (37%)
- loss of interest in sex (30.5%)
- inconvenience in obtaining medication (28.9%)
- recovery of erectile ability (15%)
- partner reluctance (14.6%)
- side effects (11.8%)
- other non-specified reasons (24%).[26]

Shortly after the widespread use of sildenafil, a few cardiovascular deaths were thought to be linked to its use, and therefore there was a push to elucidate what if any cardiovascular safety concerns there might be with its use. All three PDE5 inhibitors were examined in large randomized control trials and it was shown that there are no differences to be seen in rates of myocardial infarcts or cardiac deaths per 100 patient years.[27–29] Additionally, administering a PDE5 inhibitor to a patient with coronary artery disease or hypertension on medications had no detrimental effects. However, concomitant nitrate use is still considered a contraindication to PDE5 inhibitor use due to the risk of life-threatening hypotension. Should angina occur during sexual activity the patient should stop immediately and seek immediate emergency care. Additionally, cardiac clearance should be sought prior to initiating PDE5 inhibitor therapy on patients with aortic stenosis, left ventricular outflow obstruction, hypotension, and hypovolemia. Vardenafil should not be used in patients on type-1A or 3 antiarrhythmics or those with congenital prolonged QT syndromes.

A concern arose around non-arteritic anterior optic neuropathy (NAION) causing blindness after PDE5 inhibitor use. The review of the product by the US Food and Drug Administration (FDA), as well as retrospective database analyses, have failed to identify a causal link between PDE5 inhibitors and NAION.[30] However, it is still considered a contraindication to administer a PDE5 inhibitor to anyone with a hereditary degenerative retinal disorder such as retinitis pigmentosa. There have also been some concerns about sudden hearing loss, and potential for abnormalities in spermatogenesis; however, no causal link has been identified.

A newer vardenafil formulation (the vardenafil orodispersible tablet) has been shown to have better bioavailability and possibly an enhanced safety profile compared with the film-coated vardenafil tablet.[31] This first and only orodispersible PDE5 inhibitor does not require water for administration and appears unaffected by high-fat meals, in contrast to its oral counterparts. Efficacy has been reported with SEP3 rates of 65–70%.[32] It remains to be seen whether the differences in bioavailability have any clinical superiority.

Since tadalafil has a prolonged half-life it is possible for it to be used as a daily medication providing enhanced spontaneity to the couple. Currently tadalafil is the only PDE5 inhibitor approved for daily administration. Large multicenter randomized controlled trials have also shown that a daily 5 mg dose is equally efficacious as an on-demand 20 mg dose.[33,34] Interestingly, in patients unresponsive to PDE5 inhibitor therapy, placing them on daily PDE5 inhibitors may salvage 50% of them. The daily use of tadalafil appears to have improved tolerability compared to on-demand use.[33] Tachyphylaxis has not been experienced even with chronic use.[34] Animal models have also suggested that there may be additional benefits to chronic PDE5 inhibitor therapy. Chronic administration has been shown to induce endothelial progenitor cells to move into the circulation.[35] These cells may be a piece of the story that explains why in rabbits, chronic PDE5 inhibitor use reduces myocardial infarct size[36] and reperfusion injury after an ischemic event.[37] A new PDE5 inhibitor, udenafil, was recently reported also to have excellent efficacy, with SEP3 rate of 73%. Udenafil also has a prolonged half-life of approximately 13 hours, and appears similarly well tolerated.[38] Recently, there has been an explosion of newer PDE5 inhibitors in the market, such as mirodenafil, avanafil, and lodenafil.[39] While it may be that these second generation PDE5 inhibitors will demonstrate advantages in terms of efficacy or tolerability compared to the older PDE5 inhibitors, any differences are modest at best and they are far from replacing the original three PDE5 inhibitors. Currently they are selectively marketed to specific countries and their use is similarly restricted.

With the above mentioned changes as well as the ease of administration and tolerability there has been some investigation into using PDE5 inhibitors in a rehabilitative fashion after radical prostate cancer surgery.[40] Two large studies have attempted to look at this prospectively. The first reported that 36 weeks of sildenafil use returned potency to 27% of men in the treatment arm as compared to 4% in the placebo arm.[41] This study did receive some criticism due to the exceptionally low erectile recovery in the placebo arm. However, a follow-up study using vardenafil did not demonstrate any difference between the groups.[42] While penile rehabilitation remains an active area of research, it appears as though PDE5 inhibitors will only play a minor role.

Ultimately a proportion of the male population will not respond to PDE5 inhibitor therapy. The first distinction one must make is if the patient is in fact a true non-responder, or if they are not responding due to misinformation around how to best use the medication. Reviewing pertinent information surrounding how to take the medication may identify this population and educate them as well.[9] For example, a patient may be non-responsive because they are not allowing sufficient time for the medication to work, or consistently have a large fat-dense meal before the use of sildenafil. Should this still not improve their outcome, and they have failed four times on maximal therapy, they are then considered non-responders.[43] True non-responders typically have much more severe disease, and may require intracavernosal injection therapy or a prosthetic. The International Society of Sexual Medicine standards committee released a document reviewing the standard operating procedures surrounding conservative management of erectile dysfunction, and there is a stepwise approach to managing non-responders, which is summarized in Table 19.3.

Table 19.3 Management of phosphodiesterase-5 (PDE5) inhibitor non-responders.

1	Re-counsel and re-educate the patient/couple about appropriate PDE5 inhibitor use and the relevant pharmacokinetics[213]
2	Optimize concomitant disease states[214]
3	Treat concomitant hypogonadism[8]
4	"High-dose" (overdosing) PDE5 inhibitor therapy[9]
5	Shift patients to another PDE5 inhibitor[215]
6	Daily dosing of PDE5 inhibitors[216]

Alpha-adrenoreceptor antagonists

Adrenergic tone has a profound anti-erectile effect, a fact that has been exploited with great results in the management algorithim for priapism.[44] Elevated adrenergic tone is implicated as an etiology of certain disease states such as essential hypertension, and may be a consequence of disease such as generalized or situation anxiety disorders. If follows that a proportion of psychogenic ED may in fact be attributable to situational stress or anxiety with elevated adrenergic tone as the mechanism. Interestingly even a single stressful event has been shown in animal models to alter the spinal cord erectile reflexes.[45] Therefore adrenoreceptor antagonists would be a logical agent to exploit in order to maximize erectile capacity. One such pharmaceutical is phentolamine mesylate, a non-specific alpha-adrenergic agonist that has the unique distinction of being effective both as an oral agent[46] and an injectable agent.[9] Two oral forms have been studied, a traditional pill form[46] and a buccal application.[47] Both seem equally efficacious with potency returned in approximately 40% of men with mild ED.[47,48] Side effects are minimal with less than 10% of patients experiencing nasal congestion, facial flushing, and headaches. The mechanism of action is thought to work via a sympatholytic effect antagonizing alpha-1 and alpha-2 receptors equally, causing a decrease in adrenergic tone, corporal smooth muscle relaxation, and inhibition of noradrenaline (norepinephrine) release.[49]

Yohimbine, a plant indole alkylamine alkaloid with alpha-2 antagonistic properties,[50] had been prescribed for nearly a century for the management of erectile dysfunction.[51] Its use fell out of favor with the introduction of PDE5 inhibitors.[9] Historically it was typically prescribed at a dose of 5–10 mg daily while observing for improvements over the ensuing month. Yohimbine is generally well tolerated with minimal side effects such as hypertension, anxiety, headaches, and tachycardia. While it appeared to have a role in non-organic ED, demonstrating efficacy in up to 70%,[52] this was not seen in men with organic ED.[53] As a result, the role for yohimbine in practice today would be limited to historic interest, and in the treatment of non-organic ED.

Dopaminergic agonists

The paraventricular nucleus (PVN) had been identified in rats as an important center for the generation of erectile activity through the use of dopamine agonists selectively administered into the PVN.[54] This stimulated excitement in the sexual medicine community as the potential use of dopaminergic agonists in the treatment of psychogenic ED was evident. Apomorphine SL was subsequently developed for sublingual use and had a period of use in Europe. Oral ingested formulations were found to become inactivated.[55] Side effects included nausea, somnolence, yawning, sweating, and emesis. Apomorphine SL had demonstrated efficacy in the treatment of ED, with a responder rate of approximately 67%,[55] and interestingly with regular sequential use the number of responders would increase to approximately 75%.[56] However, after the introduction of PDE5 inhibitors, which had superior efficacy, apomorphine SL was voluntarily withdrawn from the market in Europe. It was never approved for use in North America.[9]

Melanocortin receptor agonists

Stimulation of melanocortin (MC) receptors within the central nervous system using melanotropic ligands has been shown to initiate and facilitate penile erection. Agonists likely act downstream of dopamine and oxytocin in hypothalamic centers. Five subtypes of MC receptors exist (MC1R–MC5R), of which MC4R is thought to be the most important mediator of MC-induced erection.[57] Subcutaneously administered melanotan II, a synthetic analog of alpha-melanocyte stimulating hormone (α-MSH), was shown to have pro-erectile effects in men with psychogenic impotence.[58] Diamond et al. reported on the synergistic actions of sildenafil and PT-141 (a MC receptor agonist) versus sildenafil alone.[59] Bremelanotide, a MC3-4R-specific synthetic peptide analog of α-MSH, has demonstrated efficacy in diabetic men. However, this success comes with the cost of significant adverse events such as nausea and increases in blood pressure, as well as dose-dependent discontinuation rates (4% in the placebo group up to 49% in the bremelanotide 15 mg group).[60] Interestingly, Bremelanotide has been shown to be able to salvage some PDE5 inhibitor failures.[61] While these adrenocorticotropic hormones and melanocortin activators appear promising, their side effect profile is limiting and may preclude development and commercialization of this class of drug for the treatment of ED.

Serotonin receptor effectors

Trazodone is a serotonin antagonist and reuptake inhibitor (SARI), most famous in urology for inducing particularly treatment-resistant priapisms as a rare but important adverse event.[62] Not long after this observation attempts were made to identify whether it might be useful in the treatment of ED.[63–65] Interestingly, it was also combined with yohimbine in a prospective randomized controlled trial with good effect to treat psychogenic ED.[66] While initially it was postulated that the pro-erectile activity from trazodone use leading to priapistic episodes was serotoninergic, further research has suggested that the mechanism is more in keeping with anti-adrenergic effects.[67] Even with a better understanding of the pathophysiology of trazodone-induced priapism, it still performed quite poorly as an erectogenic aid, and its future use for the treatment of ED is quite limited as other anti-adrenergics outperform it,[68] and newer agents were more efficacious.[9]

Others

Other therapies with plausible mechanisms of action have been put forward including limaprost (prostaglandin E_1), naltrexone (opioid antagonist), L-dopa (dopamine agonist), and L-arginine (NO precursor).[69] However, the efficacy of these therapies in single-center trials has not proven to be equivalent or superior to current standard therapies and therefore further study has not been ventured. L-Arginine does get some specific attention as there is the most literature behind it. A single-center trial of impotent men demonstrated that after 6 weeks of supplementation approximately 31% of men were able to participate in sexual intercourse as compared to 12% of placebo.[70] Another randomized double-blind trial of 124 patients showed an increase of nearly 10 points on the IIEF-EF after 3 months of supplementation, and 12 points after 6 months.[71] Given that the improvements seen by most PDE5 inhibitors ranged from 8 to 10,[9] there is a possibility of future interest in this product. An interesting concept that is yet to be demonstrated is whether or not L-arginine has any rehabilitative properties with chronic use.[9] Most recently a randomized, double-blind, placebo-controlled crossover study of approximately 30 participants demonstrated that a combination of L-arginine with adenosine monophosphate improved three of the domains on the IIEF, and improved scores on the EDITS questionnaires as well.[72] However, until large multicenter randomized trials can be performed to reproduce those results L-arginine will remain an interesting curiosity instead of a mainstay of therapy.

Intracavernosal injection therapy

Intracavernosal injection (ICI) therapy was first reported by Virag[73] and Brindley[74] in the early 1980s. This heralded a surge of interest in the conservative and medical management of ED. A wide spectrum of different agents have been injected into the corpora cavernosa of many patients in an effort to maximize efficacy and minimize adverse events. These include but are not limited to: prostaglandin E_1 (PGE_1, synonymous with alprostadil),[75] papaverine,[73] phentolamine,[76] phenoxybenzamine,[74] atropine,[77] nitroprusside,[78] vasoactive intestinal peptide (VIP),[79] and chlorpromazine.[80] The agents in popular use today include PGE_1, papaverine, phentolamine, and combinations thereof. Many of these therapies started as diagnostic tools to aid in the evaluation of erections for Doppler/duplex interrogation of the vascular system. Contraindications to the use of ICI therapy include men with psychological instability, history or risk for priapism, history of severe coagulopathy or unstable cardiovascular disease, reduced manual dexterity (where the partner cannot perform the procedure), and monoamine oxidase inhibitor use (as alpha-adrenergics are used in priapistic episodes and may precipitate a hypertensive crisis).[81]

1 *Papaverine/phentolamine (Bi-Mix).* Shortly after the introduction of papaverine monotherapy complications of corporal fibrosis,[82] injection site fibrosis causing curvature,[83] and subcutaneous nodules of fibrosis[84] were being reported. Papaverine is also highly metabolized in the liver and can cause hepatotoxicity. Doses greater than 4.5 mg per injection should be avoided to prevent hepatotoxicity.[85] With the intent of reducing some of these effects, papaverine was paired with phentolamine such that the agents could act synergistically at lower doses to provide robust responses. There is also demonstrated superiority of combination therapy over papaverine monotherapy[86] and over placebo.[87] Full erections have been reported to be 50–70%, 30–50%, and 10% respectively. Etiology of the erectile dysfunction seems to predict success with 100% efficacy in purely neurogenic impotence, 65.7% in vasculogenic, 64.7% in neurogenic/vasculogenic, and 90% in the undetermined group.[88] Although early data suggested there was some technical difficulty in teaching the injection skill in approximately 40% of patients,[89] more recent series have reported lower rates of difficulty and technique-related adverse events,[90] possibly related to improvements in education and dedicated ICI teaching clinics/teams. Selected studies are integrated with other intracavernosal agents in Table 19.4.
2 *Prostaglandin E_1 (PGE_1, synonymous with alprostadil, Caverject, Viridal, and Edex).* Waldhauser and Schramek[91] were first to describe ICI PGE_1 of 92% success in a small crossover cohort study, as compared to 50% with papaverine/phentolamine. When compared to papaverine monotherapy in another study the efficacy rates were similar to each other;[92] however, it should be noted that the dosage of PGE_1 used was half of that used in the study by Waldhauser and Schramek. Most of the literature published since then tends to agree with efficacy rates of PGE_1 monotherapy similar to those of papaverine monotherapy or papaverine/phentolamine therapy, of approximately 50–70%.[92–96] Kattan et al.[94] indicated that PGE_1 may have a more favorable response than papaverine in those patients with vasculogenic impotence (46% vs 14%). Additionally, those who do not respond to a "test-dose" of PGE_1 were found to have a higher association of hypogonadism-related symptoms and a higher likelihood of major adverse cardiac events.[97] Two large multicenter prospective trials investigating PGE_1 efficacy and safety have demonstrated efficacy of 93–94% with protocoled injections, and also shown that the adverse effects identified decline early with time and experience of the patient.[75,98] The large randomized trials utilized an independent assessor to evaluate success as compared to patient-reported success, and this may account for some of the discrepancy in efficacy values. Return of spontaneous erections with PGE_1 therapy has been reported,[99] and is an interesting concept that will require further investigation in order to exploit to the benefit of patients.

Table 19.4 Adverse events and efficacy reporting.

Trial	*n*	% Fibrosis	% Hematoma	% Fibrosis resolved	Agents used	Efficacy
Levine et al. (1989)[84]	111	57%	27–49%	NR	Pap+Phe	NR
Lakin et al. (1990)[217]	100	31 ± 8.6%	20.9%	NR	Pap, Pap+Phe	NR
Pery et al. (1990)[218]	120	5%	NR	NR	Pap	NR
Virag et al. (1991)[219]	615	14	39	78%	Pap, Pap+Phe, ceritine	NR
Gall (1992)[220]	172	11%	38.3%	31%	Pap+Phe	95.8%
Armstrong et al. (1993)[221]	100	3.1%	7.5%	20%	Pap+Phe	72%
Kapoor et al. (1993)[222]	101	2%	3%	NR	Pap	NR
Hirsch et al. (1995)[223]	80	16.5%	NR	NR	PGE_1	NR
Linet & Ogrinc (1996)[75]	683	3.18%	NR	NR	PGE_1	87%
Chew et al. (1997)[224]	245	23%	6%	NR	PGE_1	NR
Casabe et al. (1998)[120]	189	5%	20%	50%	Trimix	84.4%
EASG (1998)[225]	848	4%	9%	NR	PGE_1	88%
Moemen e tal. (2004)[114]	168	15% Pap 0% PGE_1 1.8% trimix	25% Pap 25% PGE_1 20.7% trimix	NR	Pap, PGE_1, trimix	NR

NR, not reported; Pap, papaverine; Phe, phentolamine; PGE_1, prostaglandin E_1.

Table 19.5 Common drug therapies for erectile dysfunction.

Class	Agent	Dose range	Route	Comment
Phosphodiesterase inhibitors	Sildenafil	25–100 mg	p.o.	Not after fatty meal, blue vision, short half-life
	Vardenafil	5–20 mg	p.o./s.l.	Not after fatty meal, interacts with antiarrhythmics
	Tadalafil	5–20 mg	p.o.	Long half-life, available in daily dosing
Intracavernosal agents	Papaverine (P)	30 mg	i.c.	May be associated with fibrosis, acidic
	Phentolamine (Ph)	1 mg	i.c.	Not as monotherapy
	Prostaglandin E_1 (PGE_1)	5–40 μg	i.c.	May inhibit fibrosis, penile pain
	Bimix (P+Ph)	30/1	i.c.	
	Trimix (P+Ph+PGE_1)	30/1/10 30/2/20	i.c.	Most commonly prescribed
Intraurethral agents	MUSE	500–1000 μg	i.u.	Penile pain, dysuria, urethral bleeding
Topical agents	PGE_1	100–300 μg	Topically to glans	Balanitis, penile pain, skin reactions

i.c., intracavernosally; i.u., intraurethrally; p.o., per os (by mouth); s.l., sublingually.

3 *PGE_1 + papaverine + phentolamine (synonymous with Trimix)*. The combination of three agents into a single use was first proposed by Goldstein et al.[100] as a means of salvaging papaverine/phentolamine failures. Several series have subsequently been published on the efficacy and tolerability of trimix.[101–105] The general consensus of these studies is that trimix appears to be a more robust agent compared to previous agents; however, this is offset by the potential for a higher incidence of priapism. Efficacy rates are reported from 50% to 90% depending on the series, the dosages of each particular formulation, and the patient population investigated. A major disadvantage to trimix therapy is that there is no standardized formulation and individual institutions have different concentrations of the three components making inter-study comparisons difficult if not impossible.[103,105,106]

4 *Vasoactive intestinal peptide + phentolamine*. Vasoactive intestinal peptide combined with phentolamine was

another combination achieving some success and enthusiasm in the pre-PDE5 inhibitor era. Despite trials demonstrating similar efficacy to PGE1 monotherapy, patients' perception of a more natural erection, and a convenient autoinjecting device, it was never marketed globally.[79,107] It is still available in some countries, although it no longer comes with the convenient autoinjector due to cost concerns. Forskolin has also been used intracavernosally in select patients refractory to trimix therapy.[108]

5 *Sodium nitroprusside.* Sodium nitroprusside is an agent that had some initial investigation but was abandoned after the investigators encountered severe hypotension and limited effect in the first few patients.[109] This was followed by some concerns that use of sodium nitroprusside was toxic to the corpora and possibly associated with increased rates of penile fibrosis and arteriogenic impotence. This was supported by some of the basic science research that demonstrated animal models having a significant inflammatory reaction after nitroprusside use as well as periarterial inflammation.[110] However, it has attracted renewed interest in some centers as new series are reporting its efficacy, which is typically similar to phentolamine/papaverine therapy.[78,111] It remains to be seen if the incidence of fibrosis or worsening erectile function requiring more aggressive therapies will be observed.

Use of a no-needle injector was proposed for administration of intracavernosal therapy. A proof of concept was performed in an animal model demonstrating penetration of the sinusoids with India ink, and this was followed by the use of vasoactive agents, which worked in animal models.[112] However, when this was used in clinical human studies, men almost uniformly preferred injection therapy as it was more consistent in its ability to deliver a robust erection, and was more comfortable than the no-needle jet injector.[113]

Adverse reactions associated with ICI therapy have been reported and more common events include hematoma, priapism, penile pain, and penile fibrosis. The definition of penile fibrosis is nebulous and is a clinical diagnosis of subcutaneous nodules, Peyronie-like plaques in the tunica causing curvature, and corporal fibrosis leading to treatment-refractory ED. As a result rates of penile fibrosis are widely reported from 2% to 50% and are summarized in Table 19.4. A complicating matter is that hematoma formation is often considered to be an event related to poor technique, and it is difficult to parse out what portion of fibrosis is technique related, and what is drug related. However, there have been case reports of treatment-refractory corporal fibrosis from ICI therapy.[82] Particular attention should be paid to the trial by Moemen et al.,[114] which had three arms comparing PGE_1, papaverine, and trimix. It was reported that the highest incidence of fibrosis occurred in the papaverine monotherapy arm, a small portion in the trimix arm, and none in the PGE_1 arm. There is basic scientific evidence to support the antifibrotic properties of PGE_1.[115] PDE5 inhibitors may also have antifibrotic effects and have been demonstrated to cause plaque resorption in clinical studies.[116] To complicate issues further, approximately half of those deemed to have some element of fibrosis resolve spontaneously. This is difficult to reconcile as fibrosis is ultimately a histopathological diagnosis, and typically an end point of inflammation that should not be easily reversible. The basic science literature is quite compelling, however, in that rat and primate models[110,117] demonstrate that papaverine-containing therapy not only seems to cause inflammatory reactions at the site of injection, but also some fibrosis proximal and distal to the injection site as well. One theory for this is that papaverine requires a fairly acidic environment in order to be stable (pH 3.5), and the acidity on the sinusoids may cause a chemical burn-like reaction leading to fibrosis. An interesting clinical study was performed in humans where trimix (pH 4.17) was injected with and without a sodium bicarbonate buffer that brought the solution to pH 7.05. Penile pain was reduced dramatically (5% vs 58% pain), which served as a proof of concept.[118]

ICI therapy is uniquely suited for rehabilitation of erection after radical pelvic surgery as there is no reliance on the neurovascular bundle to facilitate erection. Montorsi et al. were the first to report on the recovery of spontaneous erections with regular PGE_1 therapy.[119] While many rehabilitative protocols have been suggested, they have all attained varying success.[40–42] Among the challenges of ICI therapy, particularly in the rehabilitative setting, are the high dropout rates associated with it. More than half of men stop ICI within the first year. Interestingly, fibrosis is not typically the main reason listed by most studies, but can be as high as 5%.[120] The most common reasons include: inadequate response; loss of interest of partner or loss of partner; recovery of erections; cost; lack of spontaneity; and deterioration in health.[105,120–123]

Intraurethral therapy

In the pre-PDE5 inhibitor era the urethral application of PGE_1 attempted to fill the need for an intermediary step before intracavernosal injection therapy. A system was developed to allow men to apply a pellet of PGE_1 to a moistened urethral immediately after emptying their bladder. This was termed the Medicated Urethral System for Erection, or MUSE©. An initial randomized study looked both at efficacy and dose finding ($n = 68$) and demonstrated that approximately 75% of men achieved full enlargement, 49.2% felt the erection was sufficient for intercourse, and 63.6% reported successful intercourse. However, the principal adverse reaction was penile pain, which occurred 9.1–18.3% of the time depending on dose.[124]. A much larger study followed this, with 996 men who were proven responders to MUSE in the clinic randomized to four dosing strengths and placebo. This similarly demonstrated a rate of 64.9% successful intercourse vs 18.6% in the placebo arm. Again the most common side effect was penile pain, with 10.8% of PGE_1 administrations in 32.7% of men receiving PGE_1. Other adverse effects reported include minor urethral trauma (5%) and dizziness (1.9%). The next logical step was to compare intracavernous PGE_1 to MUSE, and this was done in two studies demonstrating 70–92% vs 43–61.8% response rates.[125,126] The incidence of penile pain was reported to be 10–20% in the intracavernosal group versus 25–30% in the MUSE group. Additionally, when asked which modality the men would like to continue with, the majority selected intracavernosal injection therapy. Interestingly, there have been reports indicating that of men who found ICI therapy ineffective, approximately 58% may be able to achieve an erection with MUSE therapy, and 47% of the responsive patients report successful intercourse in the home phase.[127] Unfortunately follow-up studies could not reproduce the results reported by the index trial and reported efficacy data of only 30%.[128] One possible explanation for this might be that there have been reported inconsistencies with the response of MUSE in the home phase after a confirmed response in office, and of those who do respond only 31% are continuing to use MUSE at 9 month.[129] Although a niche area, one area where MUSE has had some success is in combination with penile implants to cause glans tumescence.[130] This use may allow increased satisfaction for some men disappointed with the lack of glans tumescence and girth associated with an implant.

A problem arose for MUSE when the PDE5 inhibitors became established as they were very efficacious, with a much more tolerable side effect profile, and did not require instrumentation of the penis or urethra in order to facilitate erection. As enthusiasm built around the concept of PDE5 inhibitor use and penile rehabilitation after radical prostate surgery, some investigators looked to revive MUSE as a means of rehabilitation itself. It is uniquely suited as it does not depend on an intact neurovascular bundle to facilitate erections, and the goal was not necessarily a completely rigid response but any penile engorgement and erection. Its safety was reported with efficacies of 70% in clinic and 57% in the transition to the home phase with a rehabilitation protocol.[131] MUSE has also been reported to increase satisfaction and salvage sildenafil non-responders in a postoperative nerve-sparing radical prostatectomy scenario, allowing for 80% of couples to have erections sufficient for vaginal penetration.[132] A study looking at three times a week low-dose MUSE therapy for 9 months post-prostatectomy found that approximately 55% of men on MUSE therapy had recovery of spontaneous erections sufficient for intercourse, as compared to 11% in the untreated group.[133] Finally, in an elegant study by McCullough et al.,[134] previously potent men post-prostatectomy were randomized to nightly sildenafil or MUSE therapy for 9 months, and then proceeded to have a 1-month washout period. The patients were then re-challenged with sildenafil 100 mg and it was demonstrated that there were no differences in IIEF-EF scores, intercourse success, or GAQ. There was a significantly better GAQ at 6 months, but this had returned to the same as the sildenafil group after the washout period.

In conclusion, MUSE did not have the efficacy or tolerability to do well as a monotherapy after the introduction of PDE5 inhibitors. There may be a role for MUSE

Table 19.6 Contraindications to erectile dysfunction medications.

Phosphodiesterase Inhibitors	• Severe hepatic impairment • Dialysis-dependent renal disease • Hereditary degenerative retinal disorders (e.g., retinitis pigmentosa) • Allergy Requiring cardiologic clearance: • Ventricular outflow obstruction • Severely impaired autonomic control of blood pressure • Myocardial infarct, stroke, or life-threatening arrhythmia within previous 6 months • NYHA class II or greater heart failure • CAD causing unstable angina • Resting hypertension (>170/100 mmHg) or hypotension (<90/50 mmHg)
Intracavernosal agents	• Allergy • Psychological instability • History or risk for priapism • History of severe coagulopathy • Unstable cardiovascular disease • Reduced manual dexterity (partner may perform) • Monoamine oxidase inhibitor use
Intraurethral agents	• Partner with viable gestation • Inaccessible or absent urethra (e.g., phimosis, surgery) • Allergy or sensitivity to product • Monoamine oxidase inhibitor use • Reduced manual dexterity (partner may perform) • Unstable cardiovascular disease • History of priapism
Topical agents	• Allergy or sensitivity • Partner with viable gestation (if PGE_1-containing product) • Unstable cardiovascular disease • Monoamine oxidase inhibitor use • History of priapism

in specific niche areas, or in the context of penile rehabilitation after prostate cancer surgery. Despite the efficacy and tolerability issues associated with MUSE, it is still a useful tool to have in the armamentarium of the urologist attempting to maximize erectile capacity and sexual satisfaction.

Topical therapies

Not all men with erectile dysfunction refractory to medical management have the desire and/or dexterity to manipulate needles for injection therapy, nor are able to manipulate a device into their urethra for application of a suppository. This of course is even more challenging when it is being attempted within the contexts of a sexual encounter. As a result, there is always an interest in developing topical therapies for erectile dysfunction that could be applied easily, or as part of the sexual act by the partner. The obvious challenges include application of an agent that has minimal skin reaction, with the ability to traverse the skin, dartos fascia, Buck's fascia, and the tunica albuginea in order to reach the site of action. As there have been some described communications between the corpus cavernosum and the corpus spongiosum,[135] there have also been attempts to exploit this as there are less inactive tissues that the agent must traverse. Several agents have been tried for this including (but not limited to) prostaglandin E_1, nitroglycerin, and papaverine.[136]

Topical papaverine for ED was described by Kim et al. in 1995 in a double-blind, crossover, placebo-controlled small study, in which a 20% papaverine gel was applied to penile shaft skin and scrotum. It appeared to be well tolerated and documented increases in cavernosal arterial diameter were observed; however, efficacy was limiting as 3/14 patients had clinical erections in both the treatment and placebo phase.[136] Little was published on the topic until recently when it was described that the addition of caproic acid, ethanol, and water in a percentage volume ratio of 50:30:20 can enhance papaverine penetration in a rabbit model.[137] It remains to be seen if this will allow topical papaverine to enter the market as a feasible erectogenic aid.

Nitroglycerin (NTG) for topical treatment of erectile dysfunction was first described in 1989 in one small study,[138] which used the simple application of a traditional NTG patch to the penile shaft versus placebo. This was met with some enthusiasm and several trials were developed in response to this. A NTG paste was developed that restored potency in 4/10 men, but it gave rise to a common complaint of headaches and fell out of favor.[139] Borges had proposed a minor procedure whereby a portion of Buck's fascia was excised and replaced with a vein graft. This was marked with India ink and then after healing, the area was used as a site for topical NTG application. Of the six patients on whom this was attempted, all of which were dependent on ICI, two continued with topical treatment exclusively, three alternated between injections and topical, and one preferred injection therapy.[140] However, with a demonstrated side effect of significant headaches in 20%[141] and inferiority to both intracavernosal agents[141] and other topical agents,[142] this quickly fell out of favor as a treatment modality. Minoxidil, a nitrate agonist commonly prescribed for hair loss, also demonstrated some pro-erectile capacity and was found to be superior to NTG.[142] However, the efficacy did not approach that of intracavernosal injections or vacuum erection devices,[143] and little research has subsequently been reported. Other agents such as co-dergocrine mesylate, aminophylline, and isosorbide dinitrate have been reported to have success;[144] however, the results have not been replicated despite attempts to do so.[145]

Prostaglandin E_1 has renewed enthusiasm in the area of topical treatment of ED. Kim et al. reported that topical application of PGE_1 in a small group of men with ED secondary to spinal cord injuries or arterial insufficiency (9 and 1 respectively) demonstrated increases in cavernosal arterial diameter in all patients, and peak systolic flow velocities in 7/10 patients. Clinical erections were observed in 2/10 patients but not in the placebo application.[146] Goldstein et al. then reported on the use of a 1% PGE_1 cream formulated with an absorption-enhancing agent (Topiglan©) on 60 patients in a randomized, double-blind fashion in combination with visual and tactile stimuli.[147] They reported greater maximum rigidity in the treatment group, and a higher rate of self-perceived adequate rigidity for vaginal penetration (38.9% vs 6.9%). Penile erythema and a mild burning or cooling sensation were the reported side effects. Finally, Padma-Nathan et al. reported phase II[148] and phase III[149] data on topical PGE_1 (Alprox-TD©) cream use and integrated the results at the time of reporting. They reported on 1732 patients randomized to receive placebo (n = 434), or topical PGE_1 cream at 100 (n = 434), 200 (n = 430), or 300 (n = 434) microgram doses. The reported changes from baseline using the IIEF-EF were <minus>0.7, 1.6, 2.5, and 2.4 respectively. SEP3 rates were 30.3%, 38.9%, 41.9%, and 38.5% respectively, and demonstrated statistical significance. Main adverse reactions reported included balanitis (5%), penile pain (17.5%), penile burning (23%), penile erythema (11%), and partner-reported vaginal burning (4%). These results were confirmed by Rooney et al.,[150] with a SEP3 rate of approximately 61.1% and an IIEF-EF change from baseline of approximately 10 points.

With their limited efficacy, topical treatments are yet to find a niche in which to be incorporated into treatment algorithms as a monotherapy. Until a topical agent is efficacious enough to be a viable and reliable alternative to intracavernosal injection therapy, it is unlikely to be successful as a monotherapy. However, there may yet be roles in combination therapies to augment other conservative measures, or as an easy method of performing penile rehabilitative therapy, roles that are yet to be fully explored.

Future therapies for erectile dysfunction

RhoA/Rho-kinase

Several studies have highlighted the important roles for GTPase RhoA and its effector, Rho-associated kinase (Rho-kinase), in calcium-independent regulation of smooth muscle contraction.[151] Chitaley et al.[152] reported that Rho-kinase antagonism stimulated rat penile erection independently of nitric oxide (NO) and showed potential as an alternative therapeutic option to treat ED. Recently published literature has suggested that elevated RhoA/Rho-kinase activity contributes to the pathogenesis of ED in conditions such as diabetes, aging, and hypogonadism.[153] Vignozzi et al.[154] found that overexpression of RhoA/Rho-kinase signaling contributed to diabetes-related ED, and treating hypogonadism associated diabetes could improve the erectile function by normalizing the RhoA/Rho-kinase pathway upregulation. Several RhoA/Rho-kinase inhibitors have been tested in various animal models and have shown promising outcomes. Chronic treatment with fasudil, an oral RhoA/Rho-kinase inhibitor, prevents the development of both vasculogenic ED and pelvic atherosclerosis[155] as well as prevention of apoptosis of the corpora associated with diabetes.[156]. Rho-kinase inhibitor Y27632 appeared to generate effective human corpus cavernosum smooth muscle relaxation when given together with doxazosin in the presence of bladder outlet obstruction.[157]

Soluble guanylase cyclase (sGC) activators

Since the successful manipulation of the PDE pathway, other mechanisms have been sought to augment NO-mediated smooth muscle relaxation, and/or salvage PDE inhibitor failures. While there has been some new and novel research in the urological literature on guanylate cyclase activation/stimulation, there has been a large volume of research in the internal medicine literature. The terms stimulation and activation refer to the ability of the target pharmaceutical to activate the sGC enzyme in a heme-dependent or -independent manner respectively.[158] The sGC enzyme is a heterodimeric complex that consists of two subunits, α and β, and each one contains three common domains:

1. The N-terminal heme-binding domain that mediates the NO sensitivity of the enzyme.
2. A dimerization domain, which is found in the middle of the structure of each subunit and is required for basal or NO-stimulated sGC activity.
3. The C-terminal catalytic domain, which is the most highly conserved region between the subunits and is responsible for the conversion of GTP to the second messenger, cGMP.[159]

The reduced heme-dependent sGC is the native form and responsive to NO stimulation. However, there is evidence to suggest in animal and human studies[160] that periods of oxidative stress including congestive heart failure, diabetes, and hypertension, can produce reactive oxygen species that will push the equilibrium towards more of the sGC being oxidized and relatively insensitive to NO, so there is only basal activity for production of cGMP.[161] This may be a contributing reason for PDE5 inhibitor responsiveness and resistance in current clinical practice.

Stimulators of sGC include many different investigational compounds, including A-778935, A-344905, A-350619, CFM-1571, and YC-1.[158] YC-1 in particular has gained some attention in the erectile dysfunction literature.[162] Unfortunately its usefulness is limited by having an element of PDE5 inhibition[159] and side effect and toxicity concerns prior to clinical trials.[28,163] Other stimulators have been shown to have increased potency over YC-1, including BAY 41-2272 and BAY 41-8543, with minimal or no PDE5 inhibition and 20–92× potency over YC-1, but these are still dependent on the reduced heme component of sGC.[158] An oral stimulator, BAY 63-2521 (Riociguat), is currently in human clinical trials for hypertension; it has no significant PDE5 inhibition in concentrations used for human use and may be an interesting augmenter to existing PDE5 inhibitor therapy. However, phase III trials are ongoing for its efficacy in treating pulmonary hypertension,[164] and erectile function data have yet to be reported from previous clinical studies. Where we do have some data in the sexual medicine literature on sGC stimulators is from a recent annual meeting where some data were published on the use of BAY 60-4552 salvaging PDE5 inhibitor failures by demonstrating a synergistic response with vardenafil in a cavernosal nerve crush model.[165]

With the understanding that the heme-free oxidized sGC may in fact be the pathological form of sGC, and may be partially responsible for NO insensitivity in some patients, the ability to activate sGC in the oxidized form would be a very important and valuable asset in the medical treatment of ED. Interestingly, activators seem to be more potent on oxidized or heme-free sGC than on native reduced sGC.[166] The first activator identified, which also led to the discovery of oxidized sGC, was BAY 58-2667 (Cinaciguat). This gives a method of increasing cGMP in conditions of oxidative stress, and potentially another method of medically treating ED. Cinaciguat is currently in trials looking at potential therapeutics for acute decompensated heart failure.[167] Other activators in the literature include AMR 1766 (Ataciguat) and BAY 60-2770, but these do not have ED-related outcomes published in the literature.

Hydrogen sulfide (H_2S)

There is growing evidence that endogenous H_2S can act as a regulatory mediator similar to NO, and may have an important role in erectile function and dysfunction.[168] The importance of H_2S was first demonstrated by Srilatha et al.[169] in a rat model demonstrating increases in penile pressure similar to the prostaglandin E_1 used as the control. Interestingly, when an adenylyl cyclase inhibitor (MDL 12,330A) was used after administration of H_2S in a rabbit model of pre-contracted cavernous smooth muscle, the inhibition was incomplete suggesting that H_2S relaxation is only partially dependent on the cAMP pathway.[170] The exact mechanism for the pro-erectile effects of H_2S is still unclear; however, current theories include:

1 H_2S as a K-ATP channel opener causing vasorelaxation via hyperpolarization.[171,172]
2 H_2S as a modulator/inhibitor of the RhoA/Rho-kinase pathway.[173]
3 H_2S as an inhibitor of superoxide formation,[174] which may either increase PDE5 expression and consequently decrease the concentration of cGMP,[175] or consume NO in the formation of reactive nitrogen species.[176]
4 H_2S as a mediator of testosterone-induced relaxation.[177]
5 H_2S cross-talk with NO.[178,179]

The H_2S pathway certainly has opened up several new potential targets for upcoming oral therapies that are still not near clinical trials, but may become new targets or augments to existing therapies in the future.

Smooth muscle inhibitors

Many successful therapies for ED have focused on manipulation of intracellular calcium via the NO pathway by inhibiting cGMP breakdown, augmenting NO production, or altering smooth muscle tone via the RhoA/Rho-kinase pathway, as previously discussed. However, there is now some evidence of the capability to manipulate the contractile elements more directly via myosin II inhibition in order to induce smooth muscle relaxation and promote erection.[180] Blebbistatin, a myosin II inhibitor, does not compete with nucleotide binding to the skeletal muscle myosin subfragment-1, but preferentially binds to the ATPase intermediate with ADP and phosphate bound at the active site of myosin II[181] and slows down phosphate release by stabilization of this state.[182]. Blebbistatin does not interfere with binding of myosin to actin or with ATP-induced actomyosin dissociation.[181] In vitro studies with rat and human corporal cavernosal tissues have demonstrated that tissue precontracted with phenylephrine can be completely relaxed with blebbistatin.[180] There is also in vivo evidence in rats that precontracted cavernosal tissue can be relaxed quite significantly with expected rises in intracavernosal pressures with blebbistatin administration delivered via intracavernosal injections, with minimal effects on mean arterial pressure that are recovered within seconds of administration. However, it should be noted that two of the rats in this study did have prolonged increases in their intracavernosal pressures and concurrent erections that lasted for an hour despite corporal cavernosal washout at maximal doses.[180] This potency of inhibition speaks to blebbistatin's ability to reduce actin affinity of the myosin-ADP-Pi complex after cavernosal washout, its pro-erectile potency, and potential priapistic concerns. In vivo studies in humans are still required to address dosing, potency, and safety.

Drug-eluting stents

Penile arterial revascularization procedures are appropriate and indicated with selected patients. An ideal patient would be a healthy individual with recently acquired ED secondary to a focal arterial occlusion and in the absence of any evidence of generalized vascular disease.[183] Trauma patients with arteriogenic ED were recently identified in systematic reviews as a population that may benefit from revascularization; however, large prospective trials would be needed.[184]

Minimally invasive coronary artery stents have revolutionized the treatment of ischemic heart disease, and this procedure has given many poor surgical candidates a therapeutic option. The main adverse event has similarly been improved with the use of drug-eluting stents to prevent thrombosis. A pilot study by Rogers et al.[185] reported a significant correlation between coronary and internal pudendal arterial disease in men with ED. Coronary artery stenosis mirrored stenosis in the internal pudendal arteries (52% right, 60% left), and was typically found ideally suited for percutaneous treatment in the mid or distal artery. To answer whether percutaneous revascularization is a worthwhile endeavor, the ZEN trial (zotarolimus-eluting peripheral stent system for the treatment of erectile dysfunction in males with suboptimal response to PDE5 inhibitors) was initiated in 2009 and is the first human feasibility safety trial for this therapy. The ZEN trial may add a new interventional therapeutic arm for the management of ED, albeit for a very select group of men with recently acquired ED secondary to a focal internal pudendal arterial occlusion without evidence of generalized vascular disease. While the safety of drug-eluting stents is known for coronary revascularization, this is yet uncharted territory that will require close follow-up of all the investigators involved to identify what adverse events to monitor for. The preliminary data for the ZEN trial are promising, both as regards the radiographic normalization of angiograms post stenting, and excellent recovery of erectile function in men with discrete lesions of the internal pudendal artery. The safety and tolerability appear to be equivalent to those of coronary artery stenting, and there may be a role for routine pelvic angiography in those undergoing investigation for coronary artery disease with concurrent complaints of ED.[186]

Conclusion

In conclusion, despite the fact that the field of drug therapy for ED is still in its infancy, dramatic advances and novel therapeutics abound. Importantly, there has been a societal shift towards greater patient comfort in discussing sexual health and in pursuit of treatment. Epidemiological research has demonstrated the link between ED and hypertension, coronary artery disease, and hypogonadism. The future of ED therapy will likely be directed towards a curative approach through gene therapy or other agents where the possibility of permanent improvement would enhance the quality of life of patients and their partners.

References

1 Klotz L. How (not) to communicate new scientific information: a memoir of the famous Brindley lecture. *BJU Int* 2005;96(7):956–7.

2 Grimm RH, Grandits GA, Prineas RJ, et al. Long-term effects on sexual function of five antihypertensive drugs and nutritional hygienic treatment in hypertensive men and women. Treatment of Mild Hypertension Study (TOMHS). *Hypertension* 1997;29(1 Pt 1):8–14.

3 Greenblatt DJ, Koch-Weser J. Gynecomastia and impotence: complications of spironolactone therapy. *JAMA* 1973;223(1):82.

4 Engbaek M, Hjerrild M, Hallas J, Jacobsen IA. The effect of low-dose spironolactone on resistant hypertension. *J Am Soc Hypertens* 2010;4(6):290–4.

5 Dadkhah F, Safarinejad MR, Asgari MA, Hosseini SY, Lashay A, Amini E. Atorvastatin improves the response to sildenafil in hypercholesterolemic men with erectile dysfunction not initially responsive to sildenafil. *Int J Impot Res* 2009;22(1):51–60.

6 Corona G, Boddi V, Balercia G, et al. The effect of statin therapy on testosterone levels in subjects consulting for erectile dysfunction. *J Sex Med* 2010;7(4 Pt 1):1547–56.

7 Garcia JA, Sanchez PE, Fraile C, Escovar P. Testosterone undecanoate improves erectile dysfunction in hypogonadal men with the metabolic syndrome refractory to treatment with phosphodiesterase type 5 inhibitors alone. *Andrologia* 2011;43(5):293–6.

8 Buvat J, Montorsi F, Maggi M, et al. Hypogonadal men nonresponders to the PDE5 inhibitor tadalafil benefit from normalization of testosterone levels with a 1% hydroalcoholic testosterone gel in the treatment of erectile dysfunction (TADTEST study). *J Sex Med* 2011;8(1):284–93.

9 Porst H, Burnett A, Brock G, et al. SOP conservative (medical and mechanical) treatment of erectile dysfunction. *J Sex Med* 2013;10(1):130–71.

10 Rosen RC, Riley A, Wagner G, Osterloh IH, Kirkpatrick J, Mishra A. The international index of erectile function (IIEF): a multidimensional scale for assessment of erectile dysfunction. *Urology* 1997;49(6):822–30.

11 Rosen RC, Cappelleri JC, Smith MD, Lipsky J, Peña BM. Development and evaluation of an abridged, 5-item version of the International Index of Erectile Function (IIEF-5) as a diagnostic tool for erectile dysfunction. *Int J Impot Res* 1999;11(6):319–26.

12 Ghofrani HA, Osterloh IH, Grimminger F. Sildenafil: from angina to erectile dysfunction to pulmonary hypertension and beyond. *Nat Rev Drug Discov* 2006;5(8):689–702.

13 Boolell M, Allen MJ, Ballard SA, et al. Sildenafil: an orally active type 5 cyclic GMP-specific phosphodiesterase inhibitor for the treatment of penile erectile dysfunction. *Int J Impot Res* 1996;8(2):47–52.

14 Goldstein I, Lue TF, Padma-Nathan H, Rosen RC, Steers WD, Wicker PA. Oral sildenafil in the treatment of erectile dysfunction. Sildenafil Study Group. *N Engl J Med* 1998; 338(20):1397–404.

15 Lue TF. Erectile dysfunction. *N Engl J Med* 2000;342(24): 1802–13.

16 Carson CC, Burnett AL, Levine LA, Nehra A. The efficacy of sildenafil citrate (Viagra) in clinical populations: an update. *Urology* 2002;60(2 Suppl. 2):12–27.

17 Brock GB, McMahon CG, Chen KK, et al. Efficacy and safety of tadalafil for the treatment of erectile dysfunction: results of integrated analyses. *J Urol* 2002;168(4 Pt 1):1332–6.

18 Porst H, Rosen R, Padma-Nathan H, et al. The efficacy and tolerability of vardenafil, a new, oral, selective phosphodiesterase type 5 inhibitor, in patients with erectile

dysfunction: the first at-home clinical trial. *Int J Impot Res* 2001;13(4):192–9.

19 Rendell MS, Rajfer J, Wicker PA, Smith MD. Sildenafil for treatment of erectile dysfunction in men with diabetes: a randomized controlled trial. *Sildenafil Diabetes Study Group. JAMA* 1999;281(5):421–6.

20 Sáenz de Tejada I, Anglin G, Knight JR, Emmick JT. Effects of tadalafil on erectile dysfunction in men with diabetes. *Diabetes Care* 2002;25(12):2159–64.

21 Goldstein I, Young JM, Fischer J, Bangerter K, Segerson T, Taylor T. Vardenafil, a new phosphodiesterase type 5 inhibitor, in the treatment of erectile dysfunction in men with diabetes: a multicenter double-blind placebo-controlled fixed-dose study. *Diabetes Care* 2003;26(3):777–83.

22 Montorsi F, Nathan HP, McCullough A, et al. Tadalafil in the treatment of erectile dysfunction following bilateral nerve sparing radical retropubic prostatectomy: a randomized, double-blind, placebo controlled trial. *J Urol* 2004;172(3): 1036–41.

23 Brock G, Nehra A, Lipshultz LI, et al. Safety and efficacy of vardenafil for the treatment of men with erectile dysfunction after radical retropubic prostatectomy. *J Urol* 2003;170 (4 Pt 1):1278–83.

24 Valiquette L, Montorsi F, Auerbach S. First-dose success with vardenafil in men with erectile dysfunction and associated comorbidities: RELY-I. *Int J Clin Pract* 2006;60(11): 1378–85.

25 McCullough AR. Four-year review of sildenafil citrate. *Rev Urol* 2002;4 (Suppl. 3):S26–38.

26 Jiann B-P, Yu C-C, Su C-C, Tsai J-Y. Compliance of sildenafil treatment for erectile dysfunction and factors affecting it. *Int J Impot Res* 2006;18(2):146–9.

27 Kloner RA, Jackson G, Hutter AM, et al. Cardiovascular safety update of Tadalafil: retrospective analysis of data from placebo-controlled and open-label clinical trials of Tadalafil with as needed, three times-per-week or once-a-day dosing. *Am J Cardiol* 2006;97(12):1778–84.

28 Porst H, Kloner RA, Mohan P, et al. Cardiovascular safety of the selective PDE 5 inhibitor vardenafil in patients with erectile dysfunction: an analysis of five placebo-controlled clinical trials. *Int J Impot Res* 2002;14 (Suppl. 4):S22, abstract P-092.

29 Mittleman MA, Glasser DB, Orazem J. Clinical trials of sildenafil citrate (Viagra) demonstrate no increase in risk of myocardial infarction and cardiovascular death compared with placebo. *Int J Clin Pract* 2003;57(7):597–600.

30 Giuliano F, Jackson G, Montorsi F, Martin-Morales A, Raillard P. Safety of sildenafil citrate: review of 67 double-blind placebo-controlled trials and the postmarketing safety database. *Int J Clin Pract* 2010;64(2):240–55.

31 Gittelman M, McMahon CG, Rodríguez-Rivera JA, Beneke M, Ulbrich E, Ewald S. The POTENT II randomised trial: efficacy and safety of an orodispersible vardenafil formulation for the treatment of erectile dysfunction. *Int J Clin Pract* 2010;64(5):594–603.

32 Green R, Hicks RW. Orally disintegrating vardenafil tablets for the treatment of erectile dysfunction: efficacy, safety, and patient acceptability. *Patient Prefer Adherence* 2011;5: 181–5.

33 Porst H, Giuliano F, Glina S, et al. Evaluation of the efficacy and safety of once-a-day dosing of tadalafil 5mg and 10mg in the treatment of erectile dysfunction: results of a multicenter, randomized, double-blind, placebo-controlled trial. *Eur Urol* 2006;50(2):351–9.

34 Porst H, Rajfer J, Casabé A, et al. Long-term safety and efficacy of tadalafil 5 mg dosed once daily in men with erectile dysfunction. *J Sex Med* 2008;5(9):2160–9.

35 Foresta C, De Toni L, Di Mambro A, Garolla A, Ferlin A, Zuccarello D. The PDE5 inhibitor sildenafil increases circulating endothelial progenitor cells and CXCR4 expression. *J Sex Med* 2009;6(2):369–72.

36 Salloum FN, Takenoshita Y, Ockaili RA, et al. Sildenafil and vardenafil but not nitroglycerin limit myocardial infarction through opening of mitochondrial K(ATP) channels when administered at reperfusion following ischemia in rabbits. *J Mol Cell Cardiol* 2007;42(2):453–8.

37 Salloum FN, Ockaili RA, Wittkamp M, Marwaha VR, Kukreja RC. Vardenafil: a novel type 5 phosphodiesterase inhibitor reduces myocardial infarct size following ischemia/reperfusion injury via opening of mitochondrial K(ATP) channels in rabbits. *J Mol Cell Cardiol* 2006;40(3):405–11.

38 Zhao C, Kim SW, Yang DY, et al. Efficacy and safety of once-daily dosing of udenafil in the treatment of erectile dysfunction: results of a multicenter, randomized, double-blind, placebo-controlled trial. *Eur Urol* 2011;60(2): 380–7.

39 Palit V, Eardley I. An update on new oral PDE5 inhibitors for the treatment of erectile dysfunction. *Nat Rev Urol* 2010;7(11):603–9.

40 Garcia FJ, Brock G. Current state of penile rehabilitation after radical prostatectomy. *Curr Opin Urol* 2010;20(3): 234–40.

41 Padma-Nathan H, McCullough AR, et al. Randomized, double-blind, placebo-controlled study of postoperative nightly sildenafil citrate for the prevention of erectile dysfunction after bilateral nerve-sparing radical prostatectomy. *Int J Impot Res.* 2008;20(5):479–86.

42 Montorsi F, Brock G, Lee J, et al. Effect of nightly versus on-demand vardenafil on recovery of erectile function in men following bilateral nerve-sparing radical prostatectomy. *Eur Urol* 2008;54(4):924–31.

43 Carson C, Giuliano F, Goldstein I, et al. The "effectiveness" scale – therapeutic outcome of pharmacologic therapies for ED: an international consensus panel report. *Int J Impot Res* 2004;16(3):207–13.

44 Tay YK, Spernat D, Rzetelski-West K, Appu S, Love C. Acute management of priapism in men. *BJU Int* 2012;109 (Suppl. 3):15–21.

45 Sakamoto H. The neurobiology of psychogenic erectile dysfunction in the spinal cord. *J Androl* 2010;31(6): 519–26.

46 Becker AJ, Stief CG, Machtens S, et al. Oral phentolamine as treatment for erectile dysfunction. *J Urol* 1998;159(4):1214–6.

47 Zorgniotti AW. Experience with buccal phentolamine mesylate for impotence. *Int J Impot Res* 1994;6(1):37–41.

48 Goldstein I. Oral phentolamine: an alpha-1, alpha-2 adrenergic antagonist for the treatment of erectile dysfunction. *Int J Impot Res* 2000;12 (Suppl. 1):S75–80.

49 Traish A, Gupta S, Gallant C, Huang YH, Goldstein I. Phentolamine mesylate relaxes penile corpus cavernosum tissue by adrenergic and non-adrenergic mechanisms. *Int J Impot Res*.1998;10(4):215–23.

50 Clark JT. Suppression of copulatory behavior in male rats following central administration of clonidine. *Neuropharmacology* 1991;30(4):373–82.

51 Morales A. Yohimbine in erectile dysfunction: the facts. *Int J Impot Res* 2000;12 (Suppl. 1):S70–74.

52 Vogt HJ, Brandl P, Kockott G, et al. Double-blind, placebo-controlled safety and efficacy trial with yohimbine hydrochloride in the treatment of nonorganic erectile dysfunction. *Int J Impot Res* 1997;9(3):155–61.

53 Telöken C, Rhoden EL, Sogari P, Dambros M, Souto CA. Therapeutic effects of high dose yohimbine hydrochloride on organic erectile dysfunction. *J Urol* 1998;159(1):122–4.

54 Melis MR, Argiolas A, Gessa GL. Apomorphine-induced penile erection and yawning: site of action in brain. *Brain Res* 1987;415(1):98–104.

55 Heaton JP, Morales A, Adams MA, Johnston B, El-Rashidy R. Recovery of erectile function by the oral administration of apomorphine. *Urology* 1995;45(2):200–6.

56 Heaton JPW, Dean J, Sleep DJ. Sequential administration enhances the effect of apomorphine SL in men with erectile dysfunction. *Int J Impot Res* 2002;14(1):61–4.

57 Martin WJ, MacIntyre DE. Melanocortin receptors and erectile function. *Eur Urol* 2004;45(6):706–13.

58 Wessells H, Levine N, Hadley ME, Dorr R, Hruby V. Melanocortin receptor agonists, penile erection, and sexual motivation: human studies with Melanotan II. *Int J Impot Res* 2000;12 (Suppl. 4):S74–9.

59 Diamond LE, Earle DC, Garcia WD, Spana C. Co-administration of low doses of intranasal PT-141, a melanocortin receptor agonist, and sildenafil to men with erectile dysfunction results in an enhanced erectile response. *Urology* 2005;65(4):755–9.

60 Steidle C, Zinner N, Karlin G, Salzstein D, Fischkoff S. Phase IIB study of bremelanotide in the treatment of ED in diabetic males (abstract 1177). *J Urol* 2007;177(s4):388.

61 Safarinejad MR, Hosseini SY. Salvage of sildenafil failures with bremelanotide: a randomized, double-blind, placebo controlled study. *J Urol* 2008;179(3):1066–71.

62 Carson CC, Mino RD. Priapism associated with trazodone therapy. *J Urol* 1988;139(2):369–70.

63 Lal S, Rios O, Thavundayil JX. Treatment of impotence with trazodone: a case report. *J Urol* 1990;143(4):819–20.

64 Adaikan PG, Ng SC, Chan C, Ratnam SS. Oral trazodone in the treatment of total secondary impotence in a diabetic patient. *Br J Urol* 1991;68(2):212–3.

65 Kurt U, Ozkardeş H, Altuğ U, Germiyanoğlu C, Gürdal M, Erol D. The efficacy of anti-serotoninergic agents in the treatment of erectile dysfunction. *J Urol* 1994;152 (2 Pt 1):407–9.

66 Montorsi F, Strambi LF, Guazzoni G, et al. Effect of yohimbine-trazodone on psychogenic impotence: a randomized, double-blind, placebo-controlled study. *Urology* 1994;44(5):732–6.

67 Saenz de Tejada I, Ware JC, Blanco R, et al. Pathophysiology of prolonged penile erection associated with trazodone use. *J Urol* 1991;145(1):60–4.

68 Azadzoi KM, Payton T, Krane RJ, Goldstein I. Effects of intracavernosal trazodone hydrochloride: animal and human studies. *J Urol* 1990;144(5):1277–82.

69 Burnett AL. Oral pharmacotherapy for erectile dysfunction: current perspectives. *Urology* 1999;54(3):392–400.

70 Chen J, Wollman Y, Chernichovsky T, Iaina A, Sofer M, Matzkin H. Effect of oral administration of high-dose nitric oxide donor L-arginine in men with organic erectile dysfunction: results of a double-blind, randomized, placebo-controlled study. *BJU Int* 1999;83(3):269–73.

71 Ledda A, Belcaro G, Cesarone MR, Dugall M, Schönlau F. Investigation of a complex plant extract for mild to moderate erectile dysfunction in a randomized, double-blind, placebo-controlled, parallel-arm study. *BJU Int* 2010;106(7):1030–3.

72 Neuzillet Y, Hupertan V, Cour F, Botto H, Lebret T. A randomized, double-blind, crossover, placebo-controlled comparative clinical trial of arginine aspartate plus adenosine monophosphate for the intermittent treatment of male erectile dysfunction. *Andrology* 2013;1(2):223–8.

73 Virag R. Intracavernous injection of papaverine for erectile failure. *Lancet* 1982;2(8304):938.

74 Brindley GS. Cavernosal alpha-blockade: a new technique for investigating and treating erectile impotence. *Br J Psychiatry* 1983;143:332–7.

75 Linet OI, Ogrinc FG. Efficacy and safety of intracavernosal alprostadil in men with erectile dysfunction. The Alprostadil Study Group. *N Engl J Med* 1996;334(14):873–7.

76 Zorgniotti AW, Lefleur RS. Auto-injection of the corpus cavernosum with a vasoactive drug combination for vasculogenic impotence. *J Urol* 1985;133(1):39–41.

77 Israilov S, Niv E, Livne PM, et al. Intracavernous injections for erectile dysfunction in patients with cardiovascular diseases and failure or contraindications for sildenafil citrate. *Int J Impot Res* 2002;14(1):38–43.

78 Shamloul R, Atteya A, Elnashaar A, Gadallah A, Zohdy W, Abdelsalam W. Intracavernous sodium nitroprusside (SNP) versus papaverine/phentolamine in erectile dysfunction: a comparative study of short-term efficacy and side-effects. *J Sex Med* 2005;2(1):117–20.

79 Shah PJR, Dinsmore W, Oakes RA, Hackett G. Injection therapy for the treatment of erectile dysfunction: a comparison between alprostadil and a combination of vasoactive intestinal polypeptide and phentolamine mesilate. *Curr Med Res Opin* 2007;23(10):2577–83.

80 Shamloul R, El-Dakhly M, Ghanem H, Gadallah A, Mokhtar H. Intracavernous chlorpromazine versus phentolamine: a double-blind clinical comparative study. *J Sex Med* 2004;1(3):310–3.

81 Sharlip ID. Evaluation and nonsurgical management of erectile dysfunction. *Urol Clin North Am* 1998;25(4):647–59, ix.

82 Fuchs ME, Brawer MK. Papaverine-induced fibrosis of the corpus cavernosum. *J Urol* 1989;141(1):125.

83 Hu KN, Burks C, Christy WC. Fibrosis of tunica albuginea: complication of long-term intracavernous pharmacological self-injection. *J Urol* 1987;138(2):404–5.

84 Levine SB, Althof SE, Turner LA, et al. Side effects of self-administration of intracavernous papaverine and phentolamine for the treatment of impotence. *J Urol* 1989;141(1):54–7.

85 Anderson K, Holmquist F, Wagner G. Pharmacology of drugs used for treatment of erectile dysfunction and priapism. *Int J Impot Res* 1991;3:155–72.

86 Keogh EJ, Watters GR, Earle CM, et al. Treatment of impotence by intrapenile injections. A comparison of papaverine versus papaverine and phentolamine: a double-blind, crossover trial. *J Urol* 1989;142(3):726–8.

87 Kiely EA, Ignotus P, Williams G. Penile function following intracavernosal injection of vasoactive agents or saline. *Br J Urol* 1987;59(5):473–6.

88 Sidi AA, Cameron JS, Duffy LM, Lange PH. Intracavernous drug-induced erections in the management of male erectile dysfunction: experience with 100 patients. *J Urol* 1986; 135(4):704–6.

89 Gasser TC, Roach RM, Larsen EH, Madsen PO, Bruskewitz RC. Intracavernous self-injection with phentolamine and papaverine for the treatment of impotence. *J Urol* 1987;137(4):678–80.

90 Armstrong DK, Convery A, Dinsmore WW. Intracavernosal papaverine and phentolamine for the medical management of erectile dysfunction in a genitourinary clinic. *Int J STD AIDS* 1993;4(4):214–6.

91 Waldhauser M, Schramek P. Efficiency and side effects of prostaglandin E1 in the treatment of erectile dysfunction. *J Urol* 1988;140(3):525–7.

92 Sarosdy MF, Hudnall CH, Erickson DR, Hardin TC, Novicki DE. A prospective double-blind trial of intracorporeal papaverine versus prostaglandin E1 in the treatment of impotence. *J Urol* 1989;141(3):551–3.

93 Mahmoud KZ, el Dakhli MR, Fahmi IM, Abdel-Aziz AB. Comparative value of prostaglandin E1 and papaverine in treatment of erectile failure: double-blind crossover study among Egyptian patients. *J Urol* 1992;147(3):623–6.

94 Kattan S, Collins JP, Mohr D. Double-blind, cross-over study comparing prostaglandin E1 and papaverine in patients with vasculogenic impotence. *Urology* 1991;37(6):516–8.

95 Earle CM, Keogh EJ, Wisniewski ZS, et al. Prostaglandin E1 therapy for impotence, comparison with papaverine. *J Urol* 1990;143(1):57–9.

96 Bechara A, Casabé A, Chéliz G, Romano S, Rey H, Fredotovich N. Comparative study of papaverine plus phentolamine versus prostaglandin E1 in erectile dysfunction. *J Urol* 1997;157(6):2132–4.

97 Rastrelli G, Corona G, Monami M, et al. Poor response to alprostadil ICI test is associated with arteriogenic erectile dysfunction and higher risk of major adverse cardiovascular events. *J Sex Med* 2011;8(12):3433–45.

98 Porst H, Buvat J, Meuleman E, Michal V, Wagner G. Intracavernous Alprostadil Alfadex – an effective and well tolerated treatment for erectile dysfunction. Results of a long-term European study. *Int J Impot Res* 1998;10(4): 225–31.

99 Brock G, Tu LM, Linet OI. Return of spontaneous erection during long-term intracavernosal alprostadil (Caverject) treatment. *Urology* 2001;57(3):536–41.

100 Goldstein I, Borges F, Fitch W, et al. Rescuing the failed papaverine/phentolamine erection: A proposed synergistic action of papaverine, phentolamine and prostaglandin E1. *J Urol* 1990;143 (4 Suppl.):304A.

101 Shenfeld O, Hanani J, Shalhav A, Vardi Y, Goldwasser B. Papaverine-phentolamine and prostaglandin E1 versus papaverine-phentolamine alone for intracorporeal injection therapy: a clinical double-blind study. *J Urol* 1995; 154(3):1017–9.

102 Bechara A, Casabé A, Chéliz G, Romano S, Fredotovich N. Prostaglandin E1 versus mixture of prostaglandin E1, papaverine and phentolamine in nonresponders to high papaverine plus phentolamine doses. *J Urol* 1996;155(3):913–4.

103 Allen RP, Engel RM, Smolev JK, Brendler CB. Objective double-blind evaluation of erectile function with intracorporeal papaverine in combination with phentolamine and/or prostaglandin E1. *J Urol* 1992;148(4):1181–3.

104 Alexandre B, Lemaire A, Desvaux P, Amar E. Intracavernous injections of prostaglandin E1 for erectile dysfunction: patient satisfaction and quality of sex life on long-term treatment. *J Sex Med* 2007;4(2):426–31.

105 Mulhall JP, Jahoda AE, Cairney M, et al. The causes of patient dropout from penile self-injection therapy for impotence. *J Urol* 1999;162(4):1291–4.

106 Montorsi F, Salonia A, Zanoni M, et al. Current status of local penile therapy. *Int J Impot Res* 2002;14 (Suppl. 1):S70–81.

107 Sandhu D, Curless E, Dean J, et al. A double blind, placebo controlled study of intracavernosal vasoactive intestinal polypeptide and phentolamine mesylate in a novel auto-injector for the treatment of non-psychogenic erectile dysfunction. *Int J Impot Res* 1999;11(2):91–7.

108 Mulhall JP, Daller M, Traish AM, et al. Intracavernosal forskolin: role in management of vasculogenic impotence resistant to standard 3-agent pharmacotherapy. *J Urol* 1997;158(5):1752–8; discussion 1758–9.

109 Brock G, Breza J, Lue TF. Intracavernous sodium nitroprusside: inappropriate impotence treatment. *J Urol* 1993;150(3):864–7.

110 Sahin M, Başar MM, Bozdoğan O, Atan A. Short-term histopathologic effects of different intracavernosal agents on corpus cavernosum and antifibrotic activity of intracavernosal verapamil: an experimental study. *Urology*. 2001; 58(3):487–92.

111 Fu Q, Yao DH, Jiang YQ. A clinical comparative study on effects of intracavernous injection of sodium nitroprusside and papaverine/phentolamine in erectile dysfunction patients. *Asian J Androl* 2000;2(4):301–3.

112 Seyam RM, Bégin LR, Tu LM, Dion SB, Merlin SL, Brock GB. Evaluation of a no-needle penile injector: a preliminary study evaluating tissue penetration and its hemodynamic consequences in the rat. *Urology* 1997;50(6):994–8.

113 Harding LM, Adeniyi A, Everson R, Barker S, Ralph DJ, Baranowski AP. Comparison of a needle-free high-pressure injection system with needle-tipped injection of intracavernosal alprostadil for erectile dysfunction. *Int J Impot Res* 2002;14(6):498–501.

114 Moemen MN, Hamed HA, Kamel II, Shamloul RM, Ghanem HM. Clinical and sonographic assessment of the side effects of intracavernous injection of vasoactive substances. *Int J Impot Res* 2004;16(2):143–5.

115 Moreland RB, Traish A, McMillin MA, Smith B, Goldstein I, Saenz de Tejada I. PGE1 suppresses the induction of collagen synthesis by transforming growth factor-beta 1 in human corpus cavernosum smooth muscle. *J Urol* 1995;153(3 Pt 1):826–34.

116 Chung E, Deyoung L, Brock GB. The role of PDE5 inhibitors in penile septal scar remodeling: assessment of clinical and radiological outcomes. *J Sex Med* 2011;8(5):1472–7.

117 Aboseif SR, Breza J, Bosch RJ, et al. Local and systemic effects of chronic intracavernous injection of papaverine, prostaglandin E1, and saline in primates. *J Urol* 1989;142(2 Pt 1):403–8.

118 Moriel EZ, Rajfer J. Sodium bicarbonate alleviates penile pain induced by intracavernous injections for erectile dysfunction. *J Urol* 1993;149(5 Pt 2):1299–300.

119 Montorsi F, Guazzoni G, Strambi LF, et al. Recovery of spontaneous erectile function after nerve-sparing radical retropubic prostatectomy with and without early intracavernous injections of alprostadil: results of a prospective, randomized trial. *J Urol* 1997;158(4):1408–10.

120 Casabé A, Bechara A, Cheliz G, Romano S, Rey H, Fredotovich N. Drop-out reasons and complications in self-injection therapy with a triple vasoactive drug mixture in sexual erectile dysfunction. *Int J Impot Res* 1998; 10(1):5–9.

121 Purvis K, Egdetveit I, Christiansen E. Intracavernosal therapy for erectile failure – impact of treatment and reasons for drop-out and dissatisfaction. *Int J Impot Res* 1999;11(5):287–99.

122 Althof SE, Turner LA, Levine SB, et al. Why do so many people drop out from auto-injection therapy for impotence? *J Sex Marital Ther* 1989;15(2):121–9.

123 Sundaram CP, Thomas W, Pryor LE, Sidi AA, Billups K, Pryor JL. Long-term follow-up of patients receiving injection therapy for erectile dysfunction. *Urology* 1997; 49(6):932–5.

124 Hellstrom WJ, Bennett AH, Gesundheit N, et al. A double-blind, placebo-controlled evaluation of the erectile response to transurethral alprostadil. *Urology* 1996;48(6): 851–6.

125 Porst H. Transurethral alprostadil with MUSE (medicated urethral system for erection) vs intracavernous alprostadil – a comparative study in 103 patients with erectile dysfunction. *Int J Impot Res* 1997;9(4):187–92.

126 Shabsigh R, Padma-Nathan H, Gittleman M, McMurray J, Kaufman J, Goldstein I. Intracavernous alprostadil alfadex is more efficacious, better tolerated, and preferred over intraurethral alprostadil plus optional actis: a comparative, randomized, crossover, multicenter study. *Urology* 2000;55(1):109–13.

127 Engel JD, McVary KT. Transurethral alprostadil as therapy for patients who withdrew from or failed prior intracavernous injection therapy. *Urology* 1998;51(5):687–92.

128 Fulgham PF, Cochran JS, Denman JL, et al. Disappointing initial results with transurethral alprostadil for erectile dysfunction in a urology practice setting. *J Urol* 1998;160 (6 Pt 1):2041–6.

129 Mulhall JP, Jahoda AE, Ahmed A, Parker M. Analysis of the consistency of intraurethral prostaglandin E(1) (MUSE) during at-home use. *Urology* 2001;58(2):262–6.

130 Chew KK, Stuckey BG. Use of transurethral alprostadil (MUSE) (prostaglandin E1) for glans tumescence in a patient with penile prosthesis. *Int J Impot Res* 2000;12(3): 195–6.

131 Costabile RA, Spevak M, Fishman IJ, et al. Efficacy and safety of transurethral alprostadil in patients with erectile dysfunction following radical prostatectomy. *J Urol* 1998;160(4):1325–8.

132 Raina R, Nandipati KC, Agarwal A, Mansour D, Kaelber DC, Zippe CD. Combination therapy: medicated urethral system for erection enhances sexual satisfaction in sildenafil citrate failure following nerve-sparing radical prostatectomy. *J Androl* 2005;26(6):757–60.

133 Raina R, Pahlajani G, Agarwal A, Zippe CD. The early use of transurethral alprostadil after radical prostatectomy potentially facilitates an earlier return of erectile function and successful sexual activity. *BJU Int* 2007;100(6): 1317–21.

134 McCullough AR, Hellstrom WG, Wang R, Lepor H, Wagner KR, Engel JD. Recovery of erectile function after nerve sparing radical prostatectomy and penile rehabilitation with nightly intraurethral alprostadil versus sildenafil citrate. *J Urol* 2010;183(6):2451–6.

135 Hsieh C-H, Liu S-P, Hsu G-L, et al. Advances in understanding of mammalian penile evolution, human penile anatomy and human erection physiology: clinical implications for physicians and surgeons. *Med Sci Monit* 2012;18(7):RA118–25.
136 Kim ED, el-Rashidy R, McVary KT. Papaverine topical gel for treatment of erectile dysfunction. *J Urol* 1995;153(2): 361–5.
137 Wen MM, El-Kamel AH, Khalil SA. Systemic enhancement of papaverine transdermal gel for erectile dysfunction. *Drug Dev Ind Pharm* 2012;38(8):912–22.
138 Claes H, Baert L. Transcutaneous nitroglycerin therapy in the treatment of impotence. *Urol Int* 1989;44(5):309–12.
139 Meyhoff HH, Rosenkilde P, Bødker A. Non-invasive management of impotence with transcutaneous nitroglycerin. *Br J Urol* 1992;69(1):88–90.
140 Borges FD. A new approach to the pharmacologic treatment of impotence. *Int J Impot Res* 1994;6(3):137–43.
141 Renganathan R, Suranjan B, Kurien T. Comparison of transdermal nitroglycerin and intracavernous injection of papaverine in the treatment of erectile dysfunction in patients with spinal cord lesions. *Spinal Cord* 1997;35(2): 99–103.
142 Cavallini G. Minoxidil versus nitroglycerin: a prospective double-blind controlled trial in transcutaneous erection facilitation for organic impotence. *J Urol* 1991;146(1): 50–3.
143 Chancellor MB, Rivas DA, Panzer DE, Freedman MK, Staas WE. Prospective comparison of topical minoxidil to vacuum constriction device and intracorporeal papaverine injection in treatment of erectile dysfunction due to spinal cord injury. *Urology* 1994;43(3):365–9.
144 Gomaa A, Shalaby M, Osman M, et al. Topical treatment of erectile dysfunction: randomised double blind placebo controlled trial of cream containing aminophylline, isosorbide dinitrate, and co-dergocrine mesylate. *BMJ* 1996; 312(7045):1512–5.
145 Naude JH, Le Roux PJ. Topical treatment of erectile dysfunction did not show results. *BMJ* 1998;316(7140):1318.
146 Kim ED, McVary KT. Topical prostaglandin-E1 for the treatment of erectile dysfunction. *J Urol* 1995;153(6):1828–30.
147 Goldstein I, Payton TR, Schechter PJ. A double-blind, placebo-controlled, efficacy and safety study of topical gel formulation of 1% alprostadil (Topiglan) for the in-office treatment of erectile dysfunction. *Urology* 2001;57(2): 301–5.
148 Padma-Nathan H, Steidle C, Salem S, Tayse N, Yeager J, Harning R. The efficacy and safety of a topical alprostadil cream, Alprox-TD, for the treatment of erectile dysfunction: two phase 2 studies in mild-to-moderate and severe ED. *Int J Impot Res* 2003;15(1):10–7.
149 Padma-Nathan H, Yeager JL. An integrated analysis of alprostadil topical cream for the treatment of erectile dysfunction in 1732 patients. *Urology* 2006;68(2):386–91.
150 Rooney M, Pfister W, Mahoney M, Nelson M, Yeager J, Steidle C. Long-term, multicenter study of the safety and efficacy of topical alprostadil cream in male patients with erectile dysfunction. *J Sex Med* 2009;6(2):520–34.
151 Somlyo AP, Somlyo AV. Signal transduction by G-proteins, rho-kinase and protein phosphatase to smooth muscle and non-muscle myosin II. *J Physiol* 2000;522 Pt 2: 177–85.
152 Chitaley K, Webb RC, Mills TM. Rho-kinase as a potential target for the treatment of erectile dysfunction. *Drug News Perspect* 2001;14(10):601–6.
153 Jin L, Burnett AL. RhoA/Rho-kinase in erectile tissue: mechanisms of disease and therapeutic insights. *Clin Sci (Lond)* 2006;110(2):153–65.
154 Vignozzi L, Morelli A, Filippi S, et al. Testosterone regulates RhoA/Rho-kinase signaling in two distinct animal models of chemical diabetes. *J Sex Med* 2007;4(3):620–30; discussion 631–32.
155 Park K, Kim SW, Rhu KS, Paick J-S. Chronic administration of an oral Rho kinase inhibitor prevents the development of vasculogenic erectile dysfunction in a rat model. *J Sex Med* 2006;3(6):996–1003.
156 Li WJ, Park K, Paick J-S, Kim SW. Chronic treatment with an oral rho-kinase inhibitor restores erectile function by suppressing corporal apoptosis in diabetic rats. *J Sex Med* 2011;8(2):400–10.
157 Demir O, Murat N, Aslan G, Gidener S, Esen AA. Effect of doxazosin with and without rho-kinase inhibitor on human corpus cavernosum smooth muscle in the presence of bladder outlet obstruction. *J Urol* 2006;175(6):2345–9.
158 Stasch J-P, Pacher P, Evgenov OV. Soluble guanylate cyclase as an emerging therapeutic target in cardiopulmonary disease. *Circulation* 2011;123(20):2263–73.
159 Lucas KA, Pitari GM, Kazerounian S, et al. Guanylyl cyclases and signaling by cyclic GMP. *Pharmacol Rev* 2000; 52(3):375–414.
160 Stasch J, Schmidt PM, Nedvetsky PI, et al. Targeting the heme-oxidized nitric oxide receptor for selective vasodilatation of diseased blood vessels. *J Clin Invest* 2006;116(9):2552–61.
161 Roy B, Mo E, Vernon J, Garthwaite J. Probing the presence of the ligand-binding haem in cellular nitric oxide receptors. *Br J Pharmacol* 2008;153(7):1495–504.
162 Brioni JD, Nakane M, Hsieh GC, Moreland RB, Kolasa T, Sullivan JP. Activators of soluble guanylate cyclase for the treatment of male erectile dysfunction. *Int J Impot Res* 2002;14(1):8–14.
163 Claudino MA, Delbin MA, Franco-Penteado CF, et al. Exercise training ameliorates the impairment of endothelial and nitrergic corpus cavernosum responses in diabetic rats. *Life Sci* 2011;88(5-6):272–7.
164 Schermuly RT, Janssen W, Weissmann N, Stasch J-P, Grimminger F, Ghofrani HA. Riociguat for the treatment of pulmonary hypertension. *Expert Opin Investig Drugs* 2011;20(4):567–76.

165 Oudot A, Behr-Roussel D, Poirier S, et al. Combination of BAY 60-4552 and vardenafil exerts proerectile facilitator effects in rats with cavernous nerve injury: a proof of concept study for the treatment of phosphodiesterase type 5 inhibitor failure. *Eur Urol* 2011;60(5):1020–6.
166 Evgenov OV, Pacher P, Schmidt PM, Haskó G, Schmidt HHHW, Stasch J-P. NO-independent stimulators and activators of soluble guanylate cyclase: discovery and therapeutic potential. *Nat Rev Drug Discov* 2006;5(9):755–68.
167 Lapp H, Mitrovic V, Franz N, et al. Cinaciguat (BAY 58-2667) improves cardiopulmonary hemodynamics in patients with acute decompensated heart failure. *Circulation* 2009;119(21):2781–8.
168 Liaw RL, Srilatha B, Adaikan PG. Effects of hydrogen sulfide on erectile function and its possible mechanism(s) of action. *J Sex Med* 2011;8(7):1853–64.
169 Srilatha B, Adaikan PG, Moore PK. Possible role for the novel gasotransmitter hydrogen sulphide in erectile dysfunction – a pilot study. *Eur J Pharmacol* 2006;535(1-3):280–2.
170 Srilatha B, Adaikan PG, Li L, Moore PK. Hydrogen sulphide: a novel endogenous gasotransmitter facilitates erectile function. *J Sex Med* 2007;4(5):1304–11.
171 Zhao W, Zhang J, Lu Y, Wang R. The vasorelaxant effect of H(2)S as a novel endogenous gaseous K(ATP) channel opener. *EMBO J* 2001;20(21):6008–16.
172 Brayden JE. Functional roles of KATP channels in vascular smooth muscle. *Clin Exp Pharmacol Physiol* 2002;29(4):312–6.
173 d'Emmanuele di Villa Bianca R, Sorrentino R, Maffia P, et al. Hydrogen sulfide as a mediator of human corpus cavernosum smooth-muscle relaxation. *Proc Natl Acad Sci U S A* 2009;106(11):4513–8.
174 Shukla N, Rossoni G, Hotston M, et al. Effect of hydrogen sulphide-donating sildenafil (ACS6) on erectile function and oxidative stress in rabbit isolated corpus cavernosum and in hypertensive rats. *BJU Int* 2009;103(11):1522–9.
175 Lu Z, Xu X, Hu X, et al. Oxidative stress regulates left ventricular PDE5 expression in the failing heart. *Circulation* 2010;121(13):1474–83.
176 Jones RWA, Rees RW, Minhas S, Ralph D, Persad RA, Jeremy JY. Oxygen free radicals and the penis. *Expert Opin Pharmacother* 2002;3(7):889–97.
177 Bucci M, Mirone V, Di Lorenzo A, et al. Hydrogen sulphide is involved in testosterone vascular effect. *Eur Urol* 2009;56(2):378–83.
178 Geng B, Cui Y, Zhao J, et al. Hydrogen sulfide downregulates the aortic L-arginine/nitric oxide pathway in rats. *Am J Physiol Regul Integr Comp Physiol* 2007;293(4):R1608–18.
179 Zhao W, Ndisang JF, Wang R. Modulation of endogenous production of H2S in rat tissues. *Can J Physiol Pharmacol* 2003;81(9):848–53.
180 Zhang X-H, Aydin M, Kuppam D, Melman A, Disanto ME. In vitro and in vivo relaxation of corpus cavernosum smooth muscle by the selective myosin II inhibitor, blebbistatin. *J Sex Med* 2009;6(10):2661–71.
181 Kovács M, Tóth J, Hetényi C, Málnási-Csizmadia A, Sellers JR. Mechanism of blebbistatin inhibition of myosin II. *J Biol Chem* 2004;279(34):35557–63.
182 Xu S, White HD, Offer GW, Yu LC. Stabilization of helical order in the thick filaments by blebbistatin: further evidence of coexisting multiple conformations of myosin. *Biophys J* 2009;96(9):3673–81.
183 Sohn MH. Current status of penile revascularization for the treatment of male erectile dysfunction. *J Androl* 1994;15(3):183–6.
184 Babaei AR, Safarinejad MR, Kolahi AA. Penile revascularization for erectile dysfunction: a systematic review and meta-analysis of effectiveness and complications. *Urol J* 2009;6(1):1–7.
185 Rogers JH, Karimi H, Kao J, et al. Internal pudendal artery stenoses and erectile dysfunction: correlation with angiographic coronary artery disease. *Catheter Cardiovasc Interv* 2010;76(6):882–7.
186 Rogers JH, Goldstein I, Kandzari DE, et al. Zotarolimus-eluting peripheral stents for the treatment of erectile dysfunction in subjects with suboptimal response to phosphodiesterase-5 inhibitors. *J Am Coll Cardiol* 2012;60(25):2618–27.
187 Berlin RG in *West J Med.* 1986 Mar; 144(3): 359–361.
188 Jauhari J. Gynaecomastia, galactorrhoea and impotence – the uncommon side effects of cimetidine therapy. *J Assoc Physicians India* 1987;35(6):462.
189 Beeley L. Drug-induced sexual dysfunction and infertility. *Adverse Drug React Acute Poisoning Rev* 1984;3(1):23–42.
190 Mitchell JE, Popkin MK. Antipsychotic drug therapy and sexual dysfunction in men. *Am J Psychiatry* 1982;139(5):633–7.
191 Schmidt HM, Hagen M, Kriston L, Soares-Weiser K, Maayan N, Berner MM. Management of sexual dysfunction due to antipsychotic drug therapy. *Cochrane Database Syst Rev* 2012 Jan;11:CD003546.
192 Shamloul R, Bella AJ. Impact of cannabis use on male sexual health. *J Sex Med* 2011;8(4):971–5.
193 Abel EL. A review of alcohol's effects on sex and reproduction. *Drug Alcohol Depend* 1980;5(5):321–32.
194 George WH, Cue Davis K, Schraufnagel TJ, et al. Later that night: descending alcohol intoxication and men's sexual arousal. *Am J Mens Health* 2008;2(1):76–86.
195 Husain AM, Carwile ST, Miller PP, Radtke RA. Improved sexual function in three men taking lamotrigine for epilepsy. *South Med J* 2000;93(3):335–6.
196 Ramsey S. Opioids for back pain are linked to increased risk of erectile dysfunction. *BMJ* 2013;346:f3223.
197 Dhikav V, Gupta S, Anand KS. Erectile dysfunction induced probably by celecoxib. *Pharmacoepidemiol Drug Saf* 2008;17(2):211–2.
198 Miller LG, Rogers JC, Swee DE. Indomethacin-associated sexual dysfunction. *J Fam Pract* 1989;29(2):210–1.

199 Lin SN, Yu PC, Yang MC, Chang LS, Chiang BN, Kuo JS. Local suppressive effect of clonidine on penile erection in the dog. *J Urol* 1988;139(4):849–52.

200 Moss HB, Procci WR. Sexual dysfunction associated with oral antihypertensive medication: a critical survey of the literature. *Gen Hosp Psychiatry* 1982;4(2):121–9.

201 Gur S, Kadowitz PJ, Hellstrom WJ. Effects of 5-alpha reductase inhibitors on erectile function, sexual desire and ejaculation. *Expert Opin Drug Saf* 2013;12(1):81–90.

202 Erdemir F, Harbin A, Hellstrom WJG. 5-Alpha reductase inhibitors and erectile dysfunction: the connection. *J Sex Med* 2008;5(12):2917–24.

203 Stevens MJ, Bell DR, Blome SA, Begbie SD. Prolonged hypogonadism after pulsed gonadotropin-releasing hormone agonist for prostate cancer. *Lancet* 1994;344(8917):274–5.

204 Rösler A, Witztum E. Treatment of men with paraphilia with a long-acting analogue of gonadotropin-releasing hormone. *N Engl J Med* 1998;338(7):416–22.

205 Mazzola CR, Deveci S, Heck M, Mulhall JP. Androgen deprivation therapy before radical prostatectomy is associated with poorer postoperative erectile function outcomes. *BJU Int* 2012;110(1):112–6.

206 Moreno-Pérez O, Escoín C, Serna-Candel C, et al. Risk factors for sexual and erectile dysfunction in HIV-infected men: the role of protease inhibitors. *AIDS* 2010;24(2): 255–64.

207 Dove LM, Rosen RC, Ramcharran D, et al. Decline in male sexual desire, function, and satisfaction during and after antiviral therapy for chronic hepatitis C. *Gastroenterology* 2009;137(3):873–84, 884.e1.

208 Shabsigh R, Seftel AD, Rosen RC, et al. Review of time of onset and duration of clinical efficacy of phosphodiesterase type 5 inhibitors in treatment of erectile dysfunction. *Urology* 2006;68(4):689–96.

209 Gbekor E, Bethel S, Fawcett L, Mount N, Phillips S. Phosphodiesterase 5 inhibitor profiles against all human phosphodiesterase families: implications for use as pharmacological tools. *J Urol* 2002;167 (4 Suppl.):246.

210 Blount MA, Beasley A, Zoraghi R, et al. Binding of tritiated sildenafil, tadalafil, or vardenafil to the phosphodiesterase-5 catalytic site displays potency, specificity, heterogeneity, and cGMP stimulation. *Mol Pharmacol* 2004; 66(1):144–52.

211 Padma-Nathan H, Eardley I, Kloner RA, Laties AM, Montorsi F. A 4-year update on the safety of sildenafil citrate (Viagra). *Urology* 2002;60 (2 Suppl. 2):67–90.

212 Reffelmann T, Kloner RA. Vardenafil: a selective inhibitor of phosphodiesterase-5 for the treatment of erectile dysfunction. *Expert Opin Pharmacother* 2007;8(7):965–74.

213 Hatzimouratidis K, Moysidis K, Bekos A, Tsimtsiou Z, Ioannidis E, Hatzichristou D. Treatment strategy for "non-responders" to tadalafil and vardenafil: a real-life study. *Eur Urol* 2006;50(1):126–32; discussion 132–3.

214 Guay AT, Perez JB, Jacobson J, Newton RA. Efficacy and safety of sildenafil citrate for treatment of erectile dysfunction in a population with associated organic risk factors. *J Androl* 2001;22(5):793–7.

215 Carson CC, Hatzichristou DG, Carrier S, et al. Erectile response with vardenafil in sildenafil nonresponders: a multicentre, double-blind, 12-week, flexible-dose, placebo-controlled erectile dysfunction clinical trial. *BJU Int* 2004;94(9):1301–9.

216 McMahon C. Efficacy and safety of daily tadalafil in men with erectile dysfunction previously unresponsive to on-demand tadalafil. *J Sex Med* 2004;1(3):292–300.

217 Lakin MM, Montague DK, VanderBrug Medendorp S, Tesar L, Schover LR. Intracavernous injection therapy: analysis of results and complications. *J Urol* 1990;143(6):1138–41.

218 Pery M, Rosenberger A, Kaftori JK, Vardi Y. Intracorporeal calcifications after self-injection of papaverine. *Radiology* 1990;176(1):81–3.

219 Virag R, Shoukry K, Floresco J, Nollet F, Greco E. Intracavernous self-injection of vasoactive drugs in the treatment of impotence: 8-year experience with 615 cases. *J Urol* 1991;145(2):287–92; discussion 292–3.

220 Gall H, Sparwasser C, Bähren W, Scherb W, Irion R. Long-term results of corpus cavernosum autoinjection therapy for chronic erectile dysfunction. *Andrologia* 24(5):285–92.

221 Armstrong DK, Convery A, Dinsmore WW. Intracavernosal papaverine and phentolamine for the medical management of erectile dysfunction in a genitourinary clinic. *Int J STD AIDS* 1993;4(4):214–6.

222 Kapoor VK, Chahal a S, Jyoti SP, Mundkur YJ, Kotwal S V, Mehta VK. Intracavernous papaverine for impotence in spinal cord injured patients. *Paraplegia* 1993;31(10):675–7.

223 Hirsch IH, Schanne FJ, Carsello J, Bagley DH, Alexander AA. Sequential penile ultrasound monitoring of patients treated with chronic intracavernous prostaglandin E1. *Urology* 1995;45(6):1037–41.

224 Chew KK, Stuckey BG, Earle CM, Dhaliwal SS, Keogh EJ. Penile fibrosis in intracavernosal prostaglandin E1 injection therapy for erectile dysfunction. *Int J Impot Res* 1997;9(4):225–9; discussion 229–30.

225 The long-term safety of alprostadil (prostaglandin-E1) in patients with erectile dysfunction. The European Alprostadil Study Group. *Br J Urol* 1998;82(4):538–43.

CHAPTER 20

Priapism

Varun Sahdev, David Ralph, and Asif Muneer
University College Hospital London, London, UK

Priapism can be defined as a persistent penile erection lasting longer than 4 hours in the absence of sexual stimulation and persisting despite ejaculation or orgasm.[1] It is a urological emergency and can be subdivided into ischemic (low flow), non-ischemic (high flow), and recurrent (stuttering) subtypes.

The disease is named after Priapus, the Greek god of fertility and protector of gardens, fruit, plants, and livestock. According to Greek mythology, Priapus was cursed by the jealous goddess Hera, while still in the goddess Aphrodite's womb, leaving him with an oversized phallus, large hands, and a large tongue. Petraens's *Gonorrhoea, Satyriasis et Priapisme* represents the earliest documented account of the disease and dates back to 1666.[2]

The underlying pathophysiology of this condition is still not well understood, but renewed scientific interest in the form of clinical and laboratory research has led to significant progress in the diagnosis and management of the disease over the past 10–15 years.

Epidemiology and pathophysiology of priapism

The incidence of priapism is 0.5–0.9 cases per 100,000 person-years.[3] Priapism is known to be more common in patients with sickle-cell disease, with the quoted prevalence in this patient group being 3.6% below the age of 18 years and up to 42% in patients aged above 18 years.[3]

Non-ischemic priapism

Non-ischemic (or arterial) priapism is a relatively uncommon condition and usually occurs following blunt trauma to the perineum especially after a straddle-type injury. The mechanism involves compression of the cavernosal artery against the pubic bone resulting in a laceration to the cavernosal artery and a subsequent high-flow fistula between the artery and the lacunar spaces of the sinusoidal tissue.[4]

In this condition, patients commonly present as a delayed consultation, with a non-painful persistent, semi-rigid erection,[3] often with visible pulsation present.[5] Blood gas analysis from blood aspirated from the corpus cavernosum reveals a normal pH and a normal pO_2. As a result, the chance of irreversible smooth muscle dysfunction of the corpus cavernosum in the long term is significantly reduced compared to other forms of the disease.

Ischemic priapism

Ischemic priapism is by far the most common form of the disease and accounts for over 95% of cases.[4,6] Unsurprisingly, it is therefore the most extensively investigated subtype. When ischemic priapism persists beyond 4 hours, it is considered to be effectively a compartment syndrome of the penis.[3,7]

In terms of the etiology, the majority of cases are idiopathic;[8,9] however, it is also known to be associated with several diseases and medication regimes. These include sickle-cell anemia, hematological dyscrasias, neoplastic syndromes, malignancy, neurological conditions, and drugs such as antipsychotics and intracavernosal injections used for erectile dysfunction (Table 20.1).

From the clinical perspective, the patient typically presents with penile pain; clinical examination reveals rigidity of the corpora cavernosa.[3] Blood gas analysis from the corpora cavernosa reveals hypoxia, hypercapnia, and acidosis,[10] with prolonged cases also developing glucopenia.[11]

Male Sexual Dysfunction: A Clinical Guide, First Edition. Edited by Suks Minhas and John Mulhall.

Table 20.1 Etiology of ischemic priapism.

Idiopathic	30% risk
Hematological	
Sickle-cell disease	
Leukemia	
Polycythemia	
Thalassemia	
Fabry's disease	
Multiple myeloma	
Factor V Leiden mutation	
Antipsychotics	
Chlorpromazine	
Clozapine	
Antihypertensives	
Hydralazine	
Prazocin	
Guanethidine	
Intracavernosal injections	5% risk
Papaverine	
Prostaglandin E_1	1% risk
Malignancy	
Metastatic prostate cancer	
Bladder cancer	
Neurological	
Cauda equina	
Spinal steroids	

These ischemic parameters lead to changes within the metabolic environment of the corpora cavernosa. In addition to the aforementioned hypoxia, hypercapnia, and acidosis, further sequelae include smooth muscle dysfunction and fibrosis, which occur in a time-dependent manner. These may become irreversible if the ischemia is not promptly reversed;[11] indeed, the duration of ischemic priapism represents the most significant predictor of erectile function.

Cellular-level changes in ischemic priapism

At the cellular level, early histological alterations are observed. These include an expanded perinuclear cytoplasm, ribosomes, Golgi apparatus, and endoplasmic reticulum, which can be seen after 12 hours of ischemia.

As the ischemia continues to between 24 and 48 hours, further degradation occurs in the form of destruction of the endothelium and exposure of the basement membrane, which in turn results in the adherence of thrombocytes.

Changes also occur in a similar manner to the smooth muscle cells, leading to necrosis, which eventually culminates in the transformation of smooth muscle cells into fibroblast-like cells.[12] In practice, priapism that lasts longer than approximately 24 hours is associated with unavoidable long-term erectile dysfunction.[8]

Regarding the pathophysiology of ischemic priapism, there are several steps where neurovascular and smooth muscle dysregulation may occur along the complex pathway involved in achieving a penile erection.

The precise mechanism involved in the initiation of abnormal penile tumescence has not been fully elucidated. However, several factors are likely to be involved with a combination of central nervous system involvement, changes in the corpus cavernosal microenvironment including disrupted aberrant neurotransmitter activity, and aberrant smooth muscle contraction.

During the erectile maintenance phase, an imbalance exists between factors regulating vasoconstriction and vasorelaxation in the penis. The role of nitric oxide (NO) has also been discussed at length in the literature. It was previously thought to play little or no part in the pathophysiology of priapism;[13] however, more recent work examining endothelial NO-mediated synthase-negative mice has revealed that it may play a more significant role.[8]

The proposed mechanism suggests that a deficiency of NO results in dysregulation of phosphodiesterase-5 (PDE5), resulting in a lower PDE5 functional set point. This in turn causes an imbalance in favor of unregulated smooth muscle relaxation.[14]

Stuttering (recurrent) priapism

In stuttering priapism, there are recurrent episodes of prolonged but self-limiting erections.[15] The frequency and duration of these priapic episodes may crescendo into an acute episode of ischemic priapism. The condition occurs more often at night with a failure of detumescence on waking, with erections becoming painful if they exceed 1 hour in duration.

In patients with sickle-cell disease, the erections are associated with the development of ischemia; however, the picture is sometimes more complex. Stuttering priapism can sometimes occur in the context of short-lived high-flow episodes; and, secondly, men who have experienced an acute ischemic priapic episode lasting more than 4 hours are also at higher risk of developing stuttering priapism.[16]

Although it is often deemed idiopathic, stuttering priapism is known to be more common in patients with sickle-cell disease.[16,17] Other postulated causes include intrinsic smooth muscle dysfunction of the penis, abnormal central and peripheral nervous system regulation, and dysfunction of the hormonal axis.[3]

Malignant priapism

Malignant priapism can be described as priapism that is related to metastatic disease or its associated local invasion or infiltration. The mechanism is poorly understood, although cases reported thus far in the literature favor an infiltrative mechanism as opposed to the hemodynamic process associated with other forms of the disease.[18]

Due to the difference in the likely mechanism, pharmacological agents are not recommended in the treatment of malignant priapism and magnetic resonance imaging (MRI) is used to characterize the primary tumor, which becomes the focus of any further management.[3]

Clinical assessment of the patient with priapism

History

When faced with a patient with priapism in the acute setting, a comprehensive but focused history provides the key information required to differentiate between the different forms of the disease. The patient should be asked specifically about the duration of the erection, the severity of pain (if present), whether he has had previous priapic episodes, and how these were managed.

Specific questions related to the past medical history include inquiring about any known history of sickle-cell disease, hemoglobinopathies, hypercoagulable states, and recent pelvic trauma. A thorough drug history should be taken asking specifically whether the patient takes any erectogenic medications or recreational drugs.[19]

Examination

A full physical evaluation in the context of priapism includes an abdominal examination, with examination of the genitalia as well as the perineum.[19,20] Classically, in non-ischemic priapism, the corpora are not fully rigid whereas in ischemic priapism, the corpora are fully rigid but the glans is not.

Investigations

Blood tests

A blood profile in the context of priapism should include a full blood count, platelet count, and coagulation screen including those to assess hematological abnormalities. Blood gas analysis is essential to differentiate ischemic and non-ischemic priapism (Table 20.2).

Imaging

Several imaging modalities are helpful for both the diagnosis as well as the management of priapism. The principal modalities available for the assessment of priapism include a penile Doppler study, angiographic studies and MRI.

Doppler studies

A penile Doppler study acts as a key adjunct to the history, examination, and blood gas analysis findings and helps to differentiate between ischemic and non-ischemic priapism.[7] Standard gray-scale studies are combined with Doppler imaging, which assesses the degree of flow present in the cavernosal artery.[21]

Doppler findings in ischemic priapism

In the case of ischemic priapism, the flow within the corpora cavernosa is absent and the Doppler trace reveals high resistance with low velocity. A concurrent low diastolic pressure is found and the arterial pressure is either normal or reduced but never raised.

The sinusoids are enlarged but the echogenicity depends upon the degree of sinusoidal thrombosis and the flow in the dorsal vein is most likely reduced or unrecordable.[22,23]

According to some studies, the degree of arterial cavernosal blood flow can remain relatively high in a small percentage of patients; however, this is matched by high vascular resistance leading to non-perfusion. In the

Table 20.2 Blood gas values.

Source	pO_2 (mmHg)	pCO_2 (mmHg)	pH
Normal arterial blood (room air)	>90	<40	7.40
Normal mixed venous blood (room air)	40	50	7.35
Ischemic priapism	<30	>60	<7.25

Adapted from Broderick et al.[19]

context of ischemic priapism, Doppler studies also provide a good method of assessing resolution immediately following intervention as well as in follow-up studies.[22]

Doppler findings in non-ischemic priapism

In non-ischemic priapism, cavernosal artery flow is either elevated or normal, with a low diastolic pressure signifying low resistance. Venous changes are also seen in non-ischemic priapism in the form of high venous outflow within the dorsal vein.[24] The sinusoids in this case are often compressible with an ultrasound probe.

Doppler is extremely accurate in detecting arterio-cavernosal fistulas, and color Doppler detects abnormal turbulent flow within the fistulous tract. This may be more challenging to detect in the immediate post-traumatic stage, but becomes more apparent with time.[25]

Arteriography

An arteriogram of the pudendal artery can reveal extravasation in the context of a cavernosal artery injury in patients with arterial priapism.[26,27] According to recent guidelines, arteriography should be reserved for patients deemed to be suitable for embolization, due to the invasive nature of the study.[3] Penile Doppler study (PDS) provides a useful means of follow-up for these patients in order to accurately assess the degree of resolution of the arterio-cavernosal fistula.[23]

Magnetic resonance imaging

MRI plays an important role in ischemic priapism. It provides key information regarding the extent of infarction in the corpora cavernosa. This may influence definitive management, specifically whether to proceed with a shunting procedure versus a primary prosthesis insertion.[28] In non-ischemic priapism, MRI can also be helpful in delineating fistulous tracts. Additionally MRI can also be used to identify rarer causes of priapism such as penile metastases and malignancies as well as partial cavernosal thrombosis.[29,30]

Kirkham et al.[30] describe a specific penile protocol for the investigation of priapism, which does not require cavernosal injection of pharmacostimulant. The penis is secured to the anterior abdominal wall and sections of 4 mm or less with high-resolution images are used with a small field of view. Intravenous contrast is essential to demonstrate areas of necrosis.[22]

Management of priapism

Management of non-ischemic priapism

There is less urgency required in treating non-ischemic priapism, as by definition there is no corporal ischemia. The priority initially is therefore to differentiate this condition from ischemic priapism; this is aided by a good clinical history and blood gas analysis followed by Doppler studies that show increased arterial blood flow to the penis. As the blood is well oxygenated, the risk of ischemic damage leading to corporal fibrosis and impotence is low.

Conservative treatment is usually attempted prior to proceeding with more invasive measures. These include applying ice to the perineum or, in the presence of a fistula at the base of the corpora, duplex ultrasound-guided compression can also be successful in reversing the high-flow priapism.[31] This can be especially successful in children.[32] Aspiration of blood from the corpora is not an option for treatment, and the use of an alpha-adrenergic antagonist is contraindicated in order to avoid systemic absorption.[3]

Selective arteriography combined with arterial embolization using an autologous clot,[33] gel foam, or permanent substances such as coils,[34] is the preferred treatment modality and success rates can be as high as 89%.[3,35] Recurrence rates of non-ischemic priapism following selective artery embolization are reported to vary from 7% to 27% in the literature.[36] In some cases a repeat procedure is required.

Surgical management of non-ischemic priapism should be reserved as a last resort in cases that are refractory to the above measures. The main surgical approach is open arterial ligation with or without intra-operative ultrasound imaging.[37] Overall, potency is reported to be preserved in 77–86% of patients with non-ischemic priapism.[38]

Management of ischemic priapism

In contrast to non-ischemic priapism, acute ischemic priapism should be addressed as a urological emergency. The aim of treatment is to restore penile flaccidity, treat pain, and prevent damage to the corpora cavernosa.[3]

Conservative treatment

Conservative measures can be performed soon after onset. These comprise ejaculation, the application of ice-packs to the perineum, and gentle exercise; these may work by inducing vasoconstriction.[4] However, it is vitally important that these attempts do not under any circumstance delay corporal aspiration in ischemic priapism lasting more than 4 hours.[19]

Some authors advocate that in cases of ischemic priapism, where there is a good history of recent pharmacotherapy (e.g., in the case of intracavernosal prostaglandin injection), direct injection of a sympathomimetic can be carried out without prior aspiration.[3]

Corporal aspiration

Aspiration of stagnant corporal blood is performed under local anesthesia, either with intracorporal access via the glans or with a percutaneous needle approaching from the lateral aspects of the proximal penile shaft. The blood usually appears deoxygenated and viscous.

Aspiration itself may resolve the problem by promoting the recovery of intracorporal blood circulation and reversing veno-occlusion. Reperfusion also allows penile detumescence and hence reduction of pain.[4,39]

Medical therapy

Sympathomimetic injection

Should aspiration fail to achieve detumescence, alpha-adrenergic agonists should be injected to induce contraction of the corpus cavernosum and the helicine arteries. This can be achieved using several sympathomimetic agents including phenylephrine, etilefrine, ephedrine, epinephrine, norepinephrine, and metaraminol.[40–46]

Phenylephrine is usually deemed to be the drug of choice given its high selectivity for the $\alpha 1$-adrenergic receptor. This avoids overstimulation of the cardiovascular system, specifically the β-mediated cardiac chronotropic and inotropic effects.[47]

Despite this, careful monitoring of the patient's blood pressure is required as the adrenergic effects of the drug on the systemic circulation can lead to systemic hypertension.[47] The desired result of sympathomimetic therapy is a reduced volume of stagnated blood and relief of pressure on the subtunical venules, ultimately leading to penile detumescence.

However, the cavernosal smooth muscle may still fail to contract due to the metabolic alteration in the immediate microenvironment of the corporal smooth muscle, resulting in refractory tumescence; therefore it has been advocated in certain circumstances to titrate up to higher doses.[42]

Other medical therapies

Alternative medical treatments such as methylene blue and etilefrine have been utilized in patients who fail to respond to these measures. Sickle-cell-associated priapism also requires a slightly different approach.

Methylene blue

Methylene blue is a compound, that has several biological effects. It is known to inhibit soluble guanylate cyclase (sGC), which leads to reduced levels of cGMP and increased smooth muscle tone in the corpora cavernosa.[48] The use of methylene blue has been limited to anecdotal reports and small series.[49–51]

Medical therapies specific to patients with sickle-cell disease

Etilefrine is an alpha-adrenergic agonist that can also be administered orally. It is more commonly utilized in sickle-cell patients, where there have been reports of successful treatment.[52]

Additional measures that may be required in patients with sickle-cell-related priapism include intravenous fluids and oxygen as well as the administration of intravenous bicarbonate.[15,53] Occasionally exchange blood transfusion may be advocated with the aim of increasing oxygen delivery to tissues.

Surgical management of ischemic priapism

Acute surgical intervention for ischemic priapism should be reserved for cases where conservative and medical treatments have failed. The aim of intervention is to divert ischemic corporal blood into the venous system by developing a new channel of blood flow.

According the International Society for Sexual Medicine (2009), shunting should be considered for priapism lasting 72 hours or longer.[19] Four main shunt procedures are described:

1 **Percutaneous distal corporoglandular shunts.** The Winter shunt and the Ebbehoj procedure are the simplest methods of creating a shunt between the corpus spongiosum and the corpus cavernosum. In the Ebbehoj technique, a narrow-blade scalpel is inserted into the glans lateral to the urethral meatus into the corpus cavernosum.[1] Multiple incisions are made through the same entry site by rotating the scalpel blade by 90°. The overlying glans is then closed using sutures. In contrast, Winter's procedure uses a Tru-cut biopsy needle to remove cores of tunica

albuginea and create fistulous communications between the corpus cavernosum and the corpus spongiosum.[1,3] Several attempts may be required before detumescence occurs.

2 **Open distal (also corporoglandular) shunts.** The Al-Ghorab procedure involves creating a shunt between the glans penis and the tip of the corpus cavernosum by excising a small amount of tunica albuginea.[1,3]

3 **Open proximal (corporospongiosal) shunts.** The Quackles procedure involves a unilateral corporotomy, which is anastomosed to the corpus spongiosump; this is performed by a perineal approach in the Quackles technique. The Sacher technique is a slightly modified version and involves a penoscrotal approach.[54]

4 **Vein anastomoses/shunts.** The Grayhack procedure involves creating a shunt between the corpus cavernosum and the long saphenous vein by tunneling the vein from the upper thigh to the proximal corpus cavernosum. In the Barry technique the corpora are shunted to the dorsal penile vein.[54]

T-shunt and tunneling procedure

For those patients with priapism lasting 1–3 days, a #10 blade-scalpel is initially positioned vertically and parallel to the urethral meatus over a marked glandular incision site, after infiltration with local anesthetic or under general anesthetic.[1]

The blade is advanced to penetrate the tip of the ipsilateral corpus cavernosum and the blade is then rotated 90° laterally away from the urethra and then withdrawn. Deoxygenated blood is then milked out through the incision and the site is then closed with sutures.[1,55]

A 15-minute grace period is given in order to ensure detumescence.[55] If the priapism does not resolve, the procedure is then repeated on the contralateral side.

In ischemic priapism lasting more than 3 days, the T-shunt procedure is performed; however, tunneling is also performed with an 8–10 Fr straight urethral sound or dilator inserted through the glans incision. This is inserted as far as the penile crura of the corpora cavernosa.

The wounds are then closed with 4-0 sutures. If rigidity returns, color duplex ultrasonography is used to assess blood flow within the cavernous arteries.[1,55]

Shunt selection and postoperative care

The type of shunt procedure is usually guided by surgeon preference and familiarity with different techniques. However, as a general rule, it is preferable to try distal techniques before proceeding to proximal techniques. With regard to outcomes, it appears that patients experiencing priapism that lasts longer than 24 hours appear to have impaired erectile tissue such that any shunt procedure after this may only serve to relieve pain but not preserve potency.[19,20]

After a shunting procedure it is important to apply intermittent compression to the penis to maintain the patency of the fistula, and repeat the corpus cavernosal blood gas analysis. Doppler ultrasound may need to be performed in the context of postoperative penile edema[6] in order to exclude recurrent priapism.

Primary penile prosthesis insertion

Intractable therapy-resistant acute ischemic priapism lasting more than 48 hours usually results in complete erectile dysfunction along with possible major penile deformity. In these cases, there is an argument for proceeding directly to immediate malleable penile prosthesis surgery in order to avoid the complications that may occur by delaying surgery.[56] Complications from penile prosthesis insertion include urethral injury, tunical erosions, infection, and/or penile shortening.[57–60] At this stage there is debate in the literature whether to proceed with prosthesis insertion or to carry out a T-shunt procedure.

Management of stuttering priapism

The primary goal in the management of patients with stuttering priapism is the prevention of further episodes. The treatment is primarily pharmacological, although each acute episode should be managed as per acute ischemic priapism.[3]

Unfortunately, it is still not clear from the literature how safe or effective these pharmacotherapies are in the context of treating stuttering priapism.[15,53,61]

Hormone treatment

Hormonal therapy in priapism aims to reduce circulating testosterone levels therefore leading to fewer penile erections.[2] The main class of drugs used in this category are gonadotropin-receptor hormone agonists or antagonists. The side effects typically comprise hot flushes, gynecomastia, impaired erectile function, loss of libido, and weakness.[3]

Anti-androgen therapy in the form of drugs such as bicalutamide and estrogen treatment may also be effective.[3] In addition, there is also some evidence that 5α-reductase inhibitors such as dutasteride and finasteride may potentially be beneficial.[62]

As hormonal treatments have a contraceptive effect, and interfere with normal sexual development, they should be used with caution in boys who have not reached sexual maturity and in men trying to achieve conception.

PDE5 inhibitors

Some studies have also found that there is a paradoxical effect following the long-term administration of a phosphodiesterase type 5 inhibitor (principally in patients with idiopathic and sickle-cell disease-associated priapism[16]). It can reduce the frequency of erections in these patients according to laboratory studies.[63,64]

Phosphodiesterase type 5 inhibitors act to enhance PDE5 function by increasing the concentration of cGMP in the smooth muscle in a nitric oxide dysfunctional state. It has been shown in some studies that although PDE5 inhibitors are usually used for treating erectile dysfunction, they can be paradoxically effective in treating stuttering priapism.[9,53] Treatment should only be started in the flaccid state and there may be a delay of 1 week before the treatment is effective.

Other pharmacological treatments

Digoxin

Studies with oral alpha-adrenergics have suggested that limited daily dosing with these agents can be effective in up to 72% of cases.[65,66] Digoxin regulates smooth muscle tone through a number of different pathways leading to penile detumescence.[16,56]

There is some evidence that digoxin can decrease sexual desire and excitement with a concomitant reduction in penile rigidity.[67] Typical side effects include decreased libido, anorexia, nausea, vomiting, confusion, blurred vision, headache, gynecomastia, rash, and arrhythmia.

Terbutaline

Terbutaline is a beta-agonist that causes vasodilation resulting in smooth muscle relaxation. It has only been shown to be effective in pharmacologically induced priapism.[3] Side effects include nervousness, shakiness, drowsiness, heart palpitations, headache, dizziness, hot flushes, and nausea.

Gabapentin

Gabapentin is an anticonvulsant, antinociceptive, and an anxiolytic. It can cause penile detumescence when given at the correct dose.[3] Its side effects include erectile dysfunction and anorgasmia.

Baclofen

Baclofen is a gamma-aminobutyric acid (GABA) derivative that can inhibit penile erection and ejaculation via inhibitory pathways. It is used to prevent prolonged erections resulting from neurological diseases can be more effectively dosed when delivered intrathecally.[68,69] The side effects may include drowsiness, confusion, dizziness, weakness, fatigue, headache, hypotension, and nausea.[68]

Hydroxyurea

Hydroxyurea is an established treatment for sickle-cell disease. For patients with sickle-cell disease and recurrent priapism there is some evidence that medical prophylaxis with hydroxyurea may be effective. However, the side effects include oligospermia and leg ulcers.[65]

Intracavernosal sympathomimetics

Intracavernosal self-injections of sympathomimetic drugs can also be considered for the treatment of acute episodes on an interim basis until ischemic priapism has been alleviated.[3]

Conclusions

Although low in incidence, priapism can be a challenging condition to treat. It is a urological emergency and should be assessed in an appropriately emergent fashion. The key is to differentiate between ischemic and non-ischemic priapism in order to organize treatment in a timely manner.

There is now a better understanding of the pathophysiology, diagnosis, and the medical, radiological, and surgical treatment options. However, further scientific progress needs to be made in order to achieve the goal of preventing physical injury to the penis and preserving sexual health.

References

1 Rees R, Summerton D, Christopher N, Ralph DJ. Surgical management of genitourethral emergencies. In: Muneer A, Arya M, Jordan GH (eds), *Atlas of Male Genitourethral Surgery: The Illustrated Guide*. Oxford: Wiley-Blackwell, 2014; pp. 181–95.

2 Hinman F. Priapism: report of cases in a clinical study of the literature with reference to its pathogenesis and surgical treatments. *Ann Surg* 1914;60:689.

3 Salonia A, Eardley I, Giuliano F, et al. European Association of Urology guidelines on priapism. *Eur Urol* 2014;65 (2):480–9.

4 Tay YK, Spernat D, Rzetelski-West K, et al. Acute management of priapism in men. *BJU Int* 2012;109:15.

5 Pryor P, Akkus E, Alter G, et al. Priapism. *J Sex Med* 2004;1:116–20.

6 Song PH, Moon KH. Priapism: current updates in clinical management. Korean J Urol 2013;54(12):816–23.

7 Montague DK, Jarow J, Broderick GA, et al. American Urological Association guideline on the management of priapism. *J Urol* 2003;170:1318–24.

8 Muneer A, Ralph DJ. Management of priapism. *European Genito-Urinary Disease* 2007;(1): 60–63

9 Berger R, Billups K, Brock G, et al. Report of the American Foundation for Urologic Disease (AFUD) Thought Leader Panel for evaluation and treatment of priapism. *Int J Impot Res* 2001;13 (Suppl. 5):S39–43.

10 Broderick GA, Harkaway R. Pharmacologic erection: time-dependent changes in the corporal environment. *Int J Impot Res* 1994;6(1):9–16.

11 Muneer A, Cellek S, Dogan A, et al. Investigation of cavernosal smooth muscle dysfunction in low-flow priapism using an *in vitro* model. *Int J Impot Res* 2005;17(1):10–18.

12 Spycher MA, Hauri D. The ultrastructure of the erectile tissue in priapism. *J Urol* 1986;135(1):142–7.

13 Kim JJ, Moon DG, Koh SK. The role of nitric oxide in in vivo feline erection under hypoxia. *Int J Impot Res* 1998;10(3):145–50.

14 Champion HC, Bivalacqua TJ, Takimoto E, et al. Phosphodiesterase-5A dysregulation in penile erectile tissue is a mechanism of priapism. *Proc Natl Acad Sci U S A* 2005;102:1661–6.

15 Levey HR, Kutlu O, Bivalacqua TJ. Medical management of ischemic stuttering priapism: a contemporary review of the literature. *Asian J Androl* 2012;14:156–63.

16 Adeyoju AB, Olujohungbe AB, Morris J, et al. Priapism in sickle-cell disease; incidence, risk factors and complications – an international multicentre study. *BJU Int* 2002;90:898–902.

17 Virag R, Bachir D, Lee K, Galacteros F. Preventive treatment of priapism in sickle cell disease with oral and self-administered intracavernous injection of etilefrine. *Urology* 1996;47:777–81; discussion 781.

18 Lin YH, Kim JJ, Stein NB, Khera M. Malignant priapism secondary to metastatic prostate cancer: a case report and review of literature. *Rev Urol* 2011;13:90–4.

19 Broderick GA, Kadioglu A, Bivalacqua TJ, Ghanem H, Nehra A, Shamloul R. Priapism: pathogenesis, epidemiology, and management. *J Sex Med* 2010;7:476–500.

20 Burnett AL, Bivalacqua TJ. Priapism: new concepts in medical and surgical management. *Urol Clin North Am* 2011;38:185–94.

21 Nolan VG, Wyszynski DF, Farrer LA, Steinberg MH. Hemolysis-associated priapism in sickle cell disease. *Blood* 2005;106:3264–7.

22 Halls JE, Patel DV, Walkden M, Patel U. Priapism: pathophysiology and the role of the radiologist. *Brit J Radiol* 2012;85 (Spec. issue 1):S79–S85. doi:10.1259/bjr/62360925.

23 Halls J, Bydawell G, Patel U. Erectile dysfunction: the role of penile Doppler ultrasound in diagnosis. *Abdom Imaging* 2009;34:712–25.

24 Wilkins CJ, Sriprasad S, Sidhu PS. Colour Doppler ultrasound of the penis. *Clin Radiol* 2003;58:514–23.

25 Bertolotto M, Quaia E, Mucelli FP, Ciampalini S, Forgács B, Gattuccio I. Color Doppler imaging of posttraumatic priapism before and after selective embolization. *Radiographics* 2003;23:495–503.

26 Kolbenstvedt A, Egge T, Schultz A. Arterial high flow priapism: role of radiology in diagnosis and treatment. *Scand J Urol Nephrol Suppl* 1996;179:143–6.

27 Kang BC, Lee DY, Byun JY, Baek SY, Lee SW, Kim KW. Posttraumatic arterial priapism: colour Doppler examination and superselective arterial embolization. *Clin Radiol* 1998;53:830–4.

28 Li CY, Agrawal V, Minhas S, Ralph DJ. The penile suspensory ligament: abnormalities and repair. *BJU Int* 2007;99:117–20.

29 Pretorius ES, Siegelman ES, Ramchandani P, Banner MP. MR imaging of the penis. *Radiographics* 2001;21:S283–98; discussion S298–9.

30 Kirkham AP, Illing RO, Minhas S, Minhas S, Allen C. MR imaging of nonmalignant penile lesions. *Radiographics* 2008;28:837–53.

31 Hakim LS, Kulaksizoglu H, Mulligan R, Greenfield A, Goldstein I. Evolving concepts in the diagnosis and treatment of arterial high flow priapism. *J Urol* 1996;155:541–8.

32 Corbetta JP, Duran V, Burek C, et al. High flow priapism: diagnosis and treatment in pediatric population. *Pediatr Surg Int* 2011;27:1217–21.

33 Numan F, Cantasdemir M, Ozbayrak M, et al. Posttraumatic non-ischemic priapism treated with autologous blood clot embolization. *J Sex Med* 2008;5:173–9.

34 Liu BX, Xin ZC, Zou YH, et al. High-flow priapism: superselective cavernous artery embolization with microcoils. *Urology* 2008;72:571–3; discussion 573–4.

35 Numan F, Cakirer S, Islak C, et al. Posttraumatic high-flow priapism treated by N-butyl-cyanoacrylate embolization. *Cardiovasc Intervent Radiol* 1996;19:278–80.

36 Savoca G, Pietropaolo F, Scieri F, Bertolotto M, Mucelli FP, Belgrano E. Sexual function after highly selective embolization of cavernous artery in patients with high flow priapism: long-term followup. *J Urol* 2004;172:644–7.
37 Brock G, Breza J, Lue TF, Tanagho EA, High-flow priapism: a spectrum of disease. *J Urol* 1993;150(3):968–71.
38 Bastuba MD, Saenz DT, Dinlenc CZ, et al. Arterial priapism: diagnosis, treatment and long-term follow-up. *J Urol* 1994;151(5):1231–7.
39 Ateyah A, Rahman El-Nashar A, Zohdy W, Arafa M, Saad El-Den H. Intracavernosal irrigation by cold saline as a simple method of treating iatrogenic prolonged erection. *J Sex Med* 2005;2:248–53.
40 Burnett AL, Sharlip ID. Standard operating procedures for priapism. *J Sex Med* 2013;10:180–94.
41 Munarriz R, Wen CC, McAuley I, Goldstein I, Traish A, Kim N. Management of ischemic priapism with high-dose intracavernosal phenylephrine: from bench to bedside. *J Sex Med* 2006;3:918–22.
42 Muneer A, Minhas S, Freeman A, Kumar P, Ralph DJ. Investigating the effects of high-dose phenylephrine in the management of prolonged ischaemic priapism. *J Sex Med* 2008;5:2152–9.
43 Davila HH, Parker J, Webster JC, Lockhart JL, Carrion RE. Subarachnoid hemorrhage as complication of phenylephrine injection for the treatment of ischemic priapism in a sickle cell disease patient. *J Sex Med* 2008;5:1025–8.
44 Muruve N, Hosking DH. Intracorporeal phenylephrine in the treatment of priapism. *J Urol* 1996;155:141–3.
45 Mantadakis E, Ewalt DH, Cavender JD, Rogers ZR, Buchanan GR. Outpatient penile aspiration and epinephrine irrigation for young patients with sickle cell anemia and prolonged priapism. *Blood* 2000;95:78–82.
46 Roberts JR, Price C, Mazzeo T. Intracavernous epinephrine: a minimally invasive treatment for priapism in the emergency department. *J Emerg Med* 2009;36:285–9.
47 Bochinski DJ, Deng DY, Lue TF. The treatment of priapism – when and how? *Int J Impot Res* 2003;15 (Suppl. 5):S86–90.
48 Trigo-Rocha F, Hsu GL, Donatucci CF, Lue TF. The role of cyclic adenosine monophosphate, cyclic guanosine monophosphate, endothelium and non-adrenergic, non-cholinergic neurotransmission in canine penile erection. *J Urol* 1993;149(4):872–7.
49 deHoll JD, Shin PA, Angle JF, Steers WD. Alternative approaches to the management of priapism. *Int J Impot Res* 1998;10(1):11–14.
50 Martinez PF, Hoang-Boehm J, Weiss J, et al. Methylene blue as a successful treatment alternative for pharmacologically-induced priapism. *Eur Urol* 2001;39(1):20–3.
51 Martinez Portillo FJ, Fernandez Arancibia MI, Bach S, et al. Methylene blue: an effective therapeutic alternative for priapism induced by intracavernous injection of vasoactive agents. *Arch Esp Urol* 2002;55(3):303–8.
52 Kheirandish P, Chinegwundoh F, Kulkarni S. Treating stuttering priapism, *BJU Int* 2011;108(7):1068–72.
53 Bivalacqua TJ, Musicki B, Kutlu O, Burnett AL. New insights into the pathophysiology of sickle cell disease-associated priapism. *J Sex Med* 2012;9:79–87.
54 Shindel AW, Garcia MM, Lue TF. Priapism made easy. International Society for Sexual Medicine. Available at: http://www.issm.info/news/review-reports/priapism-made-easy
55 Garcia MM, Shindel AW, Lue TF. T-shunt with or without tunnelling for prolonged ischaemic priapism. *BJU Int* 2008;102(11):1754–64.
56 Rees RW, Kalsi J, Minhas S, et al. The management of low-flow priapism with the immediate insertion of a penile prosthesis. *BJU Int* 2002;90(9):893–7.
57 Upadhyay J, Shekarriz B, Dhabuwala CB. Penile implant for intractable priapism associated with sickle cell disease. *Urology* 1998;51:638–9.
58 Ralph DJ, Garaffa G, Muneer A, et al. The immediate insertion of a penile prosthesis for acute ischaemic priapism. *Eur Urol* 2009;56:1033–8.
59 Salem EA, El Aasser O. Management of ischemic priapism by penile prosthesis insertion: prevention of distal erosion. *J Urol* 2010;183:2300–3.
60 Sedigh O, Rolle L, Negro CL, et al. Early insertion of inflatable prosthesis for intractable ischemic priapism: our experience and review of the literature. *Int J Impot Res* 2011;23:158–64.
61 Morrison BF, Burnett AL. Stuttering priapism: insights into pathogenesis and management. *Curr Urol Rep* 2012;13:268–76.
62 Rachid-Filho D, Cavalcanti AG, Favorito LA, Costa WS, Sampaio FJ. Treatment of recurrent priapism in sickle cell anemia with finasteride: a new approach. *Urology* 2009; 74:1054–7.
63 Bivalacqua TJ, Musicki B, Hsu LL, Gladwin MT, Burnett AL, Champion HC. Establishment of a transgenic sickle-cell mouse model to study the pathophysiology of priapism. *J Sex Med* 2009;6:2494–504.
64 Burnett AL, Bivalacqua TJ, Champion HC, Musicki B. Feasibility of the use of phosphodiesterase type 5 inhibitors in a pharmacologic prevention program for recurrent priapism. *J Sex Med* 2006;3:1077–84.
65 Vaidyanathan S, Watt JW, Singh G, et al. Management of recurrent priapism in a cervical spinal cord injury patient with oral baclofen therapy. *Spinal Cord* 2004;42:134–5.
66 D'Aleo G, Rifici C, Kofler M, Saltuari L, Bramanti P. Favorable response to intrathecal, but not oral, baclofen of priapism in a patient with spinal cord injury. *Spine (Phila Pa 1976)* 2009;34:E127–9.
67 Bartolucci P, Galacteros F. Clinical management of adult sickle-cell disease. *Curr Opin Hematol* 2012;19:149–55.
68 D'Aleo G, Rifici C, Kofler M, et al.: Favorable response to intrathecal, but not oral, baclofen of priapism in a patient with spinal cord injury. Spine (Phila PA 1976) 2009, 34:E127–E129.

CHAPTER 21

Management of erectile dysfunction after pelvic surgery

Kelly A. Chiles[1] and John P. Mulhall[2]

[1] George Washington University, Washington, DC, USA

[2] Memorial Sloan Kettering Cancer Center, New York, NY, USA

Introduction

The most extensive studies examining erectile dysfunction (ED) after radical pelvic surgery are those documenting outcomes after radical prostatectomy (RP). It is likely, however, that these results are generally applicable to any surgery within the pelvis. Cystoprostatectomy, lower rectal surgery, and pelvic exenteration are all associated with the development of ED in addition to RP.

ED rates as high as 90% have been reported after RP, although there is a remarkably wide range of reported ED outcomes. This unfortunately is the direct result of variability in the study structures and definition of ED applied, and leads to unrealistic patient expectations postoperatively.[1,2] Importantly, patients should be educated regarding the chance that they will return to their baseline rigidity. Nelson et al. demonstrated that only 43% of men who underwent RP will return to their preoperative degree of rigidity, and this included men who were taking phosphodiesterase-5 inhibitors (PDE5i) in order to achieve that erectile function (EF).[3] Only 22% of men who did not require PDE5i preoperatively will not require PDE5i postoperatively in order to achieve their baseline EF, and only 4% of men over the age of 60 years will not require erectile aids after surgery to return to their baseline.

Furthermore, there is no evidence that "minimally invasive surgery" provides any benefit over open surgery regarding ED outcomes. There are no randomized trials comparing robotic versus open surgical RP that demonstrate greater efficacy of one approach over the other with regards to preservation of EF. Retrospective chart reviews and prospective non-randomized studies do not allow comparative conclusions regarding EF outcomes because of the significant inherent selection bias.[4,5]

Mechanisms of erectile dysfunction

Neurogenic ED

Appreciation of pelvic anatomy and the autonomic nervous system that innervates the penis allows an understanding of how any pelvic surgery, and not just RP, can cause neurogenic sexual dysfunction. Damage to the parasympathetic nerves at any point along their path from spinal cord (S2-4) to penis will decrease erectile function; injury to sympathetic nerves results in ejaculatory dysfunction. Parasympathetic nerves arise from S2-4 (pelvic splanchnic nerves) and converge upon the inferior hypogastric plexus located along the sides of the rectum in men. The sympathetic nerves arise from T12-L2 and join the superior hypogastric plexus found anterior to the aortic bifurcation. Upon exit from the plexus they are known as the hypogastric nerves, and they travel along the internal iliac arteries to join the inferior hypogastric plexus. Intertwined parasympathetic and sympathetic nerves exiting this plexus are known as the cavernous nerves (CN). The CN can be found running between the prostatic fascia and levator fascia, which surrounds the

Male Sexual Dysfunction: A Clinical Guide, First Edition. Edited by Suks Minhas and John Mulhall.

prostate, before diving underneath the pubic bone to innervate the penis.

Nerve damage can occur not only as a result of direct transection, but also as a result of thermal, ischemic, and traction injury.[6] The timing of nerve injury is also not isolated just to the time of surgery. Neuropraxia and Wallerian degeneration are clearly evidenced not only by the immediate degeneration of EF in the majority of men after pelvic surgery, but also by a second precipitous decline in EF that is not apparent until weeks or months immediately following surgery. Katz et al. demonstrated that 16% of men had functional erections 3 months after RP.[7] At 3–6 months, however, 20% of the same men who had functional erections immediately post-RP had a decline in EF. Ninety-one percent of this group went on to regain functional erections at 1 year, demonstrating that nerve injury and recovery extends well beyond the confines of the operating room. Importantly, even temporary damage to nerves results in increasing irreversible damage to the erectile tissue that, eventually, no degree of nerve regeneration can overcome.

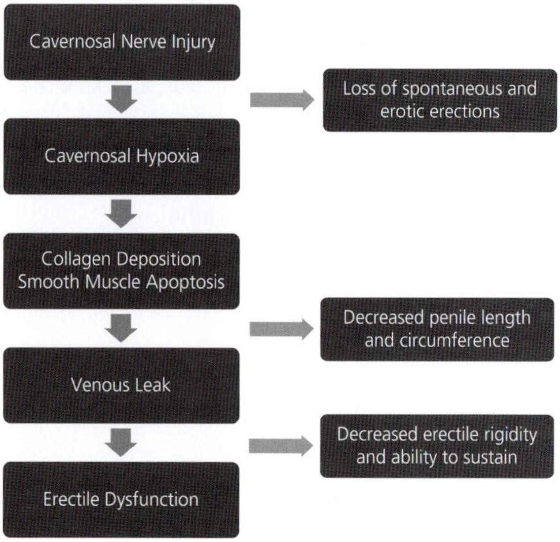

Figure 21.1 Pathophysiology of erectile dysfunction (ED) after pelvic surgery.

Vasculogenic ED

Damage to the erectile tissue ultimately causes corporal veno-occlusive dysfunction (CVOD), also known as venous leak.[6] Almost immediately postoperatively there is a total absence of nocturnal and erotic erections because of cavernosal nerve injury. Even when bilateral nerve-sparing surgery is successful macroscopically, there is an initial neuropraxia that results from any manipulation of the nerve bundles. During this time, no matter how temporary, there a loss of erections ensues. Absence of erections decreases cavernosal oxygenation and in turns promotes smooth muscle apoptosis, and these changes have been demonstrated within weeks after cavernosal injury.[8,9] In addition to the release of proapoptotic factors such as transforming growth factor-β1 (TGF-β1), collagen deposition is increased and fibrosis ensues.[6] Penile rigidity and ability to sustain an erection are largely linked to the ability of healthy tissue to expand and compress the emissary veins that run beneath Buck's fascia. As fibrosis increases, the erectile bodies no longer expand and compress these veins, so they continue to drain the corporal bodies. The resulting decrease in erectile tissue dispensability ultimately leads to CVOD and ED (Figure 21.1).

Vascular dysfunction can also result from cavernosal artery insufficiency (CAI). Damage to the arteries that feed the corpora cavernosa can result in ED. For example, Leriche syndrome – occlusion of the aorta as it bifurcates into the common iliac arteries – presents with ED in addition to gluteal claudication and absent femoral pulses. Arterial inflow to the penis continues from the internal iliac arteries to the internal pudendal arteries, and subsequently to the common penile arteries. Accessory pudendal arteries (APAs) may stem from the external iliac, obturator, vesical, and femoral arteries, and may also provide important inflow to the penis. The contribution of APAs to erection is controversial because although there are studies that demonstrate a significant prevalence of APAs in a large portion of men, very few studies have investigated the functional and clinically relevant role of APAs in EF recovery of men after pelvic surgery.[10] Doppler duplex ultrasound evaluation of accessory pudendal arteries demonstrates hemodynamic changes similar to the changes that the cavernosal arteries undergo during erection.[11] If possible, therefore, preservation of APAs during surgery should be attempted because of the possibility that they may help aid EF recovery after pelvic surgery.[12]

Treatment of erectile dysfunction

It is important to appreciate issues that confound the interpretation of ED treatment success after surgery. Of importance is how studies define their EF outcome. The gold standard study should use a validated assessment of EF both before and serially after surgery for a minimum of 24 months postoperatively, as well as a clear assessment of EF with and without erectile aids post-surgery. There must be an adequate control (baseline function prior to surgery is best), and the means of assessment should be as objective as possible. The further a study strays from appropriate control and objective outcomes, the more likely bias is introduced and the results unreliable. Unfortunately, all too often the published literature relies on patient recall and subjective determination of erectile function as an outcome, and these results must thus be interpreted cautiously. Another concern is patient selection, with only select patients (often younger patients with better preoperative function and excellent nerve-sparing surgery) being included in such an analysis. Further confounding the issue is the inclusion of penile rehabilitation (PR) strategies within the literature. Obviously PR warrants vigorous investigation because of the potential to alleviate significant surgical morbidity, but PR trials are by their very nature NOT designed to evaluate the efficacy of isolated as-needed erectile aid usage after surgery.

Oral therapy

Mechanism of action

Phosphodiesterase type 5 inhibitors (PDE5i) are considered first-line medical therapy for ED of any etiology because they are oral medications that are widely available and can be highly efficacious. Response to PDE5i after pelvic surgery is tightly linked to the degree of cavernosal (parasympathetic) nerve injury. One of the first steps in an erection is parasympathetic nerve nitric oxide release (nitrergic response); this, in turn, causes an increase in cGMP through the action of guanylate cyclase. PDE5i function by preventing the breakdown of cGMP to 3′5′-cGMP, which occurs through the enzymatic action of PDE5 enzymes. Onset of erection occurs when enough cGMP has accumulated to trigger smooth muscle relaxation and tumescence. When significant nerve injury has occurred, such as in the case of non-nerve-sparing RP, PDE5i efficacy is greatly diminished because the initial event (NO release from cavernosal nerves) that launches the signaling cascade is severely compromised (Table 21.1).

Outcomes

Because the degree of efficacy of PDE5i is directly linked to the degree of nerve preservation after pelvic surgery as well as the baseline EF of the patient, it is difficult to generalize the response rates of on-demand PDE5i. Men who have undergone an excellent nerve-sparing RP can expect response rates to PDE5i that are better than those who have experienced significant nerve trauma, assuming equivalent baseline EF. Raina et al. demonstrated a 71% response rate to sildenafil at 3 years after RP.[13] Importantly, 13% of men at one institution whom surgeons had deemed to have undergone complete non-nerve-sparing RP had EF recovery, underscoring our inability to accurately determine nerve injury in the operating room and predict nerve regeneration.[14] All men, therefore, should undertake a PDE5i challenge to assess their response regardless of their documented nerve status.[15]

Even accounting for different pharmacokinetic profiles such as onset and duration of action, there is little reason to suspect that any one PDE5i family member will be significantly more clinically effective than others in any given patient, and there are no well-designed head-to-head trials that support superiority. A recent systematic review demonstrated that all members of the

Table 21.1 Pharmacokinetics of phosphodiesterase type 5 inhibitors (PDE5i).

PDE5i	Dosing (mg)	Plasma 1/2 life (hours)	Time to max. efficacy (hours)	Duration of efficacy (hours)	Optimize efficacy
Sildenafil	25, 50, 100	4	1	8	Absorption reduced by fatty food
Tadalafil	2.5, 5, 10, 20	17.5	2	24	Fatty foods do not alter absorption
Vardenafil	2.5, 5, 10, 20	4	1	8	Absorption reduced by fatty food
Avanafil	50, 100, 200	5	0.5	8	Absorption may be affected by fatty food

PDE5i family have demonstrable improvement over placebo with regards to erectile function.[16] Patients can tailor their choice of PDE5i according to the frequency of sexual activity and degree of spontaneity they desire, as well as the side effect profile they experience.

Intracavernosal injection (ICI)

Mechanism of action

The primary goal of ICI is to achieve an erection sufficient for sexual relations that does not last for more than 1 hour. Any combination of different concentrations of prostaglandin E_1, papaverine, and/or phentolamine can be ordered from a compounding pharmacy so there is no gold standard of ICI dose or concentration. Prostaglandin E_1 functions to increase the conversion of ATP to cAMP, while papaverine is a non-specific PDE inhibitor that increases the concentration of cGMP. The accumulation of both of these metabolites decreases intracellular calcium, which causes smooth muscle relaxation and subsequent erection. Phentolamine inhibits the sympathetic response at the alpha-1 receptor level, which also serves to promote smooth muscle relaxation (Table 21.2).

Outcomes

ICI is a second-line therapy for ED only because of the notable anxiety related to injecting the penis with a needle. The remarkable efficacy of ICI in men who have failed PDE5i suggests that ICI is likely the most effective medical approach for treating ED despite its relegation to salvage therapy. All of the published ICI studies only examine efficacy in men who have failed PDE5i or who are also involved in penile rehabilitation trials, so the actual primary response rate can only be estimated. Further complicating the outcome data is the use of various combinations of intracavernosal reagents and a wide range of doses. Coombs et al. reviewed outcomes of an intracavernosal injection therapy program at Memorial Sloan Kettering Cancer Center and demonstrated a robust response to ICI.[17] The vast majority of men used a combination of 30 mg/mL papaverine, 10 μg/mL prostaglandin-E_1, and 1 mg/mL phentolamine and had failed PDE5i. Of the 1412 patients included, 89% reported achieving erections that were sufficient for intercourse; however, this outcome includes not only men who underwent pelvic surgery, but also men who underwent radiation treatment or who had organic ED from vascular disease such as diabetes. Of note, men who experience pain beyond what would normally be expected from a needlestick are likely experiencing it because of the addition of prostaglandin E_1 to their drug formula (PGE_1 hypersensitivity); prostaglandin E_1 should be eliminated in these men and replaced with a bimixture of papaverine and phentolamine.

Intraurethral suppository (IUS)

Prostaglandin E_1 can be used as an IUS that is absorbed across the urethral mucosa and is active within the corporal bodies. While a medication that is inserted into the urethral meatus appears to be more appealing to patients than a medication that requires a penile injection, there may be significant pain accompanying IU suppositories directly associated with degree of nerve injury to the neurovascular bundle (NVB) (another example of PGE_1 hypersensitivity). In fact, the attrition rate secondary to this pain is quite high. In addition, unfortunately IUS effectiveness is inconsistent. Of the 40% of men post-RP who do respond to this medication, IUS will fail to consistently achieve quality erections up to 50% of the times it is used.[18]

Vacuum erection device (VED)

VEDs rely on negative pressure pulling venous blood into the corpora cavernosa and superficial veins, and utilize a constriction band at the base of the penis to prevent venous leakage. This mechanism of action, however, results in a cold penis which is often considered unsightly because of the engorged veins which occur. In addition, the glans has no means of tumescence, so the VED has not become overwhelmingly popular as a monotherapy despite being inexpensive and relatively effective. There has been improvement in patient satisfaction when VED has been used in combination with another erectogenic aid. In conjunction with PDE5i, VEDs increased the number of patients with penetration-rigid erections to over 90% compared to 57% on PDE5i alone.[19]

Penile implant

Surgical considerations

Surgical placement of a penile implant (PI) is the final solution in the pathway of managing organic erectile dysfunction that is non-responsive to medical treatment. An important step prior to surgery is the performance of a penile doppler ultrasound (DUS). There is a significant prevalence of psychogenic ED in men who may initially appear to have factors for vascular ED, such as a history

Table 21.2 Characteristics of erectile aids.

Erectile aid	Mechanism of action	Contraindications/precautions	Adverse events	Miscellaneous
PDE5i	Prevents degradation of cGMP, which increases cavernosal smooth muscle relaxation	All PDEi: hypersensitivity to medication, using nitrate/nitrite-containing drugs, retinitis pigmentosa, macular degeneration or sudden vision loss. Vardenafil should not be taken by men with prolonged QT intervals	Headache, facial flushing, chromatopsia, dyspepsia, back pain, myalgia, dizziness, rhinitis	Patients should be stable on any alpha-blocker prior to initiating PDE5i at the lowest dose to decrease risk of hypotension
Vacuum erection device	Negative pressure pulls venous blood into the corpora cavernosa and superficial veins and a constriction band at the base of the penis maintains penile turgor	Should not be used in men on anticoagulants or men with decreased penile sensation	Discomfort from constriction band	Cyanotic penis with engorged superficial veins can result in cold, cosmetically undesirable penis
Prostaglandin E_1 urethral suppository	Stimulates adenylate cyclase, which increases cAMP and promotes smooth muscle relaxation	Hypersensitivity to medication	Penile pain, urethral bleeding, priapism	Can use up to 3 times a week; up to 50% of men who initially respond have inconsistent subsequent erections
Intracavernosal injection (ICI)	Prevents degradation of cGMP and/or increase in cAMP, which increases cavernosal smooth muscle relaxation and/or inhibits sympathetic-mediated vasoconstriction	Hypersensitivity to medication or use of monoamine oxidase inhibitors	Ecchymosis or pain at injection site, priapism	Can use up to 3 times a week

of pelvic surgery. There is no role for PI placement in men who have normal peak- and end-diastolic velocities on duplex Doppler ultrasound, as they are better served by optimizing their erectile aid usage in order to restore confidence in their erections.

After verification that the patient has organic ED, there are several important considerations. Multiple aspects of this procedure are unique to men who have undergone or will undergo pelvic surgery. For men who have severe ED who are not responsive to maximal medical therapy and who are about to undergo RP, for example, there are case reports of surgeons staging the PI placement by first placing the reservoir, with or without the pump, during the RP.[20] This serves to circumvent a blind reservoir placement in the space of Retzius at a later date, and the patient is aware that the plan is to place the remaining components, the corporal cylinders and pump, at a subsequent surgery. This option, however, is wrought with significant issues. The risk of infection of the reservoir in light of its possible exposure to urine or bowel contents during the pelvic surgery is hypothetically much greater than if placed at a later time. In addition, placing the tubing intrascrotally so that it can be easily accessed and utilized at a later date is challenging if the RP is performed via a minimally invasive approach and the pump is not placed along with the reservoir. Because the increasing popularity of ectopic reservoir placement precludes the need to always position a reservoir in the space of Retzius, there appears to be little advantage to simultaneous pelvic surgery and reservoir placement.

Another unique situation to consider is to have a three-piece inflatable implant already in place prior to pelvic surgery. In this instance, significant care must be taken to not only avoid disruption of the device itself, for example by rupture of the reservoir or tubing found in the pelvis, but also to avoid any contamination of the device.[21] No validated preoperative antibiotic regimen has been shown to decrease secondary prosthetic infection during pelvic surgery; however, the patient would likely benefit from preoperative antibiotics similar to what is chosen during an initial prosthesis implantation to cover for skin, urine, and enteric flora.

Post-pelvic surgery three-piece inflatable PI placement should be thoughtfully planned with careful consideration given to reservoir placement. As mentioned previously, classical placement of the reservoir in the space of Retzius can become complicated due to obliteration of this space or by disruption of the peritoneum associated with some surgeries, such as cystoprostatectomy or robotic-assisted RP.[22] These scenarios increase the opportunity for erroneous intra-abdominal placement of the reservoir, predisposing to adherence to and erosion of small bowel loops or a conduit that has dropped into the pelvis.[23]. Preoperative imaging of the pelvis can be considered to visualize anatomical relationships if the reservoir must be placed in the space of Retzius. Ectopic placement refers to positioning the reservoir anterior to the transversalis fascia.[24,25] The advent of low-profile reservoirs has diminished, but not eliminated, palpable or visible reservoirs in this new location. This possibility is increased in very thin men, and it is important to have a discussion preoperatively regarding this outcome in order to appropriately manage patient expectations.[26]

Outcomes

Patient satisfaction after placement of a PI generally ranges from 75 to 90% as long as recipients have been appropriately selected.[27,28] The optimal patient has clearly exhausted their medical options for return of erections, and also has realistic expectations regarding the procedure.[29] Complications specific to implant placement include the risk of urethral or corporal perforation (up to 11%).[30] As mentioned above, men who have had peritoneal disruption are not only at increased risk of intra-operative complications, but also run the risk of delayed injury to adjacent structures secondary to erosion. In addition, the risks of infection and device failure need to be clearly articulated. The risk of infection for an initial implant is expected to be about 1–3% for experienced surgeons; however, the risk of infection increases for any subsequent implant surgery regardless of reason. The most recent iterations of implants have proven to be more functionally reliable, but the risk of mechanical failure of the device is as high as 43% 15 years after implant.[28]

Conclusion

Management of realistic patient expectations regarding ED after pelvic surgery is paramount to ensuring patient satisfaction. All surgeries within the pelvis have the potential to cause ED, and patients need to be informed of the risk of ED following surgery as a mandatory component of the informed consent process. There is a multitude of treatment options that patients should try before resorting to the more invasive insertion of a penile implant.

References

1 Tal R, Alphs HH, Krebs P, Nelson CJ, Mulhall JP. Erectile function recovery rate after radical prostatectomy: a meta-analysis. *J Sex Med* 2009;6:2538–46.

2 Mulhall JP. Defining and reporting erectile function outcomes after radical prostatectomy: challenges and misconceptions. *J Urol* 2009;181:462–71.

3 Nelson CJ, Scardino PT, Eastham JA, Mulhall JP. Back to baseline: erectile function recovery after radical prostatectomy from the patients' perspective. *J Sex Med* 2013;10:1636–43.

4 Majd P, Ahmad W, Luebke T, Gawenda M, Brunkwall J. Impairment of erectile function after elective repair of abdominal aortic aneurysm. *Vascular* 2016;24:37–43.

5 Kalteis M, Gangl O, Huber F, Adelsgruber P, Kastner M, Lugmayr H. Clinical impact of hypogastric artery occlusion in endovascular aneurysm repair. *Vascular* 2015;23:575–9.

6 Mazzola C, Mulhall JP. Penile rehabilitation after prostate cancer treatment: outcomes and practical algorithm. *Urol Clin North Am* 2011;38:105–18.

7 Katz D, Bennett NE, Stasi J, et al. Chronology of erectile function in patients with early functional erections following radical prostatectomy. *J Sex Med* 2010;7:803–9.

8 Iacono F, Giannella R, Somma P, Manno G, Fusco F, Mirone V. Histological alterations in cavernous tissue after radical prostatectomy. *J Urol* 2005;173:1673–6.

9 Mulhall JP, Muller A, Donohue JF, et al. The functional and structural consequences of cavernous nerve injury are ameliorated by sildenafil citrate. *J Sex Med* 2008;5:1126–36.

10 Secin FP, Karanikolas N, Kuroiwa K, Vickers A, Touijer K, Guillonneau B. Positive surgical margins and accessory pudendal artery preservation during laparoscopic radical prostatectomy. *Eur Urol* 2005;48:786–92; discussion 93.

11 Droupy S, Benoit G, Giuliano F, Jardin A. Penile arteries in humans. Origin – distribution – variations. *Surg Radiol Anat* 1997;19:161–7.

12 Mulhall JP, Secin FP, Guillonneau B. Artery sparing radical prostatectomy – myth or reality? *J Urol* 2008;179: 827–31.

13 Raina R, Lakin MM, Agarwal A, et al. Long-term effect of sildenafil citrate on erectile dysfunction after radical prostatectomy: 3-year follow-up. *Urology* 2003;62:110–5.

14 Krishnan R, Katz D, Nelson CJ, Mulhall JP. Erectile function recovery in patients after non-nerve sparing radical prostatectomy. *Andrology* 2014;2:951–4.

15 Montorsi F, McCullough A. Efficacy of sildenafil citrate in men with erectile dysfunction following radical prostatectomy: a systematic review of clinical data. *J Sex Med* 2005;2:658–67.

16 Cui Y, Liu X, Shi L, Gao Z. Efficacy and safety of phosphodiesterase type 5 (PDE5) inhibitors in treating erectile dysfunction after bilateral nerve-sparing radical prostatectomy. *Andrologia* 2016;48:20–8.

17 Coombs PG, Heck M, Guhring P, Narus J, Mulhall JP. A review of outcomes of an intracavernosal injection therapy programme. *BJU Int* 2012;110:1787–91.

18 Costabile RA, Spevak M, Fishman IJ, et al. Efficacy and safety of transurethral alprostadil in patients with erectile dysfunction following radical prostatectomy. *J Urol* 1998; 160:1325–8.

19 Baniel J, Israilov S, Segenreich E, Livne PM. Comparative evaluation of treatments for erectile dysfunction in patients with prostate cancer after radical retropubic prostatectomy. *BJU Int* 2001;88:58–62.

20 Boyd SD. Two-stage technique for implantation of inflatable penile prosthesis in pelvic cancer surgery. *Urology* 1988; 32:1–5.

21 Tiguert R, Hurley PM, Gheiler EL, et al. Treatment outcome after radical prostatectomy is not adversely affected by a pre-existing penile prosthesis. *Urology* 1998;52:1030–3.

22 Sadeghi-Nejad H, Munarriz R, Shah N. Intra-abdominal reservoir placement during penile prosthesis surgery in post-robotically assisted laparoscopic radical prostatectomy patients: a case report and practical considerations. *J Sex Med* 2011;8:1547–50.

23 Tran CN, Boncher N, Montague DK, Angermeier KW. Erosion of inflatable penile prosthesis reservoir into neobladder. *J Sex Med* 2013;10:2343–6.

24 Perito PE, Wilson SK. Traditional (retroperitoneal) and abdominal wall (ectopic) reservoir placement. *J Sex Med* 2011;8:656–9.

25 Perito PE. Ectopic reservoir placement – no longer in the space of Retzius. *J Sex Med* 2011;8:2395–8.

26 Stember DS, Garber BB, Perito PE. Outcomes of abdominal wall reservoir placement in inflatable penile prosthesis implantation: a safe and efficacious alternative to the space of Retzius. *J Sex Med* 2014;11:605–12.

27 Trost LW, Baum N, Hellstrom WJ. Managing the difficult penile prosthesis patient. *J Sex Med* 2013;10:893–906; quiz 7.

28 Trost LW, McCaslin R, Linder B, Hellstrom WJ. Long-term outcomes of penile prostheses for the treatment of erectile dysfunction. *Expert Rev Med Devic* 2013;10:353–66.

29 Mulcahy JJ, Kramer A, Brant WO, et al. Current management of penile implant infections, device reliability, and optimizing cosmetic outcome. *Curr Urol Rep* 2014;15:413.

30 Sadeghi-Nejad H. Penile prosthesis surgery: a review of prosthetic devices and associated complications. *J Sex Med* 2007;4:296–309.

CHAPTER 22

Management of erectile dysfunction in men with diabetes

Marc Lucky[1], Suks Minhas[2], and Jas Kalsi[3]
[1] Aintree University Hospital, Liverpool, UK
[2] University College Hospital, London, UK
[3] Frimley Health NHS Foundation Trust and Imperial College Healthcare, London, UK

Introduction

Erectile dysfunction (ED) in men with diabetes mellitus is common, with a reported prevalence varying from 35% to 90%.[1] It can have a profound effect on quality of life including erectile function. Diabetes affects 246 million people worldwide, and this figure is expected to rise to 380 million by 2025, with the largest increase in incidence in developing countries.[2] The majority of men with diabetes will suffer with some degree of ED over their lifetime and this occurs more frequently compared to men without diabetes.[3] Erectile dysfunction occurs in a large proportion of both type 1 and type 2 diabetic men.[4] ED can be the initial presentation in 12% of patients subsequently diagnosed with diabetes.[5]

ED is a common issue that can cause significnt patient distress. It should be addressed early in diabetic men so that preventative strategies and early treatments can be instigated. Men who are diabetic are thought to develop ED 10–15 years earlier than men who do not have diabetes. In diabetic men over the age of 50 years, increasing duration of diabetes is associated positively with increased risk of ED.[6] The prevalence of ED in diabetic men aged 30–34 years is thought to be as high as 15%, increasing to 55% by the age of 60 years.[7] The Massachusetts Male Aging Study noted that diabetics have a three-fold increased incidence of ED as compared with non-diabetics.[8]

Advancing age, duration of diabetes, poor glycemic control, hypertension, hyperlipidemia, a sedentary lifestyle, smoking, and presence of other diabetic complications have been shown to be associated with diabetic-induced ED. In men with diabetes ED has also been shown to be associated with premature ejaculation and reduced libido.[9] The Olmstead County study showed that diabetes was associated with diminished sexual drive, ejaculatory function, and sexual satisfaction.[10] This is important to consider on initial assessment and should be addressed appropriately. Men with diabetes tend to develop ED at an earlier age and with a significantly higher prevalence, up to 75%.[11] The prevalence of men with ED and concomitant diabetes mellitus will continue to increase with time.[12]

Pathophysiology

Type 1 diabetes occurs when the body is unable to produce adequate amounts of insulin, and the affected individual therefore requires insulin replacement therapy. It is characterized by loss of the insulin-producing beta cells of the islets of Langerhans in the pancreas, leading to insulin deficiency.[13] The majority of type 1 diabetes is of an immune-mediated nature, in which beta cell loss occurs as a result of T-cell-mediated autoimmune attack.[14] Type 2 diabetes occurs when the cells of the body are unable to use insulin properly; it is sometimes referred to as non-insulin-dependent diabetes mellitus, and may have its onset in adulthood. The main problem is that of reduced insulin sensitivity. This can be treated with lifestyle modifications in mild cases and with medications that increase insulin sensitivity in more severe forms.[15]

Male Sexual Dysfunction: A Clinical Guide, First Edition. Edited by Suks Minhas and John Mulhall.

The classic signs and symptoms of diabetes develop more slowly in type 2 diabetes, and this is important as they can be easily missed resulting in the disease going undetected for some time. This may explain the fact that the prevalence of ED is higher in men with type 2 diabetes compared with men with type 1.[4] This has significant consequences as undetected and untreated disease can result in irreversible damage to the body, making it more difficult to treat ED when it arises. Untreated diabetes can affect the majority of body systems, with the cardiovascular system and kidneys being particularly affected. Diabetes doubles the risk of cardiovascular disease.[16] Early adequate treatment of this condition is essential in order to prevent progressive morbidity including ED.

The pathophysiology of ED in diabetes is complex and different to non-diabetic ED. It is multifactorial, involving endothelial and neuronal dysfunction, and is more severe and more resistant to treatment compared with non-diabetic ED.[1] There are many proposed mechanisms of ED in diabetics, which include:[17–22]

- elevated advanced glycation end-products;
- increased levels of oxygen free radicals;
- impaired nitric oxide (NO) synthesis;
- decreased and impaired cyclic guanosine monophosphate (cGMP) dependent kinase-1 (PKG-1);
- increased endothelin B receptor binding sites;
- ultrastructural changes;
- upregulated RhoA/Rho kinase pathway; and
- NO-dependent selective nitrergic nerve degeneration.

These mechanisms may interact with one another, further compounding the negative effects on erectile function. Studies have shown impaired smooth muscle relaxation in the corpus cavernosum and ED in diabetic rat penises.[18,23]

Diabetes affects the arterial blood vessels as a result of the development of atherosclerosis, and damages the capillaries supplying the penis causing microangiopathy.[24] This results in reduced blood flow to the penis during the tumescent phase resulting in decreased erection quality. Diabetes has also been shown to impair neurogenic and endothelium-mediated relaxation of penile smooth muscle.[25] This further affects erection quality as smooth muscle relaxation is a vital component of the erection mechanism. Diabetic neuropathy also significantly contributes to ED and has been shown to be one of the major factors in its pathogenesis.[26]

All of these pathogenic processes combined result in a significant detrimental effect on erectile function in diabetic patients, which can be difficult to treat and may be resistant to initial therapy.

Assessment and investigation

Diabetic patients with ED can be challenging to treat. A full medical history is necessary in the assesssment and treatment of ED in this group. Good glycemic control is essential in order to limit further damage and has been shown to correlate with ED.[27] This can be assessed by checking the serum HbA1c, which is a marker of good diabetic control.[28] Lifestyle factors such as diet, exercise, weight, smoking, and alcohol need to be discussed and counseled appropriately. Patient education plays an important role here and is vital for success of treatment.

Hormonal causes can be assessed by performing early morning determinations of serum testosterone, follicle-stimulating hormone, and luteinizing hormone levels to investigate problems with the hormonal axis. Screening for hypercholesterolemia and hypertension should be carried out if not already done. If present these need to be addressed and treated appropriately in order to halt progression and further damage. To treat these comorbidities consideration should be given to choosing the medication with the least adverse impact on erectile function. Baseline renal function and full blood count should also be carried out.

Examination of the patient is important, especially taking note of body habitus, waist circumference, and body mass index. These can be useful indicators of lifestyle, and can be used for assessing progress during follow-up of patients. Blood pressure measurement is important in order to investigate coexisting hypertension or ischemic heart disease. Neurological assessment and examination of external genitalia are also important .

Baseline erectile function should be assessed using the International Index of Erectile Function (IIEF) 5 validated assessment tool (Figure 22.1).[29] This is important as it can be used to quantify the severity of ED in order to help to direct treatment appropriately. It can also be used to objectively measure any response to treatment. It is important to enquire at initial assessment about any other associated conditions such as retrograde ejaculation or premature ejaculation, as these have been shown to be associsted with diabetes.[9,30] If these

Over the past 6 months:					
1. How do you rate your confidence that you could get and keep an erection?	Very low 1	Low 2	Moderate 3	High 4	Very high 5
2. When you had erections with sexual stimulation, how often were your erections hard enough for penetration?	Almost never or never 1	A few times (much less than half the time) 2	Sometimes (about half the time) 3	Most times (much more than half the time) 4	Almost always or always 5
3. During sexual intercourse, how often were you able to maintain your erection after you had penetrated your partner?	Almost never of never 1	A few times (much less than half the time) 2	Sometimes (About half the time) 3	Most times (much more than half the time) 4	Almost always or always 5
4. During sexual intercourse, how difficult was it to maintain your erection to completion of intercourse?	Extremely difficult 1	Very difficult 2	Difficult 3	Slightly difficult 4	Not difficult 5
5. When you attempted sexual intercourse, how often was it satisfactory for you?	Almost never or never 1	A few times (much less than half the time) 2	Sometimes (About half the time) 3	Most times (much more than half the time) 4	Almost always or always 5

Figure 22.1 The International Index of Erectile Function 5 (IIEF-5) assessment tool. Source: Feldman et al. (1994).[8] Reproduced with permission of Elsevier.

conditions are present, they will also need to be addressed and treated appropriately, and they too can have a significant effect on quality of life in this group of patients. It is also important to enquire about peripheral neuropathy and numbness as this can affect sensation and sexual function, although this is quite rare.

Psychological causes of ED are extremely important and may commonly coexist with organic ED. This can sometimes be elicited in the medical and social history – for instance, if there has been a change in personal circumstance or partner, or history of recent stress. It is important to enquire about these factors. It may be useful to see patients with their partners if possible. If necessary, psychosexual counseling should always be offered. If it is difficult to elicit a psychogenic cause from patient history, nocturnal penile tumescence testing may be a useful adjunct in order to demonstrate erectile function objectively, although this is rarely needed in diabetic patients.[31] Doppler ultrasound scanning of the penis has a useful role in cases where there is a poor response to initial treatment and can be used to delineate vascular causes of ED if suspected.[32]

Treatment

Diabetes mellitus is a chronic condition for which there is no cure. The aim of management is to keep blood glucose levels as close to the normal range as possible and minimize the risk of complications. ED is associated with a reduction in quality of life so appropriate treatment is important.[33] Patient education and awareness regarding their diabetes is important as diabetic complications are much less common and less severe in patients with well-controlled blood glucose levels.[34] With regards to treatment of the ED there are several options, which are decribed below.

Lifestyle

The first stage of the treatment of ED in diabetes is to address any adverse lifestyle factors. This is especially important in patients with type 2 diabetes where obesity, lack of physical activity, and poor diet have been implicated.[34] There is evidence that changing these factors can result in an improvement in erectile function in men at risk.[35–37] Support should be offered to patients with regard to dietary advice and exercise programs. ED has been shown to be a predictor for future cardiovascular events.[38] It can therefore be used as a marker to screen for silent coronary artery disease. Patient education regarding their condition and its management is essential. In patients with a high body mass index, dietary support and weight loss are important. Psychological support is also important, and counseling can often be a useful adjunct (Figure 22.2).

Phosphodiesterase-5 inhibitors

The management of ED in men with diabetes was revolutionized in 1999 with the introduction of phosphodiesterase-5 (PDE5) inhibitors, with good results.[39–42]

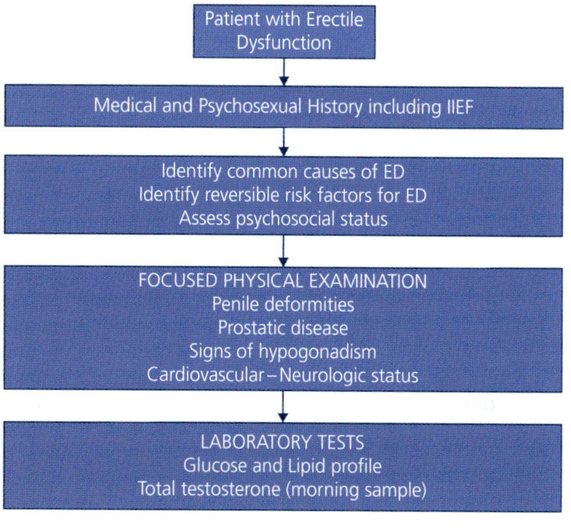

Figure 22.2 Investigation of the diabetic patient with erectile dysfunction (ED).

After conservative measures, PDE5 inhibitors are the first-line medical therapy and are safe and effective in many diabetics. These agents have been demonstrated to have a beneficial effect and have not been shown to have adverse effects on cardiovascular morbidity or mortality or on glycemic control in men with diabetes.[43] They work by inhibiting the degradation of cGMP by the phosphodiesterase type 5 enzyme. cGMP is essential for smooth muscle relaxation in blood vessels supplying the corpora cavernosa, resulting in increased blood flow and erection. PDE5 inhibitors have been shown to improve erectile function scores, penetration, and maintenance of erection, resulting in more successful intercourse.[44] Their effects are greater at higher doses, so titration of dose is recommended in order to achieve satisfactory results with minimal side effects. The pharmacokinetic data for three commonly used PDE5 inhibitors are shown in Table 22.1.

The three PDE5 inhibitors available for the treatment of ED in the UK are sildenafil, tadalafil, and vardenafil. Sildenafil and vardenafil are shorter-acting agents, while tadalafil has a longer half-life, which may provide the user with greater flexibility in sexual activity. Common adverse effects include headache, nasal congestion, and dyspepsia, all actions related to inhibition of PDE5. Tadalafil can also cause backache and muscle aches. The drugs are generally well tolerated and withdrawal rates as a result of drug-related adverse effects were rare in clinical trials.[44] The use of PDE5 inhibitors in the presence of oral nitrates is absolutely contraindicated. They are also contraindicated in men in whom sexual intercourse is inadvisable due to cardiovascular risk factors. PDE5 inhibitors can be used with caution alongside alpha-blockers for lower urinary tract symptoms, but the patient needs to be warned about the risk of hypotensive episodes.

An early study looking at the treatment with sildenafil of ED in diabetic patients showed significant improvement in erectile function and IIEF scores, with 61% of men treated with sildenafil being able to achieve penetrative intercourse.[45] Good results were also shown for tadalafil and vardenafil.[46,47] A large placebo-controlled trial showed tadalafil to be effective in improving erectile function in men with diabetes.[48] This was confirmed by a meta-analysis of 12 studies carried out by Fonseca et al., which also showed that adverse effects were similar in diabetic patients compared with non-diabetic men.[49]

Table 22.1 Pharmacokinetic data for sildenafil, tadalafil, and vardenafil.

	Maximum concentration (μg/L)	Time to maximum concentration (hours)	Half-life (hours)	Bioavailability
Sildenafil 100 mg	560	0.8–1	2.6–3.7	41%
Tadafil 20 mg	378	2	17.5	N/A
Vardenafil 20 mg	18.7	0.9	3.9	15%

The different PDE5 inhibitors all have similar mechanisms of action but with slightly different side effect profiles and durations of action. Patients should be counseled appropriately with regard to use and side effects of the PDE5 inhibitors. Tadalafil has been licensed for a once-daily dose, which may be more effective than on-demand therapy in some patients, and has been shown to be efficacious in a large, double-blinded, randomized, controlled trial.[50] Daily dosing has also been shown to be efficacious in diabetic men.[51] A meta-analysis by Shabsigh et al. looking at once-daily tadalafil use in men unable to achieve intercourse showed success rates of up to 46%.[52] This dosing regime can be a useful alternative for use in diabetic patients who do not respond to on-demand therapy initially.

Intraurethral suppositories

Alprostadil can be administered via intraurethral suppository (MUSE®).[53] This consists of a single-use pellet containing alprostadil suspended in polyethylene glycol administered using an applicator. The urethra is then gently massaged in order to dissolve the medication to allow absorption. It is then transported to the corpus cavernosum, where it causes vasodilation and relaxes smooth muscle. Studies have shown that intraurethral alprostadil has a fast onset of effect and a good safety profile, with no occurrences of priapism, fibrosis (as seen with intracavernosal injection), or the typical systemic effects observed with oral ED pharmacological treatments.[54] High patient preference, acceptance rates, and quality of life have been reported due to its ease of administration.[54] Evidence has shown that combination treatment with PDE5 inhibitors may be a possible efficient alternative when single oral or local treatment has failed.[55] Intraurethral alprostadil can be administered in patients irrespective of ED origin and is a good option in patients with ED for whom therapy with PDE5 inhibitors has failed or is contraindicated. Intraurethral alprostadil is contraindicated in patients who are predisposed to prolonged erection, such as with sickle-cell anemia, myeloma, and leukemia, as well as in men with urethral strictures, severe hypospadias, severe penile curvature, balanitis, and urethritis, and in men for whom sexual intercourse is medically inadvisable.

Intracavernosal injection

Injectable agents for ED include papaverine, phentolamine, and prostaglandin E_1 (PGE_1). They can be used alone or in combination. Papaverine is a non-specific PDE inhibitor that results in increased levels of cyclic adenosine monophosphate (cAMP) and/or cGMP, inhibition of calcium channels, and angiotensin-II secretion.[56] This results in vasodilation of penile vasculature and smooth muscle relaxation with erection. Phentolamine is a competitive antagonist of α1 and α2 adrenoreceptors. Antagonism of the α1 receptors results in vasodilation of the penile vasculature, whereas antagonism of the presynaptic α2 receptors is hypothesized to result in decreased intracorporal norepinephrine (noradrenaline) resulting in tumescence.[57]

Alprostadil is the most commonly used agent. It is a synthetic vasodilator, chemically identical to the naturally occurring PGE_1, which stimulates adenylate cyclase thereby increasing the level of cAMP, resulting in smooth muscle relaxation, vasodilation, and inhibition of platelet aggregation.[58] The vasodilation in the penis results in erection. It has been shown to have a unique role in treating ED in diabetic patients.[59] A large multicenter study analysing 336 men with type 1 and 2 diabetes demonstrated a satisfactory erectile response after 99% of injections with good tolerability.[60]

Intracavernosal injection is usually done via a small needle into the corpora of the penis. Patients are advised to alternate injection sites in order to reduce the risk of fibrosis and bruising. Patients and/or their partners are taught how to administer the injection. Side effects include prolonged erection (priapism), bruising, bleeding, and localized pain. One of the main problems with intracavernosal injection is the high dropout rate, with studies showing that 46–76% of patients discontinue its use due to various reasons, such as lack of efficacy, occurrence of side effects, and the requirement for injection of the penis, which some patients find unacceptable.[61,62] It has been shown that diabetics have an increased incidence of penile fibrosis, possibly owing to their microangiopathic disease and increased propensity for fibrosis.[63]

Vacuum devices

An alternative option for the treatment of ED in diabetic patients is the vacuum pump, which works well although patient satisfaction varies. It consists of a plastic cylinder with a pumping mechanism attached. The flaccid penis is placed inside the cylinder with the base of the cylinder placed firmly against the pubic region creating a tight seal. The pump is used to create negative pressure, which results in blood being drawn into the corpora of the penis resulting in engorgement of the penis and erection. A tight rubber ring is then placed around the base of the penis to trap the blood in the penis and maintain the erection. The cylinder and pump can then be removed. Vacuum devices can be used alongside PDE5 inhibitors and intracavernosal injection if necessary (Figure 22.3).

The main complaints are lack of spontaneity, localized bruising, and having a cold penis.[64] There can also be buckling of the penis and localized pain at the point where the constriction ring is applied. It is important that the patient is counseled regarding use of the device and warned not to leave the ring on for a prolonged period. There are no specific contraindications to using the vacuum pump but caution should be taken in patients using blood thinning medication. More than 70% of diabetic men achieve satisfactory erections; however, up to 30% of patients discontinue use as the result of inadequate rigidity, penile pain, failure to ejaculate, and appearance of the penis while using the device.[65]

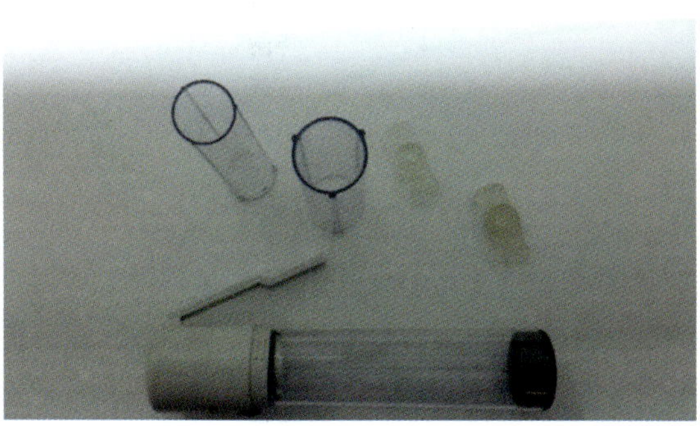

Figure 22.3 Photo of vacuum device with different sized cylinders and constriction rings.

Penile prostheses

Considerable advances have been made in the field of penile prostheses for ED. They provide a good option for diabetic patients who have failed with oral and injectable therapies or who are unwilling to use these or vacuum devices. They also have a role in patients who have coexisiting Peyronie's disease as this can be addressed simultaneously at the time of implant surgery. They are an excellent option for patients in whom the erectile mechanism is irreversibily damaged.[66] There are two main types of penile prostheses, inflatable and malleable. Inflatable prostheses consist of two cylinders that are implanted within the corpora, and are attached to a reservoir containing fluid and a pump mechanism. This allows fluid to be pumped into the cylinders to produce an erection, which can be deflated when not required. This allows the patient to achieve both an erection state and flaccidity. The malleable prostheses consist of two semi-rigid rods that are implanted into the corpora in order to make the penis rigid. The disadvantage of this is that the patient has a permanent erection and concealment may be an issue. A large study of 504 procedures using both inflatable and malleable devices showed high satisfaction rates of 81%, with dissatisfaction being largely due to complications resulting in removal of the prosthesis.[67] The main complications in this study were infection (8%) and erosion (5%), both of which were more common in diabetic patients (10%). Another large study also showed patient and partner satisfaction rates of 86.4% and 52.6% respectively (Figure 22.4).[68]

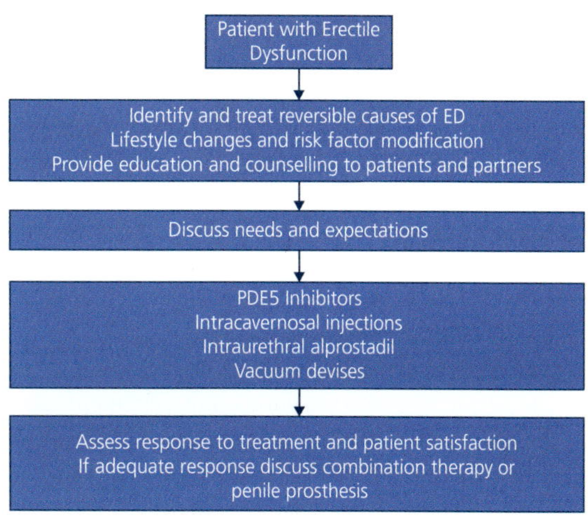

Figure 22.4 Treatment algorithm for erectile dysfunction (ED).

Infection

Infections can be more common and severe in diabetic patients. This is especially important to consider in patients who are having penile prostheses. They are thought to be at higher risk of infection at the time of surgery. Studies have documented a 2–10% incidence of penile prosthetic infection in diabetics, but there was no significant difference between diabetics and non-diabetics.[69,70] Each patient should be assessed on an individual basis, and full precautions should be taken in order to reduce the risk of infection in these cases. If infection does occur this can be catastrophic, and the implant inevitably needs to be removed in order for the infection to resolve. This can cause considerable distress to patients as well as the need for further surgery and the risks to health associated with infection and sepsis. A large study looking at 1511 patients who had the "no touch" technique of penile implant surgery reported infections in only 0.46% of patients.[71] This study also showed that infection-retardant coatings lowered the risk of infection from 5.3% to 2%.

Future treatments

The treatment of ED is an ever advancing field with improvements in both devices and medications. Research is ongoing looking at the various underlying mechanisms involved in diabetic ED, including the field of gene therapy. Areas of interest include gene therapy with neurotrophic factors, endothelial nitric oxide synthase (eNOS), neuronal NOS (nNOS), and superoxide dismutase.[72] A new class of agents called soluble guanylate cyclase stimulators like BAY 41-2272 have been shown to induce erections and smooth muscle relaxation when there is a lack of NO and also in diabetics.[73] There is also research investigating the role of Rho kinase inhibitors in the relaxation of cavernosal tissue of diabetic patients.[74] This could provide further insight to the mechanism of ED in diabetics and help to guide future therapy. Research has also been focused on the use of NO-releasing PDE5 inhibitors in patients with severe deficiency of endogenous NO, such as long-term diabetes, showing its potential use in NO-deficient conditions.[75]

Patient education plays an important role, and increased awareness and screening programs for diabetes should result in earlier diagnosis and treatment, thus preventing the associated comorbidities.

The field of penile prostheses is ever advancing, with new technologies looking at mechanized methods for cylinder inflation that would eliminate the need for the scrotal pump, which some patients find difficult to use.[68] This could also serve to more closely mimic the natural course of tumescence and detumescence. Research is also being carried out looking at rechargeable motorized pumps and incorporation of the battery, controls, and fluid transfer system within the corporal implants, obviating the need for connecting of components during surgery.[69] This could also result in lower infection rates and lower incidence of mechanical failure. Emerging advances in the field of nanotechnology could result in materials that would be useful in prosthetic design in that they demonstrate both rigidity and volume expansion properties.[70] The ideal prosthesis would have no moving parts and be constructed from material that obtained rigidity from application of heat, pressure, or electric charge.

Conclusion

Erectile dysfunction occurs commonly in diabetic patients and is often under-diagnosed. It can have a significant effect on a patient's quality of life and is easily treatable. The underlying pathophysiology is extremely complex and is still not fully understood. A holistic approach is needed in the management of diabetic ED, taking into account lifestyle factors and psychological comorbidities. A variety of treatments exist varying from medical to surgical therapies, which have been shown to work well in this patient group depending on the severity of disease. Patient education remains a priority in both prevention and treatment of this condition.

References

1 Malavige LS, Levy JC. Erectile dysfunction in diabetes mellitus. *J Sex Med* 2009;6(5):1232–47.

2 International Diabetes Federation (IDF). Diabetes Facts and Figures. Available at: http://www.idf.org/WDD15-guide/facts-and-figures.html

3 Baldé NM, Diallo AB, Baldé MC, et al. Erectile dysfunction and diabetes in Conakry (Guinea): frequency and clinical characteristics from 187 diabetic patients. *Ann Endocrinol* 2006;67(4):338–42.

4 Vickers MA, Wright EA. Erectile dysfunction in the patient with diabetes mellitus. *Am J Manag Care* 2004;10 (1 Suppl.): S3–11.

5 Lewis RW. Epidemiology of erectile dysfunction. *Urol Clin North Am* 2001;28:209–16.
6 Bacon CG, Hu FB, Giovannucci E, Glasser DB, Mittleman MA, Rimm EB. Association of type and duration of diabetes with erectile dysfunction in a large cohort of men. *Diabetes Care* 2002;25(8):1458–63.
7 Smith AD. Causes and classification of impotence. *Urol Clin North Am* 1981;8:79–89.
8 Feldman HA, Goldstein I, Hatzichristou DG, Krane RJ, McKinlay JB. Impotence and its medical and psychosocial correlates: results of the Massachusetts Male Aging Study. *J Urol* 1994;151:54–61.
9 Malavige LS, Jayaratne SD, Kathriarachchi ST, Sivayogan S, Fernando DJ, Levy JC. Erectile dysfunction among men with diabetes is strongly associated with premature ejaculation and reduced libido. *J Sex Med* 2008;5 (9):2125–34.
10 Burke FP, Jacobson DF, McGree ME, Nehra AX, Lieber MM, Jacobsen SF. Diabetes and sexual dysfunction in Olmsted County, Minnesota. *J Sex Med* 2006;3 (Suppl. 1):19.
11 Ledda A. Diabetes, hypertension and erectile dysfunction. *Curr Med Res Opin* 2000;16 (Suppl. 1):s17–20.
12 Lambert P, Bingley PJ. What is type 1 diabetes? *Medicine* 2002;30:1–5.
13 Masharani U, German MS. Pancreatic hormones and diabetes mellitus. In: Gardner D, Shoback D (eds), *Greenspan's Basic and Clinical Endocrinology*, 9th edn. New York: McGraw-Hill Medical, 2011; Chapter 17.
14 Rother KI. Diabetes treatment – bridging the divide. *N Engl J Med* 2007;356(15):1499–501.
15 Vijan S. Type 2 diabetes. *Ann Int Med* 2010;152(5):ITC31–15; quiz ITC316.
16 Emerging Risk Factors Collaboration. Diabetes mellitus, fasting blood glucose concentration, and risk of vascular disease: A collaborative meta-analysis of 102 prospective studies. *Lancet* 2010;375(9733):2215–22.
17 Seftel AD, Vaziri ND, Ni Z, et al. Advanced glycation end products in human penis: elevation in diabetic tissue, site of deposition, and possible effect through iNOS or eNOS. *Urology* 1997;50:1016–26.
18 Cartledge JJ, Eardley I, Morrison JF. Nitric oxide-mediated corpus cavernosal smooth muscle relaxation is impaired in ageing and diabetes. *BJU Int* 2001;87:394–401.
19 Christ GJ, Lerner SE, Kim DC, Melman A. Endothelin-1 as a putative modulator of erectile dysfunction: I. Characteristics of contraction of isolated corporal tissue strips. *J Urol* 1995;153:1998–2003.
20 Sullivan ME, Dashwood MR, Thompson CS, Muddle JR, Mikhailidis DP, Morgan RJ. Alterations in endothelin B receptor sites in cavernosal tissue of diabetic rabbits: potential relevance to the pathogenesis of erectile dysfunction. *J Urol* 1997;158:1966–72.
21 Buyukafsar K, Un I. Effects of the Rho-kinase inhibitors, Y-27632 and fasudil, on the corpus cavernosum from diabetic mice. *Eur J Pharmacol* 2003;472:235–8.
22 Hecht MJ, Neundorfer B, Kiesewetter F, Hilz MJ. Neuropathy is a major contributing factor to diabetic erectile dysfunction. *Neurol Res* 2001;23:651–4.
23 Usta MF, Bivalacqua TJ, Yang DY, et al. The protective effect of aminoguanidine on erectile function in streptozotocin diabetic rats. *J Urol* 2003;170:1437–42.
24 Boussageon R, Bejan-Angoulvant T, Saadatian-Elahi M, et al. (2011) Effect of intensive glucose lowering treatment on all cause mortality, cardiovascular death, and microvascular events in type 2 diabetes: meta-analysis of randomised controlled trials. *BMJ* 343:d4169.
25 Palumbo PJ. Metabolic risk factors, endothelial dysfunction, and erectile dysfunction in men with diabetes. *Am J Med Sci* 2007;334(6):466–80.
26 Zdravko A, Kamenov V, Tsanka G, Yankova M. Erectile dysfunction in diabetic men is linked more to microangiopathic complications and neuropathy than to macroangiopathic disturbances. *J Mens Health* 2007;4:64–73.
27 Romeo JH, Seftel AD, Madhun ZT, Aron DC. Sexual function in men with diabetes type 2: association with glycemic control. *J Urol* 2000;163(3):788–91.
28 Larsen ML, Hørder M, Mogensen EF. Effect of long-term monitoring of glycosylated haemoglobin levels in insulin-dependent diabetes mellitus. *N Engl J Med* 1990;323(15):1021–5.
29 Rhoden EL, Telöken C, Sogari PR, Vargas Souto CA. The use of the simplified International Index of Erectile Function (IIEF-5) as a diagnostic tool to study the prevalence of erectile dysfunction. *Int J Impot Res* 2002;14(4):245–50.
30 Fedder J, Kaspersen MD, Brandslund I, Højgaard A. Retrograde ejaculation and sexual dysfunction in men with diabetes mellitus: a prospective, controlled study. *Andrology* 2013;1(4):602–6.
31 Levine LA, Lenting EL. Use of nocturnal penile tumescence and rigidity in the evaluation of male erectile dysfunction. *Urol Clin N Am* 1995;22:775–88.
32 Sikka SC, Hellstrom WJ, Brock G, Morales AM. Standardization of vascular assessment of erectile dysfunction: standard operating procedures for duplex ultrasound. *J Sex Med* 2013;10(1):120–9.
33 Malavige LS, Jayaratne SD, Kathriarachchi ST, Sivayogan S, Ranasinghe P, Levy JC. Erectile dysfunction is a strong predictor of poor quality of life in men with Type 2 diabetes mellitus. *Diabet Med* 2014;31:699–706.
34 Nathan DM, Cleary PA, Backlund JY, et al., Diabetes Control and Complications Trial/Epidemiology of Diabetes Interventions and Complications (DCCT/EDIC) Study Research Group. Intensive diabetes treatment and cardiovascular disease in patients with type 1 diabetes. *N Engl J Med* 2005;353(25):2643–53.
35 Esposito K, Ciotola M, Giugliano F, et al. Effects of intensive lifestyle changes on erectile dysfunction in men. *J Sex Med* 2009;6(1):243–50.
36 Esposito K, Giugliano F, Di Palo C, et al. Effect of lifestyle changes on erectile dysfunction in obese men: a randomized controlled trial. *JAMA* 2004;291(24):2978–84.

37 Hannan JL, Maio MT, Komolova M, Adams MA. Beneficial impact of exercise and obesity interventions on erectile function and its risk factors. *J Sex Med* 2009;6 (Suppl. 3):254–61.

38 Risérus U, Willet W. Dietary fats and prevention of type 2 diabetes. *Prog Lipid Res* 2009;48(1):44–51.

39 Boolel M, Gepi-Attee S, Gingell JC, Allen MJ. Sildenafil, a novel effective oral therapy for male erectile dysfunction. *Br J Urol* 1996;78: 257–61.

40 Moreland RB, Goldstein I, Kim NN, Traish A. Sildenafil citrate, a selective phosphodiesterase type 5 inhibitor: research and clinical implications in erectile dysfunction. *Trends Endocrinol Metab* 1999;10:97–104.

41 Goldstein I, Young JM, Fischer J, et al. Vardenafil, a new phosphodiesterase type 5 inhibitor, in the treatment of erectile dysfunction in men with diabetes: a multicenter double-blind placebo-controlled fixed-dose study. *Diabetes Care* 2003;26(3):777–83.

42 Fink HA, MacDonald R, Rutks IR, Nelson DB, Wilt TJ. Sildenafil for male erectile dysfunction: a systematic review and meta-analysis. *Arch Intern Med* 2002;162 (12):1349–60.

43 Phé V, Rouprêt M. Erectile dysfunction and diabetes: a review of the current evidence-based medicine and a synthesis of the main available therapies. *Diabetes Metab* 2012;38(1):1–13.

44 Basu A, Ryder RE. New treatment options for erectile dysfunction in patients with diabetes mellitus. *Drugs* 2004;64(23):2667–88.

45 Rendell MS, Rajfer J, Wicker P, Smith M. Sildenafil for treatment of erectile dysfunction in men with diabetes: a randomized controlled trial. *JAMA* 1999;281:421–6.

46 Padma-Nathan H, McMurray JG, Pullman WE, et al. On demand IC351 (Cialis) enhances erectile function in patients with erectile dysfunction. *Int J Impot Res* 2001;13:2–9.

47 Porst H, Rosen R, Padma-Nathan H, et al. The efficacy and tolerability of vardenafil, a new, oral, selective phosphodiesterase type 5 inhibitor, in patients with erectile dysfunction: the first at-home clinical trial. *Int J Impot Res* 2001;13:192–9.

48 Sáenz de Tejada I, Anglin G, Knight JR, Emmick JT. Effects of tadalafil on erectile dysfunction in men with diabetes. *Diabetes Care* 2002;25(12):2159–64.

49 Fonseca V, Seftel A, Denne J, Fredlund P. Impact of diabetes mellitus on the severity of erectile dysfunction and response to treatment: analysis of data from tadalafil clinical trials. *Diabetologia* 2004;47(11):1914–23.

50 Porst H, Giuliano F, Glina S, et al. Evaluation of the efficacy and safety of once-a-day dosing of tadalafil 5 mg and 10 mg in the treatment of erectile dysfunction: results of a multicenter, randomized, double-blind, placebo-controlled trial. *Eur Urol* 2006;50(2):351–9.

51 Hatzichristou D, Gambla M, Rubio-Aurioles E, et al. Efficacy of tadalafil once daily in men with diabetes mellitus and erectile dysfunction. *Diabet Med* 2008;25(2):138–46.

52 Shabsigh R, Seftel AD, Kim ED, Ni X, Burns PR. Efficacy and safety of once-daily tadalafil in men with erectile dysfunction who reported no successful intercourse attempts at baseline. *J Sex Med* 2013;10(3):844–56.

53 Guay AT, Perez JB, Velásquez E, Newton RA, Jacobson JP. Clinical experience with intraurethral alprostadil (MUSE®) in the treatment of men with erectile dysfunction. *Eur Urol* 2000;38:671–6

54 Costa P, Potempa AJ. Intraurethral alprostadil for erectile dysfunction: a review of the literature. *Drugs* 2012;72 (17):2243–54.

55 Nehra A, Blute ML, Barrett DM, Moreland RB. Rationale for combination therapy of intraurethral prostaglandin E(1) and sildenafil in the salvage of erectile dysfunction patients desiring noninvasive therapy. *Int J Impot Res* 2002;14 (Suppl. 1):S38–42.

56 Hakenberg O, Wetterauer U, Koppermann U, Liffimann R. Systemic pharmacokinetics of papaverine and phentolamine: Comparison of intravenous and intracorporal application. *Int J Impot Res* 1990;2 (Suppl. 2):247–8.

57 Savoca G, Silvestre G, Belgrano E. Intracavernosal injection therapy and surgical therapy in diabetic patients with erectile dysfunction. *Diabetes Nutr Metab* 2002;15:53–7.

58 Tsai Y-S, Lin JS-N, Lin Y-M. Safety and efficacy of alprostadil sterile powder (S. Po., CAVERJECT®) in diabetic patients with erectile dysfunction. *Eur Urol* 2000;38:177–83.

59 Hanchanale V, Eardley I. Alprostadil for the treatment of impotence. *Expert Opin Pharmacother* 2014;15(3):421–8.

60 Heaton JP, Lording D, Liu SN, et al. Intracavernosal alprostadil is effective for the treatment of erectile dysfunction in diabetic men. *Int J Impot Res* 2001;13:317–21.

61 Irwin MB, Kata EJ. High attrition rate with intracavernous injection of prostaglandin E1 for impotency. *Urology* 1994;43:84–7.

62 Althof SE, Turner LA, Levine SB, et al. Why do so many people drop out from auto-injection therapy for impotence? *J Sex Marital Ther* 1989;15:121–9.

63 Moemen MN, Hamed HA, Kamel II, Shamloul RM, Ghanem HM. Clinical and sonographic assessment of the side effects of intracavernous injection of vasoactive substances. *Int J Impot Res* 2004;16:143–5.

64 Price DE, Cooksey G, Jehu D, Bentley S, Hearnshaw JR, Osborn DE. The management of impotence in diabetic men by vacuum tumescence therapy. *Diabet Med* 1991;8:964–7.

65 Sidi AA, Becher EF, Zhang G, Lewis JH. Patient acceptance of and satisfaction with an external negative pressure device for impotence. *J Urol* 1990;144:1154–6.

66 Moncada I, Martinez-Salamanca JI, Allona A, Hernandez C. Current role of penile implants for erectile dysfunction. *Curr Opin Urol* 2004;14:375–80.

67 Minervini A, Ralph DJ, Pryor JP. Outcome of penile prosthesis implantation for treating erectile dysfunction: experience with 504 procedures. *BJU Int* 2006;97:129–33.

68 Falcone M, Rolle L, Ceruti C, et al. Prospective analysis of the surgical outcomes and patients' satisfaction rate after

the AMS Spectra penile prosthesis implantation. *Urology* 2013;82(2):373–6.

69 Wilson SK, Carson CC, Cleves MA, Delk JR 2nd. Quantifying risk of penile prosthesis infection with elevated glycosylated hemoglobin. *J Urol* 1998;159:1537–9.

70 Montague DK, Angermeier KW, Lakin MM. Penile prosthesis infections. *Int J Impot Res* 2001;13:326–8.

71 Eid JF, Wilson SK, Cleves M, Salem EA. Coated implants and "no touch" surgical technique decreases risk of infection in inflatable penile prosthesis implantation to 0.46%. *Urology* 2012;79(6):1310–5.

72 Moore CR, Wang R. Pathophysiology and treatment of diabetic erectile dysfunction. *Asian J Androl* 2006;8(6):675–84.

73 Kalsi JS, Ralph DJ, Madge DJ, Kell PD, Cellek S. NCX-911, a novel nitric oxide-releasing PDE5 inhibitor relaxes rabbit corpus cavernosum in the absence of endogenous nitric oxide. *Int J Impot Res* 2004;16(6):479–85.

74 Toque HA, Nunes KP, Yao L, et al. Activated Rho kinase mediates diabetes-induced elevation of vascular arginase activation and contributes to impaired corpora cavernosa relaxation: possible involvement of p38 MAPK activation. *J Sex Med* 2013;10(6):1502–15.

75 Kalsi JS, Ralph DJ, Thomas P, et al. A nitric oxide-releasing PDE5 inhibitor relaxes human corpus cavernosum in the absence of endogenous nitric oxide. *J Sex Med.* 2005 Jan;2(1):53–7.

CHAPTER 23

Management of erectile dysfunction in neurological patients

Katarina Ivana Tudor[1] and Jalesh N. Panicker[2]

[1] *Department of Neurology, University Hospital Center Zagreb, Zagreb, Croatia*

[2] *The National Hospital for Neurology and Neurosurgery and UCL Institute of Neurology, London, UK*

Sexual functions comprise an important facet of human behavior.[1–3] In health, achieving an erection is dependent upon a complex interplay between vascular, neurological, and hormonal factors. Intact peripheral innervation through sympathetic and parasympathetic fibers derived from the hypogastric and pelvic plexuses conveys signals responsible for the neurological control of the erectile response. Reflex erections are mediated by sacral segmental pathways and result from genital stimulation. The reflex erection is short lived and usually inadequate for penetrative intercourse. Psychogenic erections originate from cortical and subcortical centers and are mediated through the thoracolumbar sympathetic outflow. In health, these two merge together resulting in an erectile response sufficient for penetration.[4]

Neurological lesions affecting both the peripheral and central nervous system can result in erectile dysfunction (ED). It has been estimated that 10–19% of cases of ED are from a neurogenic origin.[5] However, sexual dysfunction (SD) in neurological disorders is underreported.[6–10] In a survey of over 2000 patients with multiple sclerosis (MS) from New South Wales, Australia, only 55% of men had been able to speak to their health professional about sexual difficulties, and only 29% received help.[11] Seventy percent of respondents of a large survey of MS patients reported sexual problems, with 42% grading this as of moderate or high concern, and only 33% reported improvement with disease-specific therapy.[12] Clearly, sexual dysfunction including ED is common following neurological disorders and affects quality of life, but is underdiagnosed and undertreated.

The problem of SD (and ED) in neurological disease is multidimensional, with contributions from multiple factors. For example, in MS the demyelinating lesion affecting the neural pathways controlling sexual functions can result in ED (primary factors). Neurological deficits resulting from the disease can contribute to sexual dysfunction (secondary factors). Spasticity can result in difficulty in assuming positions conducive to intimacy and sexual intercourse. Finally, factors such as anxiety, depression, and guilt resulting from having a neurological disorder can affect the relationship and have an impact on sexual activity (tertiary factors)[6,13–19] (Table 23.1). Additionally, medications used in the management of symptoms resulting from neurological disease can affect sexual functions; examples are antidepressants, baclofen, and gabapentin[17] (Table 23.2).

Neurological disorders and sexual dysfunction

Primary brain tumors

ED is common following brain tumors. ED resulting from tumors of the hypothalamic and pituitary area may arise due to hormonal or neurological dysfunction, or both. However, a cross-sectional study in 1997 found that 47% of adult long-term survivors of primary brain tumors outside the hypothalamic-pituitary region also

Male Sexual Dysfunction: A Clinical Guide, First Edition. Edited by Suks Minhas and John Mulhall.

suffered from ED, probably due to radiation therapy or chemotherapy. Forty-two percent of the patients showed either evidence for hypothalamic hypogonadism (32%) or primary gonadal damage (10%). Nine patients (29%) presented with hyperprolactinemia. Patients reporting ED had significantly lower testosterone levels than patients with normal erectile functions.[20]

Table 23.1 The multidimensional nature of sexual dysfunction following neurological disease. Adapted from (6)

Dimensions	Factors influencing sexual functions
Primary	Neurological lesion resulting in impaired sexual functions
Secondary	Physical immobility
	Spasticity
	Tremor
	Bladder/bowel incontinence
	Difficulties in attention and concentration
	Fatigue
	Sensory symptoms – dysesthesia/ allodynia
Tertiary	Depression, anxiety
	Anger, guilt, and fear
	Altered self-image, low self-esteem
	Relationship with the partner, change in family role
	Use of urethral indwelling catheter

Source: Bronner et al. 2010.[6] Reproduced with permission of John Wiley & Sons, Ltd.

Traumatic brain injury (TBI)

Injury to limbic structures and frontal lobes may impact sexual functions. Erectile function was related to the location and severity of injury. Erectile function was related to the location and severity of injury.[21] Kreuter et al. demonstrated that after severe brain injury 26% of men and women discontinued sex with their partners, with erectile and ejaculatory dysfunction as most common cause.[22] Significant sexual changes are experienced by more than 50% of TBI individuals up to 5 years post-injury.[21] Additionally, hormonal changes may occur after hypothalamic or pituitary injury and therefore a full endocrine evaluation is sometimes necessary.[23]

Stroke

A majority of stroke patients report a marked decline in sexual functions, that is, libido, coital frequency, erectile and orgasmic ability. The observed decline in sexual functions appears to be multifactorial in nature.[24] An association has been observed between left hemispheric lesions with post-stroke SD.[25] In a study performed by Jeon and colleagues, ED was more prevalent in patients with vascular risk factors, specifically diabetes, and with thalamic stroke.[26] Concern about possible blood pressure changes that may occur related to sexual activity may have an impact on intimacy. Moreover, antihypertensive agents commonly used by stroke patients, such as beta blockers, may result in diminished cavernosal artery pressures and erectile dysfunction.[27]

Table 23.2 Medications used in the management of neurological symptoms may contribute to sexual dysfunction. Adapted from (17)

Neurological symptom	Medication	Adverse effects on sexual functions
Spasticity	Baclofen	ED, inability to ejaculate (rare)
	Dantrolene	Decreased libido, ED, retrograde ejaculation
Fatigue	Amantadine	Decreased libido
	Amphetamine, dextroamphetamine	ED, changes in libido (dose dependent)
Pain	Tricyclic antidepressants	ED, ejaculatory impairment, anorgasmia, decreased libido
	Valproic acid	ED
	Carbamazepine	ED
	Lamotrigine	ED
	Duloxetine	Decreased libido, ED, ejaculation dysfunction and anorgasmia
Depression	SSRIs	Decreased libido, anorgasmia, delayed ejaculation
	Venlafaxine	ED, anorgasmia

ED, erectile dysfunction; SSRI, selective serotonin reuptake inhibitor.
Source: Fletcher et al. (2009).[17] Reproduced with permission of Elsevier.

However with time, erectile functions may improve. In a group of men under 65 years, 82% spontaneously regained erectile function within approximately 7 weeks following the stroke.[28]

Migraine and tension type headache

Sexual dysfunction is often reported in patients with headache. Social life is affected in both headache types, due to sensitivity to stress factors, degradation in quality of life, and workforce loss in communities. Published literature indicates that depression and other psychiatric disorders (both known to be associated with SD) often accompany both types of headache. It is possible that chronic pain activates a common set of processes such as deregulation in dopamine pathways, and an increase in the amount of serotonin (5-HT), which may lead to SD. ED is usually reported in a group of patients with migraine. However, in a study done by Houle and colleagues, SD was more prevalent in patients with tension type headache compared to a group with migraine.[29] Another study found SD statistically more often in both groups compared to controls, but did not find any difference between the groups.[30]

Epilepsy and antiepileptic drugs

ED and premature ejaculation were described in 70.4% and 66.7%, respectively, of patients with epilepsy. A descriptive study evaluating sexual and reproductive health in a group of men with generalized epilepsy, by means of interviews and determination of serum hormone concentrations, demonstrated a five-fold increase of ED among this group of patients.[31,32]

Studies have shown that epileptiform discharges may disrupt the function of structures mediating sexual behavior, particularly the limbic cortex, or alter the release of hypothalamic-pituitary hormones. Assessment of the physiologic integrity of the sexual response in men with epilepsy and ED using an ambulatory nocturnal penile tumescence and rigidity monitor (NPTR) has shown an abnormal pattern to be associated with neurogenic rather than vasogenic ED. Although, temporal lobe epilepsy can present with hypersexuality and genital automatisms,[33] patients usually present with SD. Hamed et al. demonstrated a notably higher frequency of SD in men with generalized tonic-clonic convulsions. Studies have shown that the SD is more common in partial (particularly temporal) lobe epilepsy, as the limbic system is extensively interconnected with the hypothalamic nuclei involved in regulating gonadal function.[31] De Souza and colleagues reported that low desire was strongly linked to the temporal lobe origin of seizures, but more so to anxiety and depression, and loss of self-esteem.[34] A postoperative sexual change is significantly more likely to be reported by patients who had undergone temporal lobe resection (64%) than extra-temporal lobe resection (25%). This was significantly more frequent following right-sided temporal lobe resections, and more frequently reported in females than males.[35] Antiepileptic drugs are known to be associated with ED. Most cases were related to the use of traditional liver enzyme inducing antiepileptic drugs (AEDs) such as phenytoin, phenobarbitone, primidone, and carbamazepine.[36–38] AEDs induce the hepatic microsomal enzyme P450, which may in turn result in increased metabolism of sexual hormones. AEDs may also induce the synthesis of sex hormone-binding globulin resulting in reduced free and bioactive testosterone levels.

Among the newer AEDs, topiramate (TPM), which is effective in managing partial and generalized epilepsy, is associated with ED and this is related to the cumulative dosage. There is a description in the literature of one patient with partial epilepsy associated with oligoastrocytoma in whom reversible ED developed 1 month after starting therapy with zonisamide (ZNS), and which disappeared when the drug was suspended.[39] In 2012 Civardi and colleagues proposed a vasogenic mechanism as a possible cause for changes in reproductive hormone levels.[40] It is speculated that ED induced by TPM may be due to a blockade of the lumbosacral spinal cord AMPA receptors leading to an inhibition of the glutamatergic pathway. The role of serotonin in ED has been noted.[41]

Parkinson's disease

Parkinson's disease (PD) is a movement disorder associated with the degeneration of dopaminergic neurons in the substantia nigra. Though the commonest manifestations are motor disabilities resulting in slowness and falls, non-motor symptoms such as neuropsychiatric, sleep, sensory, and autonomic symptoms are recognized as being prominent complaints impacting quality of life.[42,43]

Dopaminergic mechanisms contribute to sexual desire and induction of penile erections.[27] In animal studies the medial preoptic area (MPO) of the hypothalamus has been shown to regulate sexual drive.[44] Nigral dopaminergic neurons send MPO projections, and patients with PD have changes in the hypothalamus.[4] Hyperprolactinemia, which was found in untreated patients with PD, may also contribute to ED.[45]

The prevalence of sexual symptoms in patients with PD ranges from 37% to 65%,[43] and this finding is common in both genders. Men with PD usually report sexual dissatisfaction in 65% of cases and ED in 68% of cases.[46]

Sakakibara et al. reported the prevalence of sexual symptoms in patients with PD ranging from 37% to 65%. ED was reported in 79%.[47] Wullner et al. reported ED in 50%, and Zesiewicz in 60.7% of men with PD.[48,49] In a study of 29 patients, 19 (65.5%) had difficulty in both achieving and maintaining erections and one (3.5%) had difficulty in maintaining erections. All four patients who had ejaculatory disturbance also had ED. Decreased sexual drive was described in two (4%) of the PD patients and in 6.25% of controls.[50]

Sexual dysfunction increases with age, but not with disability as measured by the Hoehn and Yahr stage. The prevalence of dissatisfaction with sexual conditions did not differ between the controls and patients with PD despite there being greater SD in the patients with PD.[4] Symptoms of ED lead to deterioration of the quality of life.[50]

Another problem of sexual functions reported in PD is hypersexuality as part of an impulse control disorder (ICD), seen in 13.6% of patients and found to be more common in patients treated with dopamine agonists. In the DOMINION study, compulsive sexual behavior was found in 3.5% of patients, as the second most common ICD, after pathological gambling.[51] Though this is not directly linked with ED, men with hypersexuality often have ED, and the combined problem can result in considerable distress for the partner.

Multiple system atrophy

There are several mimics of PD, and multiple system atrophy (MSA) is a Parkinson-plus disorder where urogenital dysfunction is often the first manifestation. ED is a widespread symptom often associated with bladder dysfunction. It is thought that in MSA, ED precedes the onset of other symptoms (including bladder dysfunction) by several years and can appear as early as 5–10 years before other clinical symptoms.[52,53] The underlying process is usually centrally originating and possibly dopamine dependent, since it occurs separately from postural hypotension.[52]

Postural hypotension in men is exacerbated by sildenafil, and when prescribing for these patients, especially with the shorter-acting type 5 phosphodiesterase inhibitor (PDE5I), caution should be exercised.[54]

Multiple sclerosis

Multiple sclerosis (MS) is an inflammatory disorder of the central nervous system that results in demyelinating lesions in the white matter of the brain and spinal cord.[10,11,55–57] It generally affects active young adults.[7,14,58] The estimated prevalence of SD in MS is between 50 and 90%.[14] Zorzon et al. in 2001 demonstrated that SD affects 73.1% of subjects affected by all types of MS.[6,10,11,59] Several papers report an ED incidence of 50% to 90% in men with MS.[55,59–61]

Men may report complete loss of erections; however, more commonly, ED is often partial.[62] Men may continue to report spontaneous erections at night, and with masturbation, especially in the early stages. SD has been correlated with lesions on MRI, Kurtzke`s Expanded Disability Status Scale (EDSS), and depression.[6,8,63–67] Identifying and treating ED can result in improvement of the quality of life (QoL) for men with MS.[60,68,69]

In most cases, ED appears during the course of the disease, a median of 8 years (range 1–30 years) after presentation of initial neurological symptoms.[70] Rarely, ED may arise early in the course; in 5.6 % of cases, ED preceded other neurological symptoms, whilst in 3.7 % of cases ED developed at the same time as other neurological symptoms.[59]

Erectile and neurogenic bladder dysfunctions are the result of spinal cord involvement, and one study also implicated the pons.[61,70,71] ED is associated with lower limb findings of pyramidal tract dysfunction and a neurogenic bladder.[70]

Spinal cord injury

Early studies of war veterans showed that, depending on the site of the injury, patients will have preserved either psychogenic or reflex erections, while ejaculation is exceptional. Patients with complete lesions above T10 have preserved reflex erections. In men who have sustained injury to the lower lumbar spine (without extensive damage to the sacral roots), psychogenic erections may be more readily induced than erection following genital stimulation. Men with a complete lesion below S2 may have psychogenic erections but no reflex erections, but damage to the cauda equina results in almost complete loss of erectile responses.[4]

In one study, about 38% of men with apparently complete lesions reported the ability to experience orgasm.[72] After complete spinal cord injury only 4% of men with high lesions and 18% of men with lower lesions of the conus and equina are able to ejaculate. Poor sperm quality after spinal cord injury is a further confounding factor.[73]

Following cauda equina injury, genital sensations are impaired, and these recover poorly. The result of impaired genital sensation and ED is orgasmic dysfunction, which was in fact the most common reported SD in men with cauda equina syndrome.[4,74]

In one published study out of 36 mostly ambulant men with longstanding cauda equina damage of various causes, 35 reported SD, which was moderate or severe in 59%.[74]

Polyneuropathy

Various polyneuropathies present with ED. Peripheral neuropathy is an important cause for ED in diabetics,[75] and this is described elsewhere. Sensory and motor neuropathies are considered important pathogenic factors for SD in patients with chronic kidney disorder, especially those having diabetes. Atherosclerosis is significantly accelerated because of hypertension, diabetes, inflammation, secondary hyperparathyroidism, and the impact of uremic toxins on the vascular endothelium. Rosas et al. reported a prevalence of 45% and Arslan et al. one of 80.7% for ED in male patients on hemodialysis.[76]

A population of heavy drinkers without liver dysfunction was assessed for autonomic neuropathy, and among 55% of symptomatic patients, impotence was the only symptom (probably due to damage of parasympathetic fibers).[77]

Guillain–Barré syndrome

Guillain–Barré syndrome (GBS) presents as acute monopathic symmetrical ascending radiculo-neuropathy, with an emphasis on the motor rather than the sensory nerve fibers. Two-thirds of cases are associated with antecedent infection, which varies by geographical location. The infective agents implicated include *Campylobacter jejuni*, cytomegalovirus, Epstein–Barr virus, and *Mycoplasma pneumoniae*. Progression between 4 and 8 weeks is termed subacute inflammatory polyradiculoneuropathy (SIDP), and progression after 8 weeks is termed chronic inflammatory demyelinating polyradiculoneuropathy (CIDP). In acute motor axonal polyneuropathy there are increased levels of antiganglioside antibodies. Despite modern treatment and improvement in intensive care facilities, the mortality remains static at 5%, with nearly 20% of patients having persistent disability.[4] Approximately two-thirds of patients will have evidence of autonomic dysfunction.[78] Residual disability from GBS was correlated with the incidence of ED in a study of 350 men.[79]

Familial amyloid polyneuropathy

Familial amyloid polyneuropathy (FAP) is a group of autosomal dominant (AD) inherited degenerative disorders caused by systemic extracellular deposition of amyloid.[80] FAP patients manifest progressive sensory-motor length-dependent polyneuropathy and severe autonomic dysfunction. The autonomic manifestations include postural hypotension, nausea and vomiting, diarrhea and constipation, and sphincter disturbances, and ED is a prominent complaint reported by most patients with the condition.[80–82]

Muscular dystrophy

Myotonic dystrophy is an AD disorder caused by unstable trinucleotide repeat expansions. ED is more common in patients with larger trinucleotide repeat expansions and longer disease duration.[4] Patients with myotonic dystrophy type 1 (DM1) also present with hypogonadism, which involves both interstitial (androgenic) and tubular (spermatogenic) gonadal functions. ED is a frequent complaint in patients with DM1.[83]

Management of ED in the neurological patient

According to Lew-Starowicz and Rola, only 2.2% of patients had ever discussed their sexual concerns with a physician.[84] A PLISSIT (permission, limited information, specific suggestions, and intensive therapy) model has been developed to help healthcare professionals address the problem of sexual dysfunction, though not specifically for neurological patients.[85] In 2005, Rubin carried out a qualitative study, with a cross-sectional design, on perceived difficulties among healthcare professionals (nurses, occupational therapists, speech and language therapists, and physiotherapists) in discussing sexual problems with male patients with MS and compared them to the patient's views. This study demonstrated that healthcare professionals were wary about giving permission to talk about sex (according to the PLISSIT model), and were worried about intrusiveness and lack of information and training, while patients wanted this permission. Nurses were considered as the most appropriate member of the healthcare team to initiate a discussion on sexuality and sexual problems.[9]

When addressing ED, primary, secondary, and tertiary factors must be addressed (see Table 23.1) and the Multiple Sclerosis Intimacy and Sexuality Questionnaire – 19 (MSISQ-19), is a validated questionnaire that assesses these factors.[14,18]

Only a few studies have evaluated the efficacy of phosphodiesterase type 5 inhibitors (PDE5I) specifically in patients with neurological disease. One of the earlier studies evaluated sildenafil in patients with Parkinson's disease. It demonstrated statistically significant improvement in total Sexual Health Inventory-M version, overall sexual satisfaction, satisfaction with sexual desire, ability to achieve erection, ability to maintain erection, and ability to reach orgasm, with use of sildenafil citrate, while the Unified Parkinson's Disease Rating Scale (UPDRS) and Beck's Depression Inventory (BDI) were not significantly changed.[48] Several studies have demonstrated superior efficacy of PDE5Is in patients with ED resulting from neurological disease over ED from vascular or mixed etiologies.[86–88]

Two studies have evaluated the safety and efficacy of sildenafil citrate for ED in men with MS. Fowler et al. demonstrated 95% improvement in erections, as well as significant improvements in both general and disease-specific QoL variables.[60,89] Whereas, Safarinejad reported little improvement on ED compared to placebo and recommended against its use in the routine management of ED in patients with MS. The reason for such divergent findings is unclear; however, differences in patient selection may have contributed. A Cochrane review from 2012 assessing the efficacy and safety of sildenafil citrate for ED in patients with MS demonstrated limited evidence to support Viagra as an effective treatment to improve erectile function and quality of life at a short-term follow-up. Patients using sildenafil citrate were more likely to improve their ability to achieve and maintain an erection and complete intercourse. Adverse events were also reported; the most common were: headache, flushing, rhinitis, visual disturbances, and dyspepsia, but two patients suffered serious adverse events including one with coronary artery disease requiring triple bypass surgery and one with a cerebrovascular accident.[90] Quality of erections and satisfaction with sex life were found to be significantly improved with 50 mg oral sildenafil taken once daily in men with ED caused by spinal cord injury between T6 and L5.[91] In 2012, Lombardi et al. reviewed the literature on oral PDE5Is – sildenafil, tadalafil, and vardenafil – in individuals with central neurological disorder. They concluded that PDE5Is represent the first-line therapy for ED in patients with SCI. Though a meta-analysis was not possible, they found encouraging results for Parkinson's and MS patients.[92] A randomized, double-blind, placebo-controlled, crossover study of sildenafil citrate in the treatment of ED in patients with PD and MSA demonstrated significant improvement, with minimal change in blood pressure in the PD group of patients. In the group of MSA patients, despite a significant postural fall in blood pressure 1 hour after taking medication in three men, all patients were reluctant to discontinue medication. Due to their potential hypotensive side effects, PDE5Is should be used with caution in patients with autonomic dysfunction and postural hypotension. Ideally blood pressure fluctuations after taking a PDE5I should be assessed on a tilt table, especially before prescribing these medications to patients with parkinsonism due to difficulty in distinguishing Parkinson's disease from multiple system atrophy in the early stages.[93] There is a case report of transient global amnesia and hemorrhage from an arteriovenous malformation after premedication with tadalafil.[94]

The evidence supporting the use of other PDE5Is such as tadalafil and vardenafil is limited; however, in clinical practice they are used with benefit in neurological patients reporting ED.

Vacuum pumps and intracavernosal injections of prostaglandin E_2 are alternative strategies to managing ED; however, the evidence supporting their use is limited. Neurological functions, such as manual dexterity, need to be considered when discussing this option with the neurological patient. Surgical implantation of a penile prosthesis should be considered with caution and a proper neurological examination is paramount as patients with perineal sensory loss are at a greater risk for complications such as skin erosion. Moreover, patients with neurological disorders, especially those with spinal cord lesions, often rely on intermittent catheterization for bladder emptying, and implanting a penile prosthesis would not be possible in such patients.

Conclusion

Sexual dysfunction is common following neurological disease. Lesions of the cortex and subcortical white matter, basal ganglia and brainstem, long tracts of the spinal cord, and pelvic nerves may affect domains of sexual functions resulting in sexual dysfunction. This chapter reviews possible neurological causes of erectile dysfunction and disorder-specific management. PDE5I are considered to be more effective for ED of neurogenic etiology compared to vascular or mixed causes for ED.

Acknowlegdements

This work was undertaken at UCLH/UCL Institute of Neurology and is supported in part by funding from the United Kingdom's Department of Health NIHR Biomedical Research Centres funding scheme.

References

1 El-Kak F, Jurdi R, Kaddour A, Zurayk H. Gender and sexual health in clinical practice in Lebanon. *Int J Gynecol Obstet* 2004;87(3):260–6.

2 Nusbaum MR, Gamble G, Skinner B, Heiman J. The high prevalence of sexual concerns among women seeking routine gynecological care. *J Fam Pract* 2000;49(3):229–32.

3 Reamy K. Sexual counseling for the nontherapist. *Clin Obstet Gynecol* 1984;27(3):781–8.

4 Fowler CJ, Panicker JN, Emmanuel A. *Pelvic Organ Dysfunction in Neurological Disease*. New York: Cambridge University Press, 2010.

5 Aboseif S, Shinohara K, Borirakchanyavat S, Deirmenjian J, Carroll PR. The effect of cryosurgical ablation of the prostate on erectile function. *Brit J Urol* 1997;80(6):918–22.

6 Bronner G, Elran E, Golomb J, Korczyn AD. Female sexuality in multiple sclerosis: the multidimensional nature of the problem and the intervention. *Acta Neurol Scand* 2010;121(5): 289–301.

7 Guo ZN, He SY, Zhang HL, Wu J, Yang Y. Multiple sclerosis and sexual dysfunction. *Asian J Androl* 2012;14(4):530–5.

8 Janardhan V, Bakshi R. Quality of life and its relationship to brain lesions and atrophy on magnetic resonance images in 60 patients with multiple sclerosis. *Arch Neurol* 2000;57(10): 1485–91.

9 Rubin R. Communication about sexual problems in male patients with multiple sclerosis. *Nursing Standard* 2005;19(24):33–7.

10 Zorzon M, Zivadinov R, Monti Bragadin L, et al. Sexual dysfunction in multiple sclerosis: a 2-year follow-up study. *J Neurol Sci* 2001;187(1-2):1–5.

11 Redelman MJ. Sexual difficulties for persons with multiple sclerosis in New South Wales, Australia. *Int J Rehab Res* 2009;32(4):337–47.

12 Hemmett L, Holmes J, Barnes M, Russell N. What drives quality of life in multiple sclerosis? *QJM* 2004;97(10): 671–6.

13 Schairer LC, Foley FW, Zemon V, et al. The impact of sexual dysfunction on health-related quality of life in people with multiple sclerosis. *Mult Scler* 2014;20:610–6.

14 Celik DB, Poyraz EC, Bingol A, Idiman E, Ozakbas S, Kaya D. Sexual dysfunction in multiple sclerosis: gender differences. *J Neurol Sci* 2013;324(1-2):17–20.

15 Dewis ME, Thornton NG. Sexual dysfunction in multiple sclerosis. *J Neurosci Nurs* 1989;21(3):175–9.

16 Demirkiran M, Sarica Y, Uguz S, Yerdelen D, Aslan K. Multiple sclerosis patients with and without sexual dysfunction: are there any differences? *Mult Scler* 2006;12(2): 209–14.

17 Fletcher SG, Castro-Borrero W, Remington G, Treadaway K, Lemack GE, Frohman EM. Sexual dysfunction in patients with multiple sclerosis: a multidisciplinary approach to evaluation and management. *Nat Clin Pract Urol* 2009;6(2):96–107.

18 Foley FW, Zemon V, Campagnolo D, et al. The Multiple Sclerosis Intimacy and Sexuality Questionnaire – re-validation and development of a 15-item version with a large US sample. *Mult Scler* 2013;19(9):1197–203.

19 Merghati-Khoei E, Qaderi K, Amini L, Korte JE. Sexual problems among women with multiple sclerosis. *J Neurol Sci* 2013;331(1-2):81–5.

20 Arlt W, Hove U, Muller B, et al. Frequent and frequently overlooked: treatment-induced endocrine dysfunction in adult long-term survivors of primary brain tumors. *Neurology* 1997;49(2):498–506.

21 Ponsford J. Sexual changes associated with traumatic brain injury. *Neuropsychol Rehabil* 2003;13(1-2):275–89.

22 Kreuter M, Dahllof AG, Gudjonsson G, Sullivan M, Siosteen A. Sexual adjustment and its predictors after traumatic brain injury. *Brain Injury* 1998;12(5):349–68.

23 Ghigo E, Masel B, Aimaretti G, et al. Consensus guidelines on screening for hypopituitarism following traumatic brain injury. *Brain Injury* 2005;19(9):711–24.

24 Korpelainen JT, Nieminen P, Myllyla VV. Sexual functioning among stroke patients and their spouses. *Stroke* 1999;30(4): 715–9.

25 Kimura M, Murata Y, Shimoda K, Robinson RG. Sexual dysfunction following stroke. *Compr Psychiat* 2001;42(3): 217–22.

26 Jeon SW, Yoo KH, Kim TH, Kim JI, Lee CH. Correlation of the erectile dysfunction with lesions of cerebrovascular accidents. *The journal of sexual medicine*. 2009;6(1):251–6.

27 Rees PM, Fowler CJ, Maas CP. Sexual function in men and women with neurological disorders. *Lancet* 2007;369(9560): 512–25.

28 Hawton K. Sexual adjustment of men who have had strokes. *J Psychosom Res* 1984;28(3):243–9.

29 Houle TT, Dhingra LK, Remble TA, Rokicki LA, Penzien DB. Not tonight, I have a headache? *Headache*. 2006;46(6):983–90.

30 Aksoy D, Solmaz V, Cevik B, Gencten Y, Erdemir F, Kurt SG. The evaluation of sexual dysfunction in male patients with migraine and tension type headache. *J Headache Pain* 2013;14:46.

31 Hamed S, Mohamed K, El-Taher A, Hamed E, Omar H. The sexual and reproductive health in men with generalized epilepsy: a multidisciplinary evaluation. *Int J Impot Res* 2006;18(3):287–95.

32 Guldner GT, Morrell MJ. Nocturnal penile tumescence and rigidity evaluation in men with epilepsy. *Epilepsia* 1996; 37(12):1211–4.

33 Panicker JN, Fowler CJ, DasGupta R. Neurourology. In: Daroff RBFGMJJMJC, editor. Bradley's Neurology in Clinical Practice, 6th edition ed. Philadelphia: Elsevier Saunders; 2012. p. 668–86.

34 Souza EA, Keiralla DM, Silveira DC, Guerreiro CA. Sexual dysfunction in epilepsy: identifying the psychological variables. *Arq Neuro Psiquiat* 2000;58(2A):214–20.

35 Baird AD, Wilson SJ, Bladin PF, Saling MM, Reutens DC. Sexual outcome after epilepsy surgery. *Epilepsy Behav* 2003;4(3):268–78.

36 Herzog AG, Fowler KM. Sexual hormones and epilepsy: threat and opportunities. *Curr Opin Neurol* 2005;18(2): 167–72.

37 Lambert MV. Seizures, hormones and sexuality. *Seizure* 2001;10(5):319–40.

38 Herzog AG, Drislane FW, Schomer DL, et al. Differential effects of antiepileptic drugs on sexual function and hormones in men with epilepsy. *Neurology* 2005;65(7): 1016–20.

39 Maschio M, Saveriano F, Dinapoli L, Jandolo B. Reversible erectile dysfunction in a patient with brain tumor-related epilepsy in therapy with zonisamide in add-on. *J Sex Med* 2011;8(12):3515–7.

40 Civardi C, Collini A, Gontero P, Monaco F. Vasogenic erectile dysfunction topiramate-induced. *Clin Neurol Neurosurg* 2012;114(1):70–1.

41 Hung LC, Chow JC, Chang CY, Tsai JJ, Huang CW. Topiramate related reversible erectile dysfunction in temporal lobe epilepsy. *Neurol Sci* 2012;33(2):331–3.

42 Chaudhuri KR, Healy DG, Schapira AH, National Institute for Clinical Excellence. Non-motor symptoms of Parkinson's disease: diagnosis and management. *Lancet Neurol* 2006;5(3):235–45.

43 Sakakibara R, Shinotoh H, Uchiyama T, et al. Questionnaire-based assessment of pelvic organ dysfunction in Parkinson's disease. *Auton Neurosci Basic Clin* 2001;92(1-2):76–85.

44 Montorsi F, Perani D, Anchisi D, et al. Apomorphine-induced brain modulation during sexual stimulation: a new look at central phenomena related to erectile dysfunction. *Int J Impot Res* 2003;15(3):203–9.

45 Bellomo G, Santambrogio L, Fiacconi M, Scarponi AM, Ciuffetti G. Plasma profiles of adrenocorticotropic hormone, cortisol, growth hormone and prolactin in patients with untreated Parkinson's disease. *J Urol* 1991;238(1):19–22.

46 Bronner G, Royter V, Korczyn AD, Giladi N. Sexual dysfunction in Parkinson's disease. *J Sex Marital Ther* 2004;30(2):95–105.

47 Sakakibara R, Uchiyama T, Yamanishi T, Kishi M. Genitourinary dysfunction in Parkinson's disease. *Movement Disord* 2010;25(1):2–12.

48 Zesiewicz TA, Helal M, Hauser RA. Sildenafil citrate (Viagra) for the treatment of erectile dysfunction in men with Parkinson's disease. *Movement Disord* 2000;15(2):305–8.

49 Wullner U, Schmitz-Hubsch T, Antony G, Fimmers R, Spottke A, Oertel WH, et al. Autonomic dysfunction in 3414 Parkinson's disease patients enrolled in the German Network on Parkinson's disease (KNP e.V.): the effect of ageing. European journal of neurology. 2007;14(12):1405–8.

50 Singer F, Zumoff B. Subnormal serum testosterone levels in male internal medicine residents. *Steroids* 1992;57(2):86–9.

51 Weintraub D, Koester J, Potenza MN, et al. Impulse control disorders in Parkinson disease: a cross-sectional study of 3090 patients. *Arch Neurol* 2010;67(5):589–95.

52 Kirchhof K, Apostolidis AN, Mathias CJ, Fowler CJ. Erectile and urinary dysfunction may be the presenting features in patients with multiple system atrophy: a retrospective study. *Int J Impot Res* 2003;15(4):293–8.

53 Beck RO, Betts CD, Fowler CJ. Genitourinary dysfunction in multiple system atrophy: clinical features and treatment in 62 cases. *J Urol* 1994;151(5):1336–41.

54 Heaton JP. Central neuropharmacological agents and mechanisms in erectile dysfunction: the role of dopamine. *Neurosci Behav Rev* 2000;24(5):561–9.

55 Kessler TM, Fowler CJ, Panicker JN. Sexual dysfunction in multiple sclerosis. *Exp Rev Neurother* 2009;9(3):341–50.

56 Burina A, Sinanovic O. [Bladder, bowel and sexual dysfunction in patient with mulitple sclerosis.] *Medicinski arhiv* 2006;60(3):182–4.

57 Crayton HJ, Rossman HS. Managing the symptoms of multiple sclerosis: a multimodal approach. *Clin Ther* 2006;28(4): 445–60.

58 Schapiro RT, Langer SL. Symptomatic therapy of multiple sclerosis. *Curr Opin Neurol* 1994;7(3):229–33.

59 Zorzon M, Zivadinov R, Bosco A, et al. Sexual dysfunction in multiple sclerosis: a case-control study. I. Frequency and comparison of groups. *Mult Scler* 1999;5(6):418–27.

60 Fowler CJ, Miller JR, Sharief MK, Hussain IF, Stecher VJ, Sweeney M. A double blind, randomised study of sildenafil citrate for erectile dysfunction in men with multiple sclerosis. *J Neurol Neurosurg Psychiat* 2005;76(5):700–5.

61 Zivadinov R, Zorzon M, Locatelli L, et al. Sexual dysfunction in multiple sclerosis: a MRI, neurophysiological and urodynamic study. *J Neurol Sci* 2003;210(1-2):73–6.

62 Tepavcevic DK, Kostic J, Basuroski ID, Stojsavljevic N, Pekmezovic T, Drulovic J. The impact of sexual dysfunction on the quality of life measured by MSQoL-54 in patients with multiple sclerosis. *Mult Scler* 2008;14(8):1131–6.

63 Barak Y, Achiron A, Elizur A, Gabbay U, Noy S, Sarova-Pinhas I. Sexual dysfunction in relapsing-remitting multiple sclerosis: magnetic resonance imaging, clinical, and psychological correlates. *J Psychiat Neurosci* 1996;21(4):255–8.
64 Forbes A, While A, Mathes L, Griffiths P. Health problems and health-related quality of life in people with multiple sclerosis. *Clin Rehabil* 2006;20(1):67–78.
65 Kurtzke JF. Rating neurologic impairment in multiple sclerosis: an expanded disability status scale (EDSS). *Neurology* 1983;33(11):1444–52.
66 Mohammadi K, Rahnama P, Moayed Mohseni S, Sahraian MA, Montazeri A. Determinants of sexual dysfunction in women with multiple sclerosis. *BMC Neurol* 2013;13(1):83.
67 Nortvedt MW, Riise T, Frugard J, et al. Prevalence of bladder, bowel and sexual problems among multiple sclerosis patients two to five years after diagnosis. *Mult Scler* 2007;13(1):106–12.
68 Vitkova M, Rosenberger J, Krokavcova M, et al. Health-related quality of life in multiple sclerosis patients with bladder, bowel and sexual dysfunction. *Disabil Rehabil* 2014;36:987–92.
69 Landtblom AM. Treatment of erectile dysfunction in multiple sclerosis. *Exp Rev Neurother* 2006;6(6):931–5.
70 Betts CD, Jones SJ, Fowler CG, Fowler CJ. Erectile dysfunction in multiple sclerosis. Associated neurological and neurophysiological deficits, and treatment of the condition. *Brain* 1994;117(Pt 6):1303–10.
71 Lottman PE, Jongen PJ, Rosier PF, Meuleman EJ. Sexual dysfunction in men with multiple sclerosis – a comprehensive pilot-study into etiology. *Int J Impot Res* 1998;10(4):233–7.
72 Alexander CJ, Sipski ML, Findley TW. Sexual activities, desire, and satisfaction in males pre- and post-spinal cord injury. *Arch Sex Behav* 1993;22(3):217–28.
73 Bors E, Turner RD. History and physical examination in neurological urology. *J Urol* 1960;83:759–67.
74 Podnar S, Oblak C, Vodusek DB. Sexual function in men with cauda equina lesions: a clinical and electromyographic study. *J Neurol Neurosurg Psychiat* 2002;73(6):715–20.
75 Sartucci F, Piaggesi A, Logi F, et al. Impaired ascendant central pathways conduction in impotent diabetic subjects. *Acta Neurol Scand* 1999;99(6):381–6.
76 Lew-Starowicz M, Gellert R. The sexuality and quality of life of hemodialyzed patients – ASED multicenter study. *J Sex Med* 2009;6(4):1062–71.
77 Ravaglia S, Marchioni E, Costa A, Maurelli M, Moglia A. Erectile dysfunction as a sentinel symptom of cardiovascular autonomic neuropathy in heavy drinkers. *J Peripher Nerv Syst* 2004;9(4):209–14.
78 Zochodne DW. Autonomic involvement in Guillain-Barré syndrome: a review. *Muscle Nerve* 1994;17(10):1145–55.
79 Burk K, Weiss A. Impotence after recovery from Guillain-Barré syndrome. *New Jersey Med* 1998;95(11):31–4.
80 Hund E. Familial amyloidotic polyneuropathy: current and emerging treatment options for transthyretin-mediated amyloidosis. *Applic Clin Genet* 2012;5:37–41.
81 Denier C, Ducot B, Husson H, et al. A brief compound test for assessment of autonomic and sensory-motor dysfunction in familial amyloid polyneuropathy. *J Neurol* 2007;254(12):1684–8.
82 Yoshioka A, Yamaya Y, Saiki S, et al. A case of familial amyloid polyneuropathy homozygous for the transthyretin Val30Met gene with motor-dominant sensorimotor polyneuropathy and unusual sural nerve pathological findings. *Arch Neurol* 2001;58(11):1914–8.
83 Antonini G, Clemenzi A, Bucci E, et al. Hypogonadism in DM1 and its relationship to erectile dysfunction. *J Neurol* 2011;258(7):1247–53.
84 Lew-Starowicz M, Rola R. Prevalence of sexual dysfunctions among women with multiple sclerosis. *Sex Disabil* 2013;31(2):141–53.
85 Annon J. PLISSIT therapy. Corsini RJ, editor. *Handbook of Innovative Psychotherapies*. New York: John Wiley & Sons, Inc., 1981; pp. 626–39.
86 Steers WD. Viagra – after one year. *Urology* 1999;54(1):12–7.
87 Rendell MS, Rajfer J, Wicker PA, Smith MD. Sildenafil for treatment of erectile dysfunction in men with diabetes: a randomized controlled trial. Sildenafil Diabetes Study Group. *JAMA* 1999;281(5):421–6.
88 Safarinejad MR, Taghva A, Shekarchi B, Safarinejad S. Safety and efficacy of sildenafil citrate in the treatment of Parkinson-emergent erectile dysfunction: a double-blind, placebo-controlled, randomized study. *Int J Impot Res* 2010;22(5):325–35.
89 Safarinejad MR. Evaluation of the safety and efficacy of sildenafil citrate for erectile dysfunction in men with multiple sclerosis: a double-blind, placebo controlled, randomized study. *J Urol* 2009;181(1):252–8.
90 Xiao Y, Wang J, Luo H. Sildenafil citrate for erectile dysfunction in patients with multiple sclerosis. *Cochrane Database Syst Rev* 2012;4:CD009427.
91 Derry FA, Dinsmore WW, Fraser M, et al. Efficacy and safety of oral sildenafil (Viagra) in men with erectile dysfunction caused by spinal cord injury. *Neurology* 1998;51(6):1629–33.
92 Lombardi G, Nelli F, Celso M, Mencarini M, Del Popolo G. Treating erectile dysfunction and central neurological diseases with oral phosphodiesterase type 5 inhibitors. Review of the literature. *J Sex Med* 2012;9(4):970–85.
93 Hussain IF, Brady CM, Swinn MJ, Mathias CJ, Fowler CJ. Treatment of erectile dysfunction with sildenafil citrate (Viagra) in parkinsonism due to Parkinson's disease or multiple system atrophy with observations on orthostatic hypotension. *J Neurol Neurosurg Psychiat* 2001;71(3):371–4.
94 Schiefer J, Sparing R. Transient global amnesia after intake of tadalafil, a PDE-5 inhibitor: a possible association? *Int J Impot Res* 2005;17(4):383–4.

CHAPTER 24

Non-surgical therapy for Peyronie's disease

Rowland Rees and Victoria Dawson
University Hospital Southampton, Southampton, UK

The first detailed description of Peyronie's disease (PD) appears in 1743, in François de la Peyronie's manuscript about erectile dysfunction. However, simplified accounts of the condition date back as far as 1687.[1] The disease is characterized by the formation of fibrotic plaques within the tunica albuginea leading to penile pain and curvature. The commonest mode of presentation is with a penile curvature preventing sexual intercourse, but men may seek medical advice for a number of reasons, such as pain, worry about a palpable lump, erectile dysfunction, or a change in shape of the penis. There may also be shortening, with attendant loss of self-esteem and sexual confidence, thus Peyronie's is often a depressing condition.

Although its etiology is not fully understood, the most widely accepted hypothesis is repeated microvascular injury or trauma to the tunica albuginea coupled with abnormal wound healing, resulting in inelastic fibrous plaque[2] (Figure 24.1). A number of associated conditions have been identified supporting the theory of microvascular insult. They include hypertension, diabetes, smoking, dyslipidemia, and obesity[3] (Table 24.1).

Broadly speaking there are two phases observed in Peyronie's disease: In the acute phase, there is active inflammation with increased proliferation of tunical fibroblasts, resulting in excessive deposition of collagen. Increasing deformity of the erect penis and penile pain occur in some, but not all patients. This initial inflammatory phase usually lasts up to 6 months, and the disease will then enter a chronic state. During this phase, there is disordered wound healing resulting in plaque stabilization and resolution of pain.[2]

A variety of molecular mechanisms have been described in connection with Peyronie's disease. Each of these processes has subsequently been targeted pharmacologically in order to improve outcomes of the disease. A well-described mechanism is the involvement of transforming growth factor-β1 (TGF-β1) in the accumulation of collagen. Ultimately activation of TGF-β1 results in an increase in connective tissue synthesis along with the inhibition of collagenases. TGF-β1 is a cytokine synthesized by a variety of cells including fibroblasts, macrophages, and platelets. Interestingly TGF-β1 has the ability to self-induce, which may underpin the development of scarring and fibrosis in PD.[2] The link between TGF-β1 and Peyronie's comes from studies showing an increase in protein expression of TGF-β1 in tunica albuginea biopsies taken from PD patients when compared to non-PD patients.[2] It has also been hypothesized that oxidative damage may be causal in the initiation and progression of the tissue fibrosis seen in PD, and thus there has also been an interest in antioxidants and their potential effect on disease progression.[2]

Treatment options will depend on the stage and severity of disease. The natural history of the disease results in spontaneous improvement in curvature in up to 13% of patients.[4] It is therefore advised that there is at least some period of observation. Surgical intervention is widely accepted as the mainstay of treatment in severe cases (once the patient has stable disease). However, the primary aim of intervention is to keep patients sexually active by restricting curvature progression. Therefore there has been a real interest in attempting to halt the disease process in the early phase with oral medications and intralesional injections, thus reducing the need for surgery.

Male Sexual Dysfunction: A Clinical Guide, First Edition. Edited by Suks Minhas and John Mulhall.

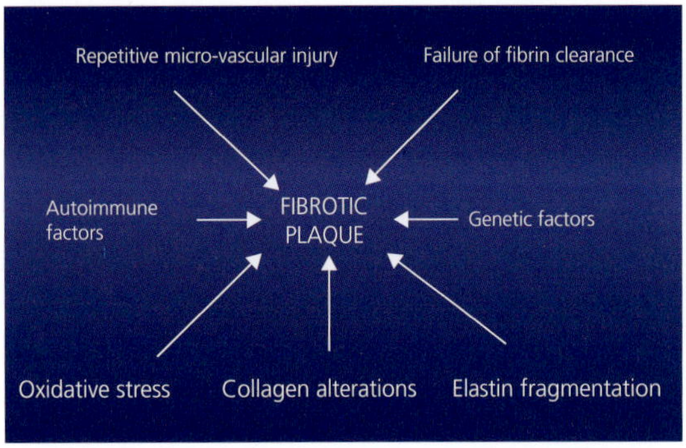

Figure 24.1 The pathophysiological theories for Peyronie's disease.

Table 24.1 Vascular risk factors in Peyronie's disease.

Risk factor	*N*	%
Hypercholesterolemia	132	43
Diabetes	102	33
Hypertriglyceridemia	87	28
Hypertension	45	15
IHD	25	8
TOTAL	307	67
ED	167	54

ED, erectile dysfunction; IHD ischemic heart disease.
Source: Kadioglu (2002).[37] Reproduced with permission of Elsevier.

Oral therapies in Peyronie's disease

The focus of oral therapies relates to the disruption of either the inflammatory process in the acute phase, or the disordered wound healing of the chronic phase in order to improve symptoms and either stabilize or reduce curvature.

The advantages of a successful oral therapy would be modified disease progression in the early phase, directly reducing morbidity due to Peyronie's disease, but also reducing the need for more invasive (surgical) therapy in a proportion of patients. It would also offer a real alternative for those not fit or keen for surgery.

A number of oral medications have been trialed on the basis of the relationship between the drug's mechanism of action and the hypothesized pathophysiology of Peyronie's disease. However, there is a lack of robust randomized controlled trials that have truly demonstrated a clear benefit for any single drug, and the US Food and Drug Administration (FDA) has only deemed potassium para-aminobenzoate (Potaba) as "possibly effective" in the treatment of Peyronie's disease.

Potassium para-aminobenzoate (Potaba)

The use of Potaba in Peyronie's disease was first introduced in 1959; however, studies have failed to show convincingly any significant improvement in symptoms, curvature, and plaque size. Its popularity is decreasing due to its high side-effect profile (mainly gastrointestinal effects and photosensitivity) and high cost.[1,4]

Mechanism of action: Thought to exert an anti-fibrotic effect; however, exact mechanism of action is unclear. It has been postulated that it rebalances the effects of serotonin and monoamine oxidases (MAO) at the tissue level through increased oxygen utilization, which in turn is thought to promote degradation of serotonin by enhancing MAO action.[5,6]

Evidence: A randomized controlled trial (RCT) in 2005 demonstrated a significant plaque-related effect of Potaba, and conclusions from the study suggested the drug may stabilize disease by preventing curvature progression.[5]

Advantages: Some evidence it improves penile pain and plaque size; however, results have not been reproducible.[5,7]

Disadvantages: Expensive. Multiple dosing. Extensive side-effect profile – nausea, anorexia, photosensitivity, anxiety, and difficulty concentrating, amongst others.

Vitamin E (tocopherol)

As both an inexpensive and safe product, the use of vitamin E by urologists for the treatment of PD has been popular since the 1940s. There was initially support in the literature for its use; however, more recent studies have failed to support this practice.[1,4] It has more recently been trialed in combination with other therapies, which has raised interest in this preparation once again. However, it somewhat "muddies the water," making it difficult to draw any clear conclusions about its individual efficacy. In these combinations it does appear to have some synergistic effect and so there may still be a place for vitamin E in the treatment of Peyronie's. However, more robust RCTs are needed to demonstrate this.

Mechanism of action: Acts as an antioxidant by scavenging oxygen free radicals, which are thought to promote fibrosis.[1]

Evidence: Conflicting results. Both Safarinejad and Hosseini[8] and Hashimoto and Hisasue[9] failed to show any statistically significant improvements in the treatment arm of their studies. There is more encouraging evidence from its use in combination with other agents.[10]

Advantages: Widely available. Low toxicity. Low cost.

Disadvantages: Minimal reproducible evidence of improvement in symptoms or penile curvature.

Tamoxifen

An initial study in the early 1990s studying the effects of tamoxifen on Peyronie's disease was performed after the drug was shown to be effective in the treatment of desmoid tumors, a condition thought to have histological similarities with Peyronie's disease.[11] Its effect on the integral TGF-β1 pathway was thought to be key to its anticipated success. Although this initial study bore positive results, subsequent research has failed to reproduce those early outcomes.

Mechanism of action: Non-steroidal antiestrogen. Thought to inhibit fibroblast proliferation as well as decrease collagen production by inhibiting the production and release of TGF-β1.[11,12]

Evidence: Main reference paper is a small RCT by Teloken et al., which demonstrated no significant improvement in plaque size, curvature or pain when compared to placebo.[12] The study was limited by its small size and poor description of randomization and blinding.

Advantages: Low side-effect profile.

Disadvantages: Poor evidence for its use.

Colchicine

More commonly seen as a treatment for gout, the interest in colchicine as a potential treatment for PD was first explored after a 1994 pilot study produced promising outcomes showing decreased plaque size and improved penile curvature.[13] More recently, robust studies have failed to reproduce these encouraging results. It has also been used in combination with vitamin E, and was initially shown to improve plaque size and penile curvature. However, there remains conflicting evidence and lack of large randomized trials to support this.[14,15] It is still, however, used widely as a medical alternative in the treatment of Peyronie's disease by American urologists.[16]

Mechanism of action: The precise mechanism of action of colchicine has not yet been completely established. It has, however, been shown to downregulate TGF-β1 in animal models.[13] Colchicine has anti-inflammatory properties that are thought to reduce collagen synthesis as well as potentiate collagenase activity.[13]

Evidence: Initially a pilot study demonstrated reductions in plaque size in 50% of patients (12/24), and 7 out of 19 patients had improvements in penile curvature.[13] A more recent RCT showed no statistically significant benefit in the treatment arm when compared to placebo.[17] Combination preparations (colchicines plus vitamin E) require further consideration as studies have failed to consistently show improvements with their use.[15] An adequately sized RCT is needed to appropriately answer this question.

Advantages: Potential improvements in plaque size and penile curvature. Has been used in combination preparations. Low side-effect profile. Once a day dosing.

Disadvantages: No clear evidence of improved outcomes.

Acetyl esters of carnitine

Carnitine, or more specifically acetyl-L-carnitine, was first trialed as an oral alternative in the treatment of PD in 2001 by Biagiotti and Cavallini after it was shown to be effective in the treatment of oxidative diseases and idiopathic infertility, where its use stems from its proposed antioxidant properties.[18] Results of this study were promising as outcomes showed it was more effective than tamoxifen at reducing pain and halting disease progression. However, more recent studies have shown no significant improvement in pain, curvature, or plaque size when compared to placebo, either on its own or in combination with vitamin E.[1,4]

Mechanism of action: It is suggested that carnitine reduces the intracellular calcium levels in endothelial cells resulting in a reduction in collagen production and fibroblast proliferation. This, in turn, is thought to reduce penile fibrosis seen in PD.

Evidence: A 2001 RCT by Biagiotti and Cavallini demonstrating statistically significant outcomes (namely halting curvature progression) in patients taking 2 g/day of acetyl-L-carnitine when compared to those taking tamoxifen.[18] More recently, Safarinejad et al. found no significant improved outcomes in penile pain, curvature, or plaque size in patients taking acetyl-L-carnitine either alone or in combination with vitamin E when compared to placebo.[19] There is some evidence that in combination with verapamil intraplaque injection, carnitine may improve disease outcomes; however, it is difficult to isolate the active drug responsible for these outcomes.[20]

Advantages: May be effective in combination with other agents.

Disadvantages: Minimal rationale and evidence for its use.

Phosphodiesterase type 5 inhibitors (PDE5i)

PDE5i have long been used by urologists in the treatment of erectile dysfunction. It has been proposed that they cause inhibition of tissue remodeling after injury and thus may be advantageous in the treatment of PD.[21]

Mechanism of action: Increase cyclic GMP levels, which prevents deposition of collagen by inhibiting TGF-β1, oxidative stress, and myofibroblast accretion.[21]

Evidence: Animal models have shown reduced plaque size and increased fibroblast apoptosis.[21] A retrospective study looking specifically at the resolution of penile septal scar with the use of PDE5i recorded significant improvements in both scar size and erectile function, neither of which are common outcomes in the assessment of oral therapies and their use in PD.[21]

Advantages: Safe. Useful in patients with coexisting erectile dysfunction.

Disadvantages: Studies yet to look at standard outcomes such as plaque size and curvature other than in rat models. Lack of prospective RCTs.

Pentoxifylline (PTX)

PTX is a methylxanthine derivative that inhibits phosphodiesterase. It is more commonly used in the treatment of arteriopathic disease, particularly in preventing atherosclerosis in hypertensive patients with type 2 diabetes mellitus, which, given the associated conditions of PD is very interesting. PTX has been shown in rat models to induce regression of collagen and TGF-β1-mediated plaque formation, and therefore has attracted interest as a potential treatment in PD.[22] It also appears to have anti-inflammatory and anti-fibrogenic properties and has been successful as an experimental treatment in a number of autoimmune diseases. With urologists still searching for the silver bullet medical alternative in the treatment of PD, PTX has been regarded in recent years as the next hopeful remedy. Results have been encouraging although outcomes are by no means cures. However, larger and repeated trials are needed to cement the use of PTX in PD.

Mechanism of action: Downregulates TGF-β1-mediated inflammation and inhibits the deposition of type 1 collagen. Increases fibrinolytic activity.[23]

Evidence: Safarinejad et al.'s 2009 RCT placebo trial is the main index study supporting the use of PTX in PD, but unfortunately this paper was retracted in 2015 due to questions over statistical methods and validity.[24] Outcomes were reduced rates of disease progression as well as improved penile curvature and plaque volume in the treatment arm. In the treatment group 40.5% of patients had a measurable improvement in penile curvature, with a mean change of 23°.[25] Unsurprisingly International Index of Erectile Function (IIEF) scores improved in patients receiving PTX.

Advantages: Safe. Some evidence suggestive of benefit, but the quality of evidence remains in question.

Disadvantages: Minimal evidence. Marginal gains. Main study looked specifically at patients with "early chronic" disease.

Coenzyme Q10 (CoQ10)

CoQ10 is fat-soluble vitamin-like quinolone. Decreased serum levels of CoQ10 have been found in diseases associated with oxidative stress.[26] It is a potent antioxidant, and the theory of its use in PD stems from speculation that the inflammation seen in the acute/early chronic stages of the disease is, in part, due to low antioxidant activity. It has also been reported that solubilized CoQ10 suppresses the expression of TGF-β1.

Mechanism of action: Hypothesized that a failure to respond to oxygen free radicals produced in the inflammatory phase of Peyronie's disease may lead to disease progression and therefore potent antioxidants such as CoQ10 may act as protection against oxidative stress.

Evidence: One RCT to date. Showed improvement in erectile function (measured via IIEF scores). Also demonstrated reduction in plaque size and penile curvature.

Advantages: Safe. Cheap. RCT showed positive outcomes.

Disadvantages: Small study (treatment group $n = 81$ who completed trial period). More studies needed to reproduce results. Improvements in penile curvature much more pronounced in patients with curvatures less than 30°.

Omega-3

Omega-3 is a polyunsaturated fatty acid that was postulated to suppress disease progression given its inhibition of inflammation. One RCT has been performed to date, which failed to show any significant improvement when used in PD.

Mechanism of action: Inhibits the release of inflammatory cytokines and increases collagenase activity.

Evidence: One RCT failed to show any significant improvements in outcomes.[27]

Advantages: Cheap. Safe.

Disadvantages: No evidence supporting its use.

Topical agents

Verapamil has been described as a topical agent for PD, applied as a gel. In one study, 15% verapamil hydrochloride was compared with placebo. There was a significantly greater improvement in curvature (43% improvement) in the treatment group versus in the treatment group at 3 months, and this was improved further at 9 months (61%). Pain and plaque size also showed significant improvement.[28] However, there are few other studies, some of which have failed to prove that verapamil reaches the plaque in a meaningful concentration, raising doubts as to its mechanism of action.

Studies examining the effect of electromotive administration (EMDA) of verapamil into the penis have shown conflicting results.[29,30]

Injectable agents

A number of agents have been developed to be injected intralesionally into the Peyronie's plaque. Interferon and collagenase are the only agents to have shown benefit.

Steroids

A single blind study using intralesional injection of betamethasone did not yield a significant improvement in deformity, plaque size, or pain. In addition, steroid injections have negative side effects such as thinning of the skin and immune suppression.[31]

Interferon

Through its actions of reducing collagen production, interferon-2α has been used as an injectable agent (5 million units twice a week for 12 weeks), with a slight improvement in curvature, plaque size, and pain as compared to placebo. However, interferon is associated with significant generalized side effects such as myalgia and flu-like symptoms.[32]

Verapamil

Verapamil has also been used as an intralesional agent due to its in vitro effect on collagenase activity and fibroblast proliferation. However, clinical studies have failed to demonstrate significant improvements in penile curvature, plaque size, or pain.[33]

Collagenase

Following the successful use of collagenase in Dupuytren's contracture, its use has recently been studied in the treatment of PD. In the IMPRESS trial, 832 men from the United States and Australia were randomized to receive either collagenase or placebo injections, and patients in the treatment arm underwent four cycles of treatment, 6 weeks apart; each cycle consisted of two injections 1–3 days apart (0.58 mg), and investigator modeling (plaque stretching) 1–3 days later.[34] The patients were also told to model their penis regularly afterwards. There was an overall 35% improvement in curvature in the treatment arm (average 17° improvement, vs −9.3° change in the placebo arm). Minor side effects such as bruising were very common, but major side effects such as penile rupture were rare (<1%).

Mechanical devices

Mechanical devices have also recently been used in the management of PD. In a comparison of a penile traction device versus no treatment, patients wore a device for an average of 4.6 hours a day for 6 months, with a mean improvement in curvature of 20° (vs a worsening of 23° in the control group).[35] The vacuum erection device has also been described as improving penile curvature in PD, but to date there are no controlled studies demonstrating superiority over conservative management.[36]

Conclusion

A number of medical treatments have been described for the treatment of PD although they have limited efficacy. Despite some that have shown some encouraging results, there is a distinct lack of powered RCTs and reproducible results. It is clear that halting disease progression and maintaining sexual function should be the aim of oral therapies; however, further analysis into those treatments that have so far produced positive outcomes is warranted. The use of CoQ10 and phosphodiesterase inhibitors may well be beneficial, although the novel collagenases appear to be promising in men with PD.

References

1 Tan RB, Sangkum P, Mitchell GC, et al. Update on medical management of Peyronie's disease. *Curr Urol Rep* 2014;15:415–23.
2 Moreland RB, Nehra A. Pathophysiology of Peyronie's disease. *Int J Impot Res* 2002;14:406–10.
3 Shaw EJ, Mitchell GC, Tan RB, et al. The non-surgical treatment of Peyronie disease: 2013 update. *World J Mens Health* 2013;31(3):183–92.
4 Hatzimouratidis K, Eardley I, Giuliano F, et al. EAU guidelines on penile curvature. *Eur Urol* 2012;62:543–52.
5 Weider W, Hauck E. Potassium paraaminobenzoate (Potaba) in the treatment of Peyronie's disease: a prospective, placebo-controlled randomized study. *Eur Urol* 2005;47: 530–6.
6 Hellstrom WJ. Medical management of Peyronie's disease. *J Androl* 2009;30(4):397–405.
7 Shah PJR, Green NA, Adib RS, et al. A multicentre double-blind controlled clinical trial of potassium para-amino-benzoate (POTABA1) in Peyronie's disease. *Progr Reprod Biol Med J* 1983;9:61–7.
8 Safarinejad M, Hosseini S. Comparison of vitamin E and propionyl-L-carnitine, separately or in combination, in patients with early chronic Peyronie's disease: a double-blind, placebo controlled, randomized study. *J Urol* 2007;178:1398–403.
9 Hashimoto K, Hisasue S. Outcome analysis for conservative management of Peyronie's disease. *Int J Urol* 2006;13:244–7.
10 Paulis G, Brancato T, D'Ascenzo R, et al. Efficacy of vitamin E in the conservative treatment of Peyronie's disease: legend or reality? A controlled study of 70 cases. *Andrology* 2013;1(1):120–8.
11 Ralph DJ, Brooks MD, Bottazzo GF, et al. The treatment of Peyronie's disease with Tamoxifen. *BJU Int*1992;70:658–51.
12 Teloken C, Rhoden EL, Grazziotin TM, et al. Tamoxifen versus placebo in the treatment of Peyronie's disease. *J Urol* 1999;162:2003–5.
13 Akkus E, Breza J, Carrie S, et al. Is colchine effective in Peyronie's disease? A pilot study. *Urology* 1994;44:291–6.
14 Prieto Castro RM, Leva Vallejo ME, Regueiro Lopez JC, et al. Combined treatment with vitamin E and colchicine in the early stages of Peyronie's disease. *BJU Int* 2003;91(6): 522–4.
15 Cortes-Gonzalez JR, Glina S. Conservative treatment of Peyronie's disease: colchicines vs colchicines plus vitamin E. *Actas Urol Esp* 2010;34(5):444–9.
16 Shindel AW, Bullock T. Urologist practice patterns in the management of Peyronie's disease: a national wide survey. *J Sex Med* 2008;5:954–64.
17 Safarinejad MR. Therapeutic effects of colchicine in the management of Peyronie's disease: a randomized double-blind, placebo-controlled study. *Int J Impot Res* 2004; 16(3):238–43.
18 Biagiotti G, Cavallini G. Acetyl-L-carnitine vs Tamoxifen in the oral therapy of Peyronie's disease: a preliminary report. *BJU Int* 2001;88:63–7.
19 Safarinejad MR, Hosseini SY, Kolahi AA. Comparison of vitamin E and propionyl-L-carnitine, separately or in combination, in patients with early chronic Peyronie's disease: a double-blind, placebo controlled, randomized study. *J Urol* 2007;178:1398–403.
20 Cavallini G, Biagiotti G. Oral propionyl-L-carnitine and intraplaque verapamil in the therapy of advanced and resistant Peyronie's disease. *BJU Int* 2002;89:895.
21 Chung E, Deyoung L. The role of PDE5 inhibitors in penile septal scar remodelling: assessment of clinical and radiological outcomes. *J Sex Med* 2011;8(5):1472–7.
22 Smith J, Shindel A, Huang YC, et al. Pentoxifylline treatment and penile calcifications in men with Peyronie's disease. *Asian J Androl* 2011;13:322–5.
23 Shindel A, Lin G, Ning H, et al. Pentoxifylline attenuates transforming growth factor-β1 stimulated collagen deposition and elastogenesis in human tunica albuginea-derived fibroblasts part 1: Impact on extracellular matrix. *J Sex Med* 2010;7(6):2077–85.
24 Safarinejad MR, Asgari MA, Hosseini SY, Dadkhah F. Retraction statement: A double-blind placebo-controlled study of the efficacy and safety of pentoxifylline in early chronic Peyronie's disease. *BJU Int* 2015;115(3):E10. doi: 10.1111/bju.13063.
25 Safarinejad MR, Asgari MA, Hosseini SY, et al. A double-blind placebo-controlled study of the efficacy and safety of pentoxifylline in early chronic Peyronie's disease. *BJU Int* 2010;106:240–8.
26 Safarinejad MR. Safety and efficacy of co-enzyme Q10 supplementation in early chronic Peyronie's disease: a double-blind placebo-controlled randomized study. *Int J Impot Res* 2010;22:298–309.
27 Safarinejad MR. Efficacy and safety of omega-3 for treatment of early-stage Peyronie's disease: a prospective, randomized, double-blind placebo-controlled study. *J Sex Med* 2009;6:1743–54.
28 Fitch 3rd WP, Easterling WJ, Talbert RL, et al. Topical verapamil HCl, topical trifluoperazine, and topical magnesium sulfate for the treatment of Peyronie's disease – a placebo-controlled pilot study. *J Sex Med* 2007;4:477–84.
29 Di Stasi SM, Giannantoni A, Stephen RL, et al. A prospective, randomized study using transdermal electromotive

administration of verapamil and dexamethasone for Peyronie's disease. *J Urol* 2004;171:1605–8.

30 Greenfield JM, Shah SJ, Levine LA. Verapamil versus saline in electromotive drug administration for Peyronie's disease: a double-blind, placebo controlled trial. *J Urol* 2007;177: 972–5.

31 Cipollone G, Nicolai M, Mastroprimiano G, et al. Betamethasone versus placebo in Peyronie's disease [in Italian]. *Arch Ital Urol Androl* 1998;70:165–8.

32 Hellstrom WJ, Kendirci M, Matern R, et al. Single-blind, multicenter, placebo controlled, parallel study to assess the safety and efficacy of intralesional interferon alpha-2B for minimally invasive treatment for Peyronie's disease. *J Urol* 2006;176:394–8.

33 Shirazi M, Haghpanah AR, Badiee M, et al. Effect of intralesional verapamil for treatment of Peyronie's disease: a randomized single-blind, placebo-controlled study. *Int Urol Nephrol* 2009;41:467–71.

34 Gelbard M, Goldstein I, Hellstrom WJ, et al. Clinical efficacy, safety and tolerability of collagenase clostridium histolyticum for the treatment of Peyronie disease in 2 large double-blind, randomized, placebo controlled phase 3 studies. *J Urol* 2013;190(1):199–207.

35 Levine LA, Newell M, Taylor FL. Penile traction therapy for treatment of Peyronie's disease: a single-center pilot study. *J Sex Med* 2008;5:1468–73.

36 Raheem AA, Garaffa G, Raheem TA, et al. The role of vacuum pump therapy to mechanically straighten the penis in Peyronie's disease. *BJU Int* 2010;106:1178–80.

37 Kadioglu A, Tefekli A, Erol B, Oktar T, Tunc M, Tellaloglu S. A retrospective review of 307 men with Peyronie's disease. *J Urol* 2002;168(3):1075–9.

CHAPTER 25

Micropenis and penile dysmorphobia: diagnosis, management, outcomes, and future developments in the field

Oliver Kayes[1], Lizzie Chandra[1], and Andrew Yates[2]

[1] St James Hospital, Leeds Teaching Hospitals NHS Trust, Leeds, UK

[2] Leeds & York Partnership NHS Foundation Trust, Leeds General Infirmary, Leeds, UK

Introduction

Although "micropenis" refers to a well-defined condition, it is a term that can be misapplied or misconstrued amongst patients and clinicians. The definition of micropenis is a stretched penile length (SPL) of 2.5 standard deviations below the mean for age and race in the absence of other genital abnormalities; this is less than 7.5 cm for Caucasian adult males and less than 1.9 cm in term neonates.[1] Micropenis can be associated with functional problems, including sexual and voiding dysfunction, and this often leads to complex psychological problems. Alongside this in clinical practice are those who present with a normal sized phallus who maintain a persistent perception of inadequate size despite counseling; they can suffer from clinically significant distress and impairment of their social functioning as a result of this perception. These patients are considered to have penile dysmorphic syndrome.[2]

Causes of micropenis

True micropenis is a congenital abnormality and is attributable to well-defined etiologies, whilst a small subset are found to be idiopathic. Despite true micropenis being an isolated finding with absence of other genital abnormalities, it can be found as part of more complex presentations, such as associated hypospadias or bladder exstrophy; it may also fall into the category of "disorders of sexual differentiation"[1] (see Chapter 31). Micropenis can also be acquired; for example, following surgical intervention for malignancy or trauma or due to skin conditions such as lichen sclerosis and following Fournier's gangrene.[3] In some cases, there can be a misdiagnosis with a buried penis and/or webbed penis presenting with clinically similar findings. Imaging such as MRI may be helpful in these cases.[1]

Congenital micropenis

The presence of congenital micropenis most commonly suggests a defect in the hypothalamic-pituitary-gonadal (HPG) axis during fetal development.[4] Genital development occurs during the first trimester under the influence of placental chorionic gonadotropins, which stimulate the Leydig cells to produce testosterone. Subsequently, this is converted to dihydrotestosterone, which stimulates penile differentiation. Penile differentiation is complete as the fetus enters its second trimester at the end of the 12th week.[5] From this point on the fetal HPG axis controls overall hormonal regulation and the placenta ceases to play a role. Pituitary gonadatropins stimulate growth of the penis, a process that continues until birth. An understanding of this process demonstrates why congenital micropenis most commonly results from a defect in the HPG axis.[4,5]

Male Sexual Dysfunction: A Clinical Guide, First Edition. Edited by Suks Minhas and John Mulhall.

Etiology of micropenis normally falls into one of three categories:

- hypogonadotropic-hypogonadism (pituitary/hypothalamic failure);
- hypergonadotropic-hypogonadism (primary testicular failure);
- idiopathic.[4]

Table 25.1 illustrates the conditions that constitute each group of disorders, which may be a result of primary hormonal/metabolic error or secondary to an underlying genetic mutation.[3] Hypogonadotropic-hypogonadism results from failure of either the hypothalamus or anterior pituitary gland. The hypothalamus produces gonadotropin-releasing hormone (GnRH), which stimulates the anterior pituitary gland to produce follicle-stimulating hormone (FSH) and luteinizing hormone (LH). LH is the primary stimulator of the Leydig cells to produce testosterone from week 12 onwards thus promoting in utero penile growth.[1] Hypergonadotropic-hypogonadism is a result of primary testicular failure despite normal or high circulating levels of the gonadatropins FSH and LH. Interestingly, it has been noted that hypergonadotropic-hypogonadism more commonly presents with concurrent hypospadias than hypogonadotropic-hypogonadism.[4] Although most patients are found to have an abnormality of the HPG axis there are a significant subset that despite thorough testing have an apparently normal hormone profile and thus are deemed to have idiopathic micropenis. This may be due to a time-limited abnormality during fetal development, such as delayed production and release of GnRH, LH, FSH, and testosterone in the second trimester; or a transient resistance to one or more of these hormones during fetal development that is no longer present at

Table 25.1 Etiology of micropenis.

Category	Cause
Deficiency of testosterone production	Hypogonadotropic hypogonadism • Isolated including Kallmann's syndrome • Associated with other pituitary hormone deficiencies • Prader–Willi syndrome • Laurence–Moon syndrome • Bardet–Biedl syndrome • Rud's syndrome Primary hypogonadism • Anorchia • Klinefelter's and poly-X syndromes • Gonadal dysgenesis • Luteinizing hormone receptor defects (incomplete forms) • Genetic defects in testosterone steroidogenesis (incomplete forms) • Noonan's syndrome • Trisomy 21 • Robinow's syndrome • Bardet–Biedl syndrome • Laurence–Moon syndrome
Defects of testosterone action	Growth hormone/insulin-like growth factor 1 deficiency Androgen receptor defects 5-Alpha reductase deficiency Fetal hydantoin syndrome
Developmental anomalies	Aphallia Cloacal exstrophy
Idiopathic	
Associated with other congenital malformations	

birth. These patients usually respond well to the same treatments as those patients with an identified HPG axis error as discussed below.[6]

Assessment

Patients who present with "micropenis" must be fully examined as the term can be used erroneously in some clinical practice. Correct and accurate measurement of SPL is essential in all age groups. This is done by using a rigid ruler to measure from the point where the penis meets the pubic bone to the distal tip of the penis whilst the penis is in the flaccid state and maximally stretched. If the measurement falls below the accepted normal limit for age and race then micropenis can be diagnosed. Table 25.2 shows the normal measurements for adult males. The length to circumference ratio is rarely affected in patients with micropenis. Penile length in childhood remains under-reported but reference values can be found in Table 25.3, and in some infants the genitalia look ambiguious. Testicular presence should be sought and measurement with an orchidometer performed if possible. Patients presenting later in life may have delayed puberty; careful assessment of secondary sexual characteristics is undertaken and the Tanner grade recorded. The presence of associated genital abnormalities should be evaluated, with some cases showing only subtle differences.[1]

Once micropenis is confirmed the patient must be investigated for a possible reversible etiology. During the examination it may become evident that micropenis forms part of a more complex condition. Patients may have syndromic features such as dysmorphic facies, abnormal stature and growth for age, and inappropriate level of development for their age. This may provide indications for an underlying diagnosis; otherwise thorough testing will be required. Diagnosis requires a multidisciplinary approach. The inputs of a geneticist and endocrinologist with the urological surgeon are essential.

The primary concern in the neonate is to establish whether micropenis is part of a presentation of panhypopituitarism. This renders the child at risk of profound hypoglycemia, which can lead to permanent damage or death. Therefore in the neonate with micropenis it is important to promptly test for growth hormone and adrenocorticotropic hormone, both of which are released from the anterior pituitary; a midline cephalic ultrasound scan(USS) may also demonstrate structural abnormality, and a urine steroid profile may also be helpful. Following this, more detailed endocrinological testing of the HPG axis can be performed. The testes' response to stimulation is important and may be ascertained by taking testosterone levels pre- and post-administration of human chorionic gonadotropin (hHCG). In some settings hormonal testicular function (and presence in cases of cryptorchidism) can be ascertained by testing for

Table 25.2 Penile dimensions for normal adults.

Study	Year	*n*	Age range	Flaccid length (cm)	Stretched length (cm)	Erect length (cm)	Flaccid girth (cm)	Erect girth (cm)
Loeb	1899	50	17–35	9.41	–	–	–	–
Schonfeld	1942	196	17–25	–	13.1	–	8.5	15.8
Kinsey	1948	2770	20–59	9.7	16.74	–	–	–
Bondil	1992	905	17–91	10.7	16.74	–	–	–
De Ros	1994	150	–	–	–	14.5	11.05	–
Wessells	1996	80	21–82	8.85	12.45	12.89	9.71	12.30
Bogaert	1999	935	–	10.41	–	16.40	9.75	12.57
		4187	–	9.83	–	15.60	9.40	12.19
Ponchietti	2001	3300	17–19	9.0	12.5	–	10.0	–
Schneider	2001	111	18–32	8.60	–	14.48	–	–
Awwad	2005	271	17–83	9.3	13.5	–	8.9	–
Promodu	2007	301	–	8.21	10.88	13.01	9.14	11.46
Mehraban	2007	1500	20–40	–	11.58	–	8.66	–
Khan	2012	609	16–90	8.7	14.3	–	–	–

Table 25.3 Mean stretched penile length (cm) in normal children.

Age range	Wang 2006	Hatipoğlu 2013	Teckchandani 2014[30]
Preterm newborns	–	2.5	–
Term newborns	3.0	3.5	–
0–5 months	–	3.9	–
5–12 months	4.0	4.3	4.02
1–2 years	–	4.7	4.50
2–3 years	–	5.1	5.01
3–4 years	–	5.5	5.52
4–5 years	5.0	5.7	5.82
5–6 years	–	6.0	6.11
6–7 years	–	6.1	6.31
7–8 years	–	6.2	6.50
8–9 years	–	6.3	6.61
9–10 years	–	6.3	6.71
10–11 years	–	6.4	–

anti-müllerian hormone and inhibin B, both of which are produced by testicular Sertoli cells. However, this is currently considered experimental and is not available at most centers. Distinguishing between hypothalamic and pituitary levels of dysfunction can be accomplished using prolactin levels, which will be high in hypothalamic dysfunction and low in pituitary dysfunction. Alongside this, most patients will require karyotyping, with particular attention to the sex chromosomes.

Acquired micropenis

The etiopathogenesis of acquired micropenis is extremely variable. It can be secondary to primary pathology or iatrogenic due to treatment of underlying conditions or surgical misadventure. Common causes include: Peyronie's disease, prostate cancer, post-priapism, and lichen sclerosis. Treatment of conditions such as genital cancers, Fournier's gangrene, trauma, and burns can also result in this state (see also Chapter 26). The underlying pathology resulting in shortening will involve a combination of: corporeal fibrosis (secondary to chronic hypoxia), anatomical shortening following surgery or trauma, graft contraction, and loss of tissue elasticity.[3] These processes result in a measurable loss in penile length, which may be minimal or profound. Patients with less severe shortening can often be successfully treated with medical therapies – most commonly phosphodiesterase-5 (PDE5) inhibitors – combined with enhancement devices such as penile vacuums and penile extension devices (e.g. Andropenis®, Jes-Extender®). Those with significant defects may be unable to have sexual intercourse and normal voiding function. This category of patient will require surgical intervention either at the time of primary surgery or at a later date. Some techniques at the time of surgery, such as glans resurfacing and advancement flaps, may be useful in preventing subsequent micropenis. Otherwise the surgical techniques discussed below may be implemented.[3]

Treating micropenis

The aim of treatment for patients with micropenis is to provide both functional and cosmetically acceptable results. Normal social drivers suggest that men will desire a normal penile length, normal penetrative sexual function, and an ability to micturate in a standing position. Treatment can be entirely non-invasive using medical therapies and counseling, with surgical intervention reserved for persistent penile deformities. Corrective surgery requires a well-informed patient who understands the potential for repeated surgeries and possible cosmetic and functional results.

Whilst this chapter concentrates on the surgical management of micropenis it is important to realize that the diagnosis of micropenis produces profound emotional and psychological responses in patients, parents, partners, and medical carers. It is best managed by a multidisciplinary team to ensure a holistic approach to patient care and a smooth transition from diagnosis to treatment.[3]

Non-invasive and medical treatments

The market for non-invasive penile enhancement devices and strategies has expanded rapidly in recent years. The offer of length and girth increases from various devices is reported but little evidence exists to support their use. Among the acclaimed enhancing approaches are: penile extenders, injectables, weights, vacuum devices, botulinum toxin, and physiotherapy. Oderda and Gontero's recent article shows that only level 4 evidence exists to support the use of penile extenders with no robust evidence available to support alternative techniques.[7] In their review article they concluded that the evidence for penile extenders was adequate to promote their use as a first-line treatment for people with small or normal penile size seeking enhancement, with 1.5–2.5 cm length increases achievable in some men. As for the other marketed strategies for penile enhancement no medical evidence exists to support their use currently.[7]

Medical therapy for micropenis involves the correction of subnormal serum testosterone levels or androgen insensitivity for men with proven HPG-axis dysfunction. This is achieved through differing protocols, but the general consensus suggests that early therapy in the months after birth is optimal. The most commonly recommended treatment regime is to use 25 mg of intramuscular testosterone monthly for 3 months. This regime can be commenced from the second postnatal month without concern for early skeletal development and growth plate fusion.[1,8] Testosterone is normally administered in its enanthate form as this has a longer duration of action. Good results have been shown following this regime, with increases of 100–150% in penile length being reported.[1,3,4,9] Alternatively, transdermal testosterone can be used: dihydrotestosterone gel is applied to the penile tip and shaft at doses of 12.5–25 mg daily for 8 weeks. This was shown to be safe in a small study by Choi et al., and showed penile length increases comparable to intramuscular testosterone administration.[9] The initial treatment phase may need supplementing with a further course of testosterone at puberty if development is delayed or penile growth is poor.[10]

Surgical treatment

Surgery can be offered to patients who fail or partially respond to medical therapy. It is important to realize that penile enhancement surgery is not a panacea, whether done for micropenis or other reasons. The procedures that have so far been developed have variable success rates and carry with them important risks, which must be discussed with all potential recipients. Alongside the usual operative risks there are specific risks such as paradoxical penile shortening, altered sensation, and postoperative erectile dysfunction; furthermore, despite careful counseling, some men will find the cosmetic results and scarring disappointing.[11] Careful patient selection and a full assessment of patient expectations are essential. Studies have shown that despite a real length or girth increase being achieved, many patients remain unsatisfied with the results.[12] The surgical options available form a spectrum of procedures from less extreme augmentation procedures to radical reconstruction such as total phalloplasty. Total phalloplasty should be reserved for the most challenging cases, with consideration of the less radical approaches in all possible cases prior to embarking on this.

It is most important to note that surgical penile enhancement and replacement techniques are considered investigational. There is a paucity of reliable and validated data in the literature regarding success, and often high levels of complications are reported. However, carefully selected patients can benefit from surgery, and this option should be discussed along with other potential treatments. With this in mind, surgical intervention should be considered carefully by all potential operating surgeons and recipient patients.

Penile lengthening

Division of the suspensory ligament is advocated by several authors to increase penile length. This is often accompanied by an inverted V-Y-plasty of the pubopenile skin. The suspensory ligament, which arises from the dorsal aspect of the penis and attaches superiorly to the pubic symphysis, is responsible in combination with the fundiform ligament for supporting the penis in the erect state. Once divided some surgeons advocate placing either a fat pad or silicone prosthesis over the pubic bone to prevent reattachment of the ligament, as this can lead to paradoxical postoperative shortening.[13] The use of postoperative penile weights and stretching exercises is also used to prevent reattachment and promote length gain, either in addition to pre-pubic bone prosthesis or independently of this. In well-selected patients there can be a length increase of 1–2 cm.[14] The main complications associated with this procedure include: paradoxical shortening, reduced angle of erection, and, in some cases, instability of the erect penis.[15] If accompanied by an inverted V-Y-plasty some patients complain of hair-bearing skin on the shaft of the penis, and hypertrophic scarring is possible.[14]

In addition to division of the suspensory ligament and V-Y-plasty; selected patients will benefit from excision of suprapubic fat pads (lipectomy) and release or excision of a penoscrotal web. This increases perceived penile length rather than providing an actual increase in penile length, but both methods are relatively simple procedures that can provide satisfaction for appropriate patients.

The literature does contain reports from other, single-center, often single-surgeon studies promoting new strategies for penile lengthening. Perovic and Djordjevic suggest using harvested autologous rib cartilage for placement between the glans cap and tip of the corpora cavernosa, which can produce a 2–4 cm length increase.[16] This technique, alongside other small studies, requires further validation and assessment before routine clinical implementation is possible.

Girth augmentation

Results for penile girth augmentation are less satisfactory than those for length enhancement. Several techniques have been attempted with varying results, and associated complications are commonly reported. The most commonly attempted approach is to inject autologous fat cells into the dartos fascia, along the length of the penis at four points around the circumference of the penis.[13] This is then massaged to produce an even spread of the injected fat cells. Results from this technique are variable secondary to multifactorial problems. Fat cells injected are subject to multiple episodes of trauma and thus there is significant cell rupture and reabsorption; up to 90% of fat cells may be lost this way. This is not a uniform process and consequently can lead to asymmetry of the penis; additionally, nodules may occur due to fat necrosis or calcification of fat cells. Conversely, if too much fat is successfully laid down then some patients complain of lack of rigidity on erection.[14,17]

In an attempt to avoid these pitfalls, several researchers have used dermal fat grafts – the success of which is reported elsewhere in plastic surgery. The dermal layer is harvested from abdominal or gluteal areas and the epidermis removed. The graft can then be placed circumferentially around the penis between the dartos and Buck's fascia. Unfortunately results with this technique are also inconsistent. Fibrosis and scarring of the fat may occur and this can lead to asymmetry and nodularity. There is also the added morbidity and scarring associated with the donor site. Providing no complications occur a girth augmentation of 2.5–5 cm can be achieved, which is a substantial increase.[14,17]

Other experimental, injectable substances such as silicone and hyaluronic acid gel have been evaluated. In order to achieve an appreciable girth increase, large volumes are required and this can lead to a number of complications including: damage to blood vessels and nerves resulting in erectile dysfunction; migration of the silicone leading to a deformed penis; and, finally, immunogenic reactions to the silicone causing granuloma formation.[14] Injection of hyaluronic acid gel for glans enhancement has achieved measurable increases in glans circumference with few complications; however, these data have not been reproduced by others to date.[18]

Austoni et al. reported a technique of saphenous vein augmentation of the corpora for girth augmentation.[19] In their technique an incision is made from the pubis to the tip of each corpus cavernosum and a saphenous vein graft inserted to the tunica albuginea. This gives good results in increasing erect penile girth but has no effect on flaccid girth. Newer techniques include using biodegradable scaffolds populated with autologous fibroblasts and AlloDerm® sheets in a similar fashion to dermal graft placement. Both these techniques are entirely experimental and have few data to support them at the current time.[13,14]

Procedures for girth augmentation are not the mainstay of treatment for the patient with micropenis; this is in part due to the relatively poor outcomes and high complication rates. These procedures may be performed for cosmetic reasons or for those with penile dysmorphic syndrome and much of the data published refers to this cohort of patients.

Penile replacement surgery (phalloplasty)

Certain patients with micropenis will require total phalloplasty. Usually, these patients have trialed less radical treatments without success or may present with concomitant genital anomalies. The main aim of phalloplasty surgery is to provide patients with a functioning and visually acceptable phallus. As previously mentioned, this includes being able to perform sexual intercourse, micturate in a standing position, and have minimal scarring or signs of surgery. Patient expectations are often high, so detailed counseling is mandatory including reference to the potential postoperative function and recovery, possible complications, and details of likely scarring. Scarring (often indicative of the procedure) is a potential source of disappointment for some patients undergoing phalloplasty surgery. The majority of evidence supporting the development and use of these techniques originates in female to male transgender surgery. Contemporary results suggest that they also remain valuable techniques for the challenging micropenis patient. Phalloplasty is a complex procedure that may require multiple operations; a number of techniques are reported.

The first phalloplasty reported was carried out by Bogaras in 1936. His technique used a tubularized abdominal pedicle flap. Other pedicle flaps were experimented with and were highly successful in terms of low rates of flap failure; however, they have limited sensation and in time have been superseded by the radial forearm free flap phalloplasty (RAFF).[3] The RAFF for total phalloplasty was developed by Song in 1982 and has become the most popular method of phalloplasty in recent years.[20] There are several advantages to the RAFF: it has a reliable arterial supply and identifiable nerves that can be anastomosed to provide potential sensation and response to erogenous stimulation.[21] Skin grafting from the thigh, buttocks, or similar areas is used to repair forearm defects; however, scarring does remain a significant feature of this surgery. Following baseline surgery, it is possible to have further procedures to place a penile implant to allow erection and sexual intercourse; surgeons advocate this stage at around 1 year from the initial phalloplasty surgery. Complications can arise with this procedure and they include: graft necrosis (complete or partial); neourethral complications such as fistula, strictures, and hair growth, which may cause urethral stones; implant infection; tissue erosion; and device failure. Despite this, outcomes are good even following treatment for complications or revision surgery.[3,21]

Alternative free flap phalloplasty techniques include: upper arm flap, latissimus dorsi flaps, anterolateral thigh flaps, and osteocutaneous fibular flaps. Those clinicians reporting these techniques are enthusiastic about their use whilst suggesting superior outcomes to traditional RAFF surgery.[3] However, wider testing in multicenter and multisurgeon studies is required to support these statements

Surgery for micropenis should be considered only after medical therapies and counseling have been provided. However, it does offer a possible solution for those in whom other strategies have completely failed or results are unsatisfactory. Those patients being considered for surgery should be counseled thoroughly regarding the risks and complications of the proposed surgery and possible need for multiple procedures. Despite the associated limitations; there is no doubt that surgery offers a valuable therapeutic option to a carefully selected patient population.

Techniques for the future

Tissue engineering

This is a rapidly expanding area of research and there has been much progress in the field of urology in recent years. The penis remains a challenging target for tissue engineering as it is composed of several tissue types with specialized functions and complex anatomy. However, progress is being made in developing tissues with the required characteristics that may at some time in the future be used therapeutically for those with penile deformities and functional problems.

There are several methods for creating specialized functional tissues for therapeutic use. These are broadly divided into acellular and cellular. In acellular techniques a scaffold of either natural or synthetic material lacking immunogenic components is implanted to promote a natural healing process in the deficient area. The cellular approach requires stem cells, which can either be used independently or "seeded" onto scaffolds (similar to those used in the acellular technique); these are then encouraged with specialized laboratory techniques to differentiate down the desired cell line route.[22]

There are a number of reports of experimental tissue engineering techniques that are relevant to this patient group. Chen and colleagues have succeeded in generating corporeal tissue with erectile function in a laboratory-based rabbit model by seeding smooth muscle and endothelial cells in a stepwise fashion onto a scaffold.[23] El-Kassaby et al. performed a clinical trial comparing buccal mucosal grafts and bladder acellular matrix in the treatment of complex urethral strictures; the success rate for the acellular matrix was lower but they concluded it was a viable option for treatment in appropriate patients and further investigation should be performed.[24] Finally, Breyer et al. attempted grafting tunica albuginea defects in patients with Peyronie's disease with porcine small bowel submucosa scaffold; despite success in previous animal studies this had high complication rates in the human trial.[25]

The above areas of experimentation show how tissue engineering is likely to provide possible future therapeutic options, but further development is necessary before these techniques become widely utilized in clinical practice.

Penile transplant

This is an area of research in which there is currently little evidence or data. Transplantation stemmed from a desire to treat life-limiting diseases that were untreatable by other means. More recently there has been experimentation with transplantation of composite tissue allografts often for conditions that do not limit life but severely effect quality of life. This raises difficult ethical questions. Furthermore, transplantation of composite grafts is more technically challenging; there are often multiple aspects to the surgical anastomosis of component parts and difficult management of immunological responses; this is especially true as skin is a highly immunogenic tissue.[26]

Penile transplantation encompasses all of the above difficulties. The penis holds significant psychosocial importance in all cultures but a deficit or absence of this organ is not life limiting.[4] This is an important consideration in the progression of penile transplantation as complications following surgery and a lifelong regime of immunosuppression are challenging. This leaves patients at risk of drug side effects, including end organ damage, opportunistic infections, and malignancy, which can in themselves be fatal. The psychological response to having donor tissue that is sensate and externally visible can be profound both in the patient and their partner.[27]

Only one attempt to date has been attempted with a complete penile transplantation undertaken in China in 2006. Although the procedure was technically successful it resulted in reversal and removal of the penis after 14 days, as the patient and his wife experienced profound psychological difficulties. As it has not been attempted again no medium- or long-term data exist; as such, the potential benefits and pitfalls of this type of surgery are unknown and, at best, can only be extrapolated from other composite tissue transplant programs.[26,28] Although this is an interesting approach, more research and further studies are required before a conclusion as to its place in the treatment of micropenis can be assessed.

Penile dysmorphobia

Penile dysmorphobia is a condition in which men have a persistent preoccupation with the physical appearance of their penis.[29] They believe the appearance and size of their penis to be abnormal or inadequate, despite normal anatomy and size. These patients become preoccupied with this thought pattern, and develop a psychological rigidity, becoming obsessed and fixated by their perceived size. They can develop clinically significant signs of depression, general and social anxiety, and even suicidal thoughts. Perceived penile inadequacy and an inability to "perform" sexually (i.e., provide sexual pleasure to a partner) commonly develop into feelings of shame, hopelessness, and negative self-belief thus resulting in avoidance of peer and sexual/intimate relationships. Distorted cognitions result in inaccurate and idealized beliefs about what partners want sexually, with sweeping generalizations about partner sexuality. The man with "small penis syndrome" typically views potential partners as judgmental, ridiculing, and threatening, which further perpetuates the cognitive rigidity and reinforces the belief.

The condition often develops in adolescence or young adulthood; boys enter and progress through sexual maturation at different times and rates, at a time when they are particularly sensitive to pressures from their contemporaries and the media. For many it becomes a lifelong affliction, which worsens without treatment. Some of these patients have more complex conditions including body dysmorphic disorder. For many, the concern is related to the size of the flaccid penis rather than the erect state. A careful history and examination of the patient is essential to ensure there is no underlying physical abnormality. Once objective penile length has been established to be normal a full picture of the patient's concerns, anxieties, and perceived inadequacies should be developed. Notably, there is a tendency for this group of men to display a cognitive bias in favor of their belief, thus readily accepting "data" that support their belief of penile inadequacy whilst rejecting information contrary to their view. There is motivation to seek out reference points that support the bias – these can be statistical data published on the internet, sites dedicated to penile size, and related discussion groups. Absorption in researching the "problem" and attempting to find a remedy paradoxically promotes and maintains the distress.

Management should revolve around psychological therapies such as psychosexual psychotherapy, psychotherapy, cognitive behavioral therapies (CBT), and sometimes antidepressant medications. Surgery in these patients should not be undertaken lightly. Satisfaction rates are low regardless of whether a good surgical outcome is achieved with objective length or girth gain. However, there is a ferocious and growing appetite for penis enhancement surgery, which is being carried out in several centers around the world. All of the surgical techniques for length and girth augmentation discussed above have reportedly been carried out for penile dysmorphic syndrome despite the variable results and possible serious complications.

Inherent in "small penis syndrome" are two central beliefs that require addressing: penile size as an outward representation of masculinity, and sufficient penile adequacy to satisfy a sexual partner (sexual performance). In many cultures the erect penis encapsulates masculinity and virility and a penis perceived to be small can trigger insecurity, shame, and embarrassment. Sex therapy clinics commonly see men who complain of subjective penile deficiency. A typical finding in this group is early and ongoing exposure to pornographic images that distort reality, and a lack of primary sex education. Early engagement with pornography becomes a reference point for sexual learning and is rich in mythical and fictional messages of biological function and sexual expectation. Addressing misbeliefs through educational material such as simplified charts and diagrams, appropriate medical illustrations of male and female genitalia, and psycho-education focused on normal sexual function with accessible reading material that normalizes sexual function is essential. Challenging the notion that penile size has a direct correlation with a partner's sexual pleasure requires careful and sensitive management as patients will often view this as a manipulative venture aimed at diverting them from their core belief. Instilling the belief that sexual intimacy is made up of much more than objectified penetration fosters an understanding that intimacy is multifactorial and, for most partners, is a combination of head, heart, and hormones that extends beyond a phallocentric model.

The psychotherapy position of working with an issue that cannot be objectively and manifestly altered is to foster acceptance and adaptation. Given that men with small penis syndrome, as a group, have an emphatic belief in their inadequate penile size, creating the merest doubt that their belief may be wrong is the starting point of treatment. Their internal dialog will be negative, and reframing these thoughts, in a more positive and adaptive way, will impact on self-worth. Achieving a more positive focus through cognitive approaches, such as CBT, hypnosis, and emotional freedom technique (EFT), all help to glimpse future possibilities of sexual fulfilment in a real-as-real way. Identifying faulty beliefs and setting them against a valid body of evidence can promote more doubt in the skewed belief and can be the portal for targeted psycho-education. Equally, spending time working on core fears of rejection, humiliation, and shame due to being an inadequate man, are central and achieved through intimacy-based interventions either as an individual or couple. Encouraging exposure to the possibility of loving and supportive relationships, free from blame and criticism, through social activities can assist in a more balanced understanding of what people look for when selecting partners.

The sexual relationship and a partner's pleasure are not premised on penile size alone, and the patient needs to learn that sex does not have to be judgmental and can be safe. In summary, treatment of this group of patients is essentially education, challenging faulty thinking through reframing negative perceptions of size, and developing improved self-worth and self-esteem by bringing about an understanding that intimacy is not premised on function and performance alone.

References

1 Wiygul J, Palmer LS. Micropenis. *Scientific World Journal* 2011;28(11):1462–9.

2 The Institute for Sexual Medicine. Penile Dysmorphic Disorder. Available from: https://sexualmed.org/known-issues/penile-dysmorphic-disorder/(accessed April 11, 2016).

3 Kayes O, Shabbir M, Ralph D, Minhas S. Therapeutic strategies for patients with micropenis or penile dysmorphic disorder. *Nat Rev Urol* 2012;9(9):499–507.

4 Ludwig G. Micropenis and apparent micropenis – a diagnostic and therapeutic challenge. *Andrologia* 1999;31 (Suppl. 1):27–30.

5 Moore KL, Persaud TVN. *Before We Are Born: Essentials of Embryology and Birth Defects*, 7th edn. Philadelphia: Saunders Elsevier, 2008; pp. 173–86.

6 Büyükgebiz A. Topical testosterone treatment in idiopathic micropenis. *Pediatr Endocrinol Rev* 2004;1(3):334–5.

7 Oderda M, Gontero P. Non-invasive methods of penile lengthening: fact or fiction? *BJU Int* 2011;107:1278–82.

8 Elder J. Abnormalities of the genitalia in boys and their surgical management. In: *Campbell-Walsh Urology*, 9th edn. Amsterdam: Elsevier, 2007; pp. 3751–4.

9 Choi SK, Han SW, Kim DH, de Lignieres B. Transdermal dihydrotestosterone therapy and its effects on patients with microphallus. *J Urol* 1993;150(2 Pt 2):657–60.

10 Bin-Abbas B, Conte FA, Grumbach MM, Kaplan SL. Congenital hypogonadotropic hypogonadism and micropenis: effect of testosterone treatment on adult penile size. Why sex reversal is not indicated. *J Pediatr* 1999;134:579–83.

11 Garaffa G, Gentile V, Antonini G, Tsafrakidis P. Penile reconstruction in the male. *Arab J Urol* 2013;11:267–71.

12 Lee PA, Houk CP. Outcome studies among men with micropenis. *J Pediatr Endocrinol Metab* 2004;17(8):1043–53.

13 Dillon BE, Chama NB, Honig SC. Penile size and penile enlargement surgery: a review. *Int J Impot Res* 2008; 20(5):519–29.

14 Vardi Y, Harshai Y, Gil T, Gruenwald I. A critical analysis of penile enhancement procedures for patients with normal penile size: Surgical techniques, success, and complications. *Eur Urol* 2008;54(5):1042–50.

15 Li CY, Kayes O, Kell PD, Christopher N, Minhas S, Ralph DJ. Penile suspensory ligament division for penile augmentation: indications and results. *Eur Urol* 2006;49:729–33.

16 Perovic SV, Djordjevic ML. Penile lengthening. *BJU Int* 2000;86:1028–33.

17 Alter GJ, Jordan GH. Penile elongation and girth enhancement. *AUA Update Series* 2007;26:229–37.

18 Kim JJ, Kwak TI, Jeon BG, Cheon J, Moon DG. Human glans penis augmentation using injectable hyaluronic acid gel. *Int J Impot Res* 2003;15:439–43.

19 Austoni E, Guarneri A, Cazzaniga A. A new technique for augmentation phalloplasty: albugineal surgery with bilateral saphenous grafts – three years of experience. *Eur Urol* 2002;42:245–53.

20 Song R, Gao Y, Song Y, Yu Y, Song Y. The forearm flap. *Clin Plast Surg* 1982;9:21–6.

21 Bluebond-Langner R, Redett RJ. Phalloplasty in complete aphallia and ambiguous genitalia. *Semin Plast Surg*. 2011 Aug;25(3):196–205

22 Shokeir AA, Harraz AM, Shehaab El-Din AB. Tissue engineering and stem cells: Basic principles and applications in urology. *Int J Urol* 2010;17(12):964–73.

23 Chen KL, Eberli D, Yoo JJ, Atala A. Bioengineered corporal tissue for structural and functional restoration of the penis. *Proc Natl Acad Sci U S A* 2010;107:3346–50.

24 El-Kassaby A, AbouShwareb T, Atala A. Randomized comparative study between buccal mucosal and acellular bladder matrix grafts in complex anterior urethral strictures. *J Urol* 2008;179:1432–6.

25 Breyer BN, Brant WO, Garcia MM, Bella AJ, Lue TF. Complications of porcine small intestine submucosa graft for Peyronie's disease. *J Urol* 2007;177:589–91.

26 Dubernard JM. Editorial, Penile transplantation? *Eur Urol* 2006;50(4):664–5.

27 Zhang LC, Zhao YB, Hu WL. Ethical issues in penile transplantation. *Asian J Androl* 2010;12:795–800.

28 Weilie Hu, Jun Lu, Lichao Zhang, et al. A preliminary report of penile transplantation. *Eur Urol* 2006;50:851–3.

29 World Health Organization. International Statistical Classification of Diseases and Related Health Problems, 10th Revision (ICD 10). WHO.

30 Teckchandani N, Bajpai M. Penile length nomogram for Asian Indian prepubertal boys. *J Pediatr Urol* 2014;10: 352–4.

CHAPTER 26

Surgical treatment of Peyronie's disease

Ates Kadioglu and Emre Salabas

Istanbul Faculty of Medicine, Istanbul University, Istanbul, Turkey

Introduction

Since Peyronie's disease (PD) was first identified in the eighteenth century, numerous medical and surgical treatment modalities have been proposed, but without reaching a definitive and final solution. It is an acquired fibrotic disease of the tunica albuginea (TA) of the penis characterized by the formation of fibrous plaques, which causes penile curvature and shortening, painful erection, loss of penile flexibility, and associated sexual dysfunction.[1] The incidence of the disease is estimated at between 3% and 9%, with a mean age of onset of 50–60 years.[2,3] This rate may increase to 20% in diabetic patients, in whom diabetic treatment reduces plaque size.[4] Furthermore, young patients (<40) who compose 10% of the total PD population, were reported to have more acute onset and lower ED rates than their older counterparts.[5,6] The disease may also occur in teenagers, who are differentiated from other age groups with high HbA1c levels in 18% of patients, non-contiguous plaques, and a subsequent ED rate of 37%.[7]

Etiology and pathogenesis

The etiology of PD is considered to be multifactorial with the interplay of a genetic predisposition, trauma, and tissue ischemia.[8] Although the exact pathogenesis is not understood, the most widely accepted theory is that PD is a wound-healing disorder, initiated by repetitive micro trauma to the penis, with subsequent scar formation. The source of the scar formation as suggested by human penile studies and experimental animal PD models appears to be extravasated fibrinogen during trauma of the penis, although there is a general lack of clinical evidence supporting the role of trauma in PD.[1] Erectile dysfunction and coital trauma were identified as independent risk factors for PD (OR 1.5 and 2.7) whereas the presence of diabetes mellitus (DM) was significant only when accompanied by ED.[9] PD has also been associated with Dupuytren's disease as 30–40% of patients with PD had both diseases, and 10% of them had a family history of Dupuytren's disease.[10] Although systemic vascular risk factors, such as DM, hyperlipidemia, hypertension, ischemic heart disease, smoking, and pelvic interventions have been hypothesized to play a role in the pathogenesis of PD, only DM has been accepted as an independent factor increasing the prevalence and the severity of PD.[1]

The initiation phase of PD is characterized by an acute inflammatory process characteristically associated with increased tunical fibroblast proliferation and abnormal presence of myofibroblasts followed by disproportionate deposition of collagen, persistence of fibrin, and elastin fragmentation in tunica albuginea of the penis. Transforming growth factor β1 (TGF-β1) is a profibrotic factor that may be harvested from plaques or other fibrotic processes in the body. It may be injected directly, together with fibrin, or may be induced with the help of adenoviral constructs to produce penile curvature and plaque in animal models.[11] Overexpression of myostatin, a member of the TGF-β family, has been found in PD plaques; it induces new plaque upon administration and can condense pre-existing plaque of TGF-β1.[12] Other profibrotic factors such as plasminogen activation inhibitor (PAI-1) and reactive oxygen species (ROS) as well as TGF-β1 are released in the acute inflammation subsequent to trauma. Following the acute stage, a chronic phase ensues, with deposition of a dense fibrotic plaque, which

Male Sexual Dysfunction: A Clinical Guide, First Edition. Edited by Suks Minhas and John Mulhall.

may be accompanied with calcification and ossification of the plaque as well as the presence of osteoblasts.[13]

NO release due to inducible nitric oxide synthase (iNOS) has been proposed as a defensive mechanism against the profibrotic factors in studies because of the increased levels of iNOS together with antioxidants in human and animal plaques leading to plaque reduction. The fibrin clot in the tunica albuginea attracts monocyte chemotactic protein 1 (MCP-1), which itself probably induces iNOS. This theory is supported by the reverse correlation of profibrotic factor levels and iNOS activity regulated by gene transfer and L-N-(1-iminoethyl) lysine acetate (L-NIL) inhibition in animal experiments.[14] It has been postulated that NO reduced by ROS activity, results in myofibroblast apoptosis with inhibition of collagen synthesis together with its end product cGMP. Reduction in plaque size, oxidative stress, and alpha smooth muscle actin (ASMA) staining was observed in PD fibroblast cultures after phosphodiesterase type 5 (PDE-5) inhibitor adminstration.[15]

The inhibition and lack of metalloproteinase and collagenases contribute to the process, while iNOS, matrix metalloproteinases (MMPs) 2 and 9, decorin (which binds TGF-β1), and thymosins are the active defense mechanisms against the disease. The positive effect of decorin on maximal cavernosal pressure and the collagen organization of the fibrotic penis has been demonstrated in a rat model and thus opens a new therapeutic gateway for the disease.[16] Furthermore MMPs 1, 8, and 13,which are inhibited by TIMP (TGF-β1 induced tissue inhibitors of metalloproteinases) in PD, are able to renovate the normally lysis-resistant collagen I and III fibers.[17] In addition, overexpression of tumor necrosis factor-related apoptosis-inducing ligand (TRAIL) and its death receptor (DR5) has been demonstrated in PD plaque when compared to normal TA, indicating the role of the external apoptotic pathway in plaque formation.[18] The persistence of myofibroblasts, which are removed by apoptosis, has been investigated in another study including apoptotic genes Fas, Fas ligand, Bcl-2, p53, and caspase 3 and 8. Despite the slight increase in expression of apoptotic genes in the Peyronie's plaque, the statistically insignificant difference between plaque and healthy tunica albuginea points to the non-localized nature of the PD.[19] In a recent study comparing tunica albuginea of PD and Congenital penile curvature (CPC) patients, the role of intrinsic pathway elements (caspase 3 and 9, Bax genes) in apoptosis, during the stable phase of the disease, has been shown.[20]

Course of the disease

Generally, PD is thought to have an acute inflammatory phase followed by a chronic phase. The acute phase is characterized by a progressive increase in plaque size or penile curvature associated with penile pain. In most cases, this phase lasts about 12 months from onset of the disease. PD progressively deteriorates if left untreated in the acute phase of the disease. The natural history of the disease was reported by Mulhall et al., who demonstrated that penile curvature worsened in almost half of the cohort: only 12% of men improved in terms of mean degree of curvature, while 40% remained stable and 48% worsened during the follow-up period.[21] The authors updated these changes in curvature (worsening, improvement, stable) as 21%, 12%, and 67%, respectively, in patients who received no treatment. Furthermore, predictive factors for stabilization were found to be presentation time (>6 months, OR 2.4), and advancing age (per decade; OR 1.5). In contrast the curvatures of young and early presenting patients improved four times greater than their older and late-presenting counterparts.[22] The chronic phase is a stable period during which penile curvature and plaque size remain the same with the absence of penile pain; this is generally accepted to start 12 months from the onset of the disease.[23]

Diagnosis and evaluation

The diagnosis of PD should be based on a comprehensive medical and sexual history and a detailed physical examination.[1] In particular, symptoms of the acute phase and erectile dysfunction (ED) should be noted. Penile pain is present in 35–45% of patients in the early phase (6 months) and resolves spontaneously in 90% of patients in the first 18 month.[3,21] The dysmorphic penis causes significant distress in these patients, as documented by validated mental health questionnaires showing depression in the 48% of patients.[24] The Center for Epidemiological Studies Depression scale (CES-D) has been used to assess the correlation between depression and PD; the rate of moderate and severe depression was observed as 26% and 21%, respectively.[25] After PD surgery significant improvement was recorded in sexual and overall relationship and confidence domains of the Self-Esteem and Relationship (SEAR) survey.[26] Using the latest PD scaling tool introduced by Hellstrom et al., the Peyronie's Disease Questionnaire (PDQ), 71% and 58% of the patients with severe and moderate/mild curvatures reported they were very/extremely bothered about the shape of their penis.[27] Correlation between ED and PD has been demonstrated in 50–60% of the patients; performance anxiety, deformity, flail penis, and impaired erection were suggested as the potential causes.[28] Erectile dysfunction should be assessed with the help of International Index of Erectile Function (IIEF-5) questionnaires and duplex ultrasonography. Ultrasonography is also a useful tool for determining plaque size and location, but is not indicated in routine clinical practice.[1]

Since progressive penile shortening is common in patients with PD, measurement of stretched penile length is an important part of the physical examination.[2] Men with PD have either a well-defined plaque or a palpable induration; for example, two-thirds of patients have a palpable induration on the dorsal aspect of the penis, with a corresponding penile curvature. Meanwhile, plaques that are ventrally or laterally located are less common, with an incidence of 10–20% and 6–10%, respectively, but cause more difficulty in penetration.[1] Assessment of curvature may be performed with the help of Intracavernosal injection (ICI), vacuum devices, or photographically but there is a significant underestimation of curvature degree (10°) in the latter technique when compared to ICI, especially in patients with ED.[29] Patient-reported curvature is unreliable, and only half of the patients are correct when compared with objective measurements.[30] Severe penile curvature (>60°) was reported as the sole reason for sexual disability.[31] In our series consisting of 1001 PD patients, independent predictors for severe curvature were identified as age, side of deformity, erectile dysfunction, and diabetes mellitus.[32] Stable curvature and resolution of pain for at least 3 months are indicators of the chronic phase, and this differentiation from the acute phase is vital because only in this phase should surgical intervention be considered.

Medical treatment

Medical therapy is an important aspect of Peyronie's disease management. Medical therapy can be undertaken depending on the phase and severity of disease. Efficacy of treatment should be assessed by the change in the curvature, as neither plaque size nor pain alterations are objective criteria. Most medical treatments lack critical evidenced-based support for their effectiveness due to the absence of randomized controlled trials (RCTs) or insignificant results in the RCTs. Iontophoresis, oral therapies (vitamin E, potassium para-aminobenzoate, tamoxifen, carnitine, and colchicine), extracorporeal, shockwave therapy, and intralesional injection with verapamil or nicardipine have shown mixed or negative results. The only treatments to decrease penile curvature deformity in placebo-controlled studies are intralesional injection with interferon α-2b or collagenase clostridium histolyticum.[33]

Surgical treatment

Surgical correction is the gold standard treatment option for PD, having the most reliable and sustained outcomes for correction of penile deformities in men with functional impairment. Surgery should only be considered:

1. After stabilization of the disease (12 months after the onset of disease or once the deformity has been stable and painless for at least 3 months, preferably 6 months).
2. In the presence of severe penile shortening or severe deformity that causes difficulty in penetration.
3. In the presence of plaque calcification.
4. After previously failed conservative treatment or when the patient wants a definitive result.[1]

Selection of the appropriate procedure for each patient depends on an intimate understanding of surgical outcomes and current status of the penile deformity. Erectile capacity should be assessed initially as it is the key determinant in selecting the surgical technique and the preference between reconstructive surgery and penile prosthesis implantation. Other important factors to be assessed are the direction and severity of the curvature, presence of destabilizing hinge effect caused by severe indentation or hourglass deformity, and the patient's expectations related to the outcomes of surgical interventions. An accepted reduction in penile length for every 30° of penile curvature is 1 cm, so the preoperative size of the penis should be measured and a lengthening operation should be preferred as reconstructive surgery for men with a short penis and greater degrees of curvature.

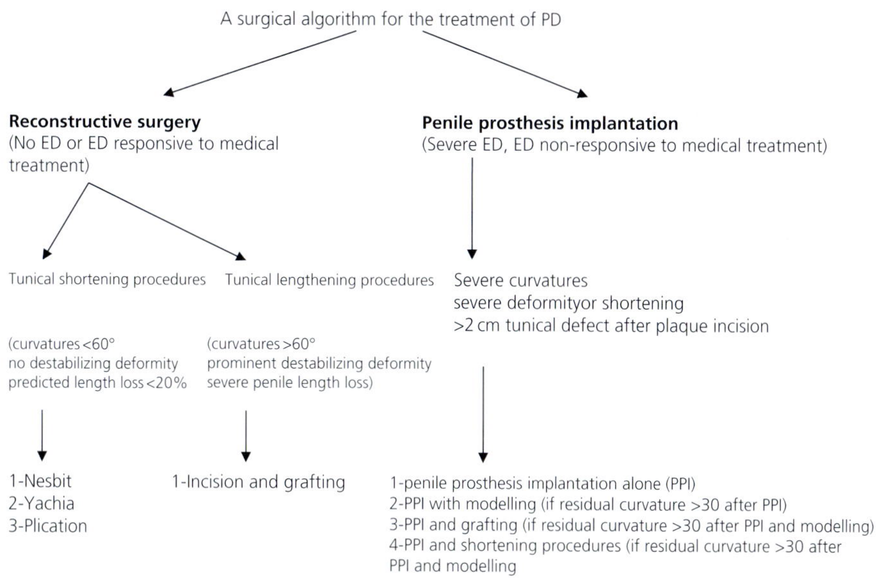

Figure 26.1 A surgical algorithm for the treatment of Peyronie's disease.

The surgical treatment options available for PD involve different techniques, which can be divided into two main categories (Figure 26.1):

1. Reconstructive surgeries are based upon either shortening the convex side or lengthening the concave side of the TA, by incision or partial excision of plaque and use of different types of grafts for closure of defect.
2. Penile prosthesis implantation with or without additional procedures such as remodeling, plication, and grafting.

Reconstructive surgery

Tunical shortening procedures

Tunical shortening procedures are recommended for men with satisfactory erectile function and curvatures less than 60–70° without any destabilizing deformities or hinge effect, and when the postoperative length loss is predicted to be less than 20% of the erect penile length as the difference in length (cm) between the concave and convex sides of the penis, measured from the peno-pubic junction to the tip of the glans penis dorsally, and from the penoscrotal junction to the tip of the glans ventrally.[1,8] Patients should be informed that penile length after surgery will be equal to the length of the concave side of the penis in all kinds of shortening procedures.

Nesbit procedure

Originally described by Nesbit in 1965, this method involves excision of an ellipsoid area of tissue from the TA at the opposite side of the penis to the most prominent point of curvature.[34] Naturally, shortening of the convex side of the penis is expected after closure of the defect. Depending on direction of the curvature, mobilization of the dorsal neurovascular bundle (NVB) or ventral corpus spongiosum is required.

Mobilization of the NVB for the correction of ventral deformities can be achieved by medial or lateral dissection of NVB depending on the experience of the surgeon. In the latter, mobilization of the NVB is performed by two longitudinal lateral incisions on Buck's fascia above the urethra at 5 and 7 o'clock positions. Alternatively, a medial dissection is performed in the bed of the previously resected deep dorsal vein.[35] A meticulous medial dissection with the help of surgical loupes should be preferred, preserving the NVB. Studies evaluating outcomes of the Nesbit procedure for different kinds of curvatures have reported success rates of penile straightening between 79% and 100%, with an overall patient satisfaction rate of 67–100%.[36–40] In these series, penile shortening of up to 2.5 cm was reported in 17.4–100% of the patients by Giammusso et al. In the largest series to date, involving 359 men who had undergone the Nesbit procedure, difficulty in achieving penetration after surgery was reported in less than 2% of the patients. All men experienced penile shortening, with an 82% overall satisfaction rate.[39] A modified Nesbit technique was described by Schwarzer et al. in which flaps of tunica albuginea, freed from the underlying corpus cavernosum after U-shaped incisions without any tunical tissue removal, were placed under the remaining TA in a watertight fashion. The authors reported penile straightness and patient satisfaction rates of 94% and 86%, respectively, in 50 patients with 27 months mean follow-up, while penile shortening and erectile dysfunction were detected in 78% and 13% of the cases.[40]

Yachia procedure

The Yachia procedure is a modification of the Nesbit technique that utilizes the Heineke–Mikulicz principle, whereby a single long incision or multiple small incisions are made longitudinally in the TA and subsequently closed horizontally to shorten the convex side of the penis.[41] Reported patient satisfaction rates after the Yachia procedure range between 78% and 100%.[42–44] Despite this, the procedure is not commonly used and the authors believe this operation should be within the surgical armamentarium of urologists dealing with sexual medicine. The major reasons for dissatisfaction with the Nesbit and Yachia procedures were the loss of penile tactile sensation (24%) and ED (12%) owing to elevation of the NVB and disruption of cavernosal integrity, respectively.[45] Nesbit surgery without circumcision has been suggested in one study with only one curvature recurrence and three paraphimoses out of 147 patients.[46]

Plication procedures

The penile plication technique, originally described by Essed and Schroeder, is the least invasive and thus the most commonly used surgical option for tunical shortening. No absorbable sutures are placed over the convex side of the TA, and there is no need for excision of TA tissue or mobilization of NVB in order to achieve a straight penis.[45] Plication procedures result in penile shortening similar to that of the Nesbit and Yachia procedures and are therefore recommended only in patients with adequate penile length and good baseline erectile function without any destabilizing deformity. Since the NVB is not mobilized, fewer complications, such as reduced penile sensation and retarded ejaculation, are seen in comparison with aforementioned techniques.

In a quality-of-life assessment performed by Van der Horst et al., 28 men with PD who underwent plication were retrospectively evaluated after 30 months.[47] Patients reported penile straightening, penile shortening, postoperative ED, and sensory changes at rates of 100%, 74%, 35.7%, and 28%, respectively, with an overall satisfaction rate of 67.8%. Similarly, Kadioglu et al. reported penile straightening in 14 of 15 men who had a preoperative mean penile curvature of 51° after a mean follow-up of 24 months.[48] All patients reported penile shortening and none complained of ED. In another series, more than 90% of patients reported penile straightening with a postoperative ED rate of approximately 10%.[49,50] Gholami and Lue reported a 16-dot (two pairs of plication) or 24-dot (three pairs of plication) plication technique, depending on the severity of the curvature, with minimal tension using multiple parallel plications.[51] After a mean follow-up of 2.6 years, 93% of 116 patients had straight erections and only 4% of them complained of decreased erectile function. However, recurrence of the curvature was observed in 15% of patients, and approximately 41% of them complained of penile shortening – the most commonly encountered adverse outcome of plication surgery. In the most recent study investigating plication, straightening and good erectile function rates of 91% and 89% were achieved, while penile shortening (1.5–3 cm) and glans sensitivity reduction rates of 22.5% and 9% were reported in 89 PD patients.[52]

The penoscrotal plication technique has been described for reconstruction of penile curvature in 45 men with PD.[53] The technique was performed with a 2-cm longitudinal incision at the penoscrotal junction opposite the direction of maximal curvature and carried down through Buck's fascia to expose the TA, where parallel sutures were placed in vertical mattress fashion parallel to the urethra. Penile straightening was achieved in all patients, with an overall satisfaction rate of 93%. Despite evaluating a relatively small cohort of patients with limited follow-up (only 34 were performed within 2 years), the technique described by the authors is promising since it is applicable for almost all curvatures, including severe or biplanar ones. The major advantage of the technique is the avoidance of circumcision to prevent distal ischemic and lymphatic complications. This technique has been performed recently for a larger patient population ($n = 102$) with a severe or biplanar curvature in 43% of them and a similar follow-up time,

15 months. The rate of patients with residual curvature, erectile dsyfunction and penile shortening were 4%, 14% and 14% respectively.[54]

Tunica albuginea plication (TAP), a modification of the Baskin–Duckett procedure, is another procedure that merits a mention. In this technique, plication was performed by using suturing in an inverted fashion after tunical shaving. The plication is subsequently reinforced with several additional interrupted sutures in a Lembert fashion. Levine et al. evaluated the outcomes of the TAP technique in a cohort including 100 patients with a median curvature angle of 49° and reported that 93% of the patients had curvatures less than 30° after a median follow-up of 72 months.[49] Postoperatively, 3 months of traction therapy prevented objective length loss of 1.5 cm, as shown in the secondary study of Levine.[55]

In summary, the major advantages of plication procedures are that they are simple, less invasive than other tunical shortening techniques, and are associated with better preservation of erectile function. However, potential disadvantages of these procedures are: penile shortening (especially after correction of curvatures greater than 60°, which may lead to shortening of up to 2 cm); the need for mobilization of NVB, which may lead to NVB injury and more length loss in ventral curvatures; and augmentation of an existing hourglass deformity or hinge effect due to the need for longer plications.[1] Consequently, plication techniques are currently more utilized because extensive surgical experience – except for ventral curvatures – is not needed.

Tunical lengthening procedures

The lengthening of the short side of curved penis is particularly suggested to patients who have normal erectile capacity together with either

1 curvature rates greater than 60 degrees,
2 hourglass deformity or
3 expected penile length loss greater than 2 cm."

Grafts are applied to the defect caused by the incision of prominent point of the convex side of the penis in which the plaque resides and thus lengthening of the penis is achieved. Plaque incision is preferred to excision because of the potential for cavernosal dysfunction with the disruption of the veno-occlusive mechanism.

Although there are several different graft materials, the surgical technique is generally uniform. Following a circumferential degloving incision of the skin of the penis to expose the entire shaft, an intraoperative artificial erection is induced to measure the penile length and curvature. Medial or lateral dissection of the neurovascular bundle (NVB) may be preferred depending on the plaque location. While medial dissection performed through the bed of the dorsal vein following the removal of deep dorsal vein at the prominent point of curvature, is preferred for isolated dorsal plaques, lateral NVB dissection may be required to achieve adequate lateral exposure in patients with lateral curvatures or hourglass deformities. NVB dissection should be carried out up to the healthy tissue (approximately 1 cm) with medial or lateral dissection off the underlying TA under loupe magnification. The absence of any plaque attachment to the NVB is vital for the prevention of curvature recurrences.

Subsequently, plaque incision is performed and graft material is positioned and sutured to restore tunical tissue integrity. Egydio et al. described the use of a single, almost complete circumferential-relaxing incision instead of the traditional H incision, applying geometric principles; this is suitable for all kinds of curvatures. Four tripod-shaped forks of 120 ° produce a simpler configuration of the tunical defect, which allows for easy suturing of the graft during the procedure. This technique has potential to become the standard technique for plaque incision in the future.[56]

Graft materials

Historically, three types of grafts have been described: autologous grafts; allografts (or xenografts); and synthetic grafts.[1] Synthetic materials, including polyester and polytetrafluoroethylene, are no longer used owing to increased rates of infection, fibrosis resulting from significant inflammation around the graft site with contracture, and risk of allergic reactions.[57]

The definition of the ideal graft material is one that is pliable, inexpensive, resistant to infection, and able to preserve erectile capacity. The graft type is also determined by the surgeon's experience, patient preference, and the type of deformity.

Although the choice of grafting material choice is associated with postoperative erectile dysfunction, preoperative erectile capacity of the patient and intervention type are closely correlated with ED. Forty-six percent of the patients who underwent grafting surgery with cadaveric pericardium had significant reductions in erectile capacity (>6-point IIEF score reduction), and independent ED risk factors were reported as: (1) degree of preoperative curvature (>60°); (2) type of plaque incision (Egydio); (3) patient age(>55); and (4) presence of cavernosal dysfunction. In another study comparing plication versus grafting, a higher ED rate in grafting procedures was shown in comparison with plication (21% vs 10%), although without statistical significance, and the only related comorbid disease was demonstrated to be DM.[57,58,59]

Autologous grafts

Autologous grafts are derived from the recipient of the graft. These grafts can provide the advantage of easy incorporation into host tissue with decreased incidence of local inflammatory reaction. A variety of materials are used including buccal mucosa, saphenous vein, preputium, dermis, tunica albuginea, tunica vaginalis, fascia lata, and rectus sheath.

Replacement of the plaque with buccal mucosa was first reported in 2005. In animal experiments, buccal mucosa was better than vein, dermis, aponeurosis, and peritoneum in terms of elasticity, lengthening, and morphological properties of the graft. Cormio et al. studied 15 patients who underwent plaque incision and buccal mucosa grafting, and reported 100% penile straightening with no postoperative ED after 13 months. However, disadvantages including oral numbness (16%) and tightness (32%) caused by tissue harvesting and potential inclusion cysts requiring secondary surgery were pitfalls in the use of this as a graft material.[57]

Tunica albuginea from the patient's own proximal crus may avoid immunogenic reactions and retraction of the graft due to fibrosis, and have potential to improve cosmesis. Schwarzer reported satisfactory penile straightening in 26 of 31 patients; four patients had minimal residual curvature. Despite immunogenic advantages, only small grafts can be obtained with this method involving surgery of the proximal crura. In a further study, 90% achieved penile straightening with a high patient satisfaction rate using crural grafts.[60]

Dermal grafts have a declining popularity as a result of high de novo veno-occlusive dysfunction rates with a reduction in tunical wall tension at the graft site. Some authors advocate the tight structure of the foreskin's keratinized squamous epithelium for the prevention of cavernosal dysfunction, but the small sample size of the study puts a limitation to the generalizability of the results.[57]

Saphenous vein is the most commonly used graft material for tunical lengthening owing to the ease and reliability of harvesting, large surface area, and increased compliance with its thin vascular walls that can be perfused from the corporal bodies. Moreover, it is hypothesized that the nitric oxide secreted from endothelium might prevent hematoma formation and improve erectile function. Since its initial application in 1993, several different groups have used this technique, with high functional and anatomical success rates of 75% and 90%, respectively. While a straight penis is achieved in 75–96% of the patients, a postoperative ED rate of up to 25% may be observed. Kalsi associated de novo ED with high curvature (mean 75°), DM, and ischemic heart disease.

In our series of 75 patients and mean curvature of 60°, penile curvature was completely straightened in 75.7% of patients with a residual curvature greater or lesser than 20° in 12.8% and 11.4% of patients, respectively. Other studies performed with saphenous vein grafting reported overall rates for successful penile straightening, penile shortening, and patient satisfaction in the following ranges: 72–96%, 17–40%, and 88–100%, respectively.[61]

The worst results using saphenous vein were reported by Montorsi, with a 22% risk of ED, 100% risk of length loss, and 12% risk of persistent or recurrent curvature. In this study (with long-term follow-up) only 60% of the patients were satisfied with the surgery. While the ED rate of 22.5% was similar in Kalsi's five year long follow-up study, length loss was reported only in 35% of the patients. In contrast 90% of the patients operated by UCSF group were satisfied with the results. Authors of this study recommend using strong non-absorbable monofilament sutures while avoiding unnecessary electrocautery, suction and extensive dissection of penile anatomic layers.[61]

Disadvantages of saphenous vein grafting include the need for a second incision, harvest site comorbidities (leg wound infection, hypoesthesia of the legs, and lymphocele), labor-intensive preparation, and penile complications (decreased penile sensation, retarded ejaculation, penile edema, bulging of the graft, and hematoma under the graft site). Advantages include: a greater general accumulation of experience; favorable tissue properties of veins; and a well-established surgical technique.[61]

Allografts and xenografts

Allografts are extracellular matrix tissues isolated from the same species as the recipient, such as human cadaveric pericardium or dermis, whereas xenografts are processed from animal tissues such as bovine pericardium or porcine small intestinal submucosa (SIS). They allow host cell ingrowth with minimal inflammatory response.

Mid-term outcomes of allograft surgery are similar to those of autologous grafts, with the advantages of a decreased operation time and the absence of tissue harvesting, meaning no harvest-site complications.[1,2] For this reason, there is a current tendency for surgeons to use allografts. Among these materials, pericardium is the most commonly used graft type.

Bovine pericardium has a rate of 88% for complete penile straightening, with 3% of recipients reporting glans hypoesthesia, and no erectile dysfunction.[62] Studies with human cadaveric pericardium reported similar penile straightening success rates of 56–98%, with penile shortening rates of 0–33%. Overall satisfaction rates in these studies ranged between 73% and 98%. In a study investigating partial plaque excision with processed cadaveric pericardial grafting (follow-up 5 years), 92% achieved penile straightening, 47% suffered penile length loss, and a 24% risk of ED was reported, leading to a satisfaction rate of 76%. Thus, pericardium, either bovine or cadaveric, is the most widely used off-the-shelf biomaterial with satisfactory short- to mid-term outcomes. These clinical results were supported by an animal study in which cadaveric pericardium, dermis, vein, and synthetic grafts were compared in terms of fibrosis and erectile dysfunction in rats; no significant difference was reported.[63]

Small intestinal submucosa (SIS) is another acellular biomaterial consisting of stratum compactum of tunica mucosa, tunica muscularis mucosa, and submucosa of porcine jejunum. Initially used by Knoll in 2001, lyophilized porcine 4-layer SIS graft achieved straightening in 92% of patients. In a study using porcine 4-layer SIS grafting, the reported rates of straightening, adequate erectile capacity, and prevention of penile length loss were 91%, 79%, and 5%, respectively, without any further complications. In contrast, high rates of recurrent curvature and plaque (37% and 25%), graft site hematomas (25%), and infection were observed after 1-layer SIS grafting by Breyer. Poor results were reported in another study investigating 4-layer SIS, with penile straightness in only 67%, with 11% experiencing ED and 25% penile shortening.[64] In another study reporting on long-term outcomes of xenografting (bovine pericardium and 4-layer SIS), the initial satisfaction rate of 80% decreased to 35% over the term.[65]

Cadaveric fascia lata is another biologically stable graft material with enough mechanical strength and available in a range of sizes. While penile straightening was achieved in 78% of the patients, penile shortening and de novo ED rates were reported to be 28% and 7%. The outcomes of autologous dermal, cadaveric fascia lata, and 4-layered SIS grafting were compared in another study. Self-reported resolution of penile curvature was noted in 60% of dermal, 100% of cadaveric fascia lata, and 76.9% of 4-layer SIS graft recipients. Meanwhile, patient satisfaction was higher in cadaveric fascia lata (92%) and 4-layer SIS (84.6%) in comparison with dermal grafts. Thus, the authors suggested using cadaveric fascia lata based on their comparative study. Accordingly, among allografts and xenografts, pericardium and 4-layer SIS are the currently available options with satisfactory clinical outcomes. Of note, among allograft materials the use of dura mater, despite its high success rates, has been abandoned due to the probability of development of slow viral and prion infections.[61]

Penile prosthesis implantation

Penile prosthesis implantation (PPI) is the standard procedure for men with PD and concomitant ED that does not respond to medical treatment.[1,61] Both malleable and inflatable implants are available, but inflatable prostheses are associated with higher functional satisfaction and lower persistent curvature rates. Indeed, Montorsi et al.[66] reported a patient satisfaction rate of only 48% in 48 men 5 years after they underwent malleable prosthesis surgery, while there are several studies of inflatable penile prostheses reporting success rates ranging between 84% and 100%.[67–71] Generally, pubic or penoscrotal incisions are preferred for the insertion of inflatable penile prostheses, according to the surgeon's experience. After cavernotomy, Hegar dilators can be used to dilate the corpora before insertion of the prosthesis.

In patients with mild curvatures (<30°), penile straightening can be achieved with the implantation of a prosthesis alone. If considerable penile curvature (>30°) persists after PPI, there are several further options, including manual modeling, plaque incision with or without grafting, and plication.[1] PPI combined with manual modeling can result in penile straightening in more than half of patients, but up to 20–30% of men with significant residual curvature require additional plaque surgery (incision with or without grafting, plication) in order to achieve a straight penis.[48,67] Grafting is generally recommended if the incision creates a tunical defect greater than 2 cm, in order to decrease the risk of contracture owing to fibrosis. However, we tend to close the tunical defect with grafted tissue, regardless of its size, in order to prevent formation of hematoma, infection, and herniation of the cylinders.

A range of autologous and allograft or xenograft tissues such as pericardium can be used in prosthetic surgery, but autologous rectus fascia and saphenous vein are the most widely used. Dermal grafts had fallen out of favor because of high infection rates in synchronous penile prosthesis implantation. Autologous rectus fascia was used in 18 men undergoing incision of plaque and grafting after PPI, and reported curvature recurrence was an acceptable rate of 5%.[48] The major advantages of autologous rectus fascia are its resistance to ischemia owing to low metabolic demands, and the fact that tissue harvesting can be performed without an additional incision if a pubic incision is used for implantation of the prosthesis. Austoni et al. reported the outcomes of 145 patients undergoing three-piece inflatable PPI using a relaxing incision and grafting with saphenous vein. After 13 months, 80 patients reported satisfaction in terms of penile straightening and sexual function.[72]

In a further study with 105 PD patients, Egydio performed penile prosthesis implantation with concomitant penile lengthening and girth restoration through circular and longitudinal incisions in the tunica albuginea followed by pericardial grafting. After a mean follow-up time of 18.2 months, a patient satisfaction rate of 89.4% was achieved, with 3.6 cm of penile lengthening, and 99% having successful sexual intercourse.[73] Meanwhile, Rolle et al. described a similar combined penile prosthesis and grafting technique called "sliding," in which porcine SIS tissue was grafted on both dorsal and ventral sides of the defect. The mean increase in penile length was reported to be 3.2 cm and all the patients were able to have sexual intercourse.[74]

Based on the results of these studies, the preference of graft material for use in conjunction with penile prostheses mostly depends on the experience of the surgeon and cost-effectiveness.

Conclusion

Medical therapy may be administered for Peyronie's disease in the early phase, and the efficacy of the treatment should be evaluated by curvature improvement. No significant improvement in curvature has been demonstrated in placebo-controlled studies for oral treatments. While interferon and collagenase treatment seems to be the best alternative in the non-surgical treatment group, with significant improvements in curvature, intralesional verapamil treatment, iontophoresis, and other options require further investigation.

Surgical treatment is the gold standard treatment option for men in the chronic phase of PD with disabling penile deformity and/or concomitant ED. Surgical approaches can be categorized as reconstructive surgeries (penile shortening or penile lengthening) or PPI. Erectile function should be assessed initially as it is the key determinant in the choice of surgical technique, followed by the direction and severity of the curvature, presence of destabilizing hinge effect caused by severe indentation or hourglass deformity, penis size, and patients' expectations related to the outcomes of surgical interventions.

Among the tunical shortening procedures, penile plication is a less invasive option that is relatively easy to perform in comparison with Nesbit and Yachia procedures. Lengthening procedures should be reserved for severe curvatures and complex deformities; saphenous vein and cadaveric pericardium are the most reliable graft materials.

For patients with PD and associated ED who are non-responsive to medical treatment, PPI is the standard of care. However, additional interventions such as manual modeling, tunical plication, plaque incision, and grafting might be required to obtain complete penile straightening. If these maneuvers fail to correct the deformity, grafting with autologous rectus fascia and cadaveric pericardium or 4-SIS can be considered. Although it is well-known that PD is a heterogeneous condition and no single procedure applies to all patients, the surgeon must choose the type of operation according to his or her own individual experiences as well as the preference of the patient. Since the ideal graft material is not available, reported outcomes are variable due to the surgeon's experience and material availability. Autologous grafts, especially saphenous vein and pericardial (both human and bovine) grafts, are the mainstream candidates for grafting, with their high success rates. Future directions of PD treatment are potentially stem-cell-enhanced grafts and other potentially minimally invasive treatments.

References

1 Ralph D, Gonzalez-Cadavid N, Mirone V, et al. The management of Peyronie's disease: Evidence-based 2010 guidelines. *J Sex Med* 2010;7:2359–74.

2 Smith JF, Walsh TJ, Lue TF. Peyronie's disease: a critical appraisal of current diagnosis and treatment. *Int J Impot Res* 2008;20:445–59.

3 Mulhall JP, Creech SD, Boorjian SA, et al. Subjective and objective analysis of the prevalence of Peyronie's disease in a population of men presenting for prostate cancer screening. *J Urol* 2004;171:2350–3.

4 Cavallini GI, Paulis G. Improvement of chronic Peyronie's disease symptoms after diabetic compensation: a retrospective study. *Urology* 2013;81(4):794–8.

5 Deveci S, Hopps CV, O'Brien K, Parker M, Guhring P, Mulhall JP. Defining the clinical characteristics of Peyronie's disease in young men. *J Sex Med* 2007;4(2):485–90.

6 Tefekli A, Kandirali E, Erol H, Alp T, Köksal T, Kadioğlu A. Peyronie's disease in men under age 40: characteristics and outcome. *Int J Impot Res* 2001;13(1):18–23.

7 Tal R, Hall MS, Alex B, Choi J, Mulhall JP. Peyronie's disease in teenagers. *J Sex Med* 2012;9(1):302–8.

8 Mulhall JP, Anderson M, Parker M. A surgical algorithm for men with combined Peyronie's disease and erectile dysfunction: Functional and satisfaction outcomes. *J Sex Med* 2005;2:132–8.

9 Casabé A, Bechara A, Cheliz G. Risk factors of Peyronie's disease. What does our clinical experience show? *J Sex Med* 2011;8(2):518–23.

10 Bjekic MD, Vlajinac HD, Sipetic SB, Marinkovic JM. Risk factors for Peyronie's disease: a case-control study. *BJU Int* 2006;97:570–4.

11 Davila H, Ferrini M, Rajfer J, et al. Fibrin induction of a Peyronie's-like plaque in the rat penile tunica albuginea. A new model for Peyronie's disease. *Br J Urol* 2003;91:830–8.

12 Cantini LP, Ferrini MG, Vernet D, et al. Pro-fibrotic role of myostatin in Peyronie's disease. *J Sex Med* 2008;5:1607–22.

13 Gonzalez-Cadavid NF, Rajfer J. Mechanisms of disease: new insights into the cellular and molecular pathology of Peyronie's disease. *Nat Clin Pract Urol* 2005;2(6):291–7.

14 Gonzalez-Cadavid NF, Rajfer J. Experimental models of Peyronie's disease. Implications for new therapies. *J Sex Med* 2009;6(2):303–13.

15 Vernet D, Ferrini MG, Valente E, et al. Effect of nitric oxide on the differentiation of fibroblasts into myofibroblasts in the Peyronie's fibrotic plaque and in its rat model. *Nitric Oxide* 2002;7:262–76.

16 Akman T, Tefekli A, Armagan A, et al. Decorin as a new treatment alternative in Peyronie's disease: preliminary results in the rat model. *Andrologia* 2013;45(2):101–6.

17 Chung E, De Young L, Solomon M, Brock GB. Peyronie's disease and mechanotransduction: an in vitro analysis of the cellular changes to Peyronie's disease in a cell-culture strain system. *J Sex Med* 2013;10:1259–67.

18 Loreto C, Barbagli G, Djinovic R, et al. Tumor necrosis factor-related apoptosis-inducing ligand (TRAIL) and its death receptor (DR5) in Peyronie's disease. A biomolecular study of apoptosis activation. *J Sex Med* 2011;8(1):109–15.

19 Zorba OU, Sirma S, Ozgon G, Salabas E, Ozbek U, Kadioglu A. Comparison of apoptotic gene expression profiles between Peyronie's disease plaque and tunica albuginea. *Adv Clin Exp Med* 2012;21(5):607–14.

20 Loreto C, La Rocca G, Anzalone R, et al. The role of intrinsic pathway in apoptosis activation and progression in Peyronie's disease. *Biomed Res Int* 2014(2014); article ID:616149.

21 Mulhall JP, Schiff J, Guhring P. An analysis of the natural history of Peyronie's disease. *J Urol* 2006;175:2115–18.

22 Berookhim BM1, Choi J, Alex B, Mulhall JP. Deformity stabilization and improvement in men with untreated Peyronie's disease. *BJU Int* 2014;113(1):133–6.

23 Hellstrom WJ, Bivalacqua TJ. Peyronie's disease: etiology, medical and surgical therapy. *J Androl* 2000;21:347–54.

24 Levine LA, Greenfield JM. Establishing a standardized evaluation of the man with Peyronie's disease. *Int J Impot Res* 2003(Suppl. 5):103–12.

25 Nelson CJ, Diblasio C, Kendirci M, Hellstrom W, Guhring P, Mulhall JP. The chronology of depression and distress in men with Peyronie's disease. *J Sex Med* 2008;5(8):1985–90.

26 Tal R, Nabulsi O, Nelson CJ, Mulhall JP. The psychosocial impact of penile reconstructive surgery for congenital penile deviation. *J Sex Med* 2010;7(1 Pt 1):121–8.

27 Gelbard M, Hellstrom WJ, McMahon CG, et al. Baseline characteristics from an ongoing phase 3 study of collagenase clostridium histolyticum in patients with Peyronie's disease. *J Sex Med* 2013;10(11):2822–31.

28 Kadioglu A, Tefekli A, Erol B, et al. A retrospective review of 307 men with Peyronie's disease. *J Urol* 2002;168(3):1075–9.

29 Ohebshalom M, Mulhall J, Guhring P, et al. Measurement of penile curvature in Peyronie's disease patients: comparison of three methods. *J Sex Med* 2007;4(1):199–203.

30 Matsushita K, Stember DS, Nelson CJ, Mulhall JP. Concordance between patient and physician assessment of the magnitude of Peyronie's disease curvature. *J Sex Med* 2014;11(1):205–10.

31 Walsh TJ, Hotaling JM, Lue TF, Smith JF. How curved is too curved? The severity of penile deformity may predict sexual disability among men with Peyronie's disease. *Int J Impot Res* 2013;25(3):109–12.

32 Kadioglu A, Sanli O, Akman T, et al. Factors affecting the degree of penile deformity in Peyronie disease: an analysis of 1001 patients. *J Androl* 2011;32(5):502–8.

33 Jordan GH, Carson CC, Lipshultz LI. Minimally invasive treatment of Peyronie's disease: evidence-based progress. *BJU Int* 2014;114(1):16–24.

34 Nesbit RM. Congenital curvature of the phallus: report of three cases with description of corrective operation. *J Urol* 1965;93:230–2.

35 Giammusso B, Burrello M, Branchina A, Nicolosi F, Motta M. Modified corporoplasty for ventral penile curvature: description of technique and initial results. *J Urol* 2004;171:1209–11.

36 Savoca G, Scieri F, Pietropaolo F, Garaffa G, Belgrano E. Straightening corporoplasty for Peyronie's disease: a review of 218 patients with median follow-up of 89 months. *Eur Urol* 2004;46:610–14.

37 Bokarica P, Parazajder J, Mazuran B, Gilja I. Surgical treatment of Peyronie's disease based on penile length and degree of curvature. *Int J Impot Res* 2005;17:170–4.

38 Licht MR, Lewis RW. Modified Nesbit procedure for the treatment of Peyronie's disease: a comparative outcome analysis. *J Urol* 1997;158:460–3.

39 Ralph DJ, al-Akraa M, Pryor JP. The Nesbit operation for Peyronie's disease: 16-year experience. *J Urol* 1995;154:1362–3.

40 Schwarzer JU, Steinfatt H. Tunica albuginea underlap—a new modification of the Nesbit procedure: description of the technique and preliminary results. *J Sex Med* 2012;9(11):2970–4.

41 Yachia, D. Modified corporoplasty for the treatment of penile curvature. *J Urol* 1990;143:80–2.

42 Daitch JA, Angermeier KW, Montague DK. Modified corporoplasty for penile curvature: long-term results and patient satisfaction. *J Urol* 1999;162:2006–9.

43 Rehman J, Benet A, Minsky LS, Melman A. Results of surgical treatment for abnormal penile curvature: Peyronie's disease and congenital deviation by modified Nesbit plication (tunical shaving and plication). *J Urol* 1997;157:1288–91.

44 Lopes I, Tomada N, Vendeira P. Penile corporoplasty with Yachia's technique for Peyronie's disease: Single center experience with 117 patients. *Urol Ann* 2013;5(3):167–71.

45 Essed E, Schroeder FH. New surgical treatment for Peyronie's disease. *Urology* 1985;25:582–7.

46 Pavone C, Abbadessa D, Usala M. Circumcision in Nesbit corporoplasty: a mandatory time? Our experience on 158 patients *Urologia.* 2012;79(1):44–8.

47 Van der Horst C, Martínez Portillo FJ, Seif C, Alken P, Juenemann KP. Treatment of penile curvature with Essed-Schröder tunical plication: aspects of quality of life from the patients' perspective. *BJU Int* 2004; 93:105–8.

48 Kadioglu A, Sanli O, Akman T, Cakan M, Erol B, Mammadov F. Surgical treatment of Peyronie's disease: A single center experience with 145 patients. *Eur Urol* 2008;53:432–40.

49 Greenfield JM, Lucas S, Levine LA. Factors affecting the loss of length associated with tunica albuginea plication for correction of penile curvature. *J Urol* 2006;175:238–41.

50 Taylor FL, Levine LA. Surgical correction of Peyronie's disease via tunica albuginea plication or partial plaque excision with pericardial graft: long-term follow-up. *J Sex Med* 2008;5:2221–8.

51 Gholami SS, Lue TF. Correction of penile curvature using the 16-dot plication technique: a review of 132 patients. *J Urol* 2002;167:2066–9.

52 Cantoro U, Polito M, Catanzariti F, et al. Penile plication for Peyronie's disease: our results with mean follow-up of 103 months on 89 patients. *Int J Impot Res* 2014;26(4):156–9.

53 Dugi DD 3rd, Morey AF. Penoscrotal plication as a uniform approach to reconstruction of penile curvature. *BJU Int* 2010;105:1440–4.

54 Adibi M, Hudak SJ, Morey AF. Penile plication without degloving enables effective correction of complex Peyronie's deformities. *Urology* 2012;79(4):831–5.

55 Rybak J, Papagiannopoulos D, Levine L. A retrospective comparative study of traction therapy vs. no traction following tunica albuginea plication or partial excision and grafting for Peyronie's disease: measured lengths and patient perceptions. *J Sex Med* 2012;9(9):2396–403.

56 Egydio PH, Lucon AM, Arap S. A single relaxing incision to correct different types of penile curvature: surgical technique based on geometrical principles. *BJU Int* 2004;94:1147–57.

57 Kadioglu A, Sanli O, Akman T, et al. Graft materials in Peyronie's disease surgery: A comprehensive review. *J Sex Med* 2007;4:581–95.

58 Flores S, Choi J, Alex B, et al. Erectile dysfunction after plaque incision and grafting: short-term assessment of incidence and predictors. *J Sex Med* 2011;8:2031–7.

59 Taylor FL, Abern MR, Levine LA. Predicting erectile dysfunction following surgical correction of Peyronie's disease without inflatable penile prosthesis placement: vascular assessment and preoperative risk factors. *J Sex Med* 2012;9:296–301.

60 Da Ros CT, Graziottin TM, Ribeiro E, Averbeck MA. Long-term follow-up of penile curvature correction utilizing autologous albugineal crural graft. *Int Braz J Urol* 2012;38(2):242–7.

61 Kadioglu A, Küçükdurmaz F, Sanli O. Current status of the surgical management of Peyronie's disease. *Nat Rev Urol* 2011;8(2):95–106.

62 Sansalone S, Garaffa G, Djinovic R. Long-term results of the surgical treatment of Peyronie's disease with Egydio's technique: a European multicentre study. *Asian J Androl* 2011;13(6):842–5.

63 Leungwattanakij SI, Bivalacqua TJ, Yang DY, Hyun JS, Hellstrom WJ. Comparison of cadaveric pericardial, dermal, vein, and synthetic grafts for tunica albuginea substitution using a rat model. *BJU Int* 2003;92(1):119–24.

64 Staerman F, Pierrevelcin J, Ripert T, et al. Medium-term follow-up of plaque incision and porcine small intestinal submucosal grafting for Peyronie's disease. *Int J Impot Res* 2010;22(6):343–8.

65 Chung E, Clendinning E, Lessard L, Brock G. Five-year follow-up of Peyronie's graft surgery: outcomes and patient satisfaction. *J Sex Med* 2011;8(2):594–600.

66 Montorsi F, Guazzoni G, Bergamaschi F, Rigatti P. Patient-partner satisfaction with semirigid penile prostheses for Peyronie's disease: a 5-year followup study. *J Urol* 1993;150:1819–21.

67 Wilson SK, Delk JR 2nd. A new treatment for Peyronie's disease: modeling the penis over an inflatable penile prosthesis. *J Urol* 1994;152:1121–3.
68 Levine LA, Dimitriou RJ. A surgical algorithm for penile prosthesis placement in men with erectile failure and Peyronie's disease. *Int J Impot Res* 2000;12:147–51.
69 Carson CC. Penile prosthesis implantation in the treatment of Peyronie's disease and erectile dysfunction. *Int J. Impot Res* 2000;12(Suppl. 4):S122–S126.
70 Chaudhary M, Sheikh N, Asterling S, Ahmad I, Greene D. Peyronie's disease with erectile dysfunction: penile modeling over inflatable penile prostheses. *Urology* 2005;65:760–4.
71 Levine LA, Benson J, Hoover C. Inflatable penile prosthesis placement in men with Peyronie's disease and drug-resistant erectile dysfunction: a single-center study. *J Sex Med* 2010; 7:3775–83.
72 Austoni E, Colombo F, Romanò A-L, et al. Soft prosthesis implant and relaxing albugineal incision with saphenous grafting for surgical therapy of Peyronie's disease: a 5-year experience and long-term follow-up on 145 operated patients. *Eur Urol* 2005;47:223–9.
73 Egydio PH, Kuehhas FE, Sansalone S. Penile length and girth restoration in severe Peyronie's disease using circular and longitudinal grafting. *BJU Int* 2013;111(4 Pt B):E213–9.
74 Rolle L, Ceruti C, Timpano M, et al. A new, innovative, lengthening surgical procedure for Peyronie's disease by penile prosthesis implantation with double dorsal-ventral patch graft: the "sliding technique". *J Sex Med* 2012;9(9):2389–95.

CHAPTER 27

Penile implant surgery

Patrick Selph[1] and Culley Carson[2]

[1] *University of Alabama at Birmingham, Birmingham, AL, USA*

[2] *University of North Carolina, Chapel Hill, NC, USA*

Introduction

It is estimated that over 15,000 penile implant surgeries are performed annually in the United States.[1] While the advent of phosphodiesterase inhibitors (PDEIs) has changed the medical management of erectile dysfunction (ED), and their use is often seen as first-line therapy, for many men, penile implant surgery is the definitive treatment for ED. Indications for penile implant surgery include men with ED refractory to medical management, severe Peyronie's disease, and recurrent ischemic priapism. Penile implants have gone through multiple iterations in the last four decades, and because of their reliability, functionality, and high patient satisfaction rates, inflatable penile prostheses (IPPs) are the most common type of implant performed today. Preoperative counseling is important for patients undergoing penile implant surgery, and a thorough discussion of risks and outcomes is warranted in order to appropriately guide a patient's expectations. Perioperative complications include infection, mechanical malfunction, erosion or perforation, incorrect sizing of the device, autoinflation, urethral injury, and, rarely, vascular or bowel injury. Reported outcomes have shown high patient and partner satisfaction rates.[2] In this chapter, we will review the indications for implant surgery, the types of implants, perioperative considerations, complications, and outcomes.

Indications

Epidemiological studies have estimated that more than 50% of men aged 40 to 70 have some form of ED, and nearly half of men in the seventh decade of life have moderate to severe ED.[3] It is estimated that nearly 620,000 Caucasian men aged 40–69 years will develop ED each year in the United States.[4] The introduction of PDEIs, beginning with sildenafil in 1998, changed the landscape of treatment for ED. While more men could be offered oral therapy for ED, an initial study showed the rates of penile implant surgery in the post-PDEI era were not significantly different, and, in fact, it was postulated that the rates of implant surgery may even rise as more men became aware of treatments for ED or failed PDEI treatment.[5]

The main indication for penile implant surgery is ED refractory to medical management. This group also includes men with ED after radical pelvic surgery, including radical prostatectomy. Medical therapies include PDEIs, intracavernosal injections (ICI), vacuum erection devices (VEDs), and/or intraurethral suppositories. While PDEIs are considered first-line treatment for ED, about 30–40% of patients will not respond to sildenafil, vardenafil, or tadalafil.[6,7] Second-line treatments often have high failure or withdrawal rates. In one recent study of discontinuation rates of ICI in men who had previously failed PDEIs, nearly 80% of men discontinued ICI treatment for a variety of reasons, including pain, inconvenience, poor response, and adverse events.[8] In one prospective study of couple satisfaction rates among 354 couples undergoing treatment for ED with either PDEIs, ICIs, VEDs, testosterone, or penile implant surgery, VEDs showed the lowest rates of mean total satisfaction score, end score, and percentage change in all domains of International Index of Erectile Function (IIEF) scores.[9] Even in patients who are post-nerve-sparing radical prostatectomy (RP) for prostate cancer, it is estimated that 20–80% will not have

Male Sexual Dysfunction: A Clinical Guide, First Edition. Edited by Suks Minhas and John Mulhall.

erections satisfactory for penetration.[10] In a SEER-Medicare database analysis of 15,811 men undergoing RP for prostate cancer, 2.3% underwent penile implant surgery.[11] Encouragingly, satisfaction rates for penile implant surgery are high in the post-RP group.[12–14]

Severe Peyronie's disease, or Peyronie's disease concomitant with ED, is also an indication for implant surgery.[15,16] In the man with significant fibrosis and curvature to the penis, penile plication or plaque incision and grafting may not provide enough correction in curvature to provide a functional outcome. In these cases, performing an IPP with associated modeling or plaque incision should be considered as first-line treatment.[16]

A more recent development has been the promotion of IPPs in men with refractory ischemic priapism. In men with recurrent episodes of ischemic priapism, or who have episodes lasting greater than 36 hours, rates of ED are high, ranging from 54% to 100% depending on duration.[17,18] While some of these men may pursue an elective penile implant in the future, scarring and fibrosis that develop in the long term in patients who have had recurrent priapism may cause penile shortening or make primary implant more difficult. In order to prevent the cycle of recurrent trips to the ER requiring procedures, limit fibrosis and penile shortening, and treat the nearly inevitable ED, immediate insertion of a penile prosthesis in cases of delayed or refractory ischemic priapism has been studied.[19–21] A study by Ralph reported a 96% satisfaction rate among 50 patients undergoing immediate insertion of a penile prosthesis (43 malleable, 7 inflatable three-piece) for delayed or refractory ischemic priapism, with a 6% infection rate.[21] Concerns over this aggressive treatment include the potential for a higher complication rate in the acute setting, and future costs associated with mechanical failure rates in what are usually young patients.

Types of prostheses

Multiple types of prostheses are available, including semirigid and malleable prostheses, two-piece inflatable prostheses, and three-piece inflatable prostheses. Since the original development of the inflatable penile prosthesis by Scott et al. in 1973 and the Small–Carrion silicone prosthesis in 1975, penile implants have gone through multiple revisions such that the three-piece inflatable penile prosthesis is the most popular device inserted today.[22,23] Table 27.1 lists the currently available penile prostheses and the two major manufacturers: American Medical Systems (AMS; Minnetonka, MN), and Coloplast Corporation (Humlebaek, Denmark).

A semirigid prosthesis can be either a malleable or mechanical device that is inserted into the penis to provide rigidity. They have the advantages of being moldable into different orientations depending on the need (e.g., intercourse, voiding, or hiding under clothes), low requirements for manual dexterity, low mechanical failures, and a simpler insertion process for the surgeon.[24] Disadvantages include the constant erect state of the penis, a less rigid erection than an inflatable device, less flaccidity, and perhaps a higher rate of erosion.[25] Older iterations of the malleable prosthesis by AMS included the 600, 650, and Dura II prostheses, but these have been discontinued in favor of the newer Spectra™

Table 27.1 Available penile prostheses.

	AMS	Coloplast	Others
Semirigid	Spectra	Genesis	Promedon Tube (Argentina)
			HR Penile Prosthesis (Brazil)
			Silimed (Brazil)
			Jonas ESKA (Germany)
			Virilis I/II (Italy)
			Shah (India)
Two-piece	Ambicor	Excel	
Three-piece	700 CX	Titan	
	700 CXR	Titan narrow base	
	700 LGX	Titan OTR	

device. The AMS Spectra is a blending of the features of the older models. Its cylinders have a durable silicone core and a spring loaded design to improve ease of use, along with the ability to conceal the device at a 7° angle. Three cylinder diameters and lengths are available, and rear tip extenders can be utilized to adjust device size based on penile length. Coloplast markets the Genesis™ malleable prosthesis, which has a hydrophilic coating that can be soaked in antibiotics in an attempt to reduce infection rates. The Promedon Tube from Argentina is another malleable prosthesis composed of a silver core that has different rigidities along its length.[26,27] The Silimed™ malleable device from Brazil is a silicone elastomer with a silver core.[27] The HR Prosthesis from Brazil comes in two models: a malleable device with a steel core and another with a silver core.[27] The Virilis implants from Italy are variations on the same theme: a soft silicone base that is slightly more rigid in the distal third of the Virilis II when compared to the Virilis I.[27] A unique feature of this model is that given the completely soft silicone elastomer and lack of a silver core, the corporal bodies can be displaced rather than destroyed during placement, which perhaps allows a more physiologic erection.[28] The Shah implant from India is a silicone non-malleable device with four distinct areas of rigidity and removable sleeves that allow diameter adjustments.[27]

The two-piece inflatable devices currently available on the market include the AMS Ambicor™ and the Coloplast Excel™. With these devices, a pump is placed in the scrotum, and inflatable cylinders are placed in each corpus. Advantages to these devices include good rigidity, more flaccidity when compared to a malleable device, and an easier insertion when compared to a three-piece implant given that no abdominal incision is needed and the device is pre-connected and prefilled. Disadvantages include less flaccidity when compared to a three-piece inflatable device, and the possibility of mechanical malfunction and the need for some manual dexterity as compared to a malleable device. The AMS Ambicor™ is inflated by squeezing on the pump, and the device is deflated by compressing the penis. The fluid reservoir is located in the base of each cylinder. Multiple diameters are available, and rear tip extenders can be used to adjust the fit for penile length. The Coloplast Excel™ is similar in its design, though the Resipump™ in the scrotum acts as both the pump and reservoir. A hydrophilic coating is present on the Bioflex polymer base that allows for soaking in antibiotic solution.

The three-piece inflatable penile prosthesis is the most commonly implanted of all types of prostheses. Given the relatively similar infection and malfunction rates of semirigid devices and three-piece IPPs, there are few advantages to placing a semirigid device over a three-piece implant. Modifications in design of three-piece IPPs, including plastic connectors replacing stainless steel connectors, non-kink tubing, Teflon input sleeves, multiple layer cylinders, and single design construction, have decreased mechanical malfunction rates from over 30% to less than 5%. These devices consist of cylinders placed into each corpus, a pump in the scrotum, and a fluid reservoir in the abdomen. Fluid (usually saline but can be a water/contrast mixture) is drawn from the reservoir into the corporal cylinders by pumping on the scrotal pump. Three-piece IPPs are able to provide a more natural appearing and feeling erection as compared to the other implants, and they are able to provide for greater flaccidity. Furthermore, they can provide girth and in some cases length expansion. The Coloplast Titan™ line (Titan, Titan OTR, Titan narrow base) and the AMS 700 MS series (CX, CXR, LGX) are the available devices. The Coloplast Titan™ consists of paired cylinders made of Bioflex attached by silicone tubing to a scrotal pump and an abdominal reservoir. The device is activated by squeezing the scrotal pump, and fluid is drawn into the cylinders to provide rigidity and girth to the penile shaft. If the corpora are narrow, the narrow base model is used. The Titan OTR™ provides for ease of deflation by allowing the patient to deflate the cylinders with one hand rather than using two hands. The device has a hydrophilic coating that allows for soaking in solutions (e.g., antibiotics) in order to reduce infection rates. A lock-out valve is present to reduce autoinflation rates. The AMS 700 MS series consists of three models: the CX, CXR, and LGX. The CX provides for girth expansion, and the CXR allows girth expansion in patients with a narrow corporal body. The LGX (formerly Ultrex) provides for girth and length expansion of 1–4 cm postoperatively.[29] Notably, the AMS 700 series is coated in a proprietary combination of rifampin and minocycline called Inhibizone™ that elutes into the peri-device space postoperatively, and this feature has helped to significantly reduce infection rates.[30] A lock-out valve is present in these models, as well as the Momentary Squeeze™ pump, which allows a user to press the release button once and then squeeze the cylinders for deflation (rather than performing both simultaneously).

Preoperative counseling and surgical planning

When discussing preoperative expectations with a patient and partner, it is important to set appropriate expectations for outcomes. Many patients see an IPP as the key to a return to a firm, natural erection they may have had in the past. Counseling a patient that the IPP produces a rigid, erection-like state is critical to improving postoperative satisfaction. Furthermore, there is no additional firmness provided to the glans penis. We are cautious in our approach to telling patients about length expansion with some models, and more often than not, a patient may notice a shortening of his penis postoperatively. Stretch penile length preoperatively is usually a good estimate of postoperative size. Being clear about the difference between erection, emission, and orgasm is paramount, as an IPP can only provide an erection-like state rather than an improvement to emission or orgasmic sensation. Regardless of these limits, overall patient and partner satisfaction with a variety of these devices remains high.[2,31–34] It is helpful to have a model of each of the implant types in order to improve patient understanding. The differences in flaccidity may also influence a patient's choice in prosthesis, as men who wear tighter clothing or shower in public may prefer the improved flaccidity of a three-piece device. Similarly, patients with severe Peyronie's disease, patients undergoing repeat implant surgery, or patients with peripheral neuropathy or other risks factors for extrusion (e.g., spinal cord injury) may be better suited for a three-piece device because of lower intracavernosal pressures during deflation that may reduce risk of erosion. A malleable device may be more suitable for a man who does not need the benefits of inflation and deflation, such as a male patient who needs the rigidity to help with placement of an external urinary collection device, a patient with poor manual dexterity, or the severely obese male.

Implantation can be done on an outpatient or overnight-stay basis under general, regional, or spinal anesthesia. The American Urological Association recommends the administration of preoperative prophylactic antibiotics during open prosthetic surgery.[35] Most patients who remain overnight are discharged the next day. Postoperative pain is usually managed with narcotics, and a dorsal penile nerve block at the time of surgery has been shown to improve postoperative pain control.[36] Patients are advised to refrain from using the device for 4 to 6 weeks and until cleared to do so at a follow-up appointment, where device activation is performed and instructions on use are given. In the case of the Ambicor and three-piece IPPs, patients are given a silicone model of the pump to go home with that allows them to better understand the anatomy of the pump and thus hopefully improve patient comfort and ease of use.

Counseling on complications is critical when discussing surgery with a patient. One of the most feared complications of penile prosthetic surgery is infection. The mechanical design improvements noted previously, along with the rise of antibiotic resistance, have now made infection a more common reason for device revision when compared to historical rates of revision for mechanical malfunction. Almost invariably, a postoperative infection requires complete explant of the device. This can be devastating for the patient. If a new prosthetic cannot be inserted at the same time as explant of the old device, then corporal fibrosis and scarring ensue that make a future reimplant more difficult. Penile shortening is typical, and more aggressive dilating maneuvers may be needed that increase the risk of associated complications like urethral injury or device erosion. Furthermore, higher rates of infection in revision surgery have been noted.[37] Prevention of infection is thus paramount to improving patient outcomes. The patient should be examined for any evidence of infection at the planned surgical site or at distant sites, and if present they should be treated. A sterile urine culture is of utmost importance, and a Foley catheter should be placed intraoperatively in patients with a risk of urine spillage. One can consider a preoperative bath with an antimicrobial agent like chlorhexidine, though most studies have shown a reduction in colony counts on the skin rather than reduced infection rates.[38,39] Hair removal, if necessary, should be done immediately prior to surgery rather than the night before based on multiple studies showing lower infection rates if performed immediately prior to surgery, and while many hospitals have mandated the use of clippers rather than straight razors, the Sexual Medicine Society of North America

(SMSNA) advises that surgeons should have a choice to use razors given the decreased tissue trauma and similar infection rates.[40–42] With regards to the preoperative skin prep agent, studies in surgery have shown a reduction in surgical site infections with chlorhexidine-alcohol-based solutions as compared to povidone-iodine solutions, and a study on infection rates in genitourinary prosthetic surgery showed reduced colony counts in patients prepped with chlorhexidine-alcohol solutions.[43,44] The "no-touch" technique has also been advocated as a stringent method to reduce infection rates: By placing a drape over the field that limits contact between skin and prosthesis, the infection rate was reduced from 2.23% to 0.73% and from 2.0% to 0.46% in two separate studies.[45,46] While most SMSNA surgeons send patients home with prophylactic antibiotics after penile implant surgery,[47] there are no studies showing a reduction in infection rates with this protocol, and certainly in the era of increasing bacterial resistance to antimicrobials, more study is needed here.

Surgical technique

Meticulous sterile prep is performed after induction of anesthesia. Many implanters use a 10-minute prep with povidone-iodine, but a 2-minute prep with chlorhexidine-alcohol scrub has been shown to reduce skin colony counts to lower levels without any increased risk of prosthetic infection or urethral or skin complications.[44]

Penile implants can be placed through a perineal, subcoronal, infrapubic, or penoscrotal approach. The perineal approach was used historically for semirigid implants, but it is rarely used today as the rate of infection is higher given the nearness to the anus and the dissection required is more significant. The subcoronal approach is typically reserved for malleable implants due to the ease of dilation, closure, and rod placement, but patients should be counseled on the risk of glans sensation loss and postoperative edema from lymphatic obstruction distal to the incision with this technique. The penoscrotal approach is used for two-piece devices because no abdominal reservoir is needed. The penoscrotal and infrapubic techniques are the most commonly used methods for implantation of three-piece IPPs.

With the subcoronal approach for a malleable implant, a Foley catheter is placed, and a 180° transverse incision is made about 1 cm proximal to the coronal sulcus on the dorsal shaft. The dartos tissues are mobilized to pull the penile skin midway down the penis. Care is taken to avoid injury to the dorsal neurovascular bundle on each side, which is present within Buck's fascia. The corpora are identified bilaterally and 2-0 absorbable, synthetic tagging sutures are placed in each corpus lateral to the neurovascular bundle. An incision can be made either longitudinally or transversely in the corporal body, with the former perhaps reducing risk of injury to the neurovascular bundle. The corpora are dilated, beginning with Metzenbaum scissors, and then moving on to Hegar, Brooks, or Dilamezinsert dilators of the appropriate diameter. A Furlow inserter is used to measure corporal length, and the implant is placed first proximally and then distally. A vein retractor placed under the distal corporal incision is helpful to allow placement of the distal cylinder. The corpora are closed with the tagging sutures, followed by the skin incision. A penile block can be performed, followed by placement of a non-compressible dressing.

The infrapubic approach has the distinct advantage of allowing the user to the place the reservoir under direct vision into the desired space. A distinct disadvantage as compared to the penoscrotal technique is the risk of injury to the dorsal neurovascular bundle and decreased distal penile sensation. If desired, a dorsal penile nerve block is performed prior to the placement of any inflatable device. A horizontal incision is made a finger breadth below the pubic symphysis. Dissection through the subcutaneous tissues is performed to the rectus fascia. The fascia is incised horizontally and the rectus muscle is split in the midline. Tagging sutures can be placed in the fascia at this time to avoid inadvertent injury to the reservoir after later placement. A pocket is bluntly created below the rectus muscle that allows for comfortable insertion of the reservoir. Dissection is now turned toward the corpora cavernosa. As dissection is performed here, it is important to identify the neurovascular bundle, which usually sits 2–3 mm lateral to the deep dorsal vein. Once dissection to the corporal bodies has been completed, tagging sutures are placed, and a corporotomy incision is made. Dilation is performed using the preferred technique, and corporal measurement with the Furlow is performed with the traction sutures as the reference point. Once cylinder size is determined, the implant is positioned, and the corporotomy is closed. The device should be inflated by

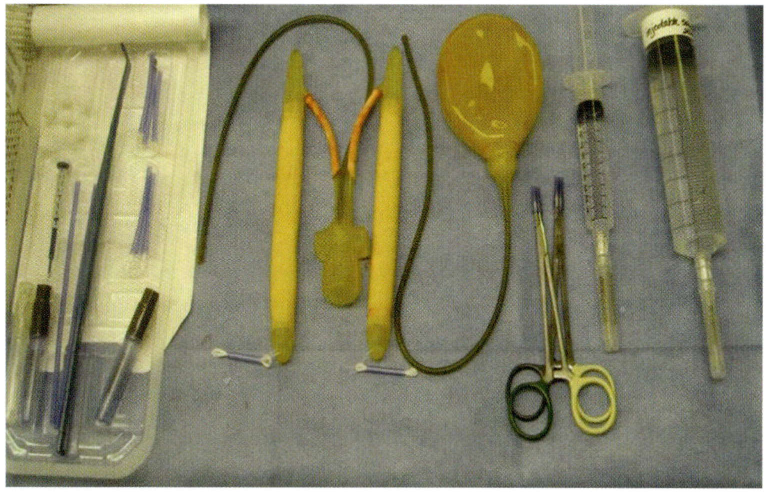

Figure 27.1 Typical setup for an inflatable penile prosthesis (IPP) placement with the AMS 700 LGX device.

instilling fluid through the cylinder input tubing to check for proper positioning, size, and inflation. The pump is placed by putting a finger in the most dependent portion of the scrotum lateral to the right or left testicle, and then pushing this skin up towards the external ring. A subcutaneous pouch is developed, the pump is placed here, and a Babcock clamp is used to hold it in place. The reservoir is positioned in the previously created pocket and filled with fluid. The tubing is then connected and the device is inflated and deflated multiple times to check for satisfactory placement. The fascial defect is closed, followed by the subcutaneous tissues and skin incision.

The penoscrotal approach is the most commonly used technique for implant placement given the comfort of most urologists with anatomy in this area. Figure 27.1 illustrates the typical setup for prosthesis placement. It has the advantages of better corporal exposure, no risk of injury to the dorsal neurovascular bundle, and ease of pump placement. The main drawback is the blind placement of the reservoir into the abdomen, especially in patients with prior abdominal or pelvic surgery. Scarring in this area can make placement more difficult or lead to untoward complications because of anatomical changes. While placing the reservoir in the prevesical space has been shown to be safe in these cases,[48] alternate reservoir placements can be utilized through separate incisions.[49–52] A Foley catheter is placed to aid in visualization of the corpus spongiosum during dissection. A transverse or longitudinal incision is made at the base of the penis on the anterior scrotum. A Scott retractor can be utilized to help with exposure. Dissection is carried out to the corporal bodies, tagging sutures are placed, and the corporotomies are made. Dilation is performed and sizing is completed. The cylinders are positioned appropriately, and the pump is placed in the dependent scrotum. The reservoir is usually placed by identifying the external inguinal ring, and staying medial to the spermatic cord, the transversalis fascia in the posterior wall of the inguinal canal is punctured. Sharp and blunt dissection is used to create a pocket in the space of Retzius, and the reservoir is placed and filled. Tubing is connected, the device is tested, and incisions are closed. It is important to ensure the tubing is dunked within the dartos tissues in order to prevent it from riding up onto the base of the penis, which for many men can cause functional penile shortening.

Postoperatively, devices are left deflated for 4 to 6 weeks. Patients are advised to massage the pump gently down into the scrotum starting 1 week after surgery in order to reduce the risk of pump migration cephalad. The device is activated in clinic and patients are educated on use. Men are advised to inflate and deflate the device at least daily for the first 4 weeks after activation in order to permit tissue expansion around the implant.

Complications

Mechanical failure

Mechanical failure is less a complication than a reflection of the mechanical nature of the device. Five-year survival rates range from about 84% to 94%, and

10-year estimates of roughly 77.6% to 85% survival have been documented.[31,33,53–58]

Infection

Mechanical failure rates have been significantly reduced by improvements in prosthesis design such that infection and erosion are more common complications.[59] Virgin implants have infection rates around 1–3%,[59] while revision surgery has a higher risk of infection: 6.7–18%.[60] The introduction of the hydrophilic coating on the Coloplast models and the Inhibizone™ coating on the AMS models has led to significant reductions in infection rates when compared to historical data.[61–63] Most infections are felt to be related to contamination of the prosthesis with skin flora at the time of surgery.[64] Other documented risk factors include spinal cord injury, diabetes mellitus, concomitant urologic surgery, urinary tract infection, immunosuppression, and distant sites of infection.[60] *Staphylococcus epidermidis* is the most common offending agent, but more virulent organisms like *Pseudomonas aeruginosa, Escherichia coli, Serratia marcescens, Enterococcus* species, *Proteus mirabilis,* and methicillin-resistant *Staphylococcus aureus* (MRSA) have been documented.[64–66] Anecdotally, we have seen more infections with fungal organisms like *Candida albicans* at our institution, especially in the revision cases.

Most infections occur within 1 year after surgery, and a majority of those are within 7 months after surgery.[67] Clinically apparent infections present with fever, induration, erythema, and purulent drainage, and eventually lead to device erosion. Infections that occur shortly after surgery are usually caused by more virulent organisms rather than *S epidermidis.* Treatment requires device explantation. More often, patients develop a subclinical infection that presents with chronic, dull pain over the device and perhaps fixation of the pump to the scrotal skin. These infections can be hard to diagnose and treat. Some groups have recommended long-term antibiotic therapy in these patients in an effort to avoid revision surgery.[68,69]

The importance of biofilm in the development of prosthetic infections has been recently elucidated. A biofilm is a survival mechanism via which organisms secrete a slimy matrix that prevents phagocytosis, inhibits antibiotic diffusion, limits the immune response to the organism, and traps nutrients.[70] Silverstein noted that 8 out of 10 clinically uninfected prostheses removed for mechanical failure had biofilm present, and a multicenter study of penile prosthesis cultures during revision surgery for reasons other than infection found that 70% of patients had positive cultures from the prosthesis.[71,72] Infections become clinically evident when the bacteria become planktonic and are released from the biofilm, and device removal is currently the only method for eradication.[70] This can clearly be a devastating complication for the patient for the reasons noted earlier.

Because of the difficulty associated with delayed replacement of a penile prosthesis after removal for infection, urologists have investigated the role of salvage surgery that involves removal of the infected device and immediate replacement of a new prosthesis. The infected device is removed, the device spaces are irrigated with a sequence of antibiotic, hydrogen peroxide, and povidone-iodine solution, gloves and instruments are changed, and a new device is implanted.[73] Long-term data with this salvage protocol showed an 84% (85/101) success rate.[74] Despite a study showing some promising results, because of the risk of bacterial migration along device components, most surgeons recommend against removing only the infected component of the device.[75–77] The critical component of this salvage procedure is felt to be the manual irrigation that breaks up the biofilm and eradicates it from the tissue. Consequently, in a study of 21 patients who had infected prostheses, one group showed that a salvage protocol using 10–12 liters of normal saline irrigated in the explanted spaces can have a 100% success rate at a median 1-year follow-up.[78]

Erosion or perforation

Perforation of the corporal bodies can occur both proximally and distally. Proximal perforation occurs during dilation when the dilator perforates the corporal body and protrudes into the perineum. In most cases dilation of the proper plane with larger dilators can correct the problem, though in other cases a synthetic graft or "plug and patch" technique can be used to correct the defect and prevent proximal cylinder migration.[79,80] Distal perforation can occur during dilation when the dilator crosses over to the other corpus. Keeping the dilator lateral during dilation can prevent this complication. If urethral injury occurs, the procedure should be aborted and a urethral catheter left in place over which the injury can heal. Implantation can then be completed at a later date.

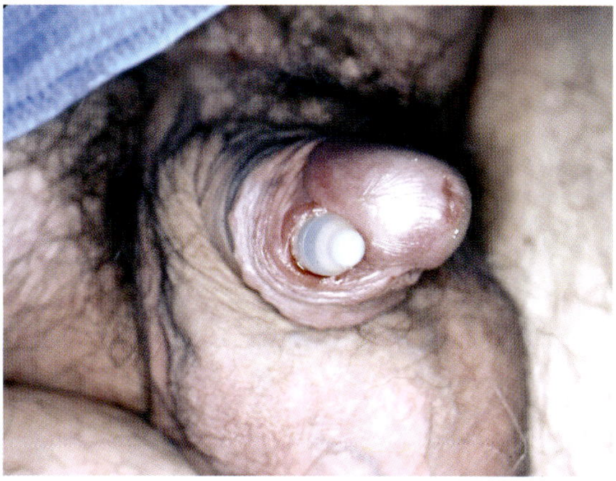

Figure 27.2 Cylinder erosion.

Erosion occurs some time after the surgery when a portion of the device becomes visible (Figure 27.2). This may be a complication of infection, trauma, decreased sensation, or improper cylinder sizing intraoperatively. In the case of a distal subcutaneous erosion, repair can be done using a "windsock" technique or with a corporoplasty.[81] A dorsal circumcising-type incision is made, the site of erosion is identified, and the corporal body can be repaired primarily or with a synthetic buttress. One case series suggested that distal corporoplasty provides better outcomes than windsock repair.[82] A "double wind-sock" technique can be used in cases of bilateral erosion or severe corporal fibrosis.[83] When the cylinder is noted to be protruding from the meatus, this usually indicates urethral erosion. Risk factors include semirigid rod implantation and neurologically impaired patients.[25,84] Often, for both malleable and inflatable devices, the affected side can be removed, leaving the contralateral cylinder in place and good function is maintained without the need to reimplant a new cylinder. A catheter is left in over which the urethra can heal.

"SST-" and "S-"shaped deformity

In the case of poor sizing of the corporal cylinders, the glans can lack good support during intercourse, causing the glans to point downwards and leading to patient discomfort (Figure 27.3). It has been dubbed the "SST" deformity because of its similarity to the supersonic transporter Concorde aircraft.[85] Classically, repair involves removal of the affected cylinders, redilation of the corpora and resizing of the corpora with longer

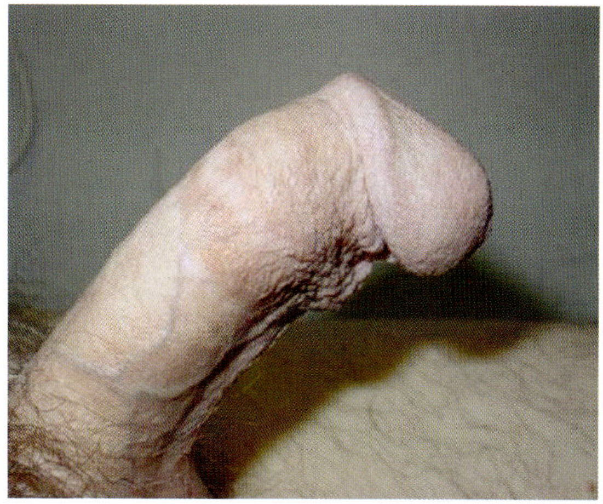

Figure 27.3 SST ("supersonic transporter")deformity.

cylinders, and placement of a new prosthesis. More minor defects can be corrected with glanuloplasty by plicating the glans onto the dorsal penile shaft.[86] In the case of the AMS 700 LGX model, which provides length and girth expansion, cylinders that are too long can cause a buckling of the penis and an "S" due to increased pressure within the device. Downsizing the cylinders can correct the problem. Furthermore, cylinders that are too long can lead to early mechanical failure through device wear and fluid loss.[87]

Autoinflation

Autoinflation occurs when pressure on the reservoir causes unwanted partial inflation of the corporal cylinders. By placing the device in the prevesical space, autoinflation is limited because abdominal pressure transmission is less. Importantly, the cylinders are left deflated immediately after surgery because this allows the reservoir to be full and create a capsule around it. If the reservoir is not completely full during the healing process, a tighter capsule may form around it and thus prevent complete filling of the reservoir when the device is deflated. Both the AMS 700 series and the Coloplast Titan models have a lockout valve that has reduced the rate of autoinflation.[88,89]

Pump migration

Pump migration can occur during the healing process when contraction of the wound occurs. This phenomenon leads to pump migration up under the base of the penis, and men can have difficulty locating

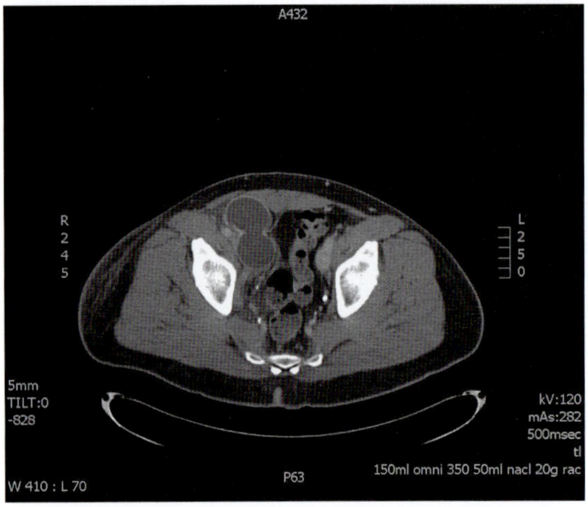

Figure 27.4 Reservoir placement in a patient with a previous robotic assisted laparoscopic prostatectomy (RALP) led to deep venous thrombosis after obstructing the right external iliac vein.

the pump and thus with inflation and deflation. In some cases, revision of the pump is needed to bring it down into the dependent scrotum. We advise patients to milk the pump down into the scrotum starting 1 week postoperatively in order to limit cephalad migration.

Vascular complications

Rarely, vascular complications can occur during reservoir placement, which is usually related to blind passage of a device through the inguinal canal to open up the space of Retzius in a patient with previous scarring in the pelvis. The iliac vessels are in close proximity here, and it is important not to direct instruments laterally so as to limit injury to the iliac vein or artery. Adequate dilation of the reservoir pocket is important to minimize impingement on the vessels, which in some cases can lead to deep venous thrombosis (Figure 27.4). Few cases have been reported in the literature, though in all of them repeat and often emergent operation was needed to replace the reservoir.[50]

Outcomes

Patient and partner satisfaction after penile prosthesis surgery is high. For malleable devices, a 75–87% satisfaction rate up to 6 years after surgery has been reported.[24,32,90,91] The Ambicor two-piece prosthesis underwent modifications in 1998 to improve durability. In a retrospective analysis of 146 patients at two centers implanted with the modified device, patient and partner satisfaction was 85% and 76%, respectively.[92] For the three-piece inflatable devices, multiple retrospective and prospective studies have shown satisfaction rates up to 97%.[2,31,33,34,57] Setting appropriate preoperative expectations has been shown to improve postoperative satisfaction rates.[93]

Conclusion

Penile implant surgery is a viable option for men who fail medical management for ED or have other comorbid conditions preventing satisfactory intercourse. Multiple types of prostheses exist, each with their own benefits and disadvantages. Advancements in technology have led to low mechanical failure rates and high satisfaction scores.

References

1 Carson C. Diagnosis, treatment and prevention of penile prosthesis infection. *Int J Impot Res* 2003;15:S139–S146.
2 Bernal RM, Henry GD. Contemporary patient satisfaction rates for three-piece inflatable penile prostheses. *Adv Urol* 2012;2012.
3 Feldman HA, Goldstein I, Hatzichristou DG, Krane RJ, McKinlay JB. Impotence and its medical and psychosocial correlates: results of the Massachusetts Male Aging Study. *J Urol* 1994;151(1):54.
4 Johannes CB, Araujo AB, Feldman HA, Derby CA, Kleinman KP, Mckinlay J. Incidence of erectile dysfunction in men 40 to 69 years old: longitudinal results from the Massachusetts male aging study. *J Urol* 2000;163(2):460–3.
5 Stanley GE, Bivalacqua TJ, Hellstrom WJ. Penile prosthetic trends in the era of effective oral erectogenic agents. *South Med J* 2000;93(12):1153.
6 Hatzimouratidis K, Hatzichristou DG. A comparative review of the options for treatment of erectile dysfunction. *Drugs* 2005;65(12):1621–50.
7 Eardley I, Donatucci C, Corbin J, et al. Pharmacotherapy for erectile dysfunction. *J Sex Med* 2010;7(1 pt 2):524–40.
8 Sung H, Ahn J, Kim J, Choo S, Han D, Lee S. The role of intracavernosal injection therapy and the reasons of withdrawal from therapy in patients with erectile dysfunction in the era of PDE5 inhibitors. *Andrology* 2014;2(1):45–50.
9 Hassan A, El-Hadidy M, El-Deeck B, Mostafa T. Couple satisfaction to different therapeutic modalities for organic erectile dysfunction. *J Sex Med* 2008;5(10):2381–91.

10 Zippe CD, Pahlajani G. Penile rehabilitation following radical prostatectomy: role of early intervention and chronic therapy. *Urol Clin North Am* 2007;34(4):601–18.

11 Tal R, Jacks LM, Elkin E, Mulhall JP. Penile implant utilization following treatment for prostate cancer: Analysis of the SEER-Medicare Database. *J Sex Med* 2011;8(6):1797–804.

12 Akin-Olugbade O, Parker M, Guhring P, Mulhall J. Determinants of patient satisfaction following penile prosthesis surgery. *J Sex Med* 2006;3(4):743–8.

13 Menard J, Tremeaux J, Faix A, Pierrevelcin J, Staerman F. Erectile function and sexual satisfaction before and after penile prosthesis implantation in radical prostatectomy patients: a comparison with patients with vasculogenic erectile dysfunction. *J Sex Med* 2011;8(12):3479–86.

14 Megas G, Papadopoulos G, Stathouros G, Moschonas D, Gkialas I, Ntoumas K. Comparison of efficacy and satisfaction profile, between penile prosthesis implantation and oral PDE5 inhibitor tadalafil therapy, in men with nerve-sparing radical prostatectomy erectile dysfunction. *BJU Int* 2013;112(2):E169–76.

15 Mulhall J, Anderson M, Parker M. A Surgical algorithm for men with combined Peyronie's disease and erectile dysfunction: functional and satisfaction outcomes. *J Sex Med* 2005;2(1):132–8.

16 Carson CC, Levine LA. Outcomes of surgical treatment of Peyronie's disease. *BJU Int* 2014;113(5):704–13.

17 Pryor J, Hehir M. The management of priapism. *Br J Urol* 1982;54(6):751–4.

18 Bennett N, Mulhall J. Sickle cell disease status and outcomes of African-American men presenting with priapism. *J Sex Med* 2008;5(5):1244–50.

19 Salem EA, El Aasser O. Management of ischemic priapism by penile prosthesis insertion: prevention of distal erosion. *J Urol* 2010;183(6):2300–3.

20 Morey AF, Tausch TJ, Evans LA. Immediate insertion of a semirigid penile prosthesis for refractory ischemic priapism. *Mil Med* 2007;172(11):1211–2.

21 Ralph DJ, Garaffa G, Muneer A, et al. The immediate insertion of a penile prosthesis for acute ischaemic priapism. *Eur Urol* 2009;56(6):1033–8.

22 Small MP, Carrion HM, Gordon JA. Small-Carrion penile prosthesis: new implant for management of impotence. *Urology* 1975;5(4):479–86.

23 Brantley Scott F, Bradley WE, Timm GW. Management of erectile impotence use of implantable inflatable prosthesis. *Urology* 1973;2(1):80–2.

24 Minervini A, Ralph DJ, Pryor JP. Outcome of penile prosthesis implantation for treating erectile dysfunction: experience with 504 procedures. *BJU Int* 2006;97(1):129–33.

25 Zermann D, Kutzenberger J, Sauerwein D, Schubert J, Loeffler U. Penile prosthetic surgery in neurologically impaired patients: long-term followup. *J Urol* 2006;175(3):1041–4.

26 Fathy A, Shamloul R, AbdelRahim A, Zeidan A, El-Dakhly R, Ghanem H. Experience with Tube® (Promedon) malleable penile implant. *Urol Int* 2007;79(3):244–7.

27 Simmons M, Montague D. Penile prosthesis implantation: past, present and future. *Int J Impot Res* 2008;20(5):437–44.

28 Bettocchi C, Palumbo F, Spilotros M, et al. Penile prostheses. *Ther Adv Urol* 2010;2(1):35–40.

29 Montague D, Lakin M. Early experience with the controlled girth and length expanding cylinder of the American Medical Systems Ultrex penile prosthesis. *J Urol* 1992;148(5): 1444–6.

30 McKim SE, Carson III CC. AMS 700™ inflatable penile prosthesis with InhibiZone®. *Expert Rev Med Devic* 2010;7(3): 311–7.

31 Carson CC, Mulcahy JJ, Govier FE. Efficacy, safety and patient satisfaction outcomes of the AMS 700CX inflatable penile prosthesis: results of a long-term multicenter study. *J Urol* 2000;164(2):376–80.

32 Falcone M, Rolle L, Ceruti C, et al. Prospective analysis of the surgical outcomes and patients' satisfaction rate after the AMS Spectra penile prosthesis implantation. *Urology* 2013;82(2):373–6.

33 Vitarelli A, Divenuto L, Fortunato F, et al. Long term patient satisfaction and quality of life with AMS700CX inflatable penile prosthesis. *Archivio Italiano di Urologia e Andrologia* 2013;85(3): 133–7.

34 Ohl DA, Brock G, Ralph D, et al. Prospective evaluation of patient satisfaction, and surgeon and patient trainer assessment of the Coloplast Titan one touch release three-piece inflatable penile prosthesis. *J Sex Med* 2012;9(9): 2467–74.

35 Wolf Jr JS, Bennett CJ, Dmochowski RR, Hollenbeck BK, Pearle MS, Schaeffer AJ. Best practice policy statement on urologic surgery antimicrobial prophylaxis. *J Urol* 2008;179(4): 1379–90.

36 Raynor MC, Smith A, Vyas SN, Selph JP, Carson III CC. Dorsal penile nerve block prior to inflatable penile prosthesis placement: a randomized, placebo-controlled trial. *J Sex Med* 2012;9(11):2975–9.

37 Selph JP, Carson III CC. Penile prosthesis infection: approaches to prevention and treatment. *Urol Clin North Am* 2011;38(2):227–35.

38 Rotter M, Larsen SO, Cooke EM, et al. A comparison of the effects of preoperative whole-body bathing with detergent alone and with detergent containing chlorhexidine gluconate on the frequency of wound infections after clean surgery. *J Hosp Infect* 1988;11(4):310–20.

39 Leigh D, Stronge J, Marriner J, Sedgwick J. Total body bathing with 'Hibiscrub'(chlorhexidine) in surgical patients: a controlled trial. *J Hosp Infect* 1983;4(3):229–35.

40 Kjønniksen I, Andersen B, Søndenaa V, Segadal L. Preoperative hair removal – a systematic literature review. *AORN J* 2002;75(5):928–40.

41 Kirby JP, Mazuski JE. Prevention of surgical site infection. *Surg Clin North Am* 2009;89(2):365–89.

42 Domes T, Grober E. Pre-operative hair removal on the male genitalia—clippers versus razors: support for the SMSNA position [abstract 104]. Program book for the 16th Annual

Fall Scientific Meeting of the Sexual Medicine Society of North America, Inc., Miami, FL, 2010.
43 Darouiche RO, Wall Jr MJ, Itani KM, et al. Chlorhexidine–alcohol versus povidone–iodine for surgical-site antisepsis. *N Engl J Med* 2010;362(1):18–26.
44 Yeung LL, Grewal S, Bullock A, Henry Lai H, Brandes SB. A comparison of chlorhexidine-alcohol versus povidone-iodine for eliminating skin flora before genitourinary prosthetic surgery: a randomized controlled trial. *J Urol* 2013;189;136–40.
45 Siegrist TC, Kwon EO, Fracchia JA, Eid J. The "no-touch" technique: a novel technique for reducing post-operative infections in patients receiving multi-component inflatable penile prostheses. *J Urol* 2008;179(4):404.
46 Eid JF, Wilson SK, Cleves M, Salem EA. Coated implants and "no touch" surgical technique decreases risk of infection in inflatable penile prosthesis implantation to 0.46%. *Urology* 2012;79(6):1310–6.
47 Wosnitzer MS, Greenfield JM. Antibiotic patterns with inflatable penile prosthesis insertion. *J Sex Med* 2011;8(5): 1521–8.
48 Lane BR, Abouassaly R, Angermeier KW, Montague DK. Three-piece inflatable penile prostheses can be safely implanted after radical prostatectomy through a transverse scrotal incision. *Urology* 2007;70(3):539–42.
49 Sadeghi-Nejad H, Munarriz R, Shah N. Intra-abdominal reservoir placement during penile prosthesis surgery in post-robotically assisted laparoscopic radical prostatectomy patients: a case report and practical considerations. *J Sex Med* 2011;8(5):1547–50.
50 Levine LA, Hoeh MP. Review of penile prosthetic reservoir: Complications and presentation of a modified reservoir placement technique. *J Sex Med* 2012;9(11):2759–69.
51 Hartman R, Helfand B, McVary K. Outcomes of lateral retroperitoneal reservoir placement of three-piece penile prosthesis in patients following radical prostatectomy. *Int J Impot Res* 2010;22(4):279–83.
52 Stember DS, Garber BB, Perito PE. Outcomes of abdominal wall reservoir placement in inflatable penile prosthesis implantation: a safe and efficacious alternative to the space of Retzius. *J Sex Med* 2014;11(2):605–12.
53 Daitch JA, Angermeier KW, Lakin MM, Ingleright BJ, Montague DK. Long-term mechanical reliability of AMS 700 series inflatable penile prostheses: comparison of CX/CXM and Ultrex cylinders. *J Urol* 1997;158(4):1400–2.
54 Dhar NB, Angermeier KW, Montague DK. Long-term mechanical reliability of AMS 700CX™/CXM inflatable penile prosthesis. *J Urol* 2006;176(6):2599–601.
55 Dubocq F, Tefilli MV, Gheiler EL, Li H, Dhabuwala C. Long-term mechanical reliability of multicomponent inflatable penile prosthesis: comparison of device survival. *Urology* 1998;52(2):277–81.
56 Kim DS, Yang KM, Chung HJ, Choi HM, Choi YD, Choi HK. AMS 700CX/CXM inflatable penile prosthesis has high mechanical reliability at long-term follow-up. *J Sex Med* 2010;7(7):2602–7.
57 Montorsi F, Rigatti P, Carmignani G, et al. AMS three-piece inflatable implants for erectile dysfunction: a long-term multi-institutional study in 200 consecutive patients. *Eur Urol* 2000;37(1):50–5.
58 Chung E, Van C, Wilson I, Cartmill R. Penile prosthesis implantation for the treatment for male erectile dysfunction: clinical outcomes and lessons learnt after 955 procedures. *World J Urol* 2013;31(3):591–5.
59 Henry GD, Wilson SK. Updates in inflatable penile prostheses. *Urol Clin North Am* 2007;34(4):535–47.
60 Selph JP, Carson III CC. Penile prosthesis infection: approaches to prevention and treatment. *Urol Clin North Am* 2011;38(2):227–35.
61 Carson III CC, Mulcahy JJ, Harsch MR. Long-term infection outcomes after original antibiotic impregnated inflatable penile prosthesis implants: up to 7.7 years of followup. *J Urol* 2011;185(2):614–8.
62 Nehra A, Carson CC, Chapin AK, Ginkel AM. Long-term infection outcomes of 3-piece antibiotic impregnated penile prostheses used in replacement implant surgery. *J Urol* 2012;188(3):899–903.
63 Serefoglu EC, Mandava SH, Gokce A, Chouhan JD, Wilson SK, Hellstrom WJ. Long-term revision rate due to infection in hydrophilic-coated inflatable penile prostheses: 11-year follow-up. *J Sex Med* 2012;9(8):2182–6.
64 Carson C. Infections in genitourinary prostheses. *Urol Clin North Am* 1989;16(1):139.
65 Licht MR, Montague DK, Angermeier KW, Lakin MM. Cultures from genitourinary prostheses at reoperation: questioning the role of Staphylococcus epidermidis in periprosthetic infection. *J Urol* 1995;154(2):387–90.
66 Mulcahy JJ. Long-term experience with salvage of infected penile implants. *J Urol* 2000;163(2):481–2.
67 Fishman I, Scott F, Selim A. Rescue procedure: an alternative to complete removal for treatment of infected penile prosthesis. *J Urol* 1987;137(4):202–8.
68 Mulcahy JJ. Penile prosthesis infection: progress in prevention and treatment. *Curr Urol Rep* 2010;11(6):400–4.
69 Parsons CL, Stein PC, Dobke MK, Virden CP, Frank DH. Diagnosis and therapy of subclinically infected prostheses. *Surg Gynecol Obstet* 1993;177(5):504–6.
70 Stewart PS, William Costerton J. Antibiotic resistance of bacteria in biofilms. *Lancet* 2001;358(9276):135–8.
71 Silverstein AD, Henry GD, Evans B, Pasmore M, Simmons CJ, Donatucci CF. Biofilm formation on clinically noninfected penile prostheses. *J Urol* 2006;176(3): 1008–11.
72 Henry GD, Wilson SK, Delk Jr JR, et al. Penile prosthesis cultures during revision surgery: a multicenter study. *J Urol* 2004;172(1):153–6.
73 Brant MD, Ludlow JK, Mulcahy JJ. The prosthesis salvage operation: immediate replacement of the infected penile prosthesis. *J Urol* 1996;155(1):155–7.
74 Mulcahy J. Treatment alternatives for the infected penile implant. *Int J Impot Res* 2003;15:S147–S149.

75 Furlow W, Goldwasser B. Salvage of the eroded inflatable penile prosthesis: a new concept. *J Urol* 1987;138(2): 312–4.

76 Carson C. Diagnosis, treatment and prevention of penile prosthesis infection. *Int J Impot Res* 2003;15:S139–S146.

77 Lue TF. Penile prosthetic infection: management by delayed and immediate salvage techniques. *J Urol* 1999;161(5): 1727–8.

78 Masson P, Eid JF. Salvage replacement of penile prosthesis with normal saline washout. *J Sex Med* 2012;9 (Suppl. 4):191.

79 Mulcahy JJ. A technique of maintaining penile prosthesis position to prevent proximal migration. *J Urol* 1987;137(2): 294–6.

80 Szostak MJ, Pizzo JJE, Sklar GN. The plug and patch: a new technique for repair of corporal perforation during placement of penile prostheses. *J Urol* 2000;163(4):1203–5.

81 Mulcahy JJ. Distal corporoplasty for lateral extrusion of penile prosthesis cylinders. *J Urol* 1999;161(1):193–5.

82 Carson C, Noh C. Distal penile prosthesis extrusion: treatment with distal corporoplasty or Gortex windsock reinforcement. *Int J Impot Res* 2002;14(2):81–4.

83 Egydio PH, Kuehhas FE. Distal penile shaft reconstruction and reinforcement: the "double-windsocks" technique. *J Sex Med* 2013;10(10):2571–8.

84 Steidle CP, Mulcahy JJ. Erosion of penile prostheses: a complication of urethral catheterization. *J Urol* 1989;142(3):736–9.

85 Ball Jr TP. Surgical repair of penile "SST" deformity. *Urology* 1980;15(6):603–4.

86 Mulhall JP, Kim FJ. Reconstructing penile supersonic transporter (SST) deformity using glanulopexy (glans fixation). *Urology* 2001;57(6):1160–2.

87 Montague D, Angermeier K. Cylinder sizing: less is more. *Int J Impot Res* 2003;15:S132–S133.

88 Wilson SK, Henry GD, Delk Jr JR, Cleves MA. The mentor Alpha 1 penile prosthesis with reservoir lock-out valve: effective prevention of auto-inflation with improved capability for ectopic reservoir placement. *J Urol* 2002;168(4): 1475–8.

89 Hollenbeck BK, Miller DC, Ohl DA. The utility of lockout valve reservoirs in preventing autoinflation in penile prostheses. *Int Urol Nephrol* 2002;34(3):379–83.

90 Ferguson KH, Cespedes RD. Prospective long-term results and quality-of-life assessment after Dura-II penile prosthesis placement. *Urology* 2003;61(2):437–41.

91 Burns-Cox N, Burston A, Gingell JC. Fifteen years experience of penile prosthesis insertion. *Int J Impot Res* 1997;9(4):211–6.

92 Lux M, Reyes-Vallejo L, Morgentaler A, Levine LA. Outcomes and satisfaction rates for the redesigned 2-piece penile prosthesis. *J Urol* 2007;177(1):262–6.

93 Kramer AC, Schweber A. Patient expectations prior to Coloplast Titan penile prosthesis implant predicts postoperative satisfaction. *J Sex Med* 2010;7(6):2261–6.

CHAPTER 28

Vascular surgery for erectile dysfunction

Ronny B.W. Tan[1] and Wayne J.G. Hellstrom[2]

[1] *Tan Tock Seng Hospital, Singapore*

[2] *Tulane University, New Orleans, LA, USA*

Introduction

Erectile function is dependent on the integrity of the vascular system, which can be categorized into the arterial and venous components. Complexity arises from the dynamic relationship between arterial inflow and the corporal veno-occlusive mechanism that occurs in the penis. Conceptually, since penile erection is a vascular perfusion event, managing the vascular inflow and outflow would be key to the success of the treatment of vasculogenic erectile dysfunction (ED). Historically, the success of bypass grafting for coronary artery disease suggested that bypassing obstructed arteries to the penis might restore normal erectile function in men suffering from vasculogenic impotence. However, a review of the literature has proven that this is not the case. This is easily explained by the fact that ED is often associated with generalized cardiovascular disease, and the majority of patients with vasculogenic impotence have intrinsic smooth muscle and endothelial dysfunction. The prevalence of vascular disease increases with age and is considered the major etiology of organic ED in men over the age of 50. Therefore, even in the face of a reduction in blood flow through the penile arterial vessels, there often coexists underlying endothelial dysfunction that limits the complete success of many penile bypass procedures. Hence, the only select group of patients in which penile revascularization surgery is likely to be successful consists of young men with isolated arterial lesions following perineal or pelvic trauma.

Penile vascular anatomy

The main source of blood supply to the penis originates from the internal pudendal artery, although accessory contributions may arise from the obturator, external iliac, vesical, and femoral arteries (Figure 28.1). The internal pudendal artery becomes the common penile artery after giving off a branch in the perineum.

The three branches from the common penile artery are termed the *dorsal, bulbourethral, and cavernous* arteries. The cavernous artery further delivers multiple helicine arteries, which supply the cavernosal tissues and sinusoids. These helicine arteries are contracted when the penis is in a flaccid state and vasodilate during erection.

The dorsal artery of the penis courses along the dorsal surface of the penis and supplies the glans penis. The bulbourethral artery supplies both the bulb and corpus spongiosum, while distally the three branches anastomose in the vicinity of the glans.

Arterial revascularization

The objective of penile arterial revascularization, as in all vascular surgeries, is to re-establish adequate arterial inflow. In the case of penile arterial revascularization, we aim to increase the inflow into the corpora cavernosa to produce rigid erections, provided the corporal

Male Sexual Dysfunction: A Clinical Guide, First Edition. Edited by Suks Minhas and John Mulhall.

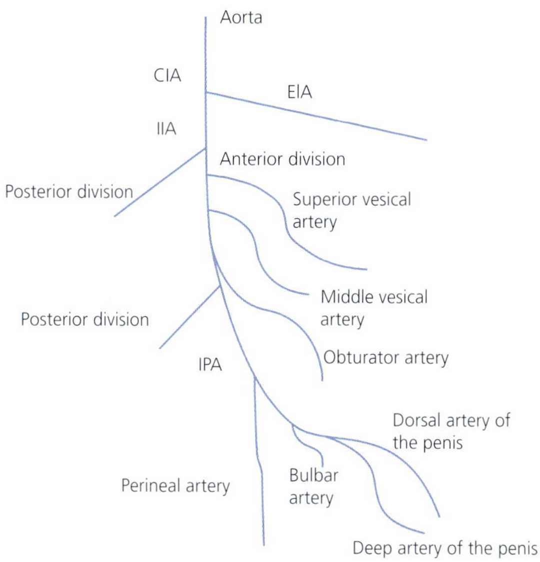

Figure 28.1 Penile vascular anatomy. CIA, common iliac artery; EIA, external iliac artery; IIA, internal iliac artery; IPA, internal pudendal artery.

veno-occlusive mechanism is intact. To achieve this, the options to consider are:

1. Direct anastomosis of an arterial donor to the corpora cavernosa.
2. Perform true revascularization.
3. Perform arterio-venous shunting.
4. Perform venous arterialization.

Direct anastomosis of an artery to the corpora cavernosa

This is the most direct approach and was described by Michal et al. in 1973,[1] where anastomosis of the inferior epigastric artery (IEA) to the corpus cavernosum was performed. This procedure unfortunately produced only short-term success with ensuing fibrosis of the smooth muscle and thrombosis of the anastomosis secondary to high-flow priapism. Attempts to anastomose the IEA as an ideal donor vessel to the intracorporal arteria profunda penis were soon abandoned due to technical obstacles and intensive intracorporal scarring. In face of these difficulties, it became necessary to anastomose the IEA to recipient vessels outside the corpora, which are in turn connected to intracorporal vessels by collateral circulation.

Revascularization

The Michal II procedure was then popularized, where the IEA was anastomosed in an end-to-side fashion to the dorsal penile artery.

Arterio-venous shunt

Hauri[2] proposed direct arterial anastomosis of the IEA to the dorsal artery, but in addition incorporating the deep dorsal vein into the anastomosis to act as an arterio-venous shunt, so as to overcome the risk of early shunt thrombosis. In principle, arterialization of the dorsal vein would improve arterial flow to the corpora cavernosa in a retrograde manner via emissary veins. However, the only experimental study[3] on postoperative flow characteristics in an animal model did not detect neoarterial flow in the dorsal arteries. All of the neoarterial runoff flowed into the venous system.

Venous arterialization

Pure venous arterialization by anastomosing the IEA only to the deep dorsal vein appeared as a viable alternative, especially in face of multiple arterial stenoses of small penile arterial vessels.

Virag and colleagues[4] described a procedure in which the IEA was anastomosed directly to the deep dorsal vein. Virag subsequently described modifications of this technique (Virag I–VI), and a number of other investigators have described other variations on this basic procedure. The principles of surgery remain the same, consisting of distal or proximal ligation of the arterialized vein, windows between the artery and vein, and ligation of the circumflex vessels (Furlow–Fischer[5]) and retrograde destruction of the valves in the dorsal vein. In theory, these modifications should improve inflow, while reducing venous outflow and also prevent glanular hyperemia, which was common in patients who had undergone the earlier Virag procedure. In concept, such procedures would be successful not only in men with pure arteriogenic ED, but also in those with a venogenic component. Unfortunately, there are no studies in peer-reviewed journals that objectively document enhanced arterial inflow into the corpora after one of these procedures.[6] In an animal model, intracorporal pressure rise was only demonstrated after creation of an artificial window between the arterialized dorsal vein and the corpus cavernosum.

In brief, the technique of penile arterial surgery can be divided into three main steps: (i) dorsal artery dissection; (ii) IEA harvesting; and (iii) microvascular anastomoses. Harvesting of the inferior epigastric vessels previously necessitated an open abdominal incision, usually vertical infra-umbilical, lower abdominal semilunar, or paramedian approaches. Recent reports have described minimally invasive vessel harvesting through laparoscopic or video-assisted endoscopic techniques,[7] including robotic-assisted harvesting of IEA prior to penile arterial microsurgery.[8]

Selection and investigation of patients with suspected arteriogenic ED

Penile arteriography is the gold standard in assessing a patient's suitability for arterial reconstructive surgery. However, prior to embarking upon this procedure, other organic causes of ED need to be excluded. For those in whom arterial surgery is contemplated, a penile duplex Doppler study confirms vascular insufficiency and may indirectly document any venous leak. A peak systolic velocity of less than 25 cm/s suggests vascular insufficiency. In patients with arteriogenic ED, it has been well documented that there is a significant improvement in surgical outcome in men with pure arteriogenic impotence as compared to those with concomitant corporal veno-occlusive dysfunction (CVOD).[9] Hence concomitant CVOD should be excluded with preoperative dynamic infusion cavernosography and cavernosometry (DICC). Younger non-diabetic men who are non-smokers have also demonstrated better outcomes after penile revascularization.

Therefore, based upon a review of the literature,[10] the following appear to be inclusion criteria in selecting patients for arterial revascularization surgery:

- Age less than 55 years
- Non-smoker
- No diabetes
- Absence of venous leakage
- Defined stenotic lesions of the internal pudendal artery.

Outcomes and complications from penile revascularization surgery

For allcomers who undergo arterial revascularization surgery for ED, a specific group who appear to have improved outcomes are young males who have sustained blunt perineal or pelvic trauma.

The most common complications from these procedures, in order of decreasing incidence, are glans hyperemia, shunt thrombosis, and inguinal hernia.

Surgery for corporal veno-occlusive dysfunction (CVOD)

The evidence for the benefits of venous surgery has more shortcomings than that for arterial surgery. Many researchers believe that this is because most techniques for penile venous surgery were invented before basic research defined the pathophysiology of CVOD.[6] It is difficult to differentiate functional abnormalities (e.g., endothelial dysfunction) from anatomical defects (e.g., tunical abnormality). The proportion of ED due to veno-occlusive ED is independent of general arterial insufficiency and is difficult to assess. Most authorities postulate that venous leakage is an effect rather than a cause and reflects underlying corporal smooth muscle dysfunction. The failure of most venous procedures is likely due to the extensive collateral venous drainage of the penis. CVOD is due to endothelial dysfunction and damage to the trabecular smooth muscle content, which in turn is often due to multiple comorbidities.[11] As with arterial surgery, there are rare cases of isolated venous leaks due to congenital or post-traumatic lesions, and targeted ligation of these venous outflow channels may yield some positive results. The position from the International Society for Sexual Medicine's (ISSM's) Standard Practice in Sexual Medicine textbook based on the review of the data and panel consensus is that "surgeries performed with the intent to limit the venous outflow of the penis are not recommended."[11]

There are many varieties of intervention for CVOD. As with all medical conditions that can be treated with a myriad of procedures, the ultimate benefits are not stellar. Types of interventions for CVOD include:

1. Superficial dorsal vein ligation
2. Deep dorsal vein ligation/excision
3. Crural vein ligation
4. Crural plication/ligation
5. Deep dorsal vein arterialization
6. Cavernosal vein arterialization
7. Spongiolysis
8. Pericavernosoplasty
9. Therapeutic embolization

10 Combinations of the above
11 Extraperitoneal laparoscopic penile vein ligation.

There is no single operative technique that proves to be superior to others. With an increase in the length of follow-up, there is an associated steep decline in success.[6] The success rates of CVOD surgery vary from 13% to 74%, with a mean of 41.4%.[12] However, crural ligation appears to be the most promising for the treatment of young men with primary venogenic ED and isolated crural leakage. The first diagnosis of crural venous leakage treated with crural ligation was performed via a perineal approach in 1987.[13] Mulhall et al. described a technique utilized at their institution in 2001.[14] In 2011 it was reported that the outcome of 14 patients with a mean age of 29 ± 7 years, with isolated crural venous leak who underwent crural ligation surgery, was a mean change of 6.5 points in the postoperative EF domain of the International Index of Erectile Function (IIEF) score per patient.[15] No patients needed intracavernosal injection therapy for ED after the surgery, and 71% reported unassisted sexual intercourse.

Complications of CVOD surgery include glanular hypoesthesia/anesthesia, glans hyperemia, skin necrosis, penile curvature, penile shortening, penile edema, hematomas (after deep dorsal vein arterialization), inguinal hernias, and pain (after embolization procedures).

The weight of the available evidence for venous procedures to treat CVOD is contrary to its routine use as a treatment option for ED. Hence its use is still considered investigational and it should be offered only in special situations,[15] for example, in young patients with site-specific congenital post-traumatic or post-inflammatory leak.

Should CVOD surgical interventions be undertaken, the recommended postoperative follow-up is at least 48 months, and this should include objective evaluation of the penile vascular and erectile status using penile color duplex Doppler ultrasound after complete cavernosal smooth muscle relaxation as well as subjective evaluation with validated questionnaires (e.g., IIEF). The penile duplex Doppler needs to be performed preoperatively and postoperatively.

In an attempt to improve the long-term outcome of venous ligation surgeries, Lewis et al.[16] promoted cavernosography using cine-taped cavernosography. The images of the origin of the veins were often not clearly identifiable due to the overlapping of other veins and the bone or cavernous body obscuring the images. Further improvement in diagnostic imaging allowed for high-resolution arterial images similar to digital subtraction angiography with a CT scanner, and images of the venous system with an MRI scanner. The advent of 3D CT allows for reconstruction of three-dimensional images. In a Japanese study,[17] 55 patients who had failed to respond to phosphodiesterase type 5 (PDE5) inhibitors underwent pharmacodynamics infusion cavernosometry and cavernosography, using 60 mg of papaverine hydrochloride. The images acquired from using a multi-slice CT scan system with 3D images reconstructed using Aquarius net station version 2 computer software were compared to images acquired using conventional cavernosography. Compared with 3D-CT cavernosography, observing cavernous veins and the proximal part of the deep dorsal veins using maximal intensity projection imaging was especially difficult because the origins of the penile veins were often obscured by the bony pelvis or the penile cavernous bodies. Of the patients who were thought to have leakage via the deep dorsal vein, 80.6% of them eventually did not in fact have leakage via this vein. The higher image resolution of 3D-CT cavernosography is definitely helpful in the diagnosis of CVOD and the assessment of the anatomy of the human penile venous system, thereby in theory improving the success rates of venous ligation surgeries.

Endovascular techniques

Current experience with transluminal angioplasty for the treatment of ED is limited. The majority of studies are case reports or case series focused on large vessel inflow disease of the iliac arteries. Only two studies evaluated the internal pudendal artery, and in many of the studies venous insufficiency was not excluded and the definition of ED was not standardized. None of the studies documented an increase in post-interventional penile blood flow. Unfortunately, there are no data on venous insufficiency or venous leak, or duration of follow-up.

Penile vasodilatation prior to angiography acts to relax the cavernosal musculature, augments blood flow and vessel caliber, and results in improved angiographic quality. This can be accomplished by an intracavernosal injection of 15 μg of prostaglandin E_1.

The Zotarolimus-Eluting Peripheral Stent System for the Treatment of ED in Males with Sub-Optimal

Response to Phosphodiesterase type 5 Inhibitors (ZEN) trial generated great interest in causing a paradigm shift in searching for an endovascular intervention to treat vasculogenic ED. A total of 30 patients with ED were enrolled and technical success was achieved in all patients with no post-procedural deaths or episodes of perineal gangrene at 30 days. At 3 months follow-up, 68% of the patients had improvement in erection function (as assessed by the IIEF). Eight patients were lost to follow-up or had angioplasty and stenting of non-pudendal vessels. This study demonstrated the short-term safety of angioplasty and stenting and improved erectile function, but demonstrated significant variant anatomy in the pelvis.[18]

The anterior division of the IIA (internal iliac artery) provides the majority of the blood supply to the genitalia whereas the posterior division supplies the gluteal and lumbosacral musculoskeletal regions. The IPA (internal pudendal artery) is the smaller of the two terminal branches of the anterior trunk of the IIA. The IPA divides into the inferior rectal artery, perineal artery, artery of the urethral bulb, urethral artery, and deep and dorsal arteries of the penis. However, there are variations in penile arterial anatomy, with the most frequent being where the IPA terminates at the artery of the urethral bulb or less frequently the perineal artery. Hence, the dorsal and the deep arteries of the penis, which supply the corporal bodies, are frequently derived from an accessory pudendal artery (APA). The APA can originate from the EIA, obturator, vesical, and femoral artery. It is not uncommon to find that the APA constitutes the dominant or only arterial supply to the corpora. There is even a classification system[19] for penile arterial supply, where type 1 is when the IPA originates from the IIA, type 2 when the IPA originates from the inferior gluteal artery, and type 3 when an accessory vessel supplies the dorsal and deep arteries of the penis.

In view of the significant variant pelvic anatomy, a second angiographic study called the Incidence of Male Pudendal Artery Stenosis in Suboptimal Erections Study (IMPASS) registry, was designed to document penile arterial insufficiency and establish an angiographic protocol. It was a multicenter trial enrolling 350 males ages 35–70 years undergoing angiography for coronary artery disease or peripheral artery disease with follow-up at 1, 2, and 3 years. Unfortunately this study has been terminated. As such, endovascular therapy for ED remains investigational.

Conclusion

Vascular surgery for ED remains a challenge to the urologist. Due to the complicated interdependence of the arterial system with the corporal veno-occlusive mechanism, as well as the systemic problem of endothelial dysfunction, which is multifactorial, careful patient selection and extensive workup to ascertain the specific problem in such patients is of extreme importance to ensure superior outcome, a satisfied patient, and an untroubled urologist.

References

1 Michal V, Kramar R, Pospichal J, Hejhal L. Direct arterial anastomosis on corpora cavernosa penis in the therapy of erective impotence. *Rozhledy v chirurgii: mesicnik Ceskoslovenske chirurgicke spolecnosti* 1973;52(9):587–90.

2 Hauri D. A new operative technique in vasculogenic erectile impotence. *World J Urol* 1986;4:237–49.

3 Floth A, Paick JS, Suh JK, Lue TF. Hemodynamics of revascularization of the corpora cavernosa in an animal model. A preliminary report. *Urol Res* 1991;19(5):281–4.

4 Virag R, Zwang G, Dermange H, Legman M. Vasculogenic impotence: A review of 92 cases with 54 surgical operations. *Vasc Surg* 1981;15:9–17.

5 Furlow WL, Fischer J. Deep dorsal vein arterialization. Clinical experience with a new technique. *J Urol* 1998; 139:289A.

6 Sohn M, Martin-Morales A. Surgical treatment of ED. In: Porst JB, Buvat J (eds), *Standard Practice in Sexual Medicine*. Hoboken, NJ: John Wiley & Sons, Inc., 2006; pp. 126–48.

7 Lund GO, Winfield HN, Donovan JF. Laparoscopically assisted penile revascularization for vasculogenic impotence. *J Urol* 1995;153(6):1923–6.

8 Raynor MC, Davis R, Hellstrom WJ. Robot-assisted vessel harvesting for penile revascularization. *J Sex Med* 2010;7(1 Pt 1):293–7.

9 Cookson MS, Phillips DL, Huff ME, Fitch WP 3rd. Analysis of microsurgical penile revascularization results by etiology of impotence. *J Urol* 1993;149(5 Pt 2):1308–12.

10 Hellstrom WJ, Montague DK, Moncada I, et al. Implants, mechanical devices, and vascular surgery for ED. *J Sex Med* 2010;7(1 Pt 2):501–23.

11 Montorsi F, Adaikan G, Becher E, et al. Summary of the recommendations on sexual dysfunctions in men. *J Sex Med* 2010;7(11):3572–88.

12 Sohn M, Hatzinger M, Goldstein I, Krishnamurti S. Standard operating procedures for vascular surgery in ED: revascularization and venous procedures. *J Sex Med* 2013;10(1): 172–9.

13 Puech-Leao P, Reis JM, Glina S, Reichelt AC. Leakage through the crural edge of corpus cavernosum. Diagnosis and treatment. *Eur Urol* 1987;13(3):163–5.
14 Mulhall JP, Martin D, Ergin E, Kim F. Crural ligation surgery for the young male with venogenic ED: technique. *Tech Urol* 2001;7(4):290–3.
15 Flores S, Tal R, O'Brien K, Mulhall JP. Outcomes of crural ligation surgery for isolated crural venous leak. *J Sex Med* 2011;8(12):3495–9.
16 Lewis RW, Puyau FA, Bell DP. Another surgical approach for vasculogenic impotence. *J Urol* 1986;136(6):1210–2.
17 Kawanishi Y, Izumi K, Muguruma H, et al. Three-dimensional CT cavernosography: reconsidering venous ligation surgery on the basis of the modern technology. *BJU Int* 2011; 107(9):1442–6.
18 Rogers JH, Goldstein I, Kandzari DE, et al. Zotarolimus-eluting peripheral stents for the treatment of ED in subjects with suboptimal response to phosphodiesterase-5 inhibitors. *J Am Coll Cardiol* 2012;60(25):2618–27.
19 Philip F, Shishehbor MH. Current state of endovascular treatment for vasculogenic ED. *Curr Cardiol Rep* 2013;15 (5):360.

CHAPTER 29

Penile cancer

Majid Shabbir[1] and Paul K. Hegarty[2]

[1] *Guy's Hospital, London, UK*

[2] *Mater Private Hospital, Mahon, Cork, Ireland*

Introduction

Progress in penile cancer has flagged behind the advances made in other malignancies. Its rarity has hampered the development of a clear understanding of many of the key aspects of the condition, from its pathogenesis and development, to its treatment. A lack of awareness of the condition among the public and clinicians alike is a major factor in its delay to presentation and appropriate treatment.

Penile cancer does not receive any significant level of media attention or public funding. As such the condition lies largely out of the public's eye. Men who develop a penile lesion present late due to fear and embarrassment and worry that the condition may relate to sexual contact in the past. When they do eventually present, they first usually see their primary care physician or attend a sexual health clinic, where there is often no experience of the condition. Due to its rarity, many clinicians may not have seen such cases previously, which makes distinguishing the worrying lesion from the more common cohort of benign penile conditions extremely difficult.

Significant delays in presentation can render simple treatable lesions into more invasive disease, requiring more emasculating surgery. While such surgery can still achieve good oncological outcomes, the poor cosmetic and functional results have a significant impact on patient well-being. Radical surgery, either with partial or total penectomy, using the traditional approach of excising the lesion with a clear surgical margin of 2 cm, provides excellent oncological control with recurrence rates of 4.6% and 0.7% respectively in pooled analysis.[1] The emasculating nature of these procedures is associated with significant psychological and sexual morbidity.[2] Romero et al. reported impaired well-being in 40% of cases, and pathological anxiety in 31% of patients after partial penectomy.[3] Ficarra et al. reported signs or symptoms of mental illness in 53% after surgery, with 25% displaying signs of avoidance behavior and 40% signs of post-traumatic stress disorder.[4] Opjordsmoen and Fossa reported that 23% would risk lower long-term survival to increase the chance of remaining sexually potent after treatment, giving an important insight into the essential need to consider the final functional outcome in penile surgery.[2] This potential impact of treatment is especially relevant when planning the management of the significant cohort of men (approximately 20%) who develop the disease at less than 40 years of age.[5]

Penile preserving surgery (PPS)

Over the last 10 years there has been a shift in the surgical management of the primary penile lesion, moving away from more radical surgery in favor of penile preserving techniques. This has been based on studies that have challenged the traditionally held beliefs supporting more extensive 2 cm margins. Agrawal et al. reviewed 64 partial and total penectomy specimens, and found only 19% of cases had microscopic extension of disease beyond the gross tumor margin. Of these, 75% were less than 5 mm.[6] Hoffman et al. reported on their experience of 14 patients who underwent conventional surgery for penile cancer.[7] Half the group had excision

Male Sexual Dysfunction: A Clinical Guide, First Edition. Edited by Suks Minhas and John Mulhall.

margins of less than 10 mm, although this had no bearing on recurrence, with no patient developing recurrence after 33 months follow-up. In a series reporting outcomes of PPS, approximately 50% of the 51 patients had clear surgical margins of less than 10 mm, including 33% with margins less than 5 mm. Despite this, the local recurrence rate in the whole series was only 4% and comparable to conventional radical surgery series despite the clearance margins of only a few millimetres.[8]

The results of these studies have led to a shift away from more radical surgery to a variety of penile preserving techniques. The use of these techniques has been more prevalent in Europe and the United States, where approximately 80% of malignant lesions present on the glans penis and prepuce and are more amenable to an organ-conserving approach.[9] Selection of the most appropriate technique is dependent on a number of factors, which can be divided into patient factors and lesion factors (Table 29.1). Individualizing treatment in this way is essential to achieve the best functional and oncological outcome. For example, high-grade distal disease poses less of a challenge than lower grade proximal disease due to the location of the lesion. An elderly patient with numerous comorbidities and no desire for sexual function is not best served by a more lengthy procedure and reconstruction with split skin graft. Such factors are best discussed with the individual and considered with a multidisciplinary team approach.

Initial experiences with PPS raised concerns of less effective oncological control. Lindegaard et al. reported 5-year actuarial cancer control rates of 69% after more "conservative" treatments compared to 100% after radical surgery.[10] However, local recurrences in this series did not affect overall survival as such cases were amenable to further salvage radical surgery. More contemporary series have reported better oncological outcomes. A large single-center series of 179 PPS cases reported local recurrence rates of only 8.9% after a mean 26 months follow-up. All those who developed local recurrence were amenable to further PPS, and even those with local recurrences had a 5-year disease-specific survival rate of 91.7%.[11] Other studies have confirmed this positive oncological outcome, with reports of falling local recurrence rates (25 to 4.8%) and mortality (20.5 to 10.7%) at a time of increasing penile preserving surgery (4.5% to 58%) in the setting of specialized supra-regional penile cancer center care.[12]

Table 29.1 Factors involved in deciding on the most appropriate method of treating the primary penile lesion tailored to the individual.

Lesion factors	Patient factors
• Site	• Age
• Size	• Comorbidity
• Stage	• Available penile length
• Grade	• Patient's functional needs

The various PPS options are divided according to the stage at presentation. There are no randomized controlled trials comparing different treatment modalities, and most guidelines are based on small retrospective case series, with low levels of evidence (mostly 2b) and low grades of recommendation (B-C).[13] Little has been done to formally study the impact of such treatments on sexual function and quality of life, but the available evidence of impact of each option is discussed.

Carcinoma in situ (Tis) and non-invasive verrucous carcinoma (Ta)

The non-invasive nature of these lesions makes them amenable to a number of different penile preserving techniques, ranging from non-surgical treatment modalities such as topical chemotherapy, topical immunotherapy, and laser ablation to surgery with glans resurfacing.

Topical therapies

Topical chemotherapy with 5% 5-fluorouracil (5-FU) is the most commonly used first-line treatment and is suitable for well-defined solitary lesions in immune-competent patients. This antimetabolite is a pyrimidine analog, which non-competitively inhibits thymidylate synthase, triggering cell cycle arrest and apoptosis. It is applied on alternate days for 4–6 weeks, and is safe, with low morbidity and systemic absorption. Non- or partial responders are often treated with topical 5% imiquimod (IQ) cream. The criteria for use remain the same. The exact mechanism of action of this novel immunomodulatory therapy is unclear. It is believed to activate the patient's own immune system via Toll-like receptors leading to secretion of cytokines such as interferon-α (IFNα), tumor necrosis factor (TNFα), and various interleukins (IL-1, -6, and -12). Imiquimod can be applied for 5 days a week for a period of 4–6 weeks,

Table 29.2 Treatment options by stage: oncological outcome and effect on sexual function.

Stage	Treatment	Oncological outcome	Sexual function	References
Tis/Ta	Topical chemotherapy	57% CR 13.5% PR 29.5% NR	Not assessed	14
Tis/Ta	Laser (CO_2/Nd:YAG)	14–26% local recurrence 5% progression	No negative effect on sexual function	16–18
Tis/Ta	TGR	0–4% local recurrence No progression	No sexual dysfunction or impaired sensitivity	24,25
T1–T2	Glansectomy	0–4% local recurrence	No reported sexual dysfunction	27–32
T2–T3	Partial penectomy	4.6% pooled local recurrence rate	21–45% unable to penetrate 66% unhappy with postop sexual function	1,3,33
T2–T3	Total penectomy	0.7% pooled local recurrence rate	N/A	1

CR, complete response; PR, partial response; NR, no response; TGR, total glans resurfacing.

although the frequency can be reduced provided that the inflammatory response is maintained. A recent study of 44 patients treated with 5-FU as first line and IQ as second line reported complete response in 57%, partial in 13%, and no response in 30%.[14] Thirteen percent suffered adverse events due to the cream, but only one patient discontinued treatment. No reports on the impact of treatment on sexual function have been made. Patients are advised against sexual activity while on therapy, and any adverse effect of treatment tends to be self-limiting, resolving 4–6 weeks after cessation of treatment.

Laser therapy

Carbon dioxide (CO_2) and neodymium:yttrium aluminum garnet (Nd:YAG) lasers have been used as first-line therapy with reasonable response rates and good cosmetic and functional results. The CO_2 laser has a tissue penetration of 2–2.5 mm. Ablation sites generally heal in 3–4 weeks. The Nd:YAG laser has a tissue penetration of 3–5 mm and causes tissue coagulation. Larger lesions can be treated using this laser, but ablation sites can take up to 2–3 months to heal. Treatment with either of these lasers is usually well tolerated, with minor complications ranging from minor pain and bleeding at treatment sites, to preputial lymphedema in those patients who have retained their foreskin.[15] Studies have reported local recurrence rates of 14–26% requiring retreatment, but reported rates of progression to invasive disease have been of more concern.[16,17] Two studies that together reported on over 250 cases, found no adverse effect of treatment on sexual function.[16,18]

Surgery

Circumcision

Circumcision forms an essential part of the management of penile cancer, both as a preventative and treatment strategy. Neonatal circumcision has a preventative effect on the development of penile cancer,[19] while circumcision is also beneficial at preventing the risk of human papillomavirus (HPV) infection,[20] HIV transmission,[21] and the development of lichen sclerosus (LS), all individually associated with penile cancer development. As a treatment strategy, it removes the lesion if confined solely to the prepuce, and can facilitate follow-up and clinical examination, which is essential with any minimally invasive approach. The effect of circumcision on sexual function has been long debated. A recent systematic review looking at over 2500 studies reporting on over 40,000 men found no evidence of adverse effect on sexual function, sensitivity, or satisfaction.[22]

Glans resurfacing

Total glans resurfacing (TGR) can be used both as a primary treatment for Tis and for cases refractory to other therapies. This technique was first described by Bracka for the management of severe LS.[23] It is the best option for patients who have extensive field change, those unlikely or unwilling to adhere to strict treatment and surveillance protocols, or failure of medical treatment. It entirely removes the epithelium and subepithelial layer, and can in theory also be used to treat patients with low risk pT1 disease (pT1a), which is well to moderately differentiated disease (Grade 1–2) confined to the subepithelial layer. It is combined with a split-thickness skin graft to achieve excellent cosmetic and functional outcomes (Figure 29.1). The two largest series have reported recurrence rates of less than 4% and no reported cases of progression.[24,25]

One of the main advantages of this surgical approach is its combined diagnostic and therapeutic ability. Whilst completely removing the diseased epithelium, total surgical excision also allows more accurate histopathological staging and diagnosis than smaller incisional biopsies used with less invasive topical therapies. In a recent series of glans resurfacing as a primary therapy for Tis, 10/25 patients (40%) had evidence of invasive carcinoma on the final pathology despite all 25 patients having had preoperative incisional biopsies confirming evidence of CIS only.[25] As most patients with CIS are treated on the basis of incisional biopsies only, and are usually treated with topical chemotherapy or laser as first line, this would not tackle any invasive element adequately. This may explain the higher recurrence rate with laser therapy (up to 26%), compared to surgical

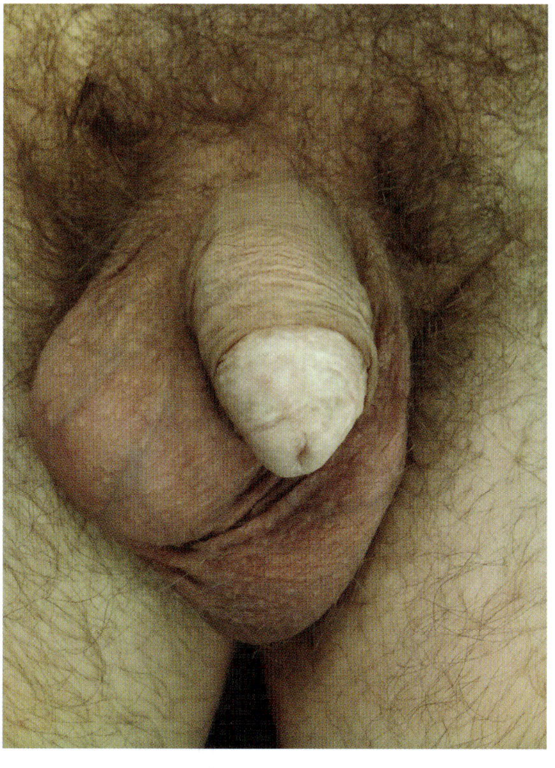

Figure 29.1 Post operative appearance after total glans resurfacing.

series (up to 4%).[16,17,24,25] These findings would favor the primary use of surgery to avoid the risk of understaging and inadequate treatment leading to subsequent progression, and may lead to a shift in our approach to managing Tis affecting the glans in the future.

In the only study to assess the effect of TGR on sexual function, 85% of patients who responded had had sexual intercourse within 3 months of surgery, with all reporting no erectile dysfunction and either no change or improvement in glans sensation postop.[24]

Partial glans resurfacing is an alternative approach and is best reserved for solitary lesions affecting less than 50% of the total glans. In the largest study to date, the risk of patients requiring a subsequent surgical procedure was up to 40%, but all were still amenable to further penile preserving techniques, with no reported progression or recurrence with this technique in this series.[25] The theoretical benefit of preserving native glans skin to allow better sensation preservation has not been demonstrated in any study. The final cosmetic appearance achieves a contour close to original glans, but with a more "patchwork" appearance due to the differential coloring of the donor skin.

Tumor invading the subepithelium (T1) or corpus spongiosum (T2)

The management of "low-risk" T1a disease (invasion into subepithelium of low or intermediate grade G1/G2 disease) can be with laser therapy or TGR as outlined above. In a series of glans resurfacing, 7/25 cases who underwent TGR for Tis, and were found to have inadvertent T1a disease that had been fully excised, were observed for a mean 29 months. None of the cases in this sub group had any recurrence or progression, further confirming the oncological safety of this approach.[25] For patients with more high-risk T1b disease (high-grade G3 or lymphovascular invasion in subepithelial disease) or disease in the corpus spongiosum (T2), glansectomy is the procedure of choice.

Glansectomy is the most commonly used PPS. This procedure utilizes knowledge of the anatomical planes between the corpora cavernosa and corpus spongiosum first described by Austoni et al.[26] In this procedure, the glans penis is dissected from the corpora cavernosa, with the subsequent formation of a new urethral meatus at the tip of the shaft. The procedure can be combined with a split-skin graft to create a "neo-glans" with excellent cosmesis and a near normal appearance, or it can utilize advancement flaps of shaft skin to cover the corporal tips to maintain a functional penis, albeit with a less satisfactory cosmetic appearance. The latter is best suited to patients who are not sexually active, or those with significant comorbidities, where a shorter anesthetic time is critical. Such patients can still achieve good urinary function, which may be all they desire.

A number of series have reported their outcomes, and recurrence rates of 4% or less have been consistently achieved, highlighting the oncological safety of this penile preserving approach.[27–31] Hatzichristou et al. reported on seven cases of glansectomy without reconstruction. All returned to normal sexual function 1 month postoperatively.[32] Morelli et al. reported on 15 patients after glansectomy with reconstruction. All were fully sexually active by 6 months after surgery, and while all had reported reduced neo-glans sensitivity, all had preserved orgasm and ejaculatory function.[27]

Tumor invading the corpus cavernosum (T2) or the urethra (T3)

Once disease extends into the corporal bodies or urethra a more extensive resection is required. Partial penectomy is the primary approach unless the disease is very proximal, where a total penectomy and perineal urethrostomy may be more appropriate. Resection margins of 2 cm are not required and excision can be combined with frozen section to ensure clear margins are achieved. Subsequent reconstructive techniques can be used to achieve a good cosmetic appearance with split-skin grafts and meatal centralization to aid urinary stream direction. If the resultant phallus post-resection is too short, lengthening procedures can be used to allow the patient to stand to void, or have penetrative sex. This may involve dividing the suspensory ligament below the pubic arch, and placing a silicone buffer to preserve the created space and prevent re-adhesions. Patients with prominent scrotal webs or suprapubic fat pads can be treated using V-Y-plasty or suprapubic fat pad excision or liposuction to improve the apparent penile length. These techniques may provide enough length gain to allow the patient to stand to pass urine comfortably, a major psychological factor for many men undergoing penile cancer surgery. In cases where reconstruction using skin graft is not used or appropriate, shaft skin advancement flaps can be used to cover the corpora and meet the spatulated urethra. This approach again suits older patients who are medically unfit, or not keen for reconstruction. It is more suited to patients where cosmesis or sexual function is less important, although erectile function and ability to penetrate are preserved. It has a significantly shorter operative time, and less need for restrictive bed rest, or complex dressings associated with reconstruction and skin graft, and remains a good option in a selected subset of patients.

Partial penectomy is a safe oncological procedure, and has a reliably low recurrence rate of 4.6% from pooled analysis.[1] Studies have reported a greater impact on sexual function after partial penectomy compared to other techniques, with between 21%[33] and 45%[3] unable to have intercourse after surgery. In the latter study, of those who were able to have sex, 72% were still able to ejaculate and orgasm as before. Overall two-thirds of patients were not satisfied with their postoperative sexual function.

Total penectomy

This is the best approach for proximal high-risk disease and avoids leaving the patient with a phallus too short to direct their urinary stream. Patients require careful counseling preoperatively about their final cosmetic and functional outcome, with the need to sit to void with a perineal urethrostomy. It has a good oncological outcome, with a recurrence rate of 0.7% from pooled analysis.[1] Selected cases will be suitable for subsequent phalloplasty reconstruction once full oncological control of the primary and regional lymph nodes has been achieved.

Total phallic reconstruction

Ideal candidates for major surgical reconstruction are healthy, young, well-motivated non-smokers who are cancer free with a good prognosis. The most common technique is the radial artery phalloplasty (RAP), made using a radial artery free flap to create a new urethra and phallus using a "tube-in-a-tube" technique,[34] giving the patient the ability to once again be able to stand to pass urine. The phallus may also have an inflatable penile prosthesis inserted at a later stage to allow return of sexual function.

Reconstruction is performed in stages, with the first being the creation from the non-dominant forearm of the new phallus, which is attached to the native urethra, and the femoral artery, saphenous veins, and ilioinguinal nerves to provide neurovascular anastomosis. Subsequent stages involve resculpting of the phallus to create a neo-glans, and insertion of an inflatable penile prosthesis, at 3-monthly intervals, with the entire reconstruction process taking up to a year to complete. In a series of 15 cases of RAP after previous total penectomy, all patients were able to stand to void after reconstruction, with 12/15 (80%) developing full sensation within the phallus. Half had insertion of a penile prosthesis, of whom 70% were using the phallus for intercourse. Subsequent complications included urethral strictures in 20%, urethral fistulae in 26%, and explant of the penile prosthesis in 14% for infection. All were happy with the final cosmetic appearance of the phalloplasty.[35]

Tumor invading adjacent structures (T4)

When treating patients with such locally advanced disease it is important to take into consideration the extent of disease, performance status, life expectancy, symptoms, and desired outcomes. If the performance status is good, the best approach is with neoadjuvant chemotherapy to downstage the disease prior to consolidative surgery in a trial setting. Those not suitable for chemotherapy or surgery are best managed with palliative radiotherapy and treatment of symptoms. The ideal regime is still unclear, but small studies using neoadjuvant combinations containing platinum-based drugs have shown some promise.[36]

Palliative surgery may have a role to play in very carefully selected advanced cases, aimed at improving the quality of the patient's remaining life. Suitable cases must have a clear understanding of the palliative intent, must be nutritionally and biochemically optimized, and managed with a multidisciplinary team approach. Surgery may range from simple urinary diversion, to more complex excisions and reconstruction, using a variety of techniques ranging from skin grafts to rectus abdominis flaps, depending on the size and nature of the defect.[37] Although only a few patients will be appropriate for surgical palliation, an understanding of the available techniques is essential to be able to offer the option in selected circumstances.

Summary

Improvements in the understanding of this rare malignancy have challenged the need for such extensive margins and allowed a move away from emasculating surgery with its significant impact on well-being and sexual function. The development of penile preserving techniques has transformed penile cancer care and reduced the impact of treatment on patients' quality of life. Treatments can be tailored to the individual dependent on the tumor characteristics and patient factors. Knowledge and expertise of the different surgical techniques is vital to ensure the best cosmetic, functional, psychological, and oncological outcome in patients who present with this potentially devastating disease.

References

1 Solsona E, Bahl A, Brandes SB, et al. New developments in the treatment of penile cancer. In: Pompeo ACL, Heyns CF, Abrams P (eds), *International Consultation on Penile Cancer*. ICUD, 2009; pp. 103–27.

2 Opjordsmoen S, Fossa SD Quality of life in patients treated for penile cancer. A follow-up study. *Br J Urol* 1994;74 (5):652–7.

3 Romero FR, Romero KR, Mattos MA, Garcia CR, Fernandes Rde C, Perez MD. Sexual function after partial penectomy for penile cancer. *Urology* 2005;66:1292–5.

4 Ficarra V, Righetti R, D'Amico A, et al. General state of health and psychological well being in patients after surgery for urological malignant neoplasms. *Urol Int* 2000;65:130–4.

5 Cancer trends in England and Wales, 1950-1999. Office for National Statistics. Available at: http://webarchive.nationalarchives.gov.uk/20160105160709/http://www.ons.gov.uk/ons/rel/cancer-unit/cancer-trends-in-england-and-wales/smps-no--66/index.html (accessed April 21, 2016).

6 Agrawal A, Pai D, Ananthakrishnan N, et al. The histological extent of the local spread of carcinoma of the penis and its therapeutic implications. *BJU Int* 2000;85(2):299–301.

7 Hoffman M, Renshaw A, Loughlin KR. Squamous cell carcinoma of the penis and microscopic pathologic margins. How much margin is needed for local cure? *Cancer* 1999;85 (7):1565–8.

8 Minhas S, Kayes O, Hegarty P, et al. What surgical resection margins are required to achieve oncological control in men with primary penile cancer? *BJU Int* 2005;96:1040–3.

9 Pietrzak P, Corbishley C, Watkin N. Organ-sparing surgery for invasive penile cancer: early follow-up data: *BJU Int* 2004;94(9):1253–7.

10 Lindegaard JC, Nielsen OS, Lundbeck FA, Mamsen A, Studstrup HN, von der Maase H. A retrospective analysis of 82 cases of cancer of the penis. *Br J Urol* 1996;77(6):883–90.

11 Philippou P, Shabbir M, Malone P, et al. Conservative surgery for squamous cell carcinoma of the penis: resection margins and long-term oncological control. *J Urol* 2012;188(3):803–8.

12 Bayles AC, Sethia KK. The impact of Improving Outcomes Guidance on the management and outcomes of patients with carcinoma of the penis. *Ann R Coll Surg Engl* 2010;92(1):44–5.

13 Pizzocaro G, Algaba F, Horenblas S, et al. EAU penile cancer guidelines 2009. *Eur Urol* 2010;57(6):1002–12.

14 Alnajjar HM, Lam W, Bolgeri M, et al. Treatment of carcinoma in situ of the glans penis with topical chemotherapy agents. *Eur Urol* 2012;62(5):923–8.

15 Tietjen DN, Malek RS. Laser therapy of squamous cell dysplasia and carcinoma of the penis. *Urology* 1998;52:559–65.

16 van Bezooijen BP, Horenblas S, Meinhardt W, Newling DW. Laser therapy for carcinoma in situ of the penis. *J Urol* 2001;166(5):1670–1.

17 Windahl T, Andersson SO. Combined laser treatment for penile carcinoma: results after long-term follow up. *J Urol* 2003;169(6):2118 21.

18 Bandieramonte G, Colecchia M, Mariani L, et al. Peniscopically controlled CO2 laser excision for conservative treatment of in situ and T1 penile carcinoma: report on 224 patients. *Eur Urol* 2008;54(4):875–82.

19 Larke NL, Thomas SL, dos Santos Silva I, Weiss HA. Male circumcision and penile cancer: a systematic review and meta-analysis *Cancer Cause Control* 2011;22:1097–110.

20 Castellsagué X, Bosch FX, Muñoz N, et al. Male circumcision, penile human papillomavirus infection, and cervical cancer in female partners. *N Engl J Med* 2002;45:1105–12.

21 Bailey RC, Moses S, Parker CB, et al. Male circumcision for HIV prevention in young men in Kisumu, Kenya: a randomised controlled trial. *Lancet* 2007;369:643–56.

22 Morris BJ, Krieger JN. Does male circumcision affect sexual function, sensitivity, or satisfaction? – a systematic review. *J Sex Med* 2013;10(11):2644–57.

23 Depasquale I, Park AJ, Bracka A. The treatment of balanitis xerotica obliterans. *BJU Int* 2000;86:459–65.

24 Hadway P, Corbishley CM, Watkin NA. Total glans resurfacing for premalignant lesions of the penis: initial outcome data. *BJU Int* 2006;98(3):532–6.

25 Shabbir M, Muneer A, Kalsi J, et al. Glans resurfacing for the treatment for carcinoma in situ of the penis: Surgical technique and outcomes. *Eur Urol* 2011;59:142–7.

26 Austoni E, Fenice O, Kartalas Goumas Y, et al. New trends in the surgical treatment of penile carcinoma. *Arch Ital Urol Androl* 1996;68:163–8.

27 Morelli G, Pagni R, Mariani C, et al. Glansectomy with split-thickness skin graft for the treatment of penile carcinoma. *Int J Impot Res* 2009;21(5):311–4.

28 Smith Y, Hadway P, Biedrzycki O, et al Reconstructive surgery for invasive squamous carcinoma of the glans penis. *Eur Urol* 52(4):1179–85.

29 Gulino G, Sasso F, Falabella R, Bassi PF. Distal urethral reconstruction of the glans for penile carcinoma: results of a novel technique at 1-year of followup. *J Urol* 2007;178(3 Pt 1):941–4.

30 Palminteri E, Berdondini E, Lazzeri M, Mirri F, Barbagli G. Resurfacing and reconstruction of the glans penis. *Eur Urol* 2007;52(3):893–8.

31 O'Kane HF, Pahuja A, Ho KJ, Thwaini A, Nambirajan T, Keane P. Outcome of glansectomy and skin grafting in the management of penile cancer. *Adv Urol* 2011; art. ID:240824.

32 Hatzichristou DG, Apostolidis A, Tzortzis V, et al Glansectomy: an alternative surgical treatment for Buschke-Lowenstein tumours of the penis. *Urology* 57:966–9.

33 D'Ancona CA, Botega NJ, De Moraes C, et al. Quality of life after partial penectomy for penile carcinoma. *Urology* 1997;50(4):593–6.

34 Chang TS, Hwang HY. Forearm flap in one-stage reconstruction of the penis. *Plast Reconstr Surg* 1984;74:251–8.

35 Garaffa G, Raheem AA, Christopher NA, Ralph DJ. Total phallic reconstruction after penile amputation for carcinoma. *BJU Int* 2009;104(6): 852–6.

36 Leijte JA, Kerst JM, Bais E, Antonini N, Horenblas S. Neoadjuvant chemotherapy in advanced penile carcinoma. *Eur Urol* 2007;52(2):488–94.

37 Shukla CJ, Shabbir M, Feneley MR, Withey S, Muneer A, Minhas S. Palliation of male genital cancers. *Clin Oncol* 2010;22(9):747–54.

CHAPTER 30

Penile reconstruction and trauma

C.J. Shukla[1] and Suks Minhas[2]

[1] *Western General Hospital, NHS Lothian, Edinburgh, UK*

[2] *University College Hospital, London, UK*

Introduction

A variety of benign conditions of the penis may necessitate surgical reconstruction. These include lichen sclerosus/balanitis xerotica obliterans (LS/BXO), buried penis, micropenis, lymphedema, Peyronie's disease, and traumatic conditions outlined in this chapter. The management of micropenis is outlined in more detail in Chapter 25, and that of Peyronie's disease in Chapter 24.

These conditions have varying effects on patients. Conditions such as LS, lymphedema, and Peyronie's disease can cause pain and difficulty in having intercourse. The etiology of pain varies due to the pathophysiology. In lichen sclerosus and lymphedema, it is the injury to the skin during intercourse that results in pain, whereas in Peyronie's disease, pain may occur in the active phase due to the initial inflammatory process affecting the tunica albuginea. In the active and quiescent phases of Peyronie's disease the patient or their partner may also experience pain from the curvature of the penis.

Voiding difficulties such as pain during voiding (from irritation) or poor stream may arise in cutaneous conditions (e.g., in LS), or from dribbling and poor stream from a shortened phallus (in buried penis, or following trauma or surgery). The effect of these conditions can impair the psychological well-being of the patient due to localized symptoms or cosmetic appearance. Additionally, patients may express concerns regarding length, which may have an impact on the patient's confidence and can manifest in erectile dysfunction.[1]

The surgical principles used to treat these conditions are very similar. Once the primary disease has been treated, the remaining phallus can be reconstructed to maintain cosmesis and function, with improvements in urinary and sexual function, in a bid to maintain psychological well-being. A number of surgical techniques exist for reconstruction in order to achieve these goals (Table 30.1).

Trauma to the urethra and reconstruction following cancer are dealt with in Chapter.

Surgical principles

The main surgical principles in reconstruction of the penis and urethra involve:

1 A designated genital/plastic surgeon.
2 Versatility and familiarity in the use of grafts or skin flaps.
3 Meticulous dressings and wound care.
4 Multidisciplinary healthcare professional involvement.

Skin grafting

Skin grafting remains of primary importance in genital reconstruction. The grafts used to reconstruct the glans penis, penile shaft, and the urethra will vary according to the recipient and donor site and underlying pathological condition. Knowledge of graft characteristics and donor site requirements dictates the choice of graft used.

Split-thickness skin grafts (SSG) consist of the entire epidermis and a dermal component of variable thickness. In a full-thickness skin graft (FTSG), the entire thickness of the dermis is also included and hence may

Male Sexual Dysfunction: A Clinical Guide, First Edition. Edited by Suks Minhas and John Mulhall.

Table 30.1 Techniques used to bridge soft tissue defects during reconstruction.

Type of defect	Technique used for reconstruction
Small with minimal gap between tissue edges	Primary closure
Superficial defect on penile shaft (e.g., after trauma, infections, Fournier's gangrene)	Full-thickness skin graft (FTSG) or thicker split-thickness skin graft (SSG)
Superficial defect on glans/corona	Split-thickness skin graft (SSG)
Tunical invasion by tumor Incision and grafting for Peyronie's disease Reconstruction of tunica/corpora after trauma	Excision of tumor and/or tunical reconstruction using biomaterials including saphenous veins, Tutoplast®, or Pelvicol®
Large defect involving deeper tissues	Standard advancement flap Vertical rectus abdominis flap Tensor fascia lata flap Rotational flap
Reconstruction of neophallus, e.g., after subtotal penile amputation for carcinoma or trauma	Rotational flap, e.g., antero-lateral thigh (ALT) Pedicled/free flap, e.g., radial artery phalloplasty (RAP)

retain sweat gland and sebaceous gland function. SSGs can be of variable thickness depending on the functional and cosmetic requirements. The choice of graft used and its thickness is dictated by the physiological needs of the recipient site and the compromises associated with either choice. The penis expands and contracts with erections and requires robust covering to withstand the trauma/shearing forces of sex. As a result, the predominant use of SSG is on the glans and corona, whereas the FTSG, being more robust to withstand shearing stresses, is usually utilized for reconstruction of the penile shaft. Although the advantage of a FTSG is that the characteristics of the donor site are maintained and there is a lower risk of secondary graft contracture, there is a higher chance of graft loss. As a result, some surgeons prefer using thicker SSGs (approximately 20–24/1000 inches on the automated air dermatome setting as opposed to approximately 12–16/1000 inches for the glans and corona) to the penile shaft as it offers the best combination of graft take and durability.[2]

Graft contracture terminology merits further elaboration as an understanding of the two main types of contracture will also dictate the choice of graft used. Primary contracture occurs due to the elastin present in the graft material and occurs at the time of surgery. This can be up to 40% with FTSGs and 10% in SSGs due to the presence of elastin in the dermis.[2]

Secondary graft contracture occurs after the healing process has occurred and is due to the presence of myofibroblasts. The propensity for secondary contracture is higher with SSGs than with FTSGs, which have more dermis that helps prevent secondary contraction. As a result, once the process of secondary contraction has completed, FTSGs have the ability to stretch making them the ideal choice for penile shaft cover.

In the cases where a FTSG is utilized for the penile shaft coverage, the donor site chosen is one that can usually be closed primarily without tension. Common donor sites include the skin over the iliac crest or groin, although other sites such as the axilla can also be used, as they are more readily concealed. The skin in this region is thinner.

Overall, for skin grafts to the glans penis, a SSG is commonly used. This can be harvested by either an automated air dermatome or a manual Humby knife. SSGs are suitably thin and improve the potential for graft take to the underlying spongiosal tissue. The donor site is usually the anterolateral aspect of the thigh, as this can be more readily concealed. Contraindications to using this donor site include cutaneous conditions that preclude harvest or healing of the donor site, including infective/inflammatory conditions such as psoriasis. Although the graft is more fragile, its thinness allows better take with a lower risk of graft loss.

Glans resurfacing of the penis

Benign conditions limited to the superficial epithelium of the glans/corona can be effectively treated by glans resurfacing. If the disease process affects the urethra, more extensive reconstructive procedures may be necessary. These are discussed in more detail below.

Male genital lichen sclerosus (LS)/ balanitis xerotica obliterans (BXO)

Male genital lichen sclerosus (LS) is a common condition that results in a progressive sclerosing inflammatory dermatosis of the prepuce and glans penis, but may also involve adjacent structures such as the urethra, scrotum,

Table 30.2 Outcomes for glans resurfacing for lichen sclerosus (LS).

Series	*n* (follow-up, months)	Complications	Recurrences	Outcomes
Palminteri	4[a]	0		Self-reported and photographs showed satisfactory outcomes
Garaffa et al.	31 (12.8)	4 (12%)	4 (12%) Persistence of LS due to positive margins – no surgery required	84% self-reported satisfied outcomes and 71% sexually active
Depasquale	5 (unknown)	0		Not reported
Campus	3 (19)	0		Satisfactory cosmesis reported by authors

[a] In this paper, due to the heterogeneous case mix, it is not possible to determine follow-up, complications, and recurrences for individual conditions, but it reported satisfactory sensation, cosmesis, and overall satisfaction by self-reported and photographic means.

perineum, and anus. Its true incidence is unknown, but it commonly affects the foreskin resulting in phimosis. In approximately 1–2% of cases it affects the glans penis and/or the urethra.

The mainstay of initial conservative treatment includes a trial of topical corticosteroids. In refractory cases, surgical reconstruction may be necessary for treatment. In most patients, where the LS is limited to the foreskin or glans penis, a circumcision will be curative in the majority of cases.[3] However, this is not always necessary and if LS and symptoms are limited to the frenulum, frenular grafting after excision of the involved frenular skin may suffice, obviating the need for circumcision.[4]

Urethral involvement of LS is variable; in a large retrospective study,[5] surgical procedures utilized included circumcision (15.8%), meatotomy (7%), circumcision and meatotomy (3.5%), and penile urethroplasty with buccal mucosa grafts (BMG) as a one- or two-stage procedure in 10.7% of cases. However, the vast majority of men (135/215 patients: 62.8%) underwent surgery for panurethral disease. This included one-stage BMG in 88 (of 135) patients and definitive perineal urethrostomy in the remaining 47 patients.

Palminteri et al.[6] and Garaffa et al.[7] reported on their experience of glans resurfacing as a technique for reconstruction of the penis affected by LS, demonstrating satisfactory outcomes (Table 30.2).

Technique of glans resurfacing and SSG

This is described in detail in a publication from the authors' institution.[5] Briefly, sharp dissection is used to elevate the involved epithelium from underlying spongiosal tissue. This may take the form of removal of only a part (partial glans resurfacing – PGR) or all (complete/total glans resurfacing – TGR) the epithelium in quadrants of the penis (Figure 30.1). The rationale for removing the epithelium in quadrants is to prevent crush injury or "buttonholing" of larger areas, and to enable labeling of the histological specimen and identification of the site of removal of tissue in case of further surgery due to concomitant malignant/premalignant changes.

In the authors' institutions, a SSG is harvested using an automated air dermatome, or it can be done manually using a Humby knife. The advantage of an automated dermatome is the short learning curve and uniformity of graft thickness: the depth of tissue harvested can be predetermined. In our experience we harvest the SSG at a thickness of 0.008 to 0.016 inches. The graft is sutured onto the edges using 4/0 or 5/0 Vicryl Rapide™ (Ethicon) and quilted with 5/0 Vicryl Rapide™. The patient is then catheterized (14-F silicone catheter), and the glans penis is dressed with a soft silicone-coated dressing (Mepitel®; Mölnlycke Health Care) and gauze, followed by a foam dressing to help immobilize the graft. The dressing is left in place for 5 days with the patient remaining on strict bed rest for the first 48 hours (to minimize slippage of dressing during the period of imbibition of graft). On the fifth day, the dressing and the catheter are removed, and the patient is discharged with wound-care advice for review in the clinic the following week. The technique for glans resurfacing for LSA is similar to that used for carcinoma in situ of the glans penis.[8]

If the distal penile urethra is also involved in the pathological process of BXO/LSA, then, in addition to the

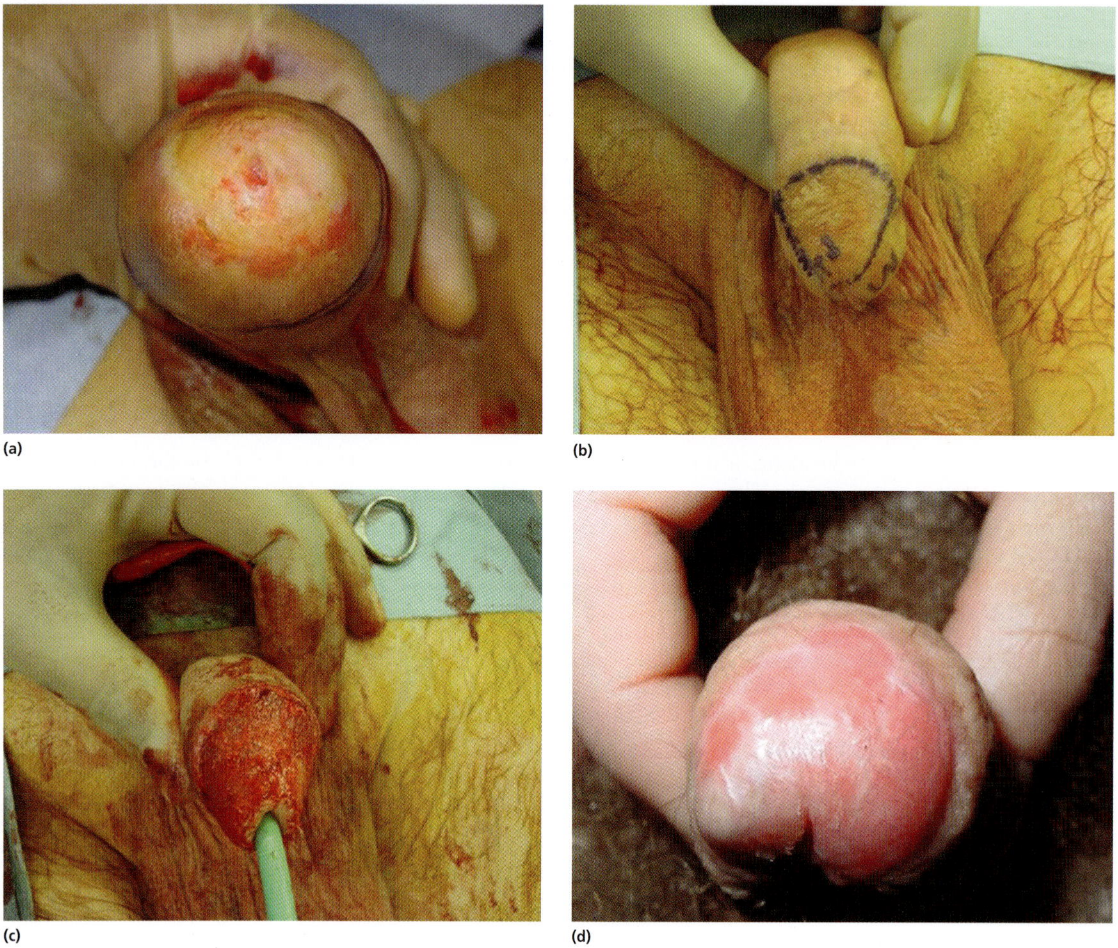

Figure 30.1 The technique of glans resurfacing for (a) balanitis xerotica obliterans (BXO) and (b) carcinoma in situ. (c) After excision of the glans epithelium. (d) Following skin grafting, the long-term outcome.

glans resurfacing to address LSA of the glans, a two-stage reconstructive procedure/urethroplasty using BMG is necessary to deal with the urethral component. There is no consensus on whether the urethra or glans are addressed first, and both practices are seen variably. In cases of extensive involvement of the penile urethra (e.g., panurethral strictures), a Kulkarni urethroplasty may be necessary using the principles of a dorsal onlay BMG into the entire strictured urethra, which is incised dorsally for the graft.[9]

Results from the largest series thus far suggest favorable outcomes, with 3% of patients being dissatisfied due to poor cosmesis and 12% being dissatisfied due to recurrence/persistence of LS.[7]

Buried penis

By definition, this condition results in at least a part of the penile shaft being buried/obscured by the overlying prepubic skin and/or scrotum due to a number of pathological conditions. This condition should be differentiated from micropenis, where the true penile length is less than 7.5 cm.

The etiology of the buried penis is multifactorial and is outlined in Table 30.3, but includes factors such as:

- Congenital causes in the pediatric population, which may be due to congenital megaprepuce, short penile shaft, abnormal attachment of the fundiform and/or supensory ligaments, or excess prepubic fat.[10]

Table 30.3 The etiology and techniques of increasing relative penile length as a treatment for buried penis.

Etiology of buried penis		Surgical corrective technique	
Shortened penis	**Increased surrounding tissue**	**Techniques for increasing relative length of penis**	**Technique for reduction of surrounding tissues**
• Post radical circumcision • Excessive skin loss post trauma/circumcision • Traumatic or surgical amputation for cancer	• Obesity • Scrotal lymphedema • Scrotal web	• Release of scar tissue • Suspensory ligament division with or without use of subpubic spacer • VY or Z plasty • Use of FTSG after degloving penis	• Reduction scrotoplasty • Abdominoplasty/lipectomy/liposuction

FTSG, full-thickness skin graft.

- Obesity.
- Excessive skin loss post-circumcision, post-trauma/self-mutilation, or due to burns.
- Lymphedema.
- After surgery for penile malignancy when a partial/subtotal penectomy is performed.

The increasing prevalence of predisposing factors such as morbid obesity and diabetes will result in an increase in prevalence of such cases, which are challenging to the urologist and plastic surgeon alike.

The consequences of this condition are that the patient is often unable to micturate in the standing position due to spraying, or he dribbles urine onto the anterior aspect of the scrotum. Additionally, the patient may find sexual intercourse difficult due to the relative size of the phallus. This can have significant physical and psychological effects on individuals.

The aims of treatment in this group of patients are to restore urinary function (ideally enabling the patient to pass urine in the standing position and without spraying of the stream), and to restore sexual function.

Although various techniques have been described to treat this condition[11] (see Table 30.3), conservative measures in the form of weight loss and psycho-sexual counseling are advocated initially in all cases. Weight loss by dieting or bariatric surgery may not suffice as skin laxity from the abdominal apron can still lead to a trapped and buried penis, requiring apronectomy.

If conservative measures fail, surgical techniques currently available to treat buried penis include:

- VY or Z plasty
- suspensory ligament division
- skin grafting (usually FTSG)
- reduction scrotoplasty
- abdominoplasty
- penile prosthesis insertion.

The choice of surgical technique must be tailored to the individual patient and his body habitus, as well as functional goals[11] and patient expectations. In many cases these techniques do not increase the true length of the penis, but can increase the relative length in relation to the abdomen/scrotum, hence providing a sense of increase in relative size. The techniques available to treat the buried penis are numerous and require versatility and often a combination of procedures, and it is not within the remit of this chapter to discuss the merits and outcomes of each individual technique. However, the reader is directed to a review by Pestana et al.,[11] who also propose an algorithm for management of the buried penis. The principles are to identify if firstly release of any scar contracture would release the penis and then tailor the use of graft/flaps to cover the defect. However, if the overriding cause is abdominal fat impingement or burying, then panniculectomy (removal of the abdominal fat) with/without division of the suspensory ligament would be the mainstay of length release. Any skin or soft tissue defects that cannot be closed without tension by primary means, will require skin graft or local flaps for coverage.

Objective outcome measures in this condition are difficult to define due to the heterogeneity of the etiology, patient body habitus, and expectations. However, long-term cosmetic results "are satisfactory."[11] Figure 30.2 illustrates a technique utilized in the authors' institution to deal with the buried penis.

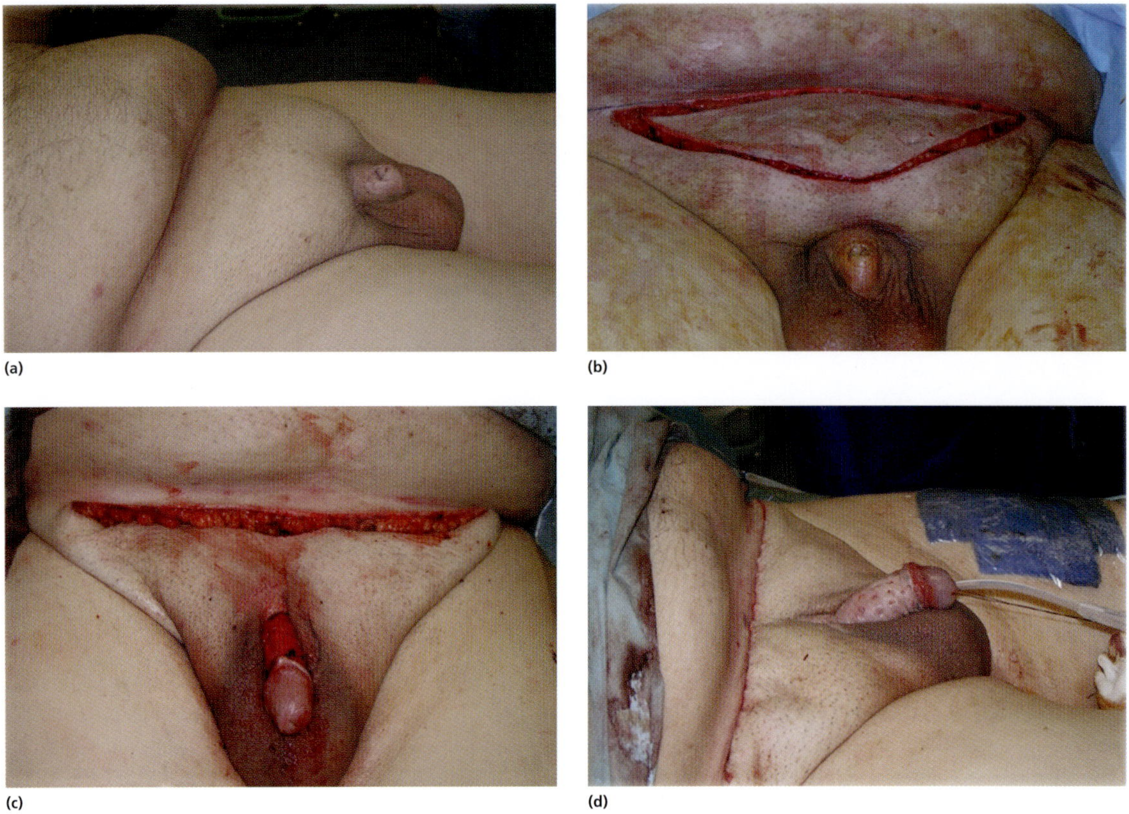

Figure 30.2 Release of the buried penis in an obese patient with phimosis due to lichen sclerosus (LS) affecting the penile shaft skin. **a)** Preoperatively, despite losing approximately 20 kg, the patient still had a significant pre-pubic fat pad. **b)** A wide incision is used to excise the pre-pubic fat pad; **c)** excision of the LS-affected skin resulted in exposure of the penile shaft, which was amenable to a thick SSG **(d)**.

Male genital lymphedema

This is an uncommon condition due to abnormal retention of lymphatic fluid in the subcutaneous tissues. Although the primary pathogenesis is a reduction in lymphatic drainage, the etiology can be primary due to an abnormal development of the subcutaneous lymphatic system, or secondary to any condition that may affect and impair the drainage of the lymphatic fluid to the inguinal lymph nodes.[12,13]

These conditions include:

- Extended inguinal and pelvic node dissections (e.g., following inguinal/groin node dissection for penile cancer surgery or melanoma surgery).
- Radiotherapy.
- Malignant infiltration of the inguinal/pelvicnodes.
- Granulomatous infiltration (e.g., Crohn's disease, sarcoidosis, and orofacial granulomatosis – granulomatous cheilitis and Melkersson–Rosenthal syndrome).
- Venereal diseases (*Chlamydia trachomatis*).
- Parasitic infections of the inguinal lymph nodes, e.g., filariasis (tropical disease caused by *Wuchereria bancrofti*, *Brugia malayi*, and *Brugia timori*).
- Patients on chronic peritoneal/ambulatory dialysis.
- Idiopathic.

Lymphedema affecting the scrotum can be treated initially by conservative methods, for example, by elevation or compression by scrotal support, treatment of primary cause if reversible, and antibiotics for suspected infectious causes.[14] In refractory cases, or in those with extremely large and debilitating lymphedema, surgical management by a reduction scrotoplasty may be necessary. A "V-" or wedge-shaped incision is used to excise the skin and subcutaneous/dartos layers (to healthy skin) and primary apposition of the remaining tissue can be used. Principles of surgical treatment of penile lymphedema include excision of all overlying skin and/or lymphedematous tissue superficial to Buck's fascia with either primary closure, FTSG, thick SSG, or local flaps to cover the remaining defect.[12,13]

Peyronie's disease

Also known as induratio penis plastic, this condition was initially described as early as 1561 by Fallopius and Ephemerides and named after François Gigot de la Peyronie, who formally described this condition in his paper "On some obstacles opposing the natural ejaculation of semen" in 1743.[15] Although non-surgical therapies may influence the progression of the disease, the definitive treatment involves surgery, the nature of which will depend on a number of factors such as the degree of curvature (<60° vs >60°), strength of erections, and compounding factors such as intracorporeal fibrosis or hour-glass deformity.[16] The surgical management of Peyronie's disease is dealt with in more detail in Chapter xx.

The indications and timing of surgery are outlined by the European Association of Urology.[17] Correction of deformity is performed after stabilization of the disease. The two main forms of surgery, which tend to correct the deformity more than non-surgical means, are described and broadly categorized as "penile shortening and penile lengthening procedures." These are described in more detail in Chapter 26.

The penile shortening procedures aim to correct the deformity by addressing the convex/non-diseased tunica albuginea using techniques of corporoplasty, excision, or 16-dot plications. The penile lengthening procedure is a misnomer as it does not "increase" length, but aims to preserve length (i.e., prevents shortening). In actual fact, the surgery reduces the degree of shortening, but due to the possibility of graft contracture, penile length may still be lost, albeit to a lesser degree. Corporoplasty procedures (e.g., Nesbit operation, Yachia or plication techniques) are suitable for lesser degrees of curvature, that is, less than 60°. In men with erectile dysfunction, other therapies may also be required at a later date to restore erectile function, such as medical therapy or even implantation of a penile prosthesis. The advantage of corporoplasty techniques is the lower risk of de novo erectile dysfunction (2–3%). However, disadvantages include shortening of the penis (approximately 1 mm for every 10° correction), palpable knots (if not buried), and recurrence (if absorbable sutures are used or if surgery is performed prior to plaque stabilization).

Plaque incision and grafting using materials such as autologus saphenous vein[18] or synthetic material such as Tutoplast®,[19] porcine small intestinal submucosa graft,[20] or Pelvicol® may be used in patients with good erectile function and greater degrees of curvature (>60°) or "hour-glass deformity."

The advantages of plaque incision and grafting include a lesser degree of shortening and maintenance of girth in cases of hour-glass deformity. However, complications such as erectile dysfunction (15–50%), glans hypoesthesia, and some loss of penile length do occur. A circumcision is not always necessary in either corporoplasty or plaque incision and grafting procedures.[21]

For patients who complain of shortening of the penis or hour-glass deformities, but have good erectile function, length and girth increases can be achieved by a combination of circular and longitudinal incisions and grafting, as described by Egydio et al.[22]

Reconstruction following trauma

Various traumatic conditions (blunt/penetrating) affecting the penis can be managed according to the common principles outlined above. We will cover the principles of management of various traumatic conditions, but this is by no means exhaustive nor prescriptive. A wide variety of techniques are available, but versatility in their use and utilizing a tailored approach (as opposed to a one size fits all) is recommended.[23]

Fractured penis

Forcibly bending the erect penis during sexual activity can result in the traumatic disruption of the tunica albuginea overlying the corpora cavernosa causing a fracture of the penis. This is particularly the case where taqaandan (a practice of forcefully detumescing an erect penis, as is performed in some Middle Eastern countries) is practiced.[24] In approximately 10% (1–38%) of cases, the urethra is also involved and disrupted to a variable degree.

Diagnosis is made on clinical grounds, with a typical history of pain, hematoma, and a snapping sound with immediate detumescence. There may be significant hematoma within the subcutaneous tissues (the so-called "aubergine" or "egg-plant sign") and a defect in the tunica may be palpable. Early surgical repair is advocated although the timing of repair has been controversial, with a common myth that immediate repair is essential. However, a large retrospective case series[25] has shown no difference in outcome in men presenting and undergoing early surgical intervention (within 24 hours) compared to those presenting late (up to 7 days).

Surgical approaches vary based on the experience of the surgeon and the location of injury or involvement of the urethra. When available, preoperative imaging in the form of ultrasound[26] or MRI[27] may not only confirm the diagnosis, but also aid localization of the defect and surface marking in order to direct the surgeon in making a short incision directly over the tunical defect.[28]

The majority of explorations are dealt with by a circumcision, degloving of the penis, and repairing the corporal defect using principles similar to corporoplasty for Peyronie's disease. However, in the authors' institution, the availability of prompt imaging in the form of ultrasound ensures the accurate localization of the corporal defect, and if a urethral injury is not suspected an incision directly over the site allows direct access to the corporal defect and closure of the tunica without the need for circumcision or degloving of the penis.[28]

In cases where a urethral injury is suspected (approximately 10%), an alternative to the conventional surgical approach is to use a midline peno-scrotal incision and dissection down to the pre-catheterized urethra and adjacent corporal defect. The urethra is dissected off the corpora and mobilized proximally and distally. The urethra is debrided and repaired over a catheter using 3/0 or 4/0 polyglactin interrupted sutures ensuring tension-free closure of the urethral mucosa and the spongiosum (Figure 30.3). This approach reduces the need to circumcise and deglove the penis, and if the urethral injury or fracture is at the base of the penis, avoids the "bunching up" of degloved skin interfering with mobilization and repair of the urethra/corpora.

Genital skin loss

Genital skin loss occurs from a host of causes, including:

- human or animal bites;
- urban road traffic accidents when loose genital skin is entangled in clothing, which is then subject to deceleration forces;
- burns;
- Fournier's gangrene.

The principles of repair are primary closure in two layers (skin and dartos) when there is no infection. Due to the elasticity and compliance of the peno-scrotal skin, the redundancy of skin allows this primary closure even with significant skin loss. In cases of suspected infection (e.g., bites, Fournier's gangrene), broad-spectrum antibiotics, wound irrigation, debridement, and even urinary or fecal diversion may be necessary prior to attempting closure – primarily or with skin grafts/local flaps. Tetanus toxoid booster or immunoglobulin prophylaxis (rabies in the case of animal bites) is necessary as per local protocol. Antibiotics should be broad spectrum to cover anaerobes as well as aerobic bacteria, and this warrants consultation with the microbiologists. *Pasteurella multocida* is of particular concern in dog bites, with *Escherichia coli, Streptococcus viridans, Staphylococcus aureus, Eikenella corrodens, Capnocytophaga canimorsus, Veillonella parvula, Bacteroides,* and *Fusobacterium* spp. also being implicated. In human bites, consideration must also be given to the risk of sexually transmitted diseases, such as syphilis, hepatitis, HIV, and herpes, as well as actinomycosis or tuberculosis.[29,30] Human or animal bites should not be closed primarily as there is almost certain infection/contamination associated, partly due to the delayed presentation, especially in the case of human bites.[31]

Burns (thermal, chemical, and electrical) affecting the genitals only are rare and comprise 1% of the surface area of the body. They are usually those concomitant to burns affecting other parts of the body. Management in a specialist unit, with resuscitation and assessment on severity (first, second or third degree), is necessary. In case of necrosis, the tissue demarcated would be debrided and grafted with SSG or FTSG as necessary.[31]

Fournier's gangrene warrants treatment in the same manner as infected genital skin loss by wide debridement into healthy bleeding tissue after resuscitation and antibiotic treatment to stabilize the patient. The superficial skin and dartos are excised removing all necrotic infected tissue. Testicles may be either placed in thigh pouches created, or may be approximated and sutured to each other and allowed to remain "loose" within the dressings.

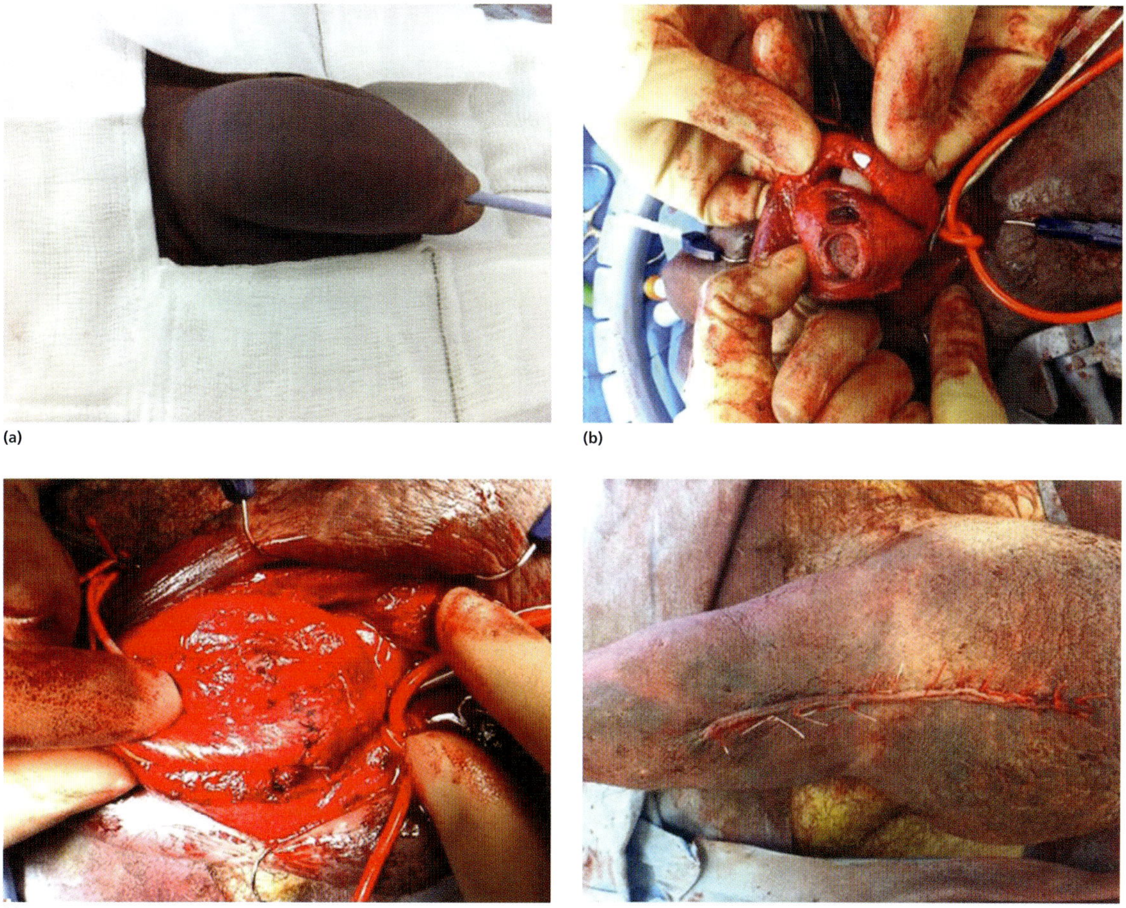

(a) (b) (c) (d)

Figure 30.3 Treatment of a fractured penis **(a)** with a bilateral corporal and urethral injury **(b)**. Repair of the corporal defect and urethra **(c)**, through the midline peno-scrotal incision **(d)** obviates the need for a circumcision and degloving of the penis.

After 24–48 hours, the wound is reinspected and debrided further if necessary. Reconstruction with skin grafting and/or local flaps can then be undertaken after approximately 7 days/or when the patient has clinically improved.

Amputation

Partial or total penile amputation, although rare, occurs following assault or is self-inflicted with patients having underlying psychological issues. Acute management requires resuscitation, management of other life-threatening injuries, and where possible/necessary a psychiatric evaluation. The amputated stump can be placed in a saline-soaked gauze within a sterile bag, which is then placed in ice.

Reconstructive/salvage options depend on the ability to retrieve and salvage the amputated appendage, the residual stump, and urinary and sexual functional needs of the patient. The three main options are closure and reconstruction (primary or delayed) of the residual stump, reimplantation, or total phallic reconstruction.

Reimplantation should be undertaken as a soon as possible. Reimplantation of the corporal structures and the urethra is undertaken first to provide a stable platform prior to anastomosis of the dorsal neurovascular structures. The neurovascular structures should be anastomosed using microsurgical techniques, which provide superior functional outcomes with respect to sensation.[29,31] Where the stump is not available, or has been dismembered beyond reconstruction/reimplantation, then the residual penile stump can be treated as if following penile cancer surgery. Complete or subtotal amputation may thus require total phalloplasty.

Reconstruction of the male genitals after total/subtotal penile loss

After surgery where the entire phallus has been excised (total/subtotal penectomy for cancer) or following amputation in trauma, and a perineal urethrostomy has been created, then surgery for reconstruction of the phallus using flaps can be contemplated in suitable individuals in order to regain sexual function as well as to allow urination in the upright position.

Rotational flaps, for example, the ALT (antero-lateral thigh), various abdominal/groin flaps, or free flaps such as the radial artery-based phalloplasty (RAP) flaps may be utilized. This operation is a staged procedure requiring creation of the sensate neophallus, glans sculpting to simulate normal glans anatomy, anastomotic urethroplasty to allow upright micturition, and then finally insertion of a penile prosthesis to allow erections for sexual intercourse. Garaffa et al.[32] describe the use of the RAP flap for treatment of penile loss from penile cancer. Of the 15 patients in this series, with a median follow-up of 20 months, all were satisfied with the cosmesis and size of the phallus, 14 were able to void while standing, and of the seven patients who had a penile prosthesis, five could engage in sexual intercourse. Urethral strictures occurred in three cases and fistulae in four, whereas one patient required penile prosthesis explantation secondary to infection. This procedure is also utilized for female-to-male transgender patients, where outcomes and complications are similar.[33]

A preliminary report of allograft penile transplant shows that this is a feasible option in patients and may avoid many of the complications of a rotational or free flap phalloplasty. Given the psychological impact of this surgery, selection and counseling of patients and their partners is likely to play a central role in the acceptance of the organ.[34,35] Use of the dorsal, cavernosal, and external pudendal vessels may further improve vascularity and outcomes should this procedure become accepted for treatment of men following loss of the phallus.[36]

Summary

In conclusion, surgical reconstructive techniques can be used to treat a number of benign and malignant diseases of the male genitals. Versatility and knowledge of the various techniques, grafts, and flaps, as well as autologus and commercially available materials available for reconstruction, are paramount for successful outcomes. It is equally important that these techniques be performed in the hands of surgeons based in centers where a high volume of cases are treated for the benefit of better outcomes.

References

1 Rybak J, Larsen S, Yu M, et al. Single center outcomes after reconstructive surgical correction of adult acquired buried penis: measurements of erectile function, depression, and quality of life. *J Sex Med* 2014;11(4):1086–91.

2 Thakar HJ, Dugi DD III. Skin grafting of the penis. *Urol Clin North Am* 2013;40(3):439–48.

3 Depasquale I, Park AJ, Bracka A. The treatment of balanitis xerotica obliterans. *BJU Int* 2000;86(4):459–65.

4 Kayes O, Li CY, Spillings A, Ralph D. Frenular grafting: an alternative to circumcision in men with a combination of tight frenulum and phimosis. *J Sex Med* 2007;4(4 Pt 1):1070–3.

5 Kulkarni S, Barbagli G, Kirpekar D, et al. Lichen sclerosus of the male genitalia and urethra: surgical options and results in a multicenter international experience with 215 patients. *Eur Urol* 2009;55(4):945–54.

6 Palminteri E, Berdondini E, Lazzeri M, et al. Resurfacing and reconstruction of the glans penis. *Eur Urol* 2007;52(3):893–8.

7 Garaffa G, Shabbir M, Christopher N, et al. The surgical management of lichen sclerosus of the glans penis: our experience and review of the literature. *J Sex Med* 2011;8(4):1246–53.

8 Shabbir M, Muneer A, Kalsi J, et al. Glans resurfacing for the treatment of carcinoma in situ of the penis: surgical technique and outcomes. *Eur Urol* 2011;59(1):142–7.

9 Kulkarni S, Barbagli G, Sansalone S, et al. One-sided anterior urethroplasty: a new dorsal onlay graft technique. *BJU Int* 2009;104(8):1150–5.

10 Hadidi AT. Buried penis: Classification surgical approach. *J Pediatr Surg* 2014;49(2):374–9.

11 Pestana IA, Greenfield JM, Walsh M, et al. Management of "buried" penis in adulthood: an overview. *Plast Reconstr Surg* 2009;124(4):1186–95.

12 Garaffa G, Sansalone S, Ralph DJ. Penile reconstruction. *Asian J Androl* 2013;15(1):16–19.

13 Garaffa G, Raheem AA, Ralph DJ. An update on penile reconstruction. *Asian J Androl* 2011;13(3):391–4.

14 Garaffa G, Christopher N, Ralph DJ. The management of genital lymphoedema. *BJU Int* 2008;102(4):480–4.

15 Androutsos G. [Francois Gigot de La Peyronie (1678–1747), benefactor of surgery and supporter of the fusion of medicine and surgery, and the disease that bears his name.] *Prog Urol* 2002;12(3):527–33.

16 Ralph DJ. The surgical treatment of Peyronie's disease. *Eur Urol* 2006;50(2):196–8.

17 Hatzimouratidis K, Eardley I, Giuliano F, et al. EAU guidelines on penile curvature. *Eur Urol* 2012;62(3):543–52.

18 Lue TF, El Sakka AI. Venous patch graft for Peyronie's disease. Part I: technique. *J Urol* 1998;160(6 Pt 1):2047–9.

19 Kalsi JS, Christopher N, Ralph DJ, et al. Plaque incision and fascia lata grafting in the surgical management of Peyronie's disease. *BJU Int* 2006;98(1):110–14.

20 Breyer BN, Brant WO, Garcia MM, et al. Complications of porcine small intestine submucosa graft for Peyronie's disease. *J Urol* 2007;177(2):589–91.

21 Garaffa G, Sacca A, Christopher AN, et al. Circumcision is not mandatory in penile surgery. *BJU Int* 2010;105(2):222–4.

22 Egydio PH, Kuehhas FE, Sansalone S. Penile length and girth restoration in severe Peyronie's disease using circular and longitudinal grafting. *BJU Int* 2013:111(4 Pt B):E213–E219.

23 Perovic SV, Djinovic RP, Bumbasirevic MZ, et al. Severe penile injuries: a problem of severity and reconstruction. *BJU Int* 2009;104(5):676–87.

24 Zargooshi J. Sexual function and tunica albuginea wound healing following penile fracture: An 18-year follow-up study of 352 patients from Kermanshah, Iran. *J Sex Med* 2009;6(4):1141–50.

25 el Assmy A, el Tholoth HS, Mohsen T, et al. Does timing of presentation of penile fracture affect outcome of surgical intervention? *Urology* 2011;77(6):1388–91.

26 Nomura JT, Sierzenski PR. Ultrasound diagnosis of penile fracture. *J Emerg Med* 2010;38(3):362–5.

27 Kirkham A. MRI of the penis. *Br J Radiol* 2012;85 (Spec. No. 1):S86–S93.

28 Abolyosr A, Moneim AE, Abdelatif AM, et al. The management of penile fracture based on clinical and magnetic resonance imaging findings. *BJU Int* 2005;96(3):373–7.

29 Morey AF, Metro MJ, Carney KJ, et al. Consensus on genitourinary trauma: external genitalia. *BJU Int* 2004;94(4):507–15.

30 van der HC, Martinez Portillo FJ, Seif C, et al. Male genital injury: diagnostics and treatment. *BJU Int* 2004;93(7):927–30.

31 Chang AJ, Brandes SB. Advances in diagnosis and management of genital injuries. *Urol Clin North Am* 2013;40(3):427–38.

32 Garaffa G, Raheem AA, Christopher NA, et al. Total phallic reconstruction after penile amputation for carcinoma. *BJU Int* 2009;104(6):852–6.

33 Garaffa G, Christopher NA, Ralph DJ. Total phallic reconstruction in female-to-male transsexuals. *Eur Urol* 2010;57(4):715–22.

34 Hu W, Lu J, Zhang L, et al. A preliminary report of penile transplantation. *Eur Urol* 2006;50(4):851–3.

35 Hu W, Lu J, Zhang L, et al. A preliminary report of penile transplantation: part 2. *Eur Urol* 2006;50(5):1115–6.

36 Tuffaha SH, Sacks JM, Shores JT, et al. Utilizing the dorsal, cavernosal and external pudendal arteries for penile transplantation: technical considerations and perfusion territories. *Plast Reconstr Surg* 2014;134(1):11e–119e.

CHAPTER 31

Disorders of sex development

Dan Wood
University College Hospital, London, UK

Introduction

This chapter presents a complex group of conditions that are rare and may be difficult for the clinician to diagnose. The care for these patients needs to be in multidisciplinary teams.

Once into adolescence and early adulthood decisions about sex of rearing will usually have been made. Occasionally, individuals may decide to change their preferred sex. Whilst no one knows the precise incidence of these decisions they do seem to be rare.

In general terms determinants of an individual's gender can be thought of as chromosomal, hormonal, or phenotypical – with the chromosomes initiating development at conception, triggering differentiation of gonads into either ovaries or testes, and the resultant hormones influencing the development of internal ducts or external genitalia.[1] Thus a failure in any of these areas can lead to disorders of sex development (DSD). Diagnosis is most commonly, but not exclusively, at birth. Where disorders are recognized, a multidisciplinary team is essential in making decisions about sex of rearing and subsequent management. Table 31.1 gives the details of an overall classification based on the work of a consensus meeting in 2006 (Chicago consensus).[2] This chapter aims to cover those aspects of DSD most relevant to a male phenotype. The division is somewhat arbitrary but a comprehensive discussion of DSD is beyond the scope of this publication.

By looking at Table 31.1 it becomes clear that to make a distinction amongst these disorders is challenging. For the purposes of this chapter we have focused on XY DSD with a male phenotype. The content will examine disorders covered by the following headings:

1 Gonadal dysgenesis
2 Failure of androgen synthesis or receptors
3 Anti-müllerian syndrome
4 Other anatomical disorders
5 Other chromosomal anomalies.

Presentation

The diagnosis of these conditions may occur in childhood and the most common presentation will be the recognition of a male infant with hypospadias and bilateral undescended testes. This should trigger a set of investigations as part of a multidisciplinary team effort, leading to a diagnosis and management plan for the patient. However, in later life the mode of presentation divides into four main groups: cyclical hematuria, infertility, gonadal/abdominal tumors, or failure of or delayed development at puberty.[3]

Common concerns

Germ cell tumors

In all DSDs the risk of germ cell tumors arises from the presence of some Y-chromosome matter and the failure of testicular development. Genes such as *PLAP*, *OCT3/4*, and *c-KIT* are upregulated in poorly developed germ cells of a DSD testis. These previously arrested germ cells then tend towards one of two premalignant states:

- Intratesticular germ cell neoplasia (ITGCN) (carcinoma in situ)
- Gonadoblastoma.

These are both non-invasive states and may be difficult to distinguish from maturation delay on histological

Male Sexual Dysfunction: A Clinical Guide, First Edition. Edited by Suks Minhas and John Mulhall.

Table 31.1 Classification of disorders of sex development (DSD).

Sex chromosome DSD	46,XY DSD	46,XX DSD
A: 45,X (Turner syndrome and variants) B: 47,XXY (Klinefelter syndrome and variants) C: 45,X/46,XY (mixed gonadal dysgenesis DSD) D: 46,XX/46,XY (chimeric ovotesticular DSD)	A: Disorders of gonadal (testicular) development **1** Complete gonadal dysgenesis (Swyer syndrome) **2** Partial gonadal dysgenesis **3** Gonadal regression **4** Ovotesticular DSD B: Disorders in androgen synthesis or effect **1** Defective androgen synthesis (e.g., 17-hydroxy-steroid dehydrogenase deficiency, 5α-reductase deficiency, stAR mutations) **2** Defect in androgen action (e.g., CAIS, PAIS) **3** LH receptor defects (Leydig cell hypoplasia, aplasia) **4** Disorders of AMH or its receptor (persistent Müllerian duct syndrome) C: Other (e.g., severe hypospadias, cloacal exstrophy)	A: Disorders of gonadal (ovarian) development **1** Ovotesticular DSD **2** Testicular DSD (e.g., SRY+, dup SOX9) **3** Gonadal dysgenesis B: Androgen excess **1** Fetal (e.g., 21-hydroxylase deficiency, 11-hydroxylase deficiency) **2** Fetoplacental (aromatase deficiency, POR) **3** Maternal (e.g., luteoma, exogenous) C: Other (e.g., cloacal exstrophy, vaginal atresia, MURCS, other syndromes)

AMH, anti-müllerian hormone; CAIS, complete androgen insensitivity syndrome; MURCS, müllerian, renal, cervicothoracic somite abnormalities; PAIS, partial androgen insensitivity syndrome; POR, cytochrome P450 oxidoreductase.
Source: Hughes et al. (2006).[2] Reproduced with permission of Elsevier.

examination. Histological staining can help with distinguishing the specific cellular characteristics. Once the premalignant state is established, current thinking is that all ITGCN cells and approximately 50% of gonadoblastomas will undergo full malignant transformation.[4]

Those at particularly high risk of tumors are patients with a combination of gonadal dysgenesis and intra-abdominal testes – with an overall risk for malignancy of between 15% and 35%. Counseling for these patients would include a recommendation for early gonadectomy. Mild gonadal genesis or partial androgen insensitivity (where a child is raised as male) represent a far more moderate risk, and when the testes are in the scrotum counseling is needed in the context of regular self-examination, with annual tumor markers and ultrasound for life, supplemented by a biopsy during early puberty.[4] The lowest risk is clearly in those with cryptorchidism, where regular testicular self-examination is all that is necessary – patients need to be informed of the importance.[5]

Tumors are classified into seminomatous and non-seminomatous tumors, with an overall survival of around 95%. Metastases, high serum markers, and non-seminomatous tumors represent high-risk elements.

Presentation is classically as a painless mass in the body of the testis. Tumor markers (α-fetoprotein, β-human chorionic gonadotropin, and lactate dehydrogenase) and an ultrasound are essential baseline investigations. Staging is performed with the use of cross-sectional imaging, most commonly a CT scan, and treatment usually begins with radical inguinal orchidectomy unless early chemotherapy is necessary.

Infertility

This is far less likely to be a concern in conditions such as isolated hypospadias or unilateral cryptorchidism. Fertility is measured by paternity rate in the normal population and is around 93%; in unilateral cryptorchidism it is 90% but drops to 65% in bilaterally affected men.[6] However, in other forms of XY DSD, fertility may be much more severely affected.

Advances in assisted reproductive technology may well offer a solution for some individuals. When the testes are biopsied or even removed for diagnosis or germ cell tumors, consideration should be given to the possibility of sperm harvest and storage. Donor sperm and adoption may be further options for families to consider.

Testicular failure, whether part of a clinical syndrome or as a result of surgical removal, needs to be managed carefully with endocrine support. The importance in achieving normal growth, bone density, and overall well-being should be discussed with both patient and parent. Where necessary periodic measurement of serum levels and end organ effect (e.g., bone densitometry) should be measured.

This begins to underline the essential requirement for a multidisciplinary team – at the heart of this is psychology. At the time of diagnosis families and patient (if they are adolescent/adult) will struggle with this and they need support in coming to terms with what it means. If diagnosed in childhood the issue of where, when, how, and by who disclosure to the child should occur is important, and psychologists play an enormous role in helping to make this judgment, begin the discussion, and manage the consequences.

Gonadal dysgenesis

The major concerns in this spectrum of disorders are around:

1 small, failing testes;
2 poor androgen production;
3 absence of anti-müllerian hormone (AMH);
4 elevated gonadotropins.

Partial and mixed gonadal dysgeneses usually result in external virilization as a result of some testicular development (in mixed there is a streak gonad on one side with a dysgenetic testis on the other). Complete gonadal dysgenesis will, as a rule, result in a female phenotype and can be diagnosed in a girl with delayed puberty when a karyotype is requested.

In partial or mixed variants the level of virilization will vary. All variants show disruption in Leydig and Sertoli cell development. Failure in Sertoli cells will result in an absence of AMH and thus the persistence of müllerian structures (uterus and fallopian tube) – the local effect of AMH means that changes may be seen on one side only, for example, a hemiuterus. If the contralateral testis is well developed then wolffian structures will persist.

Germ cell tumors may occur in any dysgenetic gonad or a streak in 46,X/46,XY; the risk is higher in a dysgenetic gonad[7] There is an associated increased risk of Wilms tumor associated with mixed gonadal dysgenesis. This is now recognized as Denys–Drash syndrome, named after the two workers credited with describing cases. Patients usually have nephropathy with proteinuria, hypertension, and progressive renal failure. Wilms tumors may be bilateral in this condition but commonly have a more favorable, triphasic histology. Thus the principles behind managing mixed gonadal dysgenesis revolve around assigning gender, gonadectomy as needed, and screening for Wilms tumor.[8]

Failure of androgen synthesis or receptors

Congenital adrenal hyperplasia

The most commonly affected enzymes are 21-hydroxylase or 11-hydroxylase. An infant male with progressive weight loss and dehydration may end up in adrenal crisis if not spotted. They may be mistaken as having pyloric stenosis as they may vomit profusely. Males will often be seen to have precocious enlargement of the penis, scrotum, and prostate in the first two to three years of life. These may be accompanied by pubic hair growth, acne, and a deeper voice. Bones will mature with early closure of the epiphyses resulting in characteristically short stature. About one-third will have nodular testes as a result of adrenal rests – these do not need intervention but regular follow-up ultrasound examination is advised.

Steroid replacement is important with hydrocortisone and mineralocorticoids. If managed well, fertility remains possible for affected boys.

There are a variety of other syndromes that may affect the synthesis of testosterone at any point in the metabolic pathway. Phenotypes may be very female in appearance or male with incompletely virilized male external genitalia. 17α-Hydroxylase deficiency may result in salt and water retention with hypertension and hypokalemia. Affected males will typically have a perineal hypospadias and chordee. There are no reports of paternity in affected males.

3β-Hydroxysteroid dehydrogenase deficiency may be female in appearance but males will have testes – often in the scrotum, a small phallus, and hypospadias. Wolffian structures are commonly present, and if Sertoli cell function is preserved müllerian structures will be absent. The condition is diagnosed on steroid profile showing raised levels of the 3β-hydroxysteroids, but it needs to be considered in undervirilized males as they may develop a salt-wasting state.

Receptor defects

Partial androgen resistance

These may present with a female phenotype but anywhere along a spectrum to a male with hypospadias – often with undescended testes, gynecomastia, and infertility. These can be managed surgically at a time judged appropriate by parent, patient, and surgical team. Receptors may be reduced in either number or affinity.[2] Men will have normal or high luteinizing hormone (LH) and testosterone levels. Sex of rearing may well be decided on the basis of the genital appearance. In a male phenotype the prostate and wolffian duct structures may be underdeveloped. Sex hormone binding globulin will decline less than expected when a patient is tested with an anabolic androgen.[9]

5α-Reductase deficiency

These individuals will have an XY karyotype and genitalia with varying degrees of ambiguity. The vasa are often blind ending, the testes may be in the groin or abdomen, and the phallus is typically small. These have low levels of dihydrotestosterone (DHT) and high testosterone (T) levels – this is demonstrated in the form of a T/DHT ratio that is much higher than normal. There will often be extensive virilization at puberty but external genitalia may be poorly developed as these seem much more dependent on DHT. These cases can be surgically reconstructed along with an orchidopexy. See "Micropenis" section below.[10]

Anti-müllerian syndrome

This is caused by either an insufficiency of anti-müllerian hormone or an insensitivity to the hormone at the point of its target organ.

The classical appearance of these patients is of a male child with normal male external genitalia but internally müllerian structures will persist – uterus, fallopian tubes, and a vagina – often draining into a urticulus masculinis. Testes may be abdominal, in a hernia sac, and may be brought into the scrotum with orchidopexy. The müllerian structures, including the fallopian tubes and uterus, may be present in the hernial sac. There is debate about removal of müllerian structures – the concern is that the vasa relate very closely to them and may be damaged in their removal, thus damaging the prospect for fertility.[11,12]

Other anatomical disorders

Hypospadias

Hypospadias is a recognizable phenotype – some would classify it amongst the DSDs. Others would recognize it as part of the manifestation of some disorders of sex development. Thus it deserves discussion here. The precise impact of hypospadias on sexual function is difficult to assess, and there are substantial variations in both the quality and interpretation of data surrounding these patients.[13,14]

There are subjective concerns – many men with hypospadias will raise concerns about cosmesis. Dissatisfaction with appearance may be based on features such as chordee, other scarring, or reduced penile length,[15] depending on the assessment and, for some, the influence of culture. The rate varies;[16,17] Rynja's review suggests that the rate may be 30% in all hypospadias rising to 54.3% in severe hypospadias.[14] Although clearly there are surgical issues that arise, the lack of prospective follow-up makes it very difficult to cite an exact incidence of concerns, and many papers do not cite a reoperation rate or a length of follow-up. The introduction of objective measures such as HOPE (Hypospadias Objective Penile Evaluation)[18] or the (pediatric penile perception score)[19] aim to achieve consistency in evaluation. These are important, and whilst no one underestimates the resource burden of prospective follow-up in such a common disorder it is essential to a true understanding of the incidence of surgical problems that arise and affect penile function in all domains.

Chordee that recurs, especially associated with the penile growth in puberty, is well recognized and is correctable with reoperation.[20] Some authors have suggested that whilst the problem may be noted at a median of 16 years, presentation is often delayed with patients presenting at a median of 21 years.[21]

Ejaculation may also be affected: in the most severe form of hypospadias anejaculation is the presentation, but more commonly spraying or lack of propulsion are noted. The basis behind this is most commonly the lack of spongiosum or a secondary urethral stricture. Other problems may include sacculation/diverticulae, or urticulus masculinus. The urethra will need evaluation and treatment in a specialist center – an ascending and descending urethrogram will give the most information if a urethral stricture is suspected. Some of these issues may affect fertility in hypospadias patients, otherwise it is difficult to explain the fact that there is a slight reduction in paternity rates and an increase in seeking infertility treatment when compared to controls. These differences were more pronounced when associated with other genital anomalies.[22]

There is a dearth of data relating to erectile dysfunction in hypospadias. Some reports have suggested a rate of up to 24%.[23] The lack of validated assessment in adult life makes it impossible to know what the real level of the problem is. Evaluation would need to take into account previous surgery but would be based along the same lines as standard guidelines for the evaluation of erectile dysfunction.

Alongside the incidence of surgical problems, concerns relating to psychological and psychosexual problems are commonly raised.[24] It is the experience of the author and reflected in the literature that many of these young men are reluctant to seek help or advice relating to problems that they encounter. Careful handling is essential. Some may need reassurance and some may need surgical or other intervention.

When evaluated, studies diverge with some showing affected men to have no difference to controls.[25,26] Others suggest a delay in sexual debut with an increase in shyness, depression, and enuresis.[14,27,28] Patients tend to view their genital outcomes more negatively than surgeons. There is a greater tendency for hypospadiac men to appraise their genitalia negatively but this does not correlate with sexual function.[26,29]

In an ideal world all these patients would feature on a prospectively compiled database and would be followed up regularly with a review into puberty and beyond. The practicalities of achieving this are huge and would overload most services. However, there is a necessity for these patients to see a surgeon familiar with the pitfalls of hypospadias surgery in adolescence. The evaluation is important and may prove reassuring. For those with surgical problems, correction should be concentrated in the hands of expert centers. Similarly, the psychosocial and psychosexual issues that arise can be significant and need handling by those expert in doing so.

Micropenis

Young adults will typically present with two principal sources of anxiety. First, the visible appearance of the penis, and second the diagnosis and treatment. Referrals may come from pediatricians, endocrinologists, or general practitioners – causation may not be clear but it remains important to seek an underlying diagnosis.[30,31]

Isolated micropenis occurs more commonly with a gonadotropin deficiency, while those associated with a lack of testosterone are often accompanied by hypospadias. Whilst micropenis may be idiopathic, recognized causes include:

- Primary testicular failure – e.g., anorchia, partial gonadal dysgenesis, Klinefelter's syndrome.
- Hypogonadotropic hypogonadism – Kallmann's syndrome, CHARGE syndrome.
- Defects in testosterone action – partial androgen insensitivity, 5α-reductase deficiency.
- Developmental anomalies – aphallia, cloacal exstrophy.

Another anxiety relates to long-term sexual function. The response of many patients and their parents is that they will simply not be able to pursue a normal sexual relationship and that an operation is the key to resolving this. The author have spent many clinic consultations discussing these anxieties and trying to find a reasonable treatment path that is acceptable to both patient and treating surgeon. The data in Table 31.2 summarize seven series and suggest that the outcome for sexual function has been favorable. In this analysis, 95% of patients were having normal erections, and 60% were engaging in regular sexual intercourse. Thirty-eight percent of those included had psychological problems, which strongly suggests that careful counseling and psychological support are essential components of management, and may allow some men to accept that they are able to achieve a meaningful and intimate relationship without surgical intervention.[32–38]

Testicular regression syndromes

These are defined by clear evidence of testicular function during development but absent testes and a 46,XY karyotype. The mechanism of the testicular absence or vanishing is not clearly understood it may have a genetic or teratogenic basis. The other possibility is bilateral torsion. It is thought that even when the testes were present they had abnormal function. At diagnosis serum follicle-stimulating hormone (FSH) and luteinizing hormone (LH) will be high but testosterone will be at castrate levels. Males will need testosterone replacement from puberty. Testicular prostheses may be helpful in managing cosmetic concerns.[8]

Other chromosomal anomalies

Klinefelter's syndrome

This has an incidence of 1 in 1000 male births. It is defined by the presence of an additional X chromosome,

Table 31.2 Sexual Function with a small penis.

	Reilly and Woodhouse[32]	Miller and Grant[33]	Money et al.[34]	Husmann[35]	Wisniewski et al.[36]	Bin-Abbas et al.[37]	Van Seters and Slob[38]	TOTAL
Number (*n*)	20	19	9	20	13	8	3	92
Gender Identity Disorders (G.I.D.)	0		2	0	0	0	0	2%
Erections	20	15	9	20	13		3	95%
Heterosexual	20		6	19	10		3	63%
Homosexual	0		3		1			4%
Bisexual				1	2			3%
Regular sexual intercourse (S.I.)	15	6		12		6	3	60%
Psychological problems		6	9	5	6	0		38%

Source: Wood and Woodhouse (2011).[39] Reproduced with permission of Hindawi Publishing Corporation.

producing a 47,XXY karyotype.[2] Diagnosis may be delayed into early adulthood and investigation initiated because of incomplete virilization. Men suffering with this are classically described as having small, firm testes, gynecomastia, and raised FSH and LH levels. Testosterone levels are normal in approximately 50%. The onset of puberty and development of secondary sexual characteristics is not usually delayed,although completion may be. Whilst virilization may be complete in some, patients may present with hypogonadism, gynecomastia, and sexual or erectile dysfunction – infertility may be the first presentation; a focused examination looking for small, firm testes and gynecomastia is important. Progressive decline in testicular function is the expected course for most patients.[40] Fertility is likely to require medical intervention for many of these patients – however there are rare cases of natural conception in the literature.[41]

Kallmann's syndrome

Kallmann's syndrome is an X-linked disorder; depending on the precise genetic anomaly it can be either autosomal dominant or recessive. There is an isolated gonadotropin-releasing hormone deficiency with an associated anosmia (hypogonadotropic hypogonadism). Males will show partial pubertal development with small testes.[42] Testosterone levels are low as are serum LH and FSH – pituitary function is otherwise normal. These boys are phenotypically characterized by a microphallus and cryptorchidism. This may be recognized in infancy if the correct hormonal profile is measured and detected – many cases are not picked up until adolescence.[43] One treatment option is with testosterone to ensure pubertal development along with normal sexual function, and bone and muscle mass. The alternative is treatment with human chorionic gonadotropin (hCG) – doses need to be carefully titrated to avoid the development of gynecomastia (estrogen may be produced as a result of stimulating the testes with hCG).

Various forms of gonadotropin therapy, including recombinant FSH, can be used to induce fertility in these men. This may be continuous or pulsatile – the aim is to induce intrinsic spermatogenesis.[44]

Smith–Lemli–Opitz syndrome

The genital anomalies seen in this rare condition are hypospadias and cryptorchidism; it is further characterized by microcephaly, hypotonia, dysmorphic facies, and syndactyly. There may be other visceral anomalies including the upper urinary tract. It is a rare condition affecting steroid metabolism and is inherited in an autosomal recessive pattern.[3]

Opitz syndrome

Again, hypospadias and cryptorchidism along with a bifid scrotum are the genital features of this condition. There is hypertelorism and abnormal separation between the respiratory bud and the foregut resulting in a cleft between the larynx and esophagus – this may result in respiratory difficulties, including aspiration for the affected infant.[3]

References

1 Jost A, Vigier B, Prépin J, Perchellet JP. Studies on sex differentiation in mammals. *Recent Prog Horm Res* 1973;29:1–41.

2 Hughes IA, Houk C, Ahmed SF, Lee PA. Consensus statement on management of intersex disorders. *J Pediatr Urol* 2006;2: 148–62.

3 Hutson JM, Warne GL, Grover SR. *Disorders of Sex Development – An Integrated Approach to Management*. Springer Verlag, 2012.

4 Looijenga L, Hersmus R, Oosterhuis JW, Cools M, Drop SL, Wolffenbuttel KP. Tumor risk in disorders of sex development (DSD). *Best Pract Res Clin Endocrinol Metab* 2007;21:480–95.

5 Schnack TH, Poulsen G, Myrup C, Wohlfahrt J, Melbye M. Familial coaggregation of cryptorchidism, hypospadias, and testicular germ cell cancer: a nationwide cohort study. *J Natl Cancer Inst* 2010;102:187–92.

6 Lee PA. Fertility after bilateral cryptorchidism. Evaluation by paternity, hormone, and semen data. *Horm Res* 2001;55: 28–32.

7 Verp MS, Simpson JL. Abnormal sexual differentiation and neoplasia. *Cancer Genet Cytogenet* 1987;25:191–218.

8 Wein AJ. In Wein AJ, Kavoussi LR, Novick AC, Partin AW, Peters CA (eds), Sexual Differentiation: Normal and Abnormal. *Campbell-Walsh Urology*, 9th edn. Elsevier-Saunders, 2007; pp. 3799–829.

9 Sinnecker GH, Hiort O, Nitsche EM, Holterhus PM, Kruse K. Functional assessment and clinical classification of androgen sensitivity in patients with mutations of the androgen receptor gene. German Collaborative Intersex Study Group. *Eur J Pediatr* 1997;156:7–14.

10 Allen L. Disorders of sexual development. *Obstet Gynecol Clin North Am* 2009;36:25–45.

11 Buchholz NP, Biyabani R, Herzig MJ, et al. Persistent mullerian duct syndrome. *Eur Urol* 1998;34:230–2.

12 Deepika, Kumar A. Persistent mullerian duct syndrome with transverse testicular ectopia: Rare entity. *J Clin Diagn Res* 2014;8:162–3.

13 Aho MO, Tammela OK, Somppi EM, Tammela TL. Sexual and social life of men operated in childhood for hypospadias and phimosis. A comparative study. *Eur Urol* 2000;37: 95–100; discussion 101.

14 Rynja SP, Wouters GA, Van Schaijik M, Kok ET, De Jong TP, De Kort LM. Long-term followup of hypospadias: functional and cosmetic results. *J Urol* 2009;182:1736–43.

15 Moriya K, Kakizaki H, Tanaka H, *et al.* Long-term cosmetic and sexual outcome of hypospadias surgery: norm related study in adolescence. *J Urol* 2006;176:1883–9.

16 Hoag CC, Gotto GT, Morrison KB, Coleman GU, Macneily AE. Long-term functional outcome and satisfaction of patients with hypospadias repaired in childhood. *Can Urol Assoc J* 2008;2:23–31.

17 Jiao C, Wu R, Xu X, Yu Q. Long-term outcome of penile appearance and sexual function after hypospadias repairs: situation and relation. *Int Urol Nephrol* 2010;43(1):47–54.

18 Van der Toorn F, de Jong TP, de Gier RP, *et al.* Introducing the HOPE (Hypospadias Objective Penile Evaluation) score: a validation study of an objective scoring system for evaluating cosmetic appearance in hypospadias patients. *J Pediatr Urol* 2013;9:1006–16.

19 Weber DM, Schonbucher VB, Landolt MA, Gobet R. The Pediatric Penile Perception Score: an instrument for patient self-assessment and surgeon evaluation after hypospadias repair. *J Urol* 2008;180:1080–4; discussion 1084.

20 Yucel S, Sanil A, Kukul E, Karaguzel G, Melikoglu M, Guntekin E. Midline dorsal plication to repair recurrent chordee at reoperation for hypospadias surgery complication. *J Urol* 2006;175:693–9.

21 Vandersteen DR, Husmann DA. Late onset recurrent penile chordee after successful correction at hypospadias repair. *J Urol* 1998;160:1131–3; discussion 1137.

22 Asklund C, Jensen TK, Main KM, Sobotka T, Skakkebaek NE, Jørgensen N. Semen quality, reproductive hormones and fertility of men operated for hypospadias. *Int J Androl* 2010;33:80–7.

23 Aho MO, Tammela OK, Tammela TL. Aspects of adult satisfaction with the result of surgery for hypospadias performed in childhood. *Eur Urol* 1997;32:218–22.

24 Mondaini N, Ponchietti R, Bonafè M, *et al.* Hypospadias: incidence and effects on psychosexual development as evaluated with the Minnesota Multiphasic Personality Inventory test in a sample of 11,649 young Italian men. *Urol Int* 2002;68:81–5.

25 Vandendriessche S, Baeyens D, Van Hoecke E, Indekeu A, Hoebeke P. Body image and sexuality in adolescents after hypospadias surgery. *J Pediatr Urol* 2010;6:54–9.

26 Mureau MA, Sliiper FM, Nijman RJ, van der Meulen JC, Verhulst FC, Slob AK. Psychosexual adjustment of children and adolescents after different types of hypospadias surgery: a norm-related study. *J Urol* 1995;154:1902–7.

27 Berg R, Berg G, Svensson J. Penile malformation and mental health. A controlled psychiatric study of men operated for hypospadias in childhood. *Acta Psychiatr Scand* 1982;66:398–416.

28 Wang W-W, Tu X-A, Deng C-H, Mo J-C, Zhao L, Chen L-W. Long-term sexual activity status and influencing factors in men after surgery for hypospadias. *Asian J Androl* 2009;11: 417–22.

29 Mureau MA, Slijper FM, Slob AK, Verhulst FC, Nijman RJ. Satisfaction with penile appearance after hypospadias surgery: the patient and surgeon view. *J Urol* 1996;155:703–6.

30 Bhangoo A, Paris F, Philibert P, Audran F, Ten S, Sultan C. Isolated micropenis reveals partial androgen insensitivity syndrome confirmed by molecular analysis. *Asian J Androl* 2010;12(4):561–6.

31 Silver RI, Yang A, Ben-Chaim J, Jeffs RD, Gearhart JP. Penile length in adulthood after exstrophy reconstruction. *J Urol* 1997;157:999–1003.

32 Reilly JM, Woodhouse CR. Small penis and the male sexual role. *J Urol* 1989;142:569–71; discussion 572.

33 Miller MA, Grant DB. Severe hypospadias with genital ambiguity: adult outcome after staged hypospadias repair. *Br J Urol* 1997;80:485–8.

34 Money J, Lehne GK, Pierre-Jerome F. Micropenis: gender, erotosexual coping strategy, and behavioral health in nine pediatric cases followed to adulthood. *Compr Psychiatry* 1985;26:29–42.

35 Husmann DA. The androgen insensitive micropenis: long-term follow-up into adulthood. *J Pediatr Endocrinol Metab* 2004;17:1037–41.

36 Wisniewski AB, Migeon CJ, Gearhart JP, *et al*. Congenital micropenis: long-term medical, surgical and psychosexual follow-up of individuals raised male or female. *Horm Res* 2001;56:3–11.

37 Bin-Abbas B, Conte FA, Grumbach MM, Kaplan SL. Congenital hypogonadotropic hypogonadism and micropenis: effect of testosterone treatment on adult penile size why sex reversal is not indicated. *J Pediatr* 1999;134:579–83.

38 Van Seters AP, Slob AK. Mutually gratifying heterosexual relationship with micropenis of husband. *J Sex Marital Ther* 1988;14:98–107.

39 Wood D, Woodhouse C. Penile anomalies in adolescence. *Scientific World Journal* 2011;11:614–23.

40 Wikström AM, Dunkel L. Testicular function in Klinefelter syndrome. *Horm Res* 2008;69:317–26.

41 Juul A, Aksglaede L, Lund AM, Duno M, Skakkebaek NE, Rajpert-De-Meyts E. Preserved fertility in a non-mosaic Klinefelter patient with a mutation in the fibroblast growth factor receptor 3 gene: case report. *Hum Reprod* 2007;22: 1907–11.

42 Pitteloud N, Boepple PA, DeCruz S, Valkenburgh SB, Crowley WF Jr, Hayes FJ. The fertile eunuch variant of idiopathic hypogonadotropic hypogonadism: Spontaneous reversal associated with a homozygous mutation in the gonadotropin-releasing hormone receptor. *J Clin Endocrinol Metab* 2001;86:2470–5.

43 Grumbach MM. Commentary: A window of opportunity: The diagnosis of gonadotropin deficiency in the male infant. *J Clin Endocrinol Metab* 2005;90:3122–7.

44 Liu PY, Baker HW, Jayadev V, Zacharin M, Conway AJ, Handelsman DJ. Induction of spermatogenesis and fertility during gonadotropin treatment of gonadotropin-deficient infertile men: Predictors of fertility outcome. *J Clin Endocrinol Metab* 2009;94:801–8.

CHAPTER 32

Sexual dysfunction and prostate cancer therapy

Ashley Ridout, Mark Emberton, and Caroline Moore
University College Hospital, London, UK

Introduction

Prostate cancer is the most common solid malignancy in men in the Western world,[1] and patients may be offered a range of treatment options. The earlier diagnosis of low-volume, low-risk prostate cancer has increased the numbers of men who have a long period of survival after diagnosis, and, therefore, health-related quality of life (HRQOL) outcomes are very important. The potential side effects of treatment for prostate cancer may be life-changing, including the risk of bladder, bowel, and sexual dysfunction, and patients must be aware of both the available treatment strategies and their potential associated side effects. A number of validated questionnaires are available to assess sexual and erectile function, which allow the ability to compare patient groups both in and between studies. Recording baseline sexual function, including pre-treatment potency and other variables of sexual function, allows more accurate comparison of functional outcomes according to baseline function. Collection of these data varies widely between published series, making comparisons difficult, as does the definition of sexual dysfunction used in each study. A comparison of patient self-reported potency and the validated International Index of Erectile Function (IIEF) measure revealed that of the men who subjectively reported full potency, only 43% measured as baseline "potent" in the sexual function domain of the IIEF,[2] highlighting the importance of using validated measures of sexual function to obtain accurate results for pre- and postoperative comparisons. Health-related quality of life outcomes are independently associated with patient satisfaction with their care,[3] and therefore considering this prior to treatment may help to manage expectations and prevent dissatisfaction.

Sexual dysfunction

Sexual dysfunction has been reported as the most common long-term side effect of prostate cancer treatment.[4] The term "sexual dysfunction" encompasses all the potential effects upon sexual function – erectile dysfunction, reduced libido, penile deformities, ejaculatory and orgasmic dysfunction, as well as changes that may occur in the relationship between the patient and his partner. Although erectile dysfunction is well documented after many methods of prostate cancer treatment, the other forms of sexual dysfunction may be equally bothersome to patients and are important to consider. Saitz et al. used the Male Sexual Health Questionnaire (MSHQ – a validated self-administered questionnaire used to assess erection, ejaculation, and sexual satisfaction in aging men[5]) to assess baseline sexual function in men in their urology clinic with a histopathologically confirmed diagnosis of prostate cancer, prior to definitive treatment.[6] They showed that decreased sexual desire and activity, erectile dysfunction, and ejaculatory dysfunction are present among men with newly diagnosed prostate cancer, prior to undergoing any treatment for the cancer. Awareness of this baseline, and individual patient expectations, may improve pre-treatment counseling.

Once oncological control is established, the functional effects of prostate cancer treatment become increasingly

Male Sexual Dysfunction: A Clinical Guide, First Edition. Edited by Suks Minhas and John Mulhall.

important and remain important to men throughout their lives, especially as survival for low-risk localized prostate cancer is excellent. The Scandinavian Prostate Cancer Group-4 (SPCG-4) randomized trial reported a cohort of 1201 men with localized prostate cancer who were randomly assigned to radical prostatectomy or watchful waiting. Johansson et al. reported the quality of life outcomes in these men and an additional 281 men as a population-based matched control group, after a median follow-up of 12.2 years (median age 77 years).[7] High self-assessed quality of life was reported in 35% of men after radical prostatectomy, 34% of men after watchful waiting, and 45% of men in the control group. Eighty-four percent of men in the radical prostatectomy group reported erectile dysfunction, 80% in the watchful waiting group, and 46% in the control group. There was also a raised level of anxiety in both the treatment groups, compared with the control group. In this study, treatment-associated morbidity was high, as was the level of anxiety and reduced quality of life. The implications of prostate cancer diagnosis and treatment are significant, and discussion about the potential risks and benefits of treatment should begin even prior to the first prostate-specific antigen (PSA) test.

Preoperative sexual function and treatment – can outcome be predicted?

The Prospective Prostate Cancer Outcomes and Satisfaction with Treatment Quality Assessment aimed to develop a model to predict longer-term erectile function for men with prostate cancer. It reports a prospective, longitudinal, multicenter cohort of men with clinical stage T1–T2 prostate cancer, who subsequently underwent primary treatment with radical prostatectomy, external beam radiotherapy, or brachytherapy. Patient-reported outcome measures were recorded, including the Expanded Prostate Cancer Index Composite (EPIC-26), as well as use of medications or devices for management of erectile dysfunction. Alemozaffar et al. reported on the 86% of these men who were followed up for at least 24 months.[8] At 2 years after surgery, functional erections were present in 37% of all men, and in 48% of men with functional erections preoperatively. Fifty-three percent (excluding those with penile prostheses) reported the use of medications or devices for their erectile dysfunction. Multivariate analyses were used to determine the risk of postoperative erectile dysfunction in individual groups, depending on preoperative factors including baseline sexual function, cancer severity, and individual clinical variables. The predicted erectile function at 2 years after treatment varied between ≤10% and >70%, depending on individual patient characteristics and the nature of their treatment.

Pre-treatment sexual function is, not surprisingly, an important predictor of post-treatment function. A systematic review of prognostic indicators for recovery of erectile function after radical retropubic prostatectomy identified that reported rates of preoperative potency ranged from 43% to 84%.[9] In addition, the importance of sexual dysfunction to patients – their "sexual bother" – is also important when considering quality of life outcomes. This may be influenced by the level of sexual activity prior to treatment for prostate cancer. Steinsvik et al.[10] showed that the level of sexual bother increased from 18% prior to radical prostatectomy, to 66% at 1 year postoperatively. This increase was more marked in the subgroup of patients who were sexually active prior to treatment (59% compared to 25%), and persisted in those who remained sexually active after prostatectomy. The importance of sexual bother is further demonstrated by Kimura et al., who retrospectively reviewed 2345 patients who underwent radical prostatectomy.[11] They noticed a subgroup of men who had a reduction in sexual bother, despite persistent sexual dysfunction. These men were more likely to be older, with higher stage disease, extracapsular extension, and seminal vesicle invasion, and not to have undergone a nerve-sparing procedure. They were also less likely to use phosphodiesterase type 5 inhibitors (PDE5Is) after surgery. Whilst sexual function is commonly measured and documented after treatment for prostate cancer, there is a group of men, as demonstrated in this study, who do not place as much importance upon post-treatment sexual function and therefore report less sexual bother.

Radical prostatectomy

Radical perineal prostatectomy was developed in 1904 at Johns Hopkins Hospital, and the retropubic approach was subsequently introduced by Millin in 1947. Both approaches were associated with significant side effects, including erectile dysfunction in almost all patients. Intraoperative and cadaveric anatomical studies revealed the dorsal vein complex, pelvic plexus, striated urethral sphincter, and lateral pelvic fascia.[12] Using this information, the "nerve-sparing" radical retropubic prostatectomy was described by Walsh and Mostwin,[13] aiming for preservation of sexual function, reduced urinary incontinence and reduced blood loss, whilst maintaining cancer control. This paper also suggested that only unilateral nerve sparing may be adequate to preserve erectile function, and Walsh et al. had previously reported that negative surgical margins, and therefore good cancer control, could be maintained with the nerve-sparing approach.[14] Anatomical observations, and subsequently surgical approaches, have been further refined – Costello et al. more precisely defined the anatomy of the neurovascular bundle and cavernosal nerves, in particular the posterolateral and posterior components.[15] Eichelberg et al. described the nerves that may be located anteriorly, and proposed an alternate, higher surgical approach to avoid these during a nerve-sparing procedure.[16] Walsh has described the "high-anterior release," aiming to avoid injury to the apical neurovascular bundle.[17] Although avoiding damage to the cavernous nerves during radical prostatectomy has greatly reduced the incidence of erectile dysfunction, this remains a significant potential side effect of the procedure. This may be due to failure of the nerve-sparing procedure, or local trauma to the nerves such as stretch, heat, ischemia, and local inflammation.[18] This temporary neuropraxia may cause structural changes in the penile tissue, due to smooth muscle apoptosis and fibrosis caused by hypoxia.[19] Therefore, even with a nerve-sparing procedure, changes in the veno-occlusive mechanism may result in erectile dysfunction. Intraoperative protection of the nerves from traction and heat exposure aims to reduce these potential side effects. Stember et al. attempted to define whether baseline erectile function was predictive for the attempted preservation of the cavernous nerve during radical prostatectomy.[20] They retrospectively reviewed a prospective database of 2323 men with localized prostate cancer who underwent radical prostatectomy at a single tertiary center, excluding those who were also treated with neoadjuvant or adjuvant hormonal therapy or radiotherapy. They reported that reduced baseline erectile function independently predicts for non-nerve-sparing procedures, presumably as the surgeon will choose not to nerve spare, and hence maximize cancer clearance, in those men with poor baseline function. Non-nerve-sparing procedures were associated with reduced urinary continence and potential cavernous venous leak, therefore they recommend that baseline erectile function, even when impaired, should not be used in deciding whether to attempt a nerve-sparing prostatectomy.

A review of oncological and functional outcomes after radical prostatectomy (RP) reported that although up to 40% of men have documented biochemical recurrence after RP, prostate cancer-related deaths occurred in less than 10% of men at 15 years after surgery.[21] With good oncological control, focus on functional outcomes aims to reduce treatment-associated morbidity. Functional outcomes vary widely and favorable outcomes have been linked to several variables including younger patient age,[22] preoperative potency,[23] and preservation of the neurovascular bundles.[9] Kundu et al.[24] reported a series of 1834 men who were potent prior to surgery, and underwent anatomical nerve-sparing (either unilateral or bilateral) radical retropubic prostatectomies without any adjuvant radiotherapy or hormone therapy. They reported that 76% of men treated with bilateral nerve-sparing and 53% with unilateral nerve-sparing procedures were able to achieve erection sufficient for intercourse. Younger men were significantly more likely to achieve erection postoperatively in this group, with 92% of men aged 40–49, 85% of men aged 50–59, 70% of men aged 60–69, and 51% of men aged 70 or over recovering erectile function. However, this group did not use a validated measure of erectile function, and most of the data were collected by the surgeon. The use of medication or devices to aid erectile function was not specifically reported. The risk of postoperative complications such as urinary incontinence and sexual dysfunction are lower in high-volume centers with experienced surgeons. This was reported by Walsh et al. in 2000,[25] and has been reliably reproduced by other groups since. There may also be a difference in quality of life outcomes between surgeons – Hartz et al. reviewed patients who had undergone prostatectomy at least 1 year previously, and showed significant variability for strength of erections, urine leakage, and length of hospital stay.[26] Patients from higher-volume surgeons reported significantly lower urinary leak and had a shorter hospital stay.

Walsh et al. reported results from a group of 64 men who underwent anatomical radical prostatectomy for localized prostate cancer, with 86% achieving erection suitable for intercourse (with or without sildenafil) at 18 months after the procedure. A prospective study of 586 men who underwent laparoscopic radical prostatectomy in a single center evaluated the erectile function of eligible men who received penile rehabilitation with medical therapy after the procedure and were followed up for 24 months.[27] At 24 months follow-up, 68% who underwent bilateral nerve-sparing surgery, and 35% who underwent unilateral nerve-sparing surgery reported erectile function suitable for intercourse, and the median IIEF-5 score for all patients was 13 (5 for unilateral nerve spare and 15 for bilateral nerve spare).

Longer-term data are now emerging: Sivarajan et al.[28] have reported outcomes from their 10-year prospective longitudinal cohort of 1836 men who underwent radical prostatectomy (mean age at surgery 59.2 years; 76.5% underwent bilateral nerve-sparing procedure, 15.1% unilateral, and 3.2% no nerve spare) at their institution between October 2000 and September 2012. They used the validated University of California, Los Angeles Prostate Cancer Index (UCLA-PCI) questionnaire, incorporating both sexual (from a composite score) and erectile function (from a single question). They reported that, after an initial decline in sexual function, the majority had improvement in both sexual and erectile function in the first 2 years after surgery. From 2 to 10 years after surgery, both sexual and erectile function remained quite stable – 58.5% of responders reported no change between 2 and 4 years after the procedure. This study also compared the age-related decline in sexual and erectile function expected in the general male population, and observed that some features of this decline were not reported in their RP population. This paper did not comment specifically on the prevalence of PDE5I use, or uptake of other treatment modalities for erectile dysfunction, and did not control for the use of either radiotherapy or androgen-deprivation therapy, although they did comment that, given the almost certain negative effect upon erectile and sexual function, exclusion of these individuals would have likely reinforced, rather than negatively affected, their conclusions. Another group, from the Memorial Sloan Kettering Cancer Center, reported a single question, five-point score (the MSKCC erectile function scale), for which they demonstrated a good correlation with the IIEF erectile function domain score,[29] suggesting that a single question may be as effective in assessing patients as a more detailed tool such as the IIEF.

A systematic review examined the other features of sexual function that may be affected after radical prostatectomy – orgasm-associated incontinence, urinary incontinence in relation to sexual stimulation, altered perception of orgasm, orgasm-associated pain, penile shortening, and penile deformity.[30] Whilst it is difficult to predict which patients will experience these side effects, all must be counseled preoperatively. A validated questionnaire would provide a framework for objective assessment and documentation, thereby potentially making comparisons easier and allowing prediction of which individuals may be affected. The lack of ejaculation ("dry ejaculation") may also affect quality of life. Dubbelman et al.[31] described a cohort of men who underwent radical retropubic prostatectomy (RRP), and who retrospectively answered questions about their sexual function pre- and postoperatively. These authors reported that 82.1% of the cohort were sexually active preoperatively, and that 32.7% of these were no longer sexually active postoperatively. Continued sexual activity was associated with age of 60 years or less, a bilateral nerve-sparing procedure, and urinary continence requiring use of two or fewer pads per day. These factors also significantly affected orgasm – prior to RRP orgasm was normal in 90% of men. This was preserved in 73.4% after bilateral nerve-sparing procedure, in 70.9% after unilateral nerve-sparing procedure, and in 54% of those with no attempted nerve spare. The loss of penile length and penile deformity, which may occur after radical prostatectomy, are likely due to penile fibrosis and apoptosis of the smooth muscle of the corpus cavernosum after cavernosal nerve injury. Preserving erectile function after RP is associated with maintenance of penile length,[32] as is postoperative use of penile vacuum devices,[33] which also conveyed an improved early sexual function.[34]

Salvage prostatectomy provides a treatment option for men with recurrent disease after initial definitive treatment. A systematic review of cancer control and functional outcomes for salvage radical prostatectomy in radiorecurrent prostate cancer[35] revealed that postoperative erectile function suitable for intercourse ranged between 0% and 20%. Thirteen studies were included, reporting open, laparoscopic, and robotic approaches.

However, the preoperative erectile dysfunction was high in some studies, with erection suitable for intercourse documented as between 9% and 90% (and between 9% and 50% if two small cohorts were excluded). Eighty percent of patients were recommended to use oral medication or other intervention for erectile dysfunction. However, oncological outcomes must be considered: 21 studies were included in the systematic review, with biochemical recurrence-free rates at 5 years ranging from 47% to 82% and 28% to 53% at 10 years, and overall survival ranging from 54% to 89% at 10 years. In some centers, the insertion of penile prostheses in these men aims to overcome the high proportion of men with erectile dysfunction after salvage treatment.

Penile rehabilitation after radical prostatectomy

Despite the use of nerve-sparing techniques, erectile and sexual dysfunction continues to be a potential side effect of radical prostatectomy, and importance is placed upon early rehabilitation after the procedure, in order to maintain long-term erectile and sexual function. The British Society for Sexual Medicine Guidelines recommend the use of both PDE5Is and a vacuum erection device for management of ED after radical prostatectomy.

The concept of penile rehabilitation was first proposed by Montorsi et al.,[36] who randomized 30 patients after nerve-sparing prostatectomy to either treatment with intracavernous alprostadil injection three times a week for 12 weeks, or no treatment. The treated group showed improvement in erections satisfactory for intercourse, nocturnal erections, and penile hemodynamics. Despite the small patient numbers, this suggested the potential importance of penile rehabilitation after prostatectomy. In animal models, PDE5Is have been shown to reduce structural changes in penile tissue after cavernous resection, through preservation of smooth muscle and inhibition of corporal fibrosis,[37] and to reduce apoptosis of penile smooth muscle and endothelial cells.[38] PDE5Is were also protective against veno-occlusive impairment after bilateral nerve resection.[18] In humans, several placebo-controlled, randomized trials have compared PDE5Is for penile rehabilitation. Padma-Nathan et al. randomized men to daily sildenafil or placebo from 4 weeks after prostatectomy.[39] This study was stopped early, due to a lack of treatment effect; however, spontaneous erectile activity occurred in 27% of the treated group, compared to only 4% of the placebo group, and nightly treatment improved nocturnal erections compared to placebo. Another study showed that, in men who were potent prior to bilateral nerve-sparing prostatectomy, vardenafil had good effect when used on demand, compared to a nightly dose and placebo.[40]

Negative pressure from a vacuum erection device (VED) draws blood into the corpora. This improves oxygenation, and, if the constriction band is not used, tissue hypoxia is prevented. Both increased IIEF scores and a marked increase in spontaneous erections have been demonstrated when used early after surgery.[34] Use of a VED has also been shown to reduce the loss of penile length that may be associated with radical prostatectomy – 5 out of 11 patients not using a VED during rehabilitation show a loss of penile length of approximately 2 cm.[41] A small group of 13 patients reported by Engel showed that men with erectile dysfunction after bilateral nerve-sparing radical prostatectomy had a more complete and quicker return of sexual function when treated with the PDE5I tadalafil and a VED (used daily for at least 5 days each week), compared to tadalafil alone.[42]

Radiotherapy and brachytherapy

Radiotherapy for prostate cancer may be associated with urinary, bowel, and sexual function side effects. Some of these effects may be due to vascular damage to the cavernosal smooth muscle nerves. Small vessel damage due to accelerated atherosclerosis has also been proposed as a potential mechanism, and other structures, such as the internal pudendal arteries, penile bulb, and crura may receive radiation during treatment. As with radical prostatectomy, patient characteristics have a large influence on post-treatment sexual outcomes. Increased patient age, use of androgen-deprivation therapy (ADT), baseline erectile function, and comorbidities, such as diabetes mellitus, are associated with reduced erectile function after treatment.[43] Potential morbidities have been reduced with more precise planning and other technical advances, such a real-time tracking, intensity-modulated radiation therapy (IMRT), and volume-modulated therapy.

The Prostate Cancer Outcomes Study (PCOS) included 3533 patients with prostate cancer diagnosed between 1 October 1994 and 31 October 1995. A cohort of 1655 of these men (aged between 55 and 74 years) underwent either surgery ($n=1164$) or radiotherapy ($n=491$).[44] Multivariate analysis demonstrated that patients who underwent prostatectomy were more likely to experience erectile dysfunction at both 2 and 5 years postoperatively, but there was no significant difference between the two groups after 15 years. However, the prevalence of erectile dysfunction in all men at 15 years was very high – 87.0% of those who underwent prostatectomy, and 93.9% of the radiotherapy group. This demonstrates the decline in sexual and urinary function over time, representative of that which also occurs in the general male population. This study represents the longer-term follow-up, which is required in studies of prostate cancer, where survival may be many years; but the small sample size at 15 years follow-up may have produced a sample-size bias, and therefore further work with long-term follow-up of larger cohorts is required.

The reported incidence of sexual dysfunction after prostate brachytherapy (both alone and in combination with other treatment modalities) ranges widely. This may be due to differences in patient population demographics (in particular patient age), differences in technique, use of additional therapies, and differing definitions of erectile and sexual dysfunction. Stone and Stock[45] reported a cohort of 325 men (mean age 67 years) with localized prostate cancer who underwent treatment with ^{125}I brachytherapy between 1990 and 2000. Median follow-up was 7 years, and 271 were evaluated at 5 years. On assessment using the Mount Sinai Erectile Sexual Function Score (MSEFS), 94.5% of men were potent prior to treatment. At 5 years follow-up, 61.5% of men who were potent prior to treatment reported the ability to maintain erections suitable for intercourse, with or without the use of PDE5Is. Buckstein et al.[46] reported on a cohort of 131 men aged less than 60 years with more than 10 years of follow-up after treatment with brachytherapy, or brachytherapy with external beam radiotherapy. Of men who were potent prior to treatment, 69% remained potent at 10 years, with or without PDE5I use, and the authors commented that those men who were not potent may reflect the 30% increased prevalence of ED in men that occurs between 60 and 70 years of age.

Pahlajani et al. reported a series of 69 men treated with ^{125}I seed implantation brachytherapy between 2002 and 2005, who had been followed up for at least 1 year with 6- and 12-month IIEF and Sexual Health Inventory for Men (SHIM) questionnaires.[47] They compared those who had chosen to take PDE5Is early (daily sildenafil, starting immediately after seed implantation, with additional doses prior to sexual activity) with those who did not use PDE5Is. In the group that did not take PDE5Is, the IIEF score dropped from 21.3 prior to treatment to 11.5 at 6 months, and to 11.2 after 12 months. This is in contrast to the PDE5I group, whose average IIEF score prior to treatment was 26.0, and then was 21.7 at 6 months, and 21.8 at 12 months. This study is limited by the non-randomized nature of the groups, and may reflect differential patient motivation and a reduced importance of remaining potent for patients in the non-PDE5I group. It does, however, demonstrate the positive effect of administering PDE5Is to patients who wish to remain potent after brachytherapy treatment.

Matsushima et al.[48] prospectively analysed change in erectile function using the IIEF questionnaire in a cohort of 119 men treated with brachytherapy (^{125}I seeds, without additional treatment with external beam radiotherapy, PDE5I, or anti-androgen therapy) between 2004 and 2010, with at least 12 months follow-up. There was a decrease in all IIEF domains at 12 months after treatment, with a gradual onset of dysfunction over time. In the group of 48 patients who were potent prior to treatment, 16 men (33.3%) were potent at 12 months after treatment; patient age (less or greater than 70 years) was the only independent predictor of erectile dysfunction after treatment. This study is more unusual in that it represents a group of patients in whom erectile function was assessed without the use of PDE5Is. However, given the widespread use of these agents, and in particular their suggested role in penile rehabilitation after treatment for prostate cancer, it may be less applicable to routine clinical practice. As with radical prostatectomy, PDE5Is have a role in the treatment and prevention of erectile dysfunction after prostate radiotherapy. Schiff et al. showed that early use after brachytherapy was associated with improved long-term erectile function.[49] They described 210 men treated with brachytherapy, of whom 85 commenced treatment with PDE5Is within a year of treatment and 125 at least a year after treatment. Those treated earlier after treatment had significantly better erectile function (both improvement and maintenance of function), compared to those treated later.

Aside from the incidence of sexual and erectile dysfunction, the impact of these difficulties is also important for patients' well-being. Cameron et al. showed that 1 month after treatment with either external beam radiation or combination treatment with brachytherapy, high-dose radiation, and external beam radiation, although sexual function was impaired, there was no change in the "bother"reported by patients.[50] This is in agreement with another study of health-related quality of life in the first year after low-dose prostate brachytherapy, which, despite a significant decrease in reported sexual function, showed no associated reduction in sexual bother score during the year.[51] It may be that patients become more concerned about their sexual function in the longer-term, once anxiety around a cancer diagnosis and treatment has receded, and longer follow-up would be required to demonstrate this.

The SPIRIT trial attempted to recruit men with favorable-risk prostate cancer to be randomized to either radical prostatectomy or brachytherapy, but closed early due to poor recruitment. Crook et al. reported HRQOL outcomes from this group, in those randomly allocated and those who subsequently chose their treatment:[52] achieving erection, erection quality and frequency, presence of morning erection, and ability for sexual function were all significantly better in men who were treated with brachytherapy. However, this group may also represent the differences conveyed by the surgeon or technician undertaking the procedure – men who underwent brachytherapy were all treated by a highly experienced technician, while those who underwent radical prostatectomy mostly returned to their local urologists, reducing the ability to compare the outcomes from the procedures. Van Tol-Geerdink et al. prospectively analysed quality of life in men with localized prostate cancer eligible for radical prostatectomy and radiotherapy (external beam or brachytherapy).[53] The radical prostatectomy group showed worse scores in the sexual domain, and were more likely to report a clinically relevant reduction from baseline than external beam radiotherapy and brachytherapy. They concluded that radiotherapy is at least as good as prostatectomy for quality of life outcomes in the treatment of localized prostate cancer.

Androgen deprivation therapy (ADT)

Androgen deprivation therapy may be used as a primary treatment, in combination with other modalities as adjuvant or neoadjuvant therapy, or as a palliative treatment for advanced disease, and the earlier diagnosis of prostate cancer has resulted in men being treated with ADT for increasing lengths of time. In addition to erectile dysfunction, men commonly report reduced libido, delayed orgasm, or inability to achieve orgasm, and these may all contribute to a feeling of reduced masculinity, in part caused by the reduction of testosterone to less than 5% of normal baseline levels. Some men who experience a reduced libido state that they want to be able to achieve erection solely for the benefit of their partner.[54] In a group of hypogonadal men, the use of testosterone replacement therapy to support morning erection significantly improved self-confidence.[55] This reflects the negative effect that erectile dysfunction may have upon quality of life, without even considering the additional effect that cancer treatment and survivorship may have. Moderate or high levels of anxiety and depression in men with localized prostate cancer are associated with both impaired sexual function and increased sexual bother.[56]

The ADT Survivorship Working Group was founded to identify and classify the problems associated with ADT in men with prostate cancer, and the implications for their partners. They identified seven domains – sexual changes, body feminization, relationship changes, cognitive and affective symptoms, fatigue, sleep disturbance, and depression.[57] They recognized the additional element of reduced libido associated with ADT, and reinforce the importance of appropriate pre-treatment counseling for both patients and their partners. They also acknowledge the significant negative impact that this may have upon quality of life, and propose strategies such as minimization of potential side effects with different treatment approaches (such as transdermal patches and gels) and individualized interventions for medical and psychological consequences of treatment. This may include sex therapy techniques such as mindfulness and cognitive awareness. PDE5Is may be less effective for these patients, and therefore psychosexual techniques may be more relevant to their functional recovery.[57] The effect of ADT upon relationships was examined by Walker and Robinson, who interviewed 18 heterosexual couples about the changes in their relationships that had occurred after ADT treatment.[58] All of the couples reported changes in their sexual relationships, including adjusting to changes in the sexual relationship, changes in their sexual dynamic, and changes in attitudes and perceptions about sexuality and their sexual relationship.

The use of ADT in conjunction with other treatment modalities can have a further detrimental effect upon sexual function. Mazzola et al.[59] reported that erectile function was more negatively affected in a cohort of 34 men who received neoadjuvant ADT prior to radical prostatectomy, compared to a matched control group of 94 men who did not receive ADT (with a significantly lower number of men with IIEF EF domain scores ≥24 after 18 months in the group treated with ADT).

In order to control and reduce the bothersome potential side effects of ADT, patients may be treated intermittently (intermittent androgen deprivation, IAD), with treatment and break length guided by PSA and testosterone levels. Phase 3 studies have demonstrated that this improves tolerability of treatment, without compromising therapeutic effectiveness, as reflected by cancer progression and survival.[60] It is hypothesized that IAD may delay the progression to castrate-resistant disease. However, investigation is still required to ascertain what PSA value should dictate restarting treatment, and for which patients this strategy is appropriate. A systematic review including over 2000 patients in phase 2 and 3 clinical trials reported that IAD was as effective as continuous androgen deprivation, with the additional advantages of improved tolerability and quality of life.[61] This approach is now included in the European Association of Urology Guidelines on Prostate Cancer, advising that, in appropriate patient groups, IAD is not oncologically inferior to continuous treatment.[62]

Active surveillance

Uptake of active surveillance as a therapeutic strategy for prostate cancer is increasing, and this choice impacts sexual function in several ways, in addition to age-related functional decline. The psychological impact of having an untreated cancer may have significant effects upon both patients and their partners. It has been hypothesized that erectile dysfunction may be associated with repeated prostate biopsy during active surveillance protocols, as a result of damage to the neurovascular bundles. This risk may continue to increase as the number of needle passes into the prostate increases – the advantage of imaging providing a more accurate representation of the whole prostate may therefore be associated with increased potential side effects. Fujita et al. described their cohort of men on active surveillance (mean age 68.7 years; range 51–83 years).[63] Men completed the 5-Item Sexual Health Inventory for Men upon entry to the active surveillance protocol, and at a single date point thereafter. All had a 10–12 core biopsy at entry, and were recommended to have yearly biopsies. They found a correlation between increasing biopsy number and erectile dysfunction, in particular those who had had three or more biopsies, compared with two or fewer. However, this is in contrast to results from Hilton et al.,[64] who found no significant association between increasing number of prostate biopsies and erectile dysfunction, once adjusted for age, sexual activity status, clinical disease stage, and time since diagnosis. A systematic review of complications of prostate biopsy concluded that any negative effect of prostate biopsy upon sexual function is likely to be transient. It may be due to a combination of local damage and temporary inflammation, in combination with anxiety about the procedure.[65]

Van den Bergh et al. compared sexual function in men on active surveillance with those treated with radical prostatectomy or radical radiotherapy.[66] They showed that more men in the active surveillance group were sexually active (65–68% vs 36–37% after radiotherapy and 36% after either radiotherapy or radical prostatectomy), and more men in the treatment groups were not sexually active as a result of erectile dysfunction, rather than other reasons. This study is limited by the numbers who dropped out of active surveillance to proceed with interventional treatments, and by the non-randomized nature of the groups. Data from the population-based Eindhoven Cancer Registry were used to match 71 men diagnosed between 1994 and 1998 who would have been suitable for active surveillance (and who had been managed expectantly) with 71 demographically and clinically matched men treated with radiotherapy.[67] Health-related quality of life data were collected at 5 and 10 years after diagnosis. Patients who underwent radiotherapy had reduced erectile function compared to those managed expectantly (68% of the radiotherapy group reported difficulty achieving erection, compared to 47% of those managed expectantly).

Ablative therapy

Ablative therapy is a minimally invasive alternative to surgery or radiotherapy for men with localized prostate cancer. Ablative therapy can be delivered in a whole gland or focal manner. Focal therapy provides an alternative strategy to avoid the longer-term morbidity of whole gland treatments, by targeting the index lesion and therefore altering the natural history of disease.

High-intensity focused ultrasound (HIFU)

Whole-gland HIFU

Berge et al. reported results from a registry of 259 patients treated with whole-gland HIFU for localized prostate cancer between October 2004 and June 2012.[68] They found no significant difference in erectile function sufficient for intercourse before and after primary whole-gland HIFU treatment (although there was a significant increased use of PDE5Is), and also reported no significant deterioration in sexual function after a repeat (redo) HIFU procedure (with no associated significant difference in PDE5I use). Multivariate analysis revealed that patient age and redo-HIFU were associated with a decline in erectile function at last follow-up. However, reporting of sexual function data was not complete (in particular relating to baseline function), and therefore this may have introduced bias. Poissonnier et al.[69] reported that 61% of men maintained erectile function after whole-gland HIFU treatment, increasing to 69% in those who underwent treatment aiming to spare the neurovascular bundles.

Focal HIFU

The team at University College London have rigorously evaluated the functional and oncological outcomes of HIFU in prospective, IRB approved studies. The first of these assessed the use of hemi-ablation (right or left lobe) for men with unilateral cancer.[70] Fifteen of 20 men had intermediate-risk disease, and all had good erectile function preoperatively (IIEF >20). After an initial reduction in erectile function (IIEF-15 reduced from >20 to 10 at 1 month), this recovered well at 3 months (men >20) with further improvement by 6 months. At 6 months, 19 of 20 men had erections sufficient for intercourse, with one in three of these men requiring the use of a PDE5 inhibitor to achieve this.

The next formal published study from this group used an index lesion approach, where indolent disease was left untreated, and treatment could be directed to less than half the gland.[71] This group included 42 men with a range of erectile function prior to treatment. Again, a reduction in potency at 1 month was noted, with recovery of erections sufficient for penetration in 80% by 3 months.

The next study in this series will be a multicenter UK evaluation of the index lesion approach.[72] This includes rigorous pre- and post-treatment evaluation of sexual function and will show whether the favorable results seen in a highly experienced center can be replicated in newer centers.

Cryotherapy

Whole-gland cryotherapy

Despite first being used in the 1960s, cryotherapy did not become a mainstream treatment strategy, in part due to severe side effects. Technical improvements have reduced potential morbidities and it is now under investigation as a focal treatment for localized prostate cancer. Asterling and Greene described 53 patients treated with an argon-based third-generation cryotherapy system.[73] They prospectively collected data at 6 weeks, then every 3 months up to 12 months, and then every 6 months, with mean follow-up of 36 months. At 6 weeks after treatment, 96.3% had ED, with two patients (3.7%) having partial erections. Only one was potent (with PDE5Is) at 9 months, and six were able to achieve partial erections. At 24 months 24% (eight men) were potent and 9% (three men) had partial erections. Of men who were potent prior to treatment, 39% regained their potency by 24 months.

Li et al. compared erectile function (in men who were potent prior to treatment, with IIEF score ≥26) and penis size in patients who had undergone either HIFU or targeted prostate cryoablation.[74] They found that those treated with cryotherapy had a significantly impaired erectile function compared to those who were treated with HIFU, with no change in penile size in either of the groups. All patients were encouraged to use both a vacuum erection device and PDE5I for rehabilitation after treatment. This study did not report full oncological outcomes, but did report no significant difference in mean PSA between the groups at each time point after the procedure (both groups showed a slowly increasing PSA).

Focal cryotherapy

A number of authors have reported hemi-ablation studies using cryotherapy.[75–77] Postoperative potency in these studies was reported between 70% and 85%, although routine reporting of medication or devices to support erections was not done. The COLD registry reported on over 1000 men treated with focal cryotherapy and analysed in a registry. In this larger, community-based group, 58% of men had spontaneous erections postoperatively.[78] This compares very favorably to men treated with whole gland cryoablation.

Conclusion

Long-term oncological and functional data for all outcomes following all modalities of prostate cancer treatment is required so that patients may be accurately counseled prior to making the important decision on which treatment to undertake. A lack of evidence for the effects of different treatment modalities in comparable groups has made pre-treatment counseling more difficult, in part due to different patient demographics in each treatment modality group. Our ability to accurately counsel patients about both the likelihood of cure, and the chance of treatment-related morbidity will allow them to make informed choices about their treatment.

References

1 Jemal A, Siegel R, Xu J, Ward E. Cancer statistics, 2010. *CA Cancer J Clin* 2010;60(5):277–300.

2 Salonia A, Zanni G, Gallina A, et al. Baseline potency in candidates for bilateral nerve-sparing radical retropubic prostatectomy. *Eur Urol* 2006;50(2):360–5.

3 Resnick MJ, Guzzo TJ, Cowan JE, Knight SJ, Carroll PR, Penson DF. Factors associated with satisfaction with prostate cancer care: Results from Cancer of the Prostate Strategic Urologic Research Endeavor (CAPSURE). *BJU Int* 2013;111 (2):213–20.

4 Baker F, Denniston M, Smith T, West MM. Adult cancer survivors: How are they faring? *Cancer* 2005;104 (11 Suppl.): 2565–76.

5 Rosen RC, Catania J, Pollack L, Althof S, O'Leary M, Seftel AD. Male sexual health questionnaire (MSHQ): Scale development and psychometric validation. *Urology* 2004;64(4):777–82.

6 Saitz TR, Serefoglu EC, Trost LW, Thomas R, Hellstrom WJ. The pre-treatment prevalence and types of sexual dysfunction among patients diagnosed with prostate cancer. *Andrology* 2013;1(6):859–63.

7 Johansson E, Steineck G, Holmberg L, et al. Long-term quality-of-life outcomes after radical prostatectomy or watchful waiting: The Scandinavian Prostate Cancer Group-4 randomised trial. *Lancet Oncol* 2011;12(9):891–9.

8 Alemozaffar M, Regan MM, Cooperberg MR, et al. Prediction of erectile function following treatment for prostate cancer. *JAMA* 2011;306(11):1205–14.

9 Dubbelman YD, Dohle GR, Schröder FH. Sexual function before and after radical retropubic prostatectomy: A systematic review of prognostic indicators for a successful outcome. *Eur Urol* 2006;50(4):711–8; discussion 718–20.

10 Steinsvik EA, Axcrona K, Dahl AA, Eri LM, Stensvold A, Fosså SD. Can sexual bother after radical prostatectomy be predicted preoperatively? Findings from a prospective national study of the relation between sexual function, activity and bother. *BJU Int* 2012;109(9):1366–74.

11 Kimura M, Bañez LL, Polascik TJ, et al. Sexual bother and function after radical prostatectomy: Predictors of sexual bother recovery in men despite persistent post-operative sexual dysfunction. *Andrology* 2013;1(2):256–61.

12 Walsh PC, Donker PJ. Impotence following radical prostatectomy: Insight into etiology and prevention. *J Urol* 1982;128(3):492–7.

13 Walsh PC, Mostwin JL. Radical prostatectomy and cystoprostatectomy with preservation of potency. Results using a new nerve-sparing technique. *Br J Urol* 1984;56(6):694–7.

14 Walsh PC, Lepor H, Eggleston JC. Radical prostatectomy with preservation of sexual function: Anatomical and pathological considerations. *Prostate* 1983;4(5):473–85.

15 Costello AJ, Brooks M, Cole OJ. Anatomical studies of the neurovascular bundle and cavernosal nerves. *BJU Int* 2004;94(7):1071–6.

16 Eichelberg C, Erbersdobler A, Michl U, et al. Nerve distribution along the prostatic capsule. *Eur Urol* 2007;51(1):105–10; discussion 110–1.

17 Nielsen ME, Schaeffer EM, Marschke P, Walsh PC. High anterior release of the levator fascia improves sexual function following open radical retropubic prostatectomy. *J Urol* 2008;180(6):2557–64; discussion 2564.

18 Fode M, Ohl DA, Ralph D, Sønksen J. Penile rehabilitation after radical prostatectomy: What the evidence really says. *BJU Int* 2013;112(7):998–1008.

19 Moreland RB. Is there a role of hypoxemia in penile fibrosis: A viewpoint presented to the society for the study of impotence. *Int J Impot Res* 1998;10(2):113–20.

20 Stember DS, Nelson CJ, Mulhall JP. Preoperative erectile function is an independent predictor for decision to spare cavernous nerves during radical prostatectomy. *J Sex Med* 2013;10(8):2101–7.

21 Boorjian SA, Eastham JA, Graefen M, et al. A critical analysis of the long-term impact of radical prostatectomy on cancer control and function outcomes. *Eur Urol* 2012;61(4):664–75.

22 Briganti A, Capitanio U, Chun FK, et al. Prediction of sexual function after radical prostatectomy. *Cancer* 2009;115 (13 Suppl.):3150–9.

23 Rabbani F, Stapleton AM, Kattan MW, Wheeler TM, Scardino PT. Factors predicting recovery of erections after radical prostatectomy. *J Urol* 2000;164(6):1929–34.

24 Kundu SD, Roehl KA, Eggener SE, Antenor JA, Han M, Catalona WJ. Potency, continence and complications in 3,477 consecutive radical retropubic prostatectomies. *J Urol* 2004;172(6 Pt 1):2227–31.

25 Walsh PC, Marschke P, Ricker D, Burnett AL. Patient-reported urinary continence and sexual function after anatomic radical prostatectomy. *Urology* 2000;55(1):58–61.

26 Hartz A, He T, Strope S, Cutler DR, Andriole G, Dechet C. Surgeon variation in patient quality of life after radical prostatectomy. *J Urol* 2013;189(4):1295–301.

27 Cathala N, Mombet A, Sanchez-Salas R, et al. Evaluation of erectile function after laparoscopic radical prostatectomy in a single center. *Can J Urol* 2012;19(4):6328–35.

28 Sivarajan G, Prabhu V, Taksler GB, Laze J, Lepor H. Ten-year outcomes of sexual function after radical prostatectomy: Results of a prospective longitudinal study. *Eur Urol* 2014;65 (1):58–65.

29 Tal R, Rabbani F, Scardino PT, Mulhall JP. Measuring erectile function after radical prostatectomy: Comparing a single question with the International Index of Erectile Function. *BJU Int* 2012;109(3):414–7.

30 Frey AU, Sønksen J, Fode M. Neglected side effects after radical prostatectomy: A systematic review. *J Sex Med* 2014;11(2):374–85.

31 Dubbelman Y, Wildhagen M, Schröder F, Bangma C, Dohle G. Orgasmic dysfunction after open radical prostatectomy: Clinical correlates and prognostic factors. *J Sex Med* 2010;7(3):1216–23.

32 Briganti A, Fabbri F, Salonia A, et al. Preserved postoperative penile size correlates well with maintained erectile function after bilateral nerve-sparing radical retropubic prostatectomy. *Eur Urol* 2007;52(3):702–7.

33 Dalkin BL, Christopher BA. Preservation of penile length after radical prostatectomy: Early intervention with a vacuum erection device. *Int J Impot Res* 2007;19(5):501–4.

34 Köhler TS, Pedro R, Hendlin K, et al. A pilot study on the early use of the vacuum erection device after radical retropubic prostatectomy. *BJU Int* 2007;100(4):858–62.

35 Chade DC, Eastham J, Graefen M, et al. Cancer control and functional outcomes of salvage radical prostatectomy for radiation-recurrent prostate cancer: A systematic review of the literature. *Eur Urol* 2012;61(5):961–71.

36 Montorsi F, Guazzoni G, Strambi LF, et al. Recovery of spontaneous erectile function after nerve-sparing radical retropubic prostatectomy with and without early intracavernous injections of alprostadil: Results of a prospective, randomized trial. *J Urol* 1997;158(4):1408–10.

37 Ferrini MG, Davila HH, Kovanecz I, Sanchez SP, Gonzalez-Cadavid NF, Rajfer J. Vardenafil prevents fibrosis and loss of corporal smooth muscle that occurs after bilateral cavernosal nerve resection in the rat. *Urology* 2006;68 (2):429–35.

38 Lysiak JJ, Yang SK, Klausner AP, Son H, Tuttle JB, Steers WD. Tadalafil increases akt and extracellular signal-regulated kinase 1/2 activation, and prevents apoptotic cell death in the penis following denervation. *J Urol* 2008;179 (2):779–85.

39 Padma-Nathan H, McCullough AR, Levine LA, et al. Randomized, double-blind, placebo-controlled study of postoperative nightly sildenafil citrate for the prevention of erectile dysfunction after bilateral nerve-sparing radical prostatectomy. *Int J Impot Res* 2008;20(5):479–86.

40 Montorsi F, Brock G, Lee J, et al. Effect of nightly versus on-demand vardenafil on recovery of erectile function in men following bilateral nerve-sparing radical prostatectomy. *Eur Urol* 2008;54(4):924–31.

41 Lehrfeld T, Lee DI. The role of vacuum erection devices in penile rehabilitation after radical prostatectomy. *Int J Impot Res* 2009;21(3):158–64.

42 Engel JD. Effect on sexual function of a vacuum erection device post-prostatectomy. *Can J Urol* 2011;18(3):5721–5.

43 Budäus L, Bolla M, Bossi A, et al. Functional outcomes and complications following radiation therapy for prostate cancer: A critical analysis of the literature. *Eur Urol* 2012; 61(1):112–27.

44 Resnick MJ, Koyama T, Fan KH, et al. Long-term functional outcomes after treatment for localized prostate cancer. *N Engl J Med* 2013;368(5):436–45.

45 Stone NN, Stock RG. Long-term urinary, sexual, and rectal morbidity in patients treated with iodine-125 prostate brachytherapy followed up for a minimum of 5 years. *Urology* 2007;69(2):338–42.

46 Buckstein M, Carpenter TJ, Stone NN, Stock RG. Long-term outcomes and toxicity in patients treated with brachytherapy for prostate adenocarcinoma younger than 60 years of age at treatment with minimum 10 years of follow-up. *Urology* 2013;81(2):364–8.

47 Pahlajani G, Raina R, Jones JS, et al. Early intervention with phosphodiesterase-5 inhibitors after prostate brachytherapy improves subsequent erectile function. *BJU Int* 2010; 106(10):1524–7.

48 Matsushima M, Kikuchi E, Maeda T, et al. A prospective longitudinal survey of erectile dysfunction in patients with localized prostate cancer treated with permanent prostate brachytherapy. *J Urol* 2013;189(3):1014–8.

49 Schiff JD, Bar-Chama N, Cesaretti J, Stock R. Early use of a phosphodiesterase inhibitor after brachytherapy restores and preserves erectile function. *BJU Int* 2006;98(6): 1255–8.

50 Cameron S, Springer C, Fox-Wasylyshyn S, El-Masri MM. A descriptive study of functions, symptoms, and perceived health state after radiotherapy for prostate cancer. *Eur J Oncol Nurs* 2012;16(3):310–4.

51 Tanaka N, Fujimoto K, Asakawa I, et al. Variations in health-related quality of life in Japanese men who underwent iodine-125 permanent brachytherapy for localized prostate cancer. *Brachytherapy* 2010;9(4):300–6.

52 Crook JM, Gomez-Iturriaga A, Wallace K, et al. Comparison of health-related quality of life 5 years after SPIRIT: Surgical prostatectomy versus interstitial radiation intervention trial. *J Clin Oncol* 2011;29(4):362–8.

53 van Tol-Geerdink JJ, Leer JW, van Oort IM, et al. Quality of life after prostate cancer treatments in patients comparable at baseline. *Br J Cancer* 2013;108(9):1784–9.

54 Fisher WA, Eardley I, McCabe M, Sand M. Erectile dysfunction (ED) is a shared sexual concern of couples II: Association of female partner characteristics with male partner ED treatment seeking and phosphodiesterase type 5 inhibitor utilization. *J Sex Med* 2009;6(11):3111–24.

55 Jockenhövel F, Minnemann T, Schubert M, et al. Timetable of effects of testosterone administration to hypogonadal men on variables of sex and mood. *Aging Male* 2009;12 (4):113–8.

56 Punnen S, Cowan JE, Dunn LB, Shumay DM, Carroll PR, Cooperberg MR. A longitudinal study of anxiety, depression and distress as predictors of sexual and urinary quality of life in men with prostate cancer. *BJU Int* 2013;112(2):E67–75.

57 Elliott S, Latini DM, Walker LM, Wassersug R, Robinson JW, ADT Survivorship Working Group. Androgen deprivation therapy for prostate cancer: Recommendations to improve patient and partner quality of life. *J Sex Med* 2010;7(9): 2996–3010.

58 Walker LM, Robinson JW. Sexual adjustment to androgen deprivation therapy: Struggles and strategies. *Qual Health Res* 2012;22(4):452–65.

59 Mazzola CR, Deveci S, Heck M, Mulhall JP. Androgen deprivation therapy before radical prostatectomy is associated with poorer postoperative erectile function outcomes. *BJU Int* 2012;110(1):112–6.

60 Schulman C, Irani J, Aapro M. Improving the management of patients with prostate cancer receiving long-term androgen deprivation therapy. *BJU Int* 2012;109 (Suppl. 6):13–21.

61 Abrahamsson PA. Potential benefits of intermittent androgen suppression therapy in the treatment of prostate cancer: A systematic review of the literature. *Eur Urol* 2010;57(1):49–59.

62 Heidenreich A, Bastian PJ, Bellmunt J, et al. EAU guidelines on prostate cancer. Part II: Treatment of advanced, relapsing, and castration-resistant prostate cancer. *Eur Urol* 2014;65 (2):467–79.

63 Fujita K, Landis P, McNeil BK, Pavlovich CP. Serial prostate biopsies are associated with an increased risk of erectile dysfunction in men with prostate cancer on active surveillance. *J Urol* 2009;182(6):2664–9.

64 Hilton JF, Blaschko SD, Whitson JM, Cowan JE, Carroll PR. The impact of serial prostate biopsies on sexual function in men on active surveillance for prostate cancer. *J Urol* 2012;188(4):1252–8.

65 Loeb S, Vellekoop A, Ahmed HU, et al. Systematic review of complications of prostate biopsy. *Eur Urol* 2013;64(6) 876–92.

66 van den Bergh RC, Korfage IJ, Roobol MJ, et al. Sexual function with localized prostate cancer: Active surveillance vs radical therapy. *BJU Int* 2012;110(7):1032–9.

67 Thong MS, Mols F, Kil PJ, Korfage IJ, van de Poll-Franse LV. Prostate cancer survivors who would be eligible for active surveillance but were either treated with radiotherapy or managed expectantly: Comparisons on long-term quality of life and symptom burden. *BJU Int* 2010;105(5):652–8.

68 Berge V, Dickinson L, McCartan N, et al. Morbidity associated with primary HIFU and redo-HIFU for the treatment of localized prostate cancer. *J Urol* 2014;191(6):1764–9.

69 Poissonnier L, Chapelon JY, Rouvière O, et al. Control of prostate cancer by transrectal HIFU in 227 patients. *Eur Urol* 2007;51(2):381–7.

70 Ahmed HU, Freeman A, Kirkham A, et al. Focal therapy for localized prostate cancer: A phase I/II trial. *J Urol* 2011;185 (4):1246–54.

71 Ahmed HU, Hindley RG, Dickinson L, et al. Focal therapy for localised unifocal and multifocal prostate cancer: A prospective development study. *Lancet Oncol* 2012;13(6): 622–32.

72 Dickinson L, Ahmed HU, Kirkham AP, et al. A multi-centre prospective development study evaluating focal therapy using high intensity focused ultrasound for localised prostate cancer: The INDEX study. *Contemp Clin Trials* 2013;36(1):68–80.

73 Asterling S, Greene DR. Prospective evaluation of sexual function in patients receiving cryosurgery as a primary radical treatment for localized prostate cancer. *BJU Int* 2009;103(6):788–92.

74 Li LY, Lin Z, Yang M, Gao X, Xia TL, Ding T. Comparison of penile size and erectile function after high-intensity focused ultrasound and targeted cryoablation for localized prostate cancer: A prospective pilot study. *J Sex Med* 2010;7(9): 3135–42.

75 Onik G, Vaughan D, Lotenfoe R, Dineen M, Brady J. The "male lumpectomy": Focal therapy for prostate cancer using cryoablation results in 48 patients with at least 2-year follow-up. *Urol Oncol* 2008;26(5):500–5.

76 Lambert EH, Bolte K, Masson P, Katz AE. Focal cryosurgery: Encouraging health outcomes for unifocal prostate cancer. *Urology* 2007;69(6):1117–20.

77 Bahn D, de Castro Abreu AL, Gill IS, et al. Focal cryotherapy for clinically unilateral, low-intermediate risk prostate cancer in 73 men with a median follow-up of 3.7 years. *Eur Urol* 2012;62(1):55–63.

78 Ward JF, Jones JS. Focal cryotherapy for localized prostate cancer: A report from the National Cryo On-line Database (COLD) registry. *BJU Int* 2012;109(11):1648–54.

CHAPTER 33

Assessment and management of the male to female transgender patient

Tina G. Rashid[1], Phillip Thomas[2,3], and James Bellringer[3]

[1] Charing Cross Hospital, London, UK

[2] Brighton and Sussex University Hospitals NHS Trust, Brighton, UK

[3] Parkside Hospital, London, UK

Background

Terminology

Whether gender identity issues have their basis in a psychiatric disorder, an intersex disorder, or a "disorder" at all is greatly debated and generates huge public and political fascination. In 2013, in a bid to abandon a psychopathological model and diminish stigma, the term "gender identity disorder" was replaced with "gender dysphoria" in the 5th edition of the *Diagnostic and Statistical Manual of Mental Disorders* (DSM-5).[1]

For an individual to be diagnosed with gender dysphoria (GD), there must be a marked difference between that individual's expressed or experienced gender and the gender others would assign him or her. This must be present for at least 6 months. Transsexual people or trans people have strong and long-lasting feelings of gender dysphoria. This is different to "transvestitism," which refers to those where intense relief (often sexual), is obtained by dressing in clothes of the opposite gender. Transvestites do not wish to undergo gender reassignment, and indeed are predominantly heterosexual males with stable gender and sexual identity.

GD remains a unique diagnosis that is reached by mental health professionals but for which treatment often involves endocrinologists, surgeons, and other professionals. Medical intervention can significantly improve the quality of life of an individual with GD, at very little relative cost.

Incidence

The prevalence of GD is difficult to estimate at best. Studies relating to GD epidemiology use indirect measures of prevalence, usually the number of people who attend specialty hospital and university-based clinics serving as gateways for surgical and hormonal gender reassignment. Inclusion criteria in studies vary, and may include those who have been granted legal name change or gender status; those receiving hormones; those who have had full gender reassignment surgery; or those who have been diagnosed with GD. By counting only those people who present at clinics for a specific type of treatment, an unspecified number of gender dysphoric individuals may be overlooked. In actual fact, it is likely that those who seek formal medical help are only the tip of the iceberg, that is, the ones who are most severely affected.

Most studies report that three times more men than women seek gender reassignment.[2] Estimates for male-to-female (MtF) GD range from 1 in 7400 in Scotland,[3] to 1 in 42,000 in Germany.[4] In the UK, the estimate is 1 in 10,000 for MtF GD, with an estimated doubling in referrals to specialist centers every 5–6 years.[5]

History

GD, as it is now known, was first formally recognized in 1950s by the American psychiatrist Harry Benjamin, who formalized diagnostic criteria in 1966; these have subsequently been refined in 2001, and most recently in

Male Sexual Dysfunction: A Clinical Guide, First Edition. Edited by Suks Minhas and John Mulhall.

2011 (World Professional Association for Transgender Health Society version 7).

In the second half of the 20th century, awareness of the phenomenon of GD increased and health professionals began to provide assistance to alleviate the disorder by supporting changes in primary and secondary sex characteristics through hormone therapy and surgery, along with a change in gender role. The initial clinical approach largely focused on identifying who was an appropriate candidate for gender reassignment to facilitate a physical change from male to female or female to male as completely as possible. As the field matured, health professionals recognized that while many individuals need both hormone therapy and surgery to alleviate their GD, others need only one of these treatment options and some need neither. The World Professional Association for Transgender Health, or WPATH (formerly known as the Harry Benjamin International Gender Dysphoria Association), is a professional organization dedicated to understanding GD. It provides information for professionals and consumers, offers ethical guidelines, and publishes the Standards of Care for the Health of Transsexual, Transgender, and Gender Non-conforming People, with the most recent version being published in 2011.[6]

Nature or nurture?

The exact etiology of GD is a much-pondered area of research. Early theories were based mainly on psychological perspectives, without supportive evidence-based data. These theories focused on the role of nurture (environmental and external psychological factors) as the cause. The earliest psychodynamic literature considered that GD was due to a growing boy's overly close relationship with his mother, compounded by an emotionally absent father.[7]

Others considered that there was an extraordinary surge of female hormones in the fetal brain at a crucial time of development, resulting in a biologically normal male child but with a female identity.[8]

By contrast studies over the past two decades from the Swaab group in Amsterdam advocate a neurological basis for gender identity with sexual morphological differentiation of the brain.[9–11] They proposed that there is a region of the hypothalamus, known as the bed nucleus of the stria terminalis (BSTc), responsible for sexual behavior. This area is always larger in men than in women. The initial study of six MtF GD individuals was corroborated by a further study in 2000 on 42 MtF GD individuals.[10] The group confirmed that a female-sized BSTc was present in the MtF GD subjects. In addition the size of the BSTc was not influenced by taking sex hormones in adulthood, implying that these individuals had a powerful biological force compelling them to be female, rather than just a psychological conviction. In a 2008, a study by the same group demonstrated another sex-differentiated area in the brain, the hypothalamic uncinate nucleus, to have a relationship with gender identity.[12]

Studies showing a higher proportion of left-handed individuals suffering from GD than right handed,[13] dermatoglyphics (fingerprint studies assessing total finger ridge count), and other studies including the use of functional MRI and positron emission tomography (PET), suggest that GD is probably best considered within the realm of intersex, and this is recognized in the most recent DSM classification.

Legislation and guidelines

International treatment guidelines are disseminated by the US-based World Professional Association for Transgender Health[6] (www.wpath.org). It is clear, however, that implementation will vary in different national healthcare and legislative circumstances. In the UK, the Royal College of Psychiatrists guidelines apply.[14]

In 2004, the Gender Recognition Act was passed. It states that transsexuals and people with gender dysphoria can:

- apply to change their birth certificate to reflect their chosen gender;
- marry in their chosen gender after acquiring their new birth certificate.

The UK pathway

Successful management of GD relies on a properly functioning multidisciplinary team. The process in the UK is generally initiated by the patient's general practitioner (GP), who must recognize the condition and refer to a specialist gender identity service. This service will include a psychiatrist, psychologist, endocrinologist, reconstructive surgeons (ear, nose, and throat, plastic, and urological), speech therapist, specialist nurse practitioner, and counselors, all with specific expertise in GD.

Mental health professionals are central to the process, providing support and treatment through each stage. Initial assessment includes a full psychiatric history with emphasis on psychosexual development, orientation, history, and current functioning.[15] Childhood gender-type behaviors and a history of cross-gender dressing are probed. Attempts to conform to cultural gender expectations are explored and the current marital or relationship status is noted. Pre-existing psychological disorder and substance abuse is also recorded. It is important to identify and/or exclude mental illness: at least 1 in 10 GD patients suffer from mental illness, genital mutilation, and attempted suicide.[16] This may be an underestimation: a study of 51 patients requesting gender reassignment surgery demonstrated that 92% of males had psychiatric diagnoses other than GD, usually character disorders, with 8% suffering from schizophrenia.[17]

Finally, the psychiatrist will explain the transition process. Reversible changes are addressed before irreversible ones, and no step should be undertaken unless the preceding steps have been accompanied by psychological and social improvement. Early and prompt treatment seems to be associated with better outcomes.[18]

Social transition (ST)

Once accepted into the gender identity service, patients are expected to function full time in their communities in their chosen gender. They will be expected to demonstrate:

1. Maintaining employment OR functioning as a student OR as a community-based volunteer.
2. Acquiring a new (legal) first or last name.
3. Providing documentation that persons other than the therapist know that the individual functions in the new gender role.

Support from family, friends, and employers is paramount to success in ST and may enable the patient to "pass" comfortably in the chosen role without "being read."

The ST tests resolve the capacity to function in the aspired-to gender, and the alignment of social, economic, and psychological supports. Some begin the ST and decide that this oft-imagined life direction is not in their best interest. However, in those individuals who feel otherwise, once agreed by appropriate professionals in the gender identity clinic, speech therapy, hair removal, and hormonal therapy may commence.

Speech therapy

Speech therapy focuses on raising pitch and modulating resonance to emulate the female voice. Instruction is also offered on establishing verbal and non-verbal cues. This is sometimes combined with surgery to alter the tension of the vocal cords and pitch, and a laryngeal shave to reduce the size of the "Adam's apple."

Hair removal

Formal medical approval is not required for general depilation, and this can be started whenever the patient feels it is prudent. Depilation of the face and body (including the scrotum if a scrotal flap is to be used for the neovagina) is arduous and expensive. Beard density is a genetically determined secondary sex characteristic and is not significantly slowed by cross-sex hormone administration. Most commonly employed options are electrolysis and laser, which are safe but time-consuming, often taking up to 2 years of regular treatments to be effective. Side effects include discomfort during and immediately after the procedure, and, less frequently, hypo- or hyperpigmentation, scarring, and folliculitis.

Options for thinning hair on the head may include wigs, hair extensions, and medical therapy such as finasteride and minoxidil.

Hormones

Hormone therapy for MtF transition is unlicensed, and prior to starting therapy it is imperative that the individual understands the desired and unwanted effects and undertakes to comply with monitoring.

Prior to commencement, general advice is given regarding a sensible diet, weight maintenance within normal limits, reduction of alcohol, smoking cessation, and the importance of regular exercise. Patients should be counseled regarding future fertility, and the opportunity for sperm storage before hormone treatment should be offered. A signed consent from the patient is obtained.

General practitioners, working under the guidance of the gender identity service, may prescribe hormone therapy from the outset and should continue to do so after patients are discharged from the gender identity service.[18]

Endocrinological feminization is achieved by androgen suppression, which can be achieved by:

1. Agents that suppress the production of gonadotropin-releasing hormone (GnRH).
2. Suppression of luteinizing hormone (LH) production.

3 Inhibiting the production of testosterone or its metabolism to dihydrotestosterone (DHT).
4 Blocking the binding of androgens to receptors in target tissues.

Commonly used agents include: cyproterone acetate (androgen receptor blocker); spironolactone (interferes with testosterone production); finasteride (prevents conversion of testosterone to potent metabolite DHT); LH releasing hormone (LHRH) analogs (continuous production of LH from stimulation of the pituitary gland results in testosterone inhibition via negative feedback); and estrogen (direct stimulation of receptors in target tissues).

Feminization effects achieved include: breast growth, some redistribution of body fat to approximate a female body habitus, decreased upper body strength, softening of skin, reduction in body hair, slowing or stopping the loss of scalp hair, decreased fertility and reduction in testicular size, and less frequent, less firm erections. Most of these changes are reversible, although breast enlargement will not completely reverse after discontinuation of treatment. The degree of desired effects actually attained varies with heredity and the individual, and the maximal effect may not be appreciated until there has been 2 years of continuous treatment. Hormones alone often generate adequate breast development and may preclude the need for augmentation mammoplasty. The chance of successful breast development is maximized if native testosterone is first ablated with LHRH analogs, and estrogens are then introduced gradually. (L. Seal, personal communication, 2011). It follows then that some patients who receive hormonal treatment will not desire surgical interventions.

Estrogen is the principal agent used. Typical doses of estrogens are two to three times higher than the recommended dose for natal women, unless testosterone is ablated by other means, with a subsequent 20-fold increase in venous thrombosis for MtF patients on feminizing hormones.[19] Cigarette smoking and estrogen therapy in combination substantially increase thrombosis risk, and smoking cessation is strongly recommended. There is also a reported risk of raised prolactin levels and symptomatic prolactinomas.[20,21] Other unwanted effects include infertility, weight gain, emotional lability, and liver disease. There are often important social effects from taking hormones, which the patient must consider, primarily relationship changes with family members, friends, and employers.

Anti-androgens may be used as adjunctive treatments in those receiving estrogens to more profoundly suppress the production of testosterone, enabling a lower dose of estrogen to be used, especially when adverse estrogen side effects are anticipated.

Viable options for delivery of the hormones include oral, injectable, and transdermal systems. Topically applied hormonal creams have not been shown to produce adequate feminization effects, but the use of transdermal estrogen patches should be considered for males over 40 years of age or those with clotting abnormalities or a history of venous thrombosis.

Relative contraindications for hormone therapy include cigarette smoking, obesity, advanced age, heart disease, hypertension, clotting abnormalities, malignancy, and some endocrine abnormalities.

Even in healthy individuals, monitoring is required: enquiring about treatment effects and side effects, blood pressure measurements before and during treatment, and weight measurements are essential. For those receiving estrogens, a pre-treatment free testosterone level, fasting glucose, liver function tests, and full blood count with reassessment at 6 and 12 months and annually thereafter are required. A pre-treatment prolactin level should be obtained and repeated at 1, 2, and 3 years. If hyperprolactinemia does not occur during this time, no further measurements are necessary.

Estrogens are usually discontinued 6 weeks before genital surgery to minimize the thrombosis risk. In patients who were taking LHRH analogs, their original dose of estrogen may usually be recommenced 2 weeks after gender reassignment surgery. Where estrogen is used in isolation, the dose after surgery is typically one-third to one-half of the preoperative dose. Lifelong maintenance treatment is usually required

Male-to-female genital reconstructive surgery

The operation of MtF genital reconstruction has the following components:

- Penectomy and bilateral orchidectomy
- Formation of a cavity for the vagina
- Sourcing an epithelial lining for the vaginal cavity
- Urethrostomy
- Clitoroplasty
- Labioplasty.

There are numerous techniques for achieving these, the commonest of which will be discussed here.

Penectomy and orchidectomy

The technique for orchidectomy is very simple; the spermatic cords are ligated at the level of the inguinal canal and the testes removed. It is important, in the authors' experience, to ensure that the ligated cord lies within the inguinal canal, and does not become tethered to skin and subcutaneous tissues in the new labia, where a painful neuroma may subsequently become apparent. The skin of the penis is used elsewhere in the operation, and part of the glans is used by most surgeons to form a clitoris (see below). The bulbar urethra, and part of the penile urethra, are separated from the degloved penis. The remaining penile tissue is excised. Some surgeons advocate complete removal of the cavernosal bodies from the ischial tuberosities, but the authors have not experienced any problems in patients where this tissue is left in place. In any case, the natal female has erectile tissue in this site: the corpora clitoridis.

Formation of the vaginal cavity

Two approaches are commonly used. In the first, the bulbospongiosus muscle is dissected from the corpus spongiosum back to the perineal body. A small incision at the insertion of the bulbospongiosus into the perineal body allows the surgeon's finger to enter the plane between the prostate and rectum. A finger of the other hand in the rectum is then used as a guide to deepen this cavity by blind blunt dissection, before retractors can be inserted to demonstrate the new space. Alternatively, a urethral sound (or Lowsley prostatic retractor) is placed in the bladder, and used to push the prostate down towards the perineum. The apex of the prostate is identified by palpation, and the perineal muscles and perineal body are divided by sharp dissection under vision until the plane of Denonvilliers (which is continuous with the pelvic peritoneum) is entered at the apex of the prostate. Vaginal retractors may then be inserted to open the cavity between the rectum and prostate. This latter technique is favored by the authors.

Lining the vaginal cavity

The need for a vagina is linked to personal identity rather than the need to be sexually active. In the UK, the penile skin tube is most commonly used to form the lining of the neovagina. It is ideal because it is smooth, hairless, elastic, and has only thin connective tissue. When the penis is of normal adult dimensions and uncircumcised, the penile skin tube can be used exclusively for the lining of the vagina and is the technique of choice. The technique described may provide a neovaginal depth of up to 18 cm.

If the penile skin tube is deemed inadequate or where penile skin is used to produce labia, scrotal skin may be used either as a vascularized flap or as a free skin graft. If scrotal skin is to be used, this must be identified preoperatively as depilation should be organized to reduce the risk of future development of "hairballs" within the vagina, although it is possible to scrape hair follicles from the back of a free graft peroperatively. Other problems with scrotal skin is that it is rugose and has a fatty layer that may predispose to vaginal tube prolapse, forming a less secure bond to surrounding tissues than skin alone. Scrotal skin may be used as a pedicled flap on the posterior scrotal arteries. Alternatively, it may be used as a free flap, in which the skin is denuded of its fat and dartos layer; however, the risk of graft failure is higher in comparison to a pedicled flap. Free skin grafts derived from the abdominal wall or thigh may also be used to augment skin tubes when the depth of the resulting vagina is inadequate, but these may display shrinkage or lack of sensation.

The sigmoid colon, right colon, or ileum may be used to provide an epithelial lining for the neovagina. The bowel segment can be obtained either using a Pfannenstiel or lower midline incision, or laparoscopically. The disadvantage of bowel segment vaginoplasty is the continuous production of mucus (which if not excessive has the advantage of providing lubrication), sometimes requiring pad usage, the future risk of defunction colitis, and stenosis at the muco-cutaneous junction.[22,23] Although bowel segment is used as a primary source of vaginal lining in Iran, in our center it is used principally as a salvage technique when skin tube vaginoplasty has failed. The increasing number of adolescent patients who undergo puberty arrest before developing adult genitalia, in whom genital skin is relatively deficient, makes it likely that bowel segment surgery will increase in the future.

Sacrospinous ligament fixation has been shown to reduce the risk of vaginal skin tube prolapse,[24] but is not universally used. In the authors' center, the rate of prolapse is below 1% without using fixation.

Clitoroplasty

Rubin first described the use of the glans penis as the neoclitoris in gender reassignment surgery.[25] Although this was cosmetically and functionally adequate, Rubin used the corpus spongiosum as the pedicle and the technique was thwarted by development of urethral fistulae. Fang et al. subsequently described the preservation of the dorsal neurovascular bundle to the glans,[26] with excellent rates of preservation of tactile and erogenous sensitivity.[27] This neurovascular bundle lies between the tunica albuginea and Buck's fascia, and may be dissected free with relative ease, giving a vascularized, sensate piece of glans penis that can then form the clitoris.

Labioplasty

The techniques available for realistic labia minora very much depend on the tissues that have been used for vaginoplasty. If the vagina is formed entirely (or mainly) of scrotal skin or bowel segment, the entire skin of the penis may be used to create labia minora, a technique adopted by most Thai surgeons. Other surgeons preserve part of the prepuce attached to the glans penis used in clitoroplasty to achieve a similar effect.[28] Both of these techniques reduce the quantity of penile skin available for vaginoplasty and may make the use of a scrotal flap essential when it might not otherwise have been. Even when the entire penile skin tube is used for the vagina, small labia minora may be produced, with or without a second stage.

Urethrostomy

The simplest way of forming the urethrostomy is to divide the urethra in the bulb, and anastomose the skin to the urothelium. This, however, has a high incidence of subsequent urethral meatal stenosis, and also tends to result in antegrade micturition. The other drawback is that the corpus spongiosum is largely untouched, which results in a bulge behind the urethra, which grows on arousal. In addition to looking unsightly, this can obstruct the vaginal introitus during sex. For this reason, most surgeons will spatulate the urethra, and resect some of the erectile tissue that surrounds it. The resulting wide anastomosis to the perineal skin has a much lower rate of stenosis, and the moist urethral epithelium gives a very satisfactory cosmetic result. This comes with an increased risk of bleeding in the 48 hours after surgery, but this can almost always be managed conservatively.

Surgical complications

Thromboembolic complications

Thromboembolic complications may occur following genital reconstructive surgery, with risk factors including: prolonged surgery, pelvic surgery, prior use of thrombotic agents such as estrogen, immobilization postoperatively in some units, in addition to normal risk factors (e.g. smoking). Prevention of such complications involves pre- and postoperative low molecular weight heparin, thromboembolic deterrent stockings (TEDS), pneumatic calf compression intraoperatively, early mobilization, and careful patient positioning. Despite this, pulmonary emboli,[28] deep vein thrombosis (DVT),[2] cerebral ischemia,[23] and compartment syndrome[29] have been reported.

Perineal nerve damage

This can be prevented with careful patient positioning.

Bleeding and labial hematoma

Bleeding occurs in 10% of cases,[29] despite meticulous technique, and usually arises from the corpus spongiosum surrounding the urethra. Bleeding can be arrested by manual pressure and only rarely requires return to theater but may necessitate administration of blood products. It may also manifest as a labial hematoma, which can be managed conservatively but may increase the risk of wound dehiscence.

Rectovaginal fistula

Rectal laceration has been reported in 0.75–2% of cases,[30–34] and may predispose to the formation of a fistulous connection between the rectum and neovagina. It is difficult to estimate the true incidence of this devastating complication and it is probable that it is, in actual fact, under-reported.

The etiology is poorly understood, and when a rectal injury is not seen at the time of dissection, we propose that fistula development results from vascular injury to the front wall of the rectum. During creation of the neovagina cavity, connective tissue is stripped from the front wall of the rectum at the junction between two arterial supplies: the inferior mesenteric artery above and the hemorrhoidal vessels below. Damage to this "watershed" region may cause breakdown or thinning of rectal mucosa in this area. This would explain why a misdirected dilator pushed by a patient into an otherwise normal rectum has been reported to result in rectovaginal fistula. As a result, a dilator with a ventrally pointing tip has been recommended to avoid this problem.[35]

If there is a small breach of the rectal mucosa at the time of surgery, primary closure may be adequate to allow healing without a covering colostomy, which may be required if an extensive injury is evident. If a fistula does develop, a defunctioning colostomy will allow 50% of fistulae to heal, the remainder requiring further surgery, with a few difficult cases requiring removal of the neovagina.[30]

Prevention of a rectovaginal fistula is only by meticulous dissection dorsally from the perineal body to the prostate along Denonvilliers fascia up to the tip of the seminal vesicles, as suggested by Amend *et al.*,[24] combined with a high index of suspicion.

Lower urinary tract complications

Commonly reported functional urinary problems after vaginoplasty include stress urinary incontinence or urgency symptoms (66%), obstruction (33%), and urinary tract infections (2%);[24,34,36–39] these may be treated as in natal females.

Urethral meatus stenosis occurs in 3–4% of cases (G. Selvaggi and J. Bellringer, unpublished work), with patients typically presenting 2 months after primary surgery, initially with reduction in urine flow, and then dribbling incontinence from chronic retention of urine. These patients require revision of the meatus, which is usually effective, although a few do go on to long-term intermittent catheterization. Progressive obstructive voiding disorder due to meatal stenosis was reported as a major complication of penile inversion vaginoplasty.[40]

Vaginal complications

Vaginal complications, including loss of depth and/or width, prolapse of the neovagina, and hair growth are probably markedly under-reported, as up to two-thirds of patients are not sexually active or do not need much vaginal depth and width for their chosen sexual activities.

Loss of depth may result from skin loss, and correction of this usually necessitates enterovaginoplasty. Some centers use abdominal skin grafts in this circumstance, and a modification of the Davidov technique (originally described for the treatment of vaginal agenesis in natal women) has also been described. Failure to follow a proper dilation regime may also result in loss of both vaginal width and depth.

Hair growth will occur if scrotal skin is used and the skin has not been subjected to depilation, either pre- or perioperatively. Once hair growth is seen in the vault of the neovagina, little can be done to prevent its continued growth, and a number of patients will have to return at intervals for removal of hairballs.

Neovaginal stenosis is reported in 4–10% of patients after a combined penile-scrotal-skin-inversion technique.[24,31,34]

Neovaginal prolapse can occur immediately postoperatively on removal of the vaginal pack or at a later date. Sacrospinous ligament fixation has been reported to prevent this at 5-year follow-up,[41] but this does require careful preparation and placement of the anchoring sutures to prevent rectal and vascular injury.

Hyposensation of the neoclitoris[34] and neoclitoral necrosis[42] have been reported in the literature.

Non-genital surgery

Non-genital surgery may include: facial feminization (brow elevation, rhinoplasty, ear pinning, cheek augmentation, chin and jaw reduction); breast augmentation; hair transplantation; vocal cord and laryngeal surgery; as well as non-surgical procedures.

Follow-up and patient satisfaction

Satisfaction in a sometimes demanding patient population needs to fulfill both cosmetic and functional criteria: esthetic appearances similar to the natal female genitalia; adequate neovaginal depth and neoclitoral sensation to achieve orgasm; lubrication and lack of neovaginal pain[43] – these are all factors that must be considered. Satisfying the patient's esthetic goals is as important as achieving vaginal capacity.[33] Factors that positively correlate with long-term satisfaction include: young age, supportive family, and adequate social support.[16] In contrast, postoperative dissatisfaction is more likely in those in whom there is personal and social instability before surgery, poor body image, and age over 30 years.[44]

Retrospective follow-up studies suggest that about 80% of patients undergoing the procedure are pleased with the functioning and cosmetic appearance of their genitalia.[2] In the account by Amend et al. of 24 patients who underwent MtF reconstruction, the mean post-operative vaginal depth was 11 cm (range: 10–14 cm), with a diameter of 3–4 cm. Eight patients (33%) reported regular sexual intercourse, and 100% of their patients were satisfied with neovaginal functionality, outcome, and cosmetic results. Neoclitoral sensation was excellent in 18 patients (78%), good in five (19%), and unsatisfactory in one patient.[24] Only 1–1.5% of MtFs experienced persistent regret following gender realignment surgery.[45] Our experience would support these findings.

References

1 American Psychiatric Association. *Diagnostic and Statistical Manual of Mental Disorders, 5th Edition* (DSM-5). American Psychiatric Association, 2013.

2 Tugnet N, Goddard JC, Vickery RM, Khoosal D, Terry TR. Current management of male-to-female gender identity disorder in the UK. *Postgrad Med J* 2007;83(984):638–42.

3 Wilson P, Sharp C, Carr S. The prevalence of gender dysphoria in Scotland: a primary care study. *Br J Gen Pract* 1999;49(449):991–2.

4 Weitze C, Osburg S. Transsexualism in Germany: empirical data on epidemiology and application of the German Transsexuals' Act during its first ten years. *Arch Sex Behav* 1996;25(4):409–25.

5 Reed B, Rhodes S, Schofield P, Wylie K. Gender variance in the UK : Prevalence, incidence, growth and geographic distribution. *Gend Identity Res Educ Soc* 2009;June:1–36.

6 Standards of Care for the Health of Transsexual, Transgender, and Gender-Nonconforming People, 7th version. World Professional Association for Transgender Health, 2012.

7 Stoller R. *Sex and Gender: On the Development of Masculinity and Femininity*. Hogarth Press, 1968.

8 Benjamin H. *The Transsexual Phenomenon*. New York: Julian Press, 1966.

9 Swaab D, Chung W, Kruijver F, Hofman M, Ishunina T. Sexual differentiation of the human hypothalamus. *Adv Exp Med Biol* 2002;511:75–105.

10 Kruijver F, Zhou J, Pool C, Hofman M, Gooren L, Swaab D. Male-to-female transsexuals have female neuron numbers in a limbic nucleus. *J Clin Endocrinol Metab* 2000;85(5):2034–41.

11 Zhou J, Hofman M, Gooren L, Swaab D. A sex difference in the human brain and its relation to transsexuality. *Nature* 1995;378:68–70.

12 Garcia-Falgueras A, Swaab D. A sex difference in the hypothalamic uncinate nucleus: relationship to gender identity. *Brain* 2008;131(Pt 12):3132–46.

13 Zucker K, Beaulieu N, Bradley S, Grimshaw G, Wilcox A. Handedness in boys with gender identity disorder. *J Child Psychol Psychiatry* 2001;42(6):767–76.

14 Good Practice Guidelines for the Assessment and Treatment of Adults with Gender Dysphoria. London: Royal College of Psychiatrists, 2013.

15 Wylie K. Good Practice Guidelines for the Assessment & Treatment of Gender Dysphoria. Royal College of Psychiatrists, 2006.

16 Wylie K. Gender related disorders. *BMJ* 2004;329(7466):615–7.

17 Levine S. Psychiatric diagnosis of patients requesting sex reassignment surgery. *J Sex Marital Ther* 1980;6(3):164–73.

18 Barrett J. Disorders of gender identity: what to do and who should do it? *Br J Psychiatry* 2014;204:96–7.

19 Meriggiola MC, Berra M. Long-term cross-sex hormone treatment is safe in transsexual subjects. *Asian J Androl* 2012;14(6):813–4.

20 Asscheman H, Gooren L, Assies J, Smits J, de Siegte R. Prolactin levels and pituitary enlargement in hormone-treated male-to-female transsexuals. *Clin Endocrinol (Oxf)* 1998;28(6):583–8.

21 Gooren L, Assies J, Asscheman H, de Siegte R, van Kessel H. Estrogen-induced prolactinoma in a man. *J Clin Endocrinol Metab* 1988;66(2):444–6.

22 Franz R. Sigmoid colon vaginoplasty: a modified method. *Br J Obstet Gynaecol* 1996;103(11):1148–55.

23 Sukumaran S, Moran P, Makar A. An unusual cause of vaginal discharge following gender reassignment. *Int Urogynecology J Pelvic Floor Dysfunct* 2009;20(2):253–4.

24 Amend B, Seibold J, Toomey P, Stenzl A, Sievert K-D. Surgical reconstruction for male-to-female sex reassignment. *Eur Urol* 2013;64(1):141–9.

25 Rubin S. A method of preserving the glans penis as a clitoris in sex conversion operations in male transsexuals. *Scand J Urol Nephrol* 1980;14(3):215–7.

26 Fang R, Chen C, Ma S. A new method for clitoroplasty in male-to-female sex reassignment surgery. *Plast Reconstr Surg* 1992;89(4):679–82.

27 Selvaggi G, Monstrey S, Ceulemans P, T'Sjoen G, De Cuypere G, Hoebeke P. Genital sensitivity after sex reassignment surgery in transsexual patients. *Ann Plast Surg* 2007;58(4):427–33.

28 Selvaggi G, Ceulemans P, De Cuypere G, et al. Gender identity disorder: general overview and surgical treatment for vaginoplasty in male-to-female transsexuals. *Plast Reconstr Surg* 2005;116(6):135e–145e.

29 Gilleard O, Qureshi M, Thomas P, Bellringer J. Urethral bleeding following male to female gender reassignment surgery. In: World Professional Association for Transgender Health Biennial Meeting, 2009.

30 Beckley I, Thomas P, Bellringer J. Aetiology and management of recto-vaginal fistulas following male to female gender reassignment. In: EAU Section of Genitourinary Surgeons and EAU Section of Andrological Urology Meeting, Madrid, 2008.

31 Karim R, Hage J, Bouman F, de Ruyter R, van Kesteren P. Refinements of pre-, intra-, and postoperative care to prevent complications of vaginoplasty in male transsexuals. *Ann Plast Surg* 1995;35(3):279–84.
32 Perovic S, Stanojevic D, Djordevic M. Vaginoplasty in male transsexuals using penile skin and a urethral flap. *BJU Int* 2000;86(7):843–50.
33 Jarolim L. Surgical conversion of genitalia in transsexual patients. *BJU Int* 2000;85(7):851–6.
34 Goddard J, Vickery R, Qureshi A, Summerton D, Khoosal D, Terry T. Feminizing genitoplasty in adult transsexuals: early and long-term surgical results. *BJU Int* 2007;100(3):607–13.
35 Melzer T. Managing complications of male to female surgery. In: World Professional Association for Transgender Health Biennial Meeting, Chicago, 2007.
36 Kuhn A, Hiltebrand R, Birkhauser M. Do transsexuals have micturition disorders? *Eur J Obstet Gynecol Reprod Biol* 2007;131(2):226–30.
37 Lawrence A. Patient-reported complications and functional outcomes of male-to-female sex reassignment surgery. *Arch Sex Behav* 2006;35(6):717–27.
38 Dangle P, Harrison S. Stress urinary incontinence after male to female gender reassignment surgery: Successful use of a pubo-vaginal sling. *Indian J Urol* 2007;23(3):311–3.
39 Jain A, Bradbeer C. A case of successful management of recurrent bacterial vaginosis of neovagina after male to female gender reassignment surgery. *Int J STD AIDS* 2007;18(2):140–1.
40 Rossi Neto R, Hintz F, Krege S, Rubben H, Vom Dorp F. Gender reassignment surgery – a 13 year review of surgical outcomes. *Int Braz J Urol* 2012;38(1):97–107.
41 Stanojevic D, Djordevic M, Milosevic A, et al. Sacrospinous ligament fixation for neovaginal prolapse prevention in male-to-female surgery. *Urology* 2007;70(4):767–71.
42 Giraldo F, Esteva I, Bergero T, et al. Corona glans clitoroplasty and urethropreputial vestibuloplasty in male-to-female transsexuals: the vulval aesthetic refinement by the Andalusia Gender Team. *Plast Reconstr Surg* 2004;114(6):1543–50.
43 Weyers S, Elaut E, De Sutter P, et al. Long-term assessment of the physical, mental, and sexual health among transsexual women. *J Sex Med* 2009;6(3):752–60.
44 Eldh J, Berg A, Gustafsson M. Long-term follow up after sex reassignment surgery. *Scand J Plast Reconstr Surg Hand Surg* 1997;31(1):39–45.
45 Pfafflin F, Junge A. *Thirty years of International Follow-up Studies after Sex Reassignment Surgery: A Comprehensive Review, 1961–1991*. Düsseldorf: Symposion, 1998.

Index

Note: Pages in *italics* refer to Figures; those in **bold** refer to Tables

Male Sexual Dysfunction: A Clinical Guide, First Edition. Edited by Suks Minhas and John Mulhall.